Multi-Objective Optimization in Computational Intelligence:
Theory and Practice

Lam Thu Bui
University of New South Wales, Australia

Sameer Alam
University of New South Wales, Australia

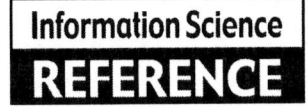

INFORMATION SCIENCE REFERENCE

Hershey · New York

Acquisitions Editor:	Kristin Klinger
Development Editor:	Kristin Roth
Senior Managing Editor:	Jennifer Neidig
Managing Editor:	Jamie Snavely
Assistant Managing Editor:	Carole Coulson
Copy Editor:	Erin Meyer
Typesetter:	Amanda Appicello
Cover Design:	Lisa Tosheff
Printed at:	Yurchak Printing Inc.

Published in the United States of America by
Information Science Reference (an imprint of IGI Global)
701 E. Chocolate Avenue, Suite 200
Hershey PA 17033
Tel: 717-533-8845
Fax: 717-533-8661
E-mail: cust@igi-global.com
Web site: http://www.igi-global.com

and in the United Kingdom by
Information Science Reference (an imprint of IGI Global)
3 Henrietta Street
Covent Garden
London WC2E 8LU
Tel: 44 20 7240 0856
Fax: 44 20 7379 0609
Web site: http://www.eurospanbookstore.com

Copyright © 2008 by IGI Global. All rights reserved. No part of this publication may be reproduced, stored or distributed in any form or by any means, electronic or mechanical, including photocopying, without written permission from the publisher.

Product or company names used in this set are for identification purposes only. Inclusion of the names of the products or companies does not indicate a claim of ownership by IGI Global of the trademark or registered trademark.

Library of Congress Cataloging-in-Publication Data

Multi-objective optimization in computational intelligence : theory and practice / Lam Thu Bui and Ricardo Sameer Alam, editors.

  p. cm.

 Summary: "This book explores the theoretical, as well as empirical, performance of MOs on a wide range of optimization issues including combinatorial, real-valued, dynamic, and noisy problems. It provides scholars, academics, and practitioners with a fundamental, comprehensive collection of research on multi-objective optimization techniques, applications, and practices"--Provided by publisher.

  ISBN-13: 978-1-59904-498-9 (hardcover)

  ISBN-13: 978-1-59904-500-9 (e-book)

 1. Computational intelligence. 2. Evolutionary computation. 3. Mathematical optimization. 4. Artificial intelligence. I. Bui, Lam Thu. II. Alam, Ricardo Sameer.

 Q342.M85 2008

 519.6--dc22

                              2007040640

British Cataloguing in Publication Data
A Cataloguing in Publication record for this book is available from the British Library.

All work contributed to this book set is original material. The views expressed in this book are those of the authors, but not necessarily of the publisher.

> *If a library purchased a print copy of this publication, please go to http://www.igi-global.com/agreement for information on activating the library's complimentary electronic access to this publication.*

Reviewer List

Carlos A. Coello Coello
INVESTAV-IPN, Evolutionary Computation Group (EVOCINV), México

Alessandro G. Di Nuovo
Università degli Studi di Catania, Italy

Maoguo Gong
Xidian University, P.R. China

Mark P. Kleeman
Air Force Institute of Technology, USA

Saku Kukkonen
Lappeenranta University of Technology, Finland

Andrew Lewis
Griffith University, Australia

Luis Martí
Universidad Carlos III de Madrid, Spain

Minh H. Nguyen
University of New South Wales, Australia

K.E. Parsopoulos
University of Patras, Greece

Ramesh Rajagopalan
Syracuse University, USA

Marcus Randall
Bond University, Australia

Soo-Yong Shin
National Institute of Standards and Technology, USA

Jason Teo
Universiti Malaysia Sabah, Malaysia

Andrea Toffolo
University of Padova, Italy

Lam Thu Bui
University of New South Wales, Australia

Sameer Alam
University of New South Wales, Australia

Table of Contents

Foreword xiv
Preface xv
Acknowledgment xix

Section I
Fundamentals

Chapter I
An Introduction to Multi-Objective Optimization 1
    Lam Thu Bui, University of New South Wales, Australia
    Sameer Alam, University of New South Wales, Australia

Chapter II
Multi-Objective Particles Swarm Optimization Approaches.. 20
    Konstantinos E. Parsopoulos, University of Patras, Greece
    Michael N. Vrahatis, University of Patras, Greece

Chapter III
Generalized Differential Evolution for Constrained Multi-Objective Optimization 43
    Saku Kukkonen, Lappeenranta University of Technology, Finland
    Jouni Lampinen, University of Vaasa, Finland

Chapter IV
Towards a More Efficient Multi-Objective Particle Swarm Optimizer.............................. 76
    Luis V. Santana-Quintero, CINVESTAV-IPN, Evolutionary Computation Group
        (EVOCINV), Mexico
    Noel Ramírez-Santiago, CINVESTAV-IPN, Evolutionary Computation Group
        (EVOCINV), Mexico
    Carlos A. Coello Coello, CINVESTAV-IPN, Evolutionary Computation Group
        (EVOCINV), Mexico

Chapter V
Multi-Objective Optimization Using Artificial Immune Systems 106
    Licheng Jiao, Xidian University, P.R. China
    Maoguo Gong, Xidian University, P.R. China
    Wenping Ma, Xidian University, P.R. China
    Ronghua Shang, Xidian University, P.R. China

Chapter VI
Lexicographic Goal Programming and Assessment Tools for a
Combinatorial Production Problem 148
    Seamus M. McGovern, U.S. DOT National Transportation Systems Center, USA
    Surendra M. Gupta, Northeastern University, USA

Chapter VII
Evolutionary Population Dynamics and Multi-Objective Optimisation Problems 185
    Andrew Lewis, Griffith University, Australia
    Sanaz Mostaghim, University of Karlsruhe, Germany
    Marcus Randall, Bond University, Australia

Section II
Applications

Chapter VIII
Multi-Objective Evolutionary Algorithms for Sensor Network Design 208
    Ramesh Rajagopalan, Syracuse University, USA
    Chilukuri K. Mohan, Syracuse University, USA
    Kishan G. Mehrotra, Syracuse University, USA
    Pramod K. Varshney, Syracuse University, USA

Chapter IX
Evolutionary Multi-Objective Optimization for DNA Sequence Design 239
    Soo-Yong Shin, Seoul National University, Korea
    In-Hee Lee, Seoul National University, Korea
    Byoung-Tak Zhang, Seoul National University, Korea

Chapter X
Computational Intelligence to Speed-Up Multi-Objective Design Space
Exploration of Embedded Systems 265
    Giuseppe Ascia, Università degli Studi di Catania, Italy
    Vincenzo Catania, Università degli Studi di Catania, Italy
    Alessandro G. Di Nuovo, Università degli Studi di Catania, Italy
    Maurizio Palesi, Università degli Studi di Catania, Italy
    Davide Patti, Università degli Studi di Catania, Italy

Chapter XI
Walking with EMO: Multi-Objective Robotics for Evolving Two, Four,
and Six-Legged Locomotion 300
    Jason Teo, Universiti Malaysia Sabah, Malaysia
    Lynnie D. Neri, Universiti Malaysia Sabah, Malaysia
    Minh H. Nguyen, University of New South Wales, Australia
    Hussein A. Abbass, University of New South Wales, Australia

Chapter XII
Evolutionary Multi-Objective Optimization in Energy Conversion Systems:
From Component Detail to System Configuration 333
    Andrea Toffolo, University of Padova, Italy

Chapter XIII
Evolutionary Multi-Objective Optimization for Assignment Problems 364
    Mark P. Kleeman, Air Force Institute of Technology, USA
    Gary B. Lamont, Air Force Institute of Technology, USA

Chapter XIV
Evolutionary Multi-Objective Optimization in Military Applications 388
    Mark P. Kleeman, Air Force Institute of Technology, USA
    Gary B. Lamont, Air Force Institute of Technology, USA

Compilation of References 430

About the Contributors 461

Index 469

Detailed Table of Contents

Foreword xiv
Preface xv
Acknowledgment xix

Section I
Fundamentals

Chapter I
An Introduction to Multi-Objective Optimization 1
    Lam Thu Bui, University of New South Wales, Australia
    Sameer Alam, University of New South Wales, Australia

This chapter is devoted to summarize all common concepts related to multiobjective optimization (MO). An overview of *"traditional"* as well as CI-based MO is given. Further, all aspects of performance assessment for MO techniques are discussed. Finally, challenges facing MO techniques are addressed. All of these description and analysis give the readers basic knowledge for understandings the rest of the book.

Chapter II
Multi-Objective Particles Swarm Optimization Approaches 20
    Konstantinos E. Parsopoulos, University of Patras, Greece
    Michael N. Vrahatis, University of Patras, Greece

The multiple criteria nature of most real world problems has boosted research on multiobjective algorithms that can tackle such problems effectively, with the smallest possible computational burden. Particle Swarm Optimization has attracted the interest of researchers due to its simplicity, effectiveness and efficiency in solving numerous single-objective optimization problems. Up-to-date, there are a significant number of multiobjective Particle Swarm Optimization approaches and applications reported in the literature. This chapter aims at providing a review and discussion of the most established results on this field, as well as exposing the most active research topics that can give initiative for future research.

Chapter III
Generalized Differential Evolution for Constrained Multi-Objective Optimization 43
    Saku Kukkonen, Lappeenranta University of Technology, Finland
    Jouni Lampinen, University of Vaasa, Finland

Multiobjective optimization with Evolutionary Algorithms has been gaining popularity recently because its applicability in practical problems. Many practical problems contain also constraints, which must be taken care of during optimization process. This chapter is about Generalized Differential Evolution, which is a general-purpose optimizer. It is based on a relatively recent Evolutionary Algorithm, Differential Evolution, which has been gaining popularity because of its simplicity and good observed performance. Generalized Differential Evolution extends Differential Evolution for problems with several objectives and constraints. The chapter concentrates on describing different development phases and performance of Generalized Differential Evolution but it also contains a brief review of other multiobjective DE approaches. Ability to solve multiobjective problems is mainly discussed, but constraint handling and the effect of control parameters are also covered. It is found that GDE versions, in particular the latest version, are effective and efficient for solving constrained multiobjective problems.

Chapter IV
Towards a More Efficient Multi-Objective Particle Swarm Optimizer 76
    Luis V. Santana-Quintero, CINVESTAV-IPN, Evolutionary Computation Group
        (EVOCINV), Mexico
    Noel Ramírez-Santiago, CINVESTAV-IPN, Evolutionary Computation Group
        (EVOCINV), Mexico
    Carlos A. Coello Coello, CINVESTAV-IPN, Evolutionary Computation Group
        (EVOCINV), Mexico

This chapter presents a hybrid between a particle swarm optimization (PSO) approach and scatter search. The main motivation for developing this approach is to combine the high convergence rate of the PSO algorithm with a local search approach based on scatter search, in order to have the main advantages of these two types of techniques. We propose a new leader selection scheme for PSO, which aims to accelerate convergence by increasing the selection pressure. However, this higher selection pressure reduces diversity. To alleviate that, scatter search is adopted after applying PSO, in order to spread the solutions previously obtained, so that a better distribution along the Pareto front is achieved. The proposed approach can produce reasonably good approximations of multiobjective problems of high dimensionality, performing only 4,000 fitness function evaluations. Test problems taken from the specialized literature are adopted to validate the proposed hybrid approach. Results are compared with respect to the NSGA-II, which is an approach representative of the state-of-the-art in the area.

Chapter V
Multi-Objective Optimization Using Artificial Immune Systems 106
    Licheng Jiao, Xidian University, P.R. China
    Maoguo Gong, Xidian University, P.R. China
    Wenping Ma, Xidian University, P.R. China
    Ronghua Shang, Xidian University, P.R. China

This chapter focuses on extending Artificial Immune Systems (AIS) to solve multiobjective problems. It introduces two multiobjective optimization algorithms using AIS, the Immune Dominance Clonal Multi-objective Algorithm (IDCMA), and the Non-dominated Neighbour Immune Algorithm (NNIA). IDCMA is unique in that its fitness values of current dominated individuals are assigned as the values of a custom distance measure, termed as Ab-Ab affinity, between the dominated individuals and one of the nondominated individuals found so far. Meanwhile, NNIA solves multiobjective optimization problems by using a non-dominated neighbour-based selection technique, an immune inspired operator, two heuristic search operators and elitism. The unique selection technique of NNIA only selects minority isolated nondominated individuals in population. The selected individuals are then cloned proportionally to their crowding-distance values before heuristic search. By using the nondominated neighbor-based selection and proportional cloning, NNIA pays more attention to the less-crowded regions of the current trade-off front.

Chapter VI
Lexicographic Goal Programming and Assessment Tools for a
Combinatorial Production Problem 148
    Seamus M. McGovern, U.S. DOT National Transportation Systems Center, USA
    Surendra M. Gupta, Northeastern University, USA

NP-complete combinatorial problems often necessitate the use of near-optimal solution techniques including heuristics and metaheuristics. The addition of multiple optimization criteria can further complicate comparison of these solution techniques due to the decision-maker's weighting schema potentially masking search limitations. In addition, many contemporary problems lack quantitative assessment tools, including benchmark data sets. This chapter proposes the use of lexicographic goal programming for use in comparing combinatorial search techniques. These techniques are implemented here using a recently formulated problem from the area of production analysis. The development of a benchmark data set and other assessment tools is demonstrated, and these are then used to compare the performance of a genetic algorithm and an H-K general-purpose heuristic as applied to the production-related application.

Chapter VII
Evolutionary Population Dynamics and Multi-Objective Optimisation Problems 185
    Andrew Lewis, Griffith University, Australia
    Sanaz Mostaghim, University of Karlsruhe, Germany
    Marcus Randall, Bond University, Australia

Problems for which many objective functions are to be simultaneously optimised are widely encountered in science and industry. These multiobjective problems have also been the subject of intensive investigation and development recently for metaheuristic search algorithms such as ant colony optimisation, particle swarm optimisation and extremal optimisation. In this chapter, a unifying framework called evolutionary programming dynamics (EPD) is examined. Using underlying concepts of self organised criticality and evolutionary programming, it can be applied to many optimisation algorithms as a controlling metaheuristic, to improve performance and results. We show this to be effective for both continuous and combinatorial problems.

Section II
Applications

Chapter VIII
Multi-Objective Evolutionary Algorithms for Sensor Network Design 208
    Ramesh Rajagopalan, Syracuse University, USA
    Chilukuri K. Mohan, Syracuse University, USA
    Kishan G. Mehrotra, Syracuse University, USA
    Pramod K. Varshney, Syracuse University, USA

Many sensor network design problems are characterized by the need to optimize multiple conflicting objectives. However, existing approaches generally focus on a single objective (ignoring the others), or combine multiple objectives into a single function to be optimized, to facilitate the application of classical optimization algorithms. This restricts their ability and constrains their usefulness to the network designer. A much more appropriate and natural approach is to address multiple objectives simultaneously, applying recently developed *multi-objective evolutionary algorithms (MOEAs)* in solving sensor network design problems. This chapter describes and illustrates this approach by modeling two sensor network design problems (mobile agent routing and sensor placement), as multiobjective optimization problems, developing the appropriate objective functions and discussing the tradeoffs between them. Simulation results using two recently developed MOEAs, viz., EMOCA (Rajagopalan, Mohan, Mehrotra, & Varshney, 2006) and NSGA-II (Deb, Pratap, Agarwal, & Meyarivan, 2000), show that these MOEAs successfully discover multiple solutions characterizing the tradeoffs between the objectives.

Chapter IX
Evolutionary Multi-Objective Optimization for DNA Sequence Design 239
    Soo-Yong Shin, Seoul National University, Korea
    In-Hee Lee, Seoul National University, Korea
    Byoung-Tak Zhang, Seoul National University, Korea

Finding reliable and efficient DNA sequences is one of the most important tasks for successful DNA-related experiments such as DNA computing, DNA nano-assembly, DNA microarrays and polymerase chain reaction. Sequence design involves a number of heterogeneous and conflicting design criteria. Also, it is proven as a class of NP problems. These suggest that multiobjective evolutionary algorithms (MOEAs) are actually good candidates for DNA sequence optimization. In addition, the characteristics of MOEAs including simple addition/deletion of objectives and easy incorporation of various existing tools and human knowledge into the final decision process could increase the reliability of final DNA sequence set. In this chapter, we review multiobjective evolutionary approaches to DNA sequence design. In particular, we analyze the performance of ε-multiobjective evolutionary algorithms on three DNA sequence design problems and validate the results by showing superior performance to previous techniques.

Chapter X
Computational Intelligence to Speed-Up Multi-Objective Design Space
Exploration of Embedded Systems.. 265
    Giuseppe Ascia, Università degli Studi di Catania, Italy
    Vincenzo Catania, Università degli Studi di Catania, Italy
    Alessandro G. Di Nuovo, Università degli Studi di Catania, Italy
    Maurizio Palesi, Università degli Studi di Catania, Italy
    Davide Patti, Università degli Studi di Catania, Italy

Multi-Objective Evolutionary Algorithms (MOEAs) have received increasing interest in industry, because they have proved to be powerful optimizers. Despite the great success achieved, MOEAs have also encountered many challenges in real-world applications. One of the main difficulties in applying MOEAs is the large number of fitness evaluations (objective calculations) that are often needed before a well acceptable solution can be found. In fact, there are several industrial situations in which both fitness evaluations are computationally expensive and, meanwhile, time available is very low. In this applications efficient strategies to approximate the fitness function have to be adopted, looking for a trade-off between optimization performances and efficiency. This is the case of a complex embedded system design, where it is needed to define an optimal architecture in relation to certain performance indexes respecting strict time-to-market constraints. This activity, known as Design Space Exploration (DSE), is still a great challenge for the EDA (Electronic Design Automation) community. One of the most important bottlenecks in the overall design flow of an embedded system is due to the simulation. Simulation occurs at every phase of the design flow and it is used to evaluate a system candidate to be implemented. In this chapter we focus on system level design proposing an hybrid computational intelligence approach based on fuzzy approximation to speed up the evaluation of a candidate system. The methodology is applied to a real case study: optimization of the performance and power consumption of an embedded architecture based on a Very Long Instruction Word (VLIW) microprocessor in a mobile multimedia application domain. The results, carried out on a multimedia benchmark suite, are compared, in terms of both performance and efficiency, with other MOGAs strategies to demonstrate the scalability and the accuracy of the proposed approach.

Chapter XI
Walking with EMO: Multi-Objective Robotics for Evolving Two, Four,
and Six-Legged Locomotion.. 300
    Jason Teo, Universiti Malaysia Sabah, Malaysia
    Lynnie D. Neri, Universiti Malaysia Sabah, Malaysia
    Minh H. Nguyen, University of New South Wales, Australia
    Hussein A. Abbass, University of New South Wales, Australia

This chapter will demonstrate the various robotics applications that can be achieved using evolutionary multiobjective optimization (EMO) techniques. The main objective of this chapter is to demonstrate practical ways of generating simple legged locomotion for simulated robots with two, four and six legs using EMO. The operational performance as well as complexities of the resulting evolved Pareto solutions that act as controllers for these robots will then be analyzed. Additionally, the operational dynamics of these evolved Pareto controllers in noisy and uncertain environments, limb dynamics and effects of using a different underlying EMO algorithm will also be discussed.

Chapter XII
Evolutionary Multi-Objective Optimization in Energy Conversion Systems:
From Component Detail to System Configuration 333
Andrea Toffolo, University of Padova, Italy

The research field on energy conversion systems presents a large variety of multiobjective optimization problems that can be solved taking full advantage of the features of evolutionary algorithms. In fact, design and operation of energy systems can be considered in several different perspectives (e.g., performance, efficiency, costs, environmental aspects). This results in a number of objective functions that should be simultaneously optimized, and the knowledge of the Pareto optimal set of solutions is of fundamental importance to the decision maker. This chapter proposes a brief survey of typical applications at different levels, ranging from the design of component detail to the challenge about the synthesis of the configuration of complex energy conversion systems. For sake of simplicity, the proposed examples are grouped into three main categories: design of components/component details, design of overall energy system and operation of energy systems. Each multiobjective optimization problem is presented with a short background and some details about the formulation. Future research directions in the field of energy systems are also discussed at the end of the chapter.

Chapter XIII
Evolutionary Multi-Objective Optimization for Assignment Problems 364
Mark P. Kleeman, Air Force Institute of Technology, USA
Gary B. Lamont, Air Force Institute of Technology, USA

Assignment problems are used throughout many research disciplines. Most assignment problems in the literature have focused on solving a single objective. This chapter focuses on assignment problems that have multiple objectives that need to be satisfied. In particular, this chapter looks at how multiobjective evolutionary algorithms have been used to solve some of these problems. Additionally, this chapter examines many of the operators that have been utilized to solve assignment problems and discusses some of the advantages and disadvantages of using specific operators.

Chapter XIV
Evolutionary Multi-Objective Optimization in Military Applications 388
Mark P. Kleeman, Air Force Institute of Technology, USA
Gary B. Lamont, Air Force Institute of Technology, USA

This chapter attempts to provide a spectrum of military multiobjective optimization problems whose characteristics imply that an MOEA approach is appropriate. The choice of selected operators indicates that good results can be achieved for these problems. Selection and testing of other operators and associated parameters may generate "better" solutions. It is not intended that these problems represent the totality or even the complete spectrum of all military optimization problems. However, the examples discussed are very complex with high-dimensionality and therefore reflect the many difficulties the military faces in achieving their goals. MOEAs with local search are another method of attacking theslems that should provide effective and efficient solutions.

Compilation of References 430

About the Contributors 461

Index 469

Foreword

The topic of multiobjective optimization is of utmost importance to most practitioners who deal with a variety of optimization tasks in real-world settings. The reason is that most real-world problems involve more than one objective. It is quite unusual to optimize along one dimension, whether this would be the cost of production, inventory levels or total profits. Rather, real-world problems involve multiple conflicting objectives (e.g., minimizing the weight of a battery while maximizing its life). Because of this, no one solution can be termed "the best"—and it is necessary to consider a set of trade-off optimal solutions.

Many classic optimization methods have been proposed to address multiobjective optimization problems. Most of these methods convert such problems into single objective formulations, which suffer from a few disadvantages. These include the necessity of making a variety of adjustments to a method and also the return of a single solution at the end of each run.

Hence, there is a huge interest in applications of computational intelligence methods for multiobjective optimization problems. Indeed, it is one of the hottest topics at present, so this book is coming out at the right time. The first part of the book deals with issues of applicability of various techniques, like particle swarm optimization, differential evolution, artificial immune systems, evolutionary algorithms, and multiobjective optimization problems. The second part of the book concentrates on various applications (e.g., wireless sensor network design, DNA sequence design, assignment problems, and military applications).

I am sure you will find this book quite useful and interesting, as it presents a variety of available techniques and some areas of potential applications.

Enjoy.

Zbigniew Michalewicz
University of Adelaide

Preface

Solving multiobjective optimization (MO) problems using computational intelligence (CI) techniques, such as genetic algorithms, particle swam optimization, artificial immune systems, is a fast-developing field of research. Similar to other optimization techniques, MO algorithms using CI techniques (or we simply call *CI-based MO algorithms*) are employed to find feasible solutions for a particular problem. In contrast to their single objective optimization counterparts, they are associated with multiobjective fitness functions, which complicate the multi-dimensional fitness landscape. With CI-based MO algorithms, there exists a set of trade-off optimal solutions. It thus gives decision makers more options to choose the best solution according to post-analysis preference information. At the current state, CI-based MO algorithms have developed to become competent with an increasingly large number of CI-based MO applications in real life. Researchers have been investigating theoretically as well as empirically the performance of CI-based MO algorithms on a wide range of optimization problems including combinatorial, real-valued to dynamic and noisy problems.

The application of MO as well as CI-based MO for real-world problems is obvious since real-world problems are hardly single-objective. Because of tremendous practical demands, the research in CI-based MO has developed quickly with diverse methods. As a result, there are massive numbers of research papers published in the format of journals as well as conferences. However, most papers on CI-based MO are scattered around in different journals and conference proceedings focussed on very special and narrow topics. Although a few books exist on evolutionary MO, there is no publication to provide readers an understanding through all these diverse CI-based MO techniques. Further, due to the practical usefulness of CI-based MO, there is an increasing demand to have separate subject of CI-based MO in the educational plan of universities worldwide for: undergraduate and postgraduate students to provide them a broad knowledge on a wide range of CI-based MO techniques. It is therefore vital to have editions of chapters across areas of MO in order to summarize the most important CI-based MO techniques as well as their specialized applications.

This edition is expected to meet the demand to have separate subject of CI-based MO in the educational plan of universities. It consists of open-solicited and invited chapters written by leading researchers in the field of computational intelligence. All papers went through a peer review process by at least two experts in the field and one of the editors. Our goal is to provide lecture notes that representatively cover the foundation as well as the practical side of the topic. This represents a responsibility from our end to balance between technicality of specialists, and readability of a larger audience. The book is organized in such a way that it is primarily used for teaching under graduate and post-graduate levels. Meanwhile, it can be a reference of CI-based MO techniques for researchers and practitioners.

For the foundation part, the book includes a description of common concepts of MO, a survey of the MO literature, and several work on hot topics such as extending genetic algorithms, differential evolution, particle swarm optimization, and artificial immune systems to the MO domain. Meanwhile, the application part covers a quite wide range of work from DNA design, network installation to the defence and security domain. Because of the space constraints, this book just contains a small collection of the work in the field. However, they are representatives for most of current topics in the CI-based MO.

There are XIV chapters total. Chapter I is devoted to summarize common concepts related to MO. A description of traditional as well as CI-based MO is given. Further, various aspects of performance assessment for MO techniques are discussed. Finally, challenges facing MO techniques are addressed. All of these descriptions and analysis give the readers basic knowledge for understanding the rest of the book.

In Chapter II, a survey of particle swarm optimization (PSO) is given. PSO has attracted the interest of researchers due to its simplicity, effectiveness and efficiency in solving numerous single-objective optimization problems. Up-to-date, there is a significant number of multiobjective PSO approaches and applications reported in the literature. This chapter aims at providing a review and discussion of the most established results on this field, as well as exposing the most active research topics that can give initiative for future research.

Chapter III discusses generalized differential evolution (GDE), which is a general-purpose optimizer. It is based on a relatively recent Evolutionary Algorithm, Differential Evolution, which has been gaining popularity because of its simplicity and good observed performance. GDE extends differential evolution for problems with several objectives and constraints. The chapter concentrates on describing different development phases and performance of GDE. The ability to solve multiobjective problems is mainly discussed, but constraint handling and the effect of control parameters are also covered as well as other relevant studies. It is found that the GDE versions, in particular the latest version, are effective and efficient for solving constrained multiobjective problems.

Chapter IV presents a hybrid between a PSO approach and scatter search. The main motivation for developing this approach is to combine the high convergence rate of the PSO algorithm with a local search approach based on scatter search, in order to have the main advantages of these two types of techniques. It proposes a new leader selection scheme for PSO, which aims to accelerate convergence by increasing the selection pressure. However, this higher selection pressure reduces diversity. To alleviate that, scatter search is adopted after applying PSO, in order to spread the solutions previously obtained, so that a better distribution along the Pareto front is achieved. The proposed approach can produce reasonably good approximations of multiobjective problems of high dimensionality, performing only a few thousnads of fitness function evaluations. Test problems taken from the specialized literature are adopted to validate the proposed hybrid approach. Results are compared with respect to the NSGA-II, which is an approach representative of the state-of-the-art in the area.

Chapter V focuses on extending artificial immune systems (AIS) to solve multiobjective problems. It introduces two multiobjective optimization algorithms using AIS, the immune dominance clonal multi-objective algorithm (IDCMA), and the non-dominated neighbour immune algorithm (NNIA). IDCMA is unique in that its fitness values of current dominated individuals are assigned as the values of a custom distance measure, termed as Ab-Ab affinity, between the dominated individuals and one of the non-dominated individuals found so far. Meanwhile, NNIA solves multiobjective optimization problems by using a nondominated neighbor-based selection technique, an immune inspired operator, two heuristic search operators and elitism. The unique selection technique of NNIA only selects minority isolated non-dominated individuals in population. The selected individuals are then cloned proportionally to their crowding-distance values before heuristic search. By using the nondominated neighbor-based selection and proportional cloning, NNIA pays more attention to the less-crowded regions of the current trade-off front.

Chapter VI proposes the use of lexicographic goal programming for use in comparing combinatorial search techniques. These techniques are implemented here using a recently formulated and multiobjective problem from the area of production analysis. The development of a benchmark data set and other assessment tools is demonstrated, and these are then used to compare the performance of a genetic algorithm and an H-K general-purpose heuristic as applied to the production-related application.

In Chapter VII, a unifying framework called evolutionary programming dynamics (EPD) is examined. Using underlying concepts of self organised criticality and evolutionary programming, it can be applied to many optimisation algorithms as a controlling meta-heuristic, to improve performance and results. The chapter shows this to be effective for both continuous and combinatorial problems.

Chapter VIII describes and illustrates this approach by modeling two sensor network design problems (mobile agent routing and sensor placement), as multiobjective optimization problems, developing the appropriate objective functions and discussing the tradeoffs between them. Simulation results using two recently developed multiobjective evolutionary algorithms (MOEAs) show that these MOEAs successfully discover multiple solutions characterizing the tradeoffs between the objectives.

Chapter IX presents a possibility to apply evolutionary multiobjective optimization in designing DNA sequences. It performs a review on multiobjective evolutionary approaches to DNA sequence design. In particular, it analyzes the performance of ε-multiobjective evolutionary algorithms on three DNA sequence design problems and validates the results by showing superior performance to previous techniques.

Chapter X describes an approach to speed up the evolutionary design of application- specific embedded systems by means of fuzzy approximation. The methodology uses a MOEA for heuristic exploration of the design space and a fuzzy system to evaluate the candidate system configurations to be visited. The proposed methodology works in two phases: firstly all configurations are evaluated using computationally expensive simulations and their results are used to train the fuzzy system until it becomes reliable; in the second phase the accuracy of the fuzzy system is refined using results obtained by simulating promising configurations. Although the methodology was applied to the design of an embedded architecture based on a very long instruction word (VLIW) microprocessor in a mobile multimedia application domain, it is of general applicability.

Chapter XI demonstrates the various robotics applications that can be achieved using MOEAs. The main objective of this chapter is to demonstrate practical ways of generating simple legged locomotion for simulated robots with two, four and six legs using MOEAs. The operational performance as well as complexities of the resulting evolved Pareto solutions that act as controllers for these robots will then be analyzed. Additionally, the operational dynamics of these evolved Pareto controllers in noisy and uncertain environments, limb dynamics and effects of using a different underlying MOEA will also be discussed.

Chapter XII proposes a brief survey of typical applications of MOEAs in the field of design energy systems at different levels, ranging from the design of component detail to the challenge about the synthesis of the configuration of complex energy conversion systems. For sake of simplicity, the proposed examples are grouped into three main categories: design of components/component details, design of overall energy system and operation of energy systems. Each multiobjective optimization problem is presented with a short background and some details about the formulation. Future research directions in the field of energy systems are also discussed at the end of the chapter.

Chapter XIII discusses assignment problems which are used throughout many research disciplines. Most assignment problems in the literature have focused on solving a single objective. This chapter focuses on assignment problems that have multiple objectives that need to be satisfied. In particular, this chapter looks at how multiobjective evolutionary algorithms have been used to solve some of these problems.

Additionally, this chapter examines many of the operators that have been utilized to solve assignment problems and discusses some of the advantages and disadvantages of using specific operators.

Chapter XIV attempts to provide a spectrum of military multiobjective optimization problems whose characteristics imply that an MOEA approach is appropriate. The choice of selected operators indicates that good results can be achieved for these problems. Selection and testing of other operators and associated parameters may generate "better" solutions. It is not intended that these problems represent the totality or even the complete spectrum of all military optimization problems. However, the examples discussed are very complex with high-dimensionality and therefore reflect the many difficulties the military faces in achieving their goals. MOEAs with local search are another method of attacking these complex problems that should provide effective and efficient solutions.

In summary, this book intends to promote the role of CI-based multiobjective optimization in solving practical problems. It is also expected to provide students with enough knowledge to be able to identify suitable techniques for their particular problems. Furthermore, it encourages deeper research into this field and the practical implementation of the results derived from this field.

Acknowledgment

The editors would like to acknowledge the help of all involved in the collation and review process of the book, without whose support the project could not have been satisfactorily completed. Deep appreciation and gratitude is due to the School of ITEE, UNSW@ADFA, for ongoing sponsorship in terms of generous allocation of Internet, hardware and software resources and other editorial support services for coordination of this year-long project.

Most of the authors of chapters included in this book also served as referees for chapters written by other authors. Thanks go to all those who provided constructive and comprehensive reviews. However, some of the reviewers must be mentioned as their reviews set the benchmark. Reviewers who provided the most comprehensive, critical and constructive comments include: Saku Kukkonen, Jason Teo, Minh Ha Nguyen, Maoguo Gong, Soo-Yong Shin, Ramesh Rajagopalan, Konstantinos E. Parsopoulos, Andrea Toffolo, Andrew Lewis, Carlos A. Coello Coello, Alessandro Di Nuovo, Mark Kleeman, Marcus Randall, and Luis Martí.

Special thanks go to the publishing team at IGI Global, whose contributions throughout the whole process from the inception of the initial idea to final publication have been invaluable. In particular, we own a great deal for Deborah Yahnke, Kristin Roth, and Ross Miller, who continuously supported us via e-mail for keeping the project on schedule.

Special thanks go to Professor Hussein Abbass for his helpful discussions on materializing this book project. And last but not least, our families, for their unfailing support and encouragement during the months it took to give birth to this book.

In closing, we wish to thank all of the authors for their insights and excellent contributions to this book.

Lam Thu Bui and Sameer Alam,
Editors,
School of ITEE, UNSW@ADFA, University of New South Wales, Australia
August 2007

Section I
Fundamentals

Chapter I
An Introduction to Multi-Objective Optimization

Lam Thu Bui
University of New South Wales, Australia

Sameer Alam
University of New South Wales, Australia

ABSTRACT

This chapter is devoted to summarize common concepts related to multi-objective optimization (MO). An overview of "traditional" as well as CI-based MO is given. Further, all aspects of performance assessment for MO techniques are discussed. Finally, challenges facing MO techniques are addressed. All of these description and analysis give the readers basic knowledge for understandings the rest of the book.

OVERVIEW

Real-world problems often have multiple conflicting objectives. For example, when purchasing computing equipments, we would usually like to have a high-performance system, but we also want to spend less money buying it (see Figure 1). Obviously, in these problems, there is no single solution that is the best when measured on all objectives (note that the terms *solution, individual* and *point* are used interchangeably in this book). These problems are examples of a special class of optimization problems called multi-objective optimization problems (MOPs). The question is what is an optimal solution for a multi-objective problem? In general, it is called a Pareto optimal solution if there exists no other feasible solution which would decrease some objectives (suppose a minimization problem) without causing a simultaneous increase in at least one other objective (Coello, 2006b).

With this definition of optimality, we usually find several trade-off solutions (called the *Pareto optimal set* to honor Vilfredo Pareto (Pareto,

Figure 1. An example of cost-performance problem

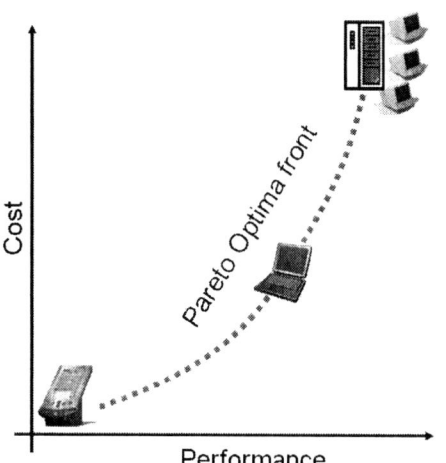

1896), or *Pareto optimal front* (POF) for the plot of the vectors corresponding to these solutions). In that sense, the search for an optimal solution has fundamentally changed from what we see in the case of single-objective problems. The task of solving MOPs is called *multi-objective optimization*.

However, users practically need only one solution from the set of optimal trade-off solutions. Therefore, solving MOPs can be seen as the combination of both searching and decision-making (Horn, 1997). In order to support this, there are four main approaches in the literature (Miettinen, 1999). The first one does not use preference information (called *no-preference*). These methods solve a problem and give a solution directly to the decision maker. The second one is to find all possible solutions of the nondominated set and to then use the user preference to determine the most suitable one (called *decision making after search*, or *posterior*). Meanwhile, the third approach is to incorporate the use of preference before the optimization process; and hence it will result in only one solution at the end (called *deci-sion making before search*, or *priori*). With this approach, the bias (from the user preference) is imposed all the time. The fourth approach (called *decision making during search*, or *interactive*) is to hybridize the second and third ones in which a human decision making is periodically used to refine the obtained trade-off solutions and thus to guide the search. In general, the second one is mostly preferred within the research community since it is less subjective than the other two.

Evolutionary algorithms (EAs) (Back, 1996; Goldberg, 1989; Michalewicz, 1996) have emerged as heuristic and global alternatives with their most striking characteristic being: using a population for the search in each iteration. This makes them suitable for solving multi-objective problems. That is why they have attracted significant attention from the research community over the last two decades. Today, the rise of evolutionary multi-objective optimization can be seen by the number of publications produced over time (Coello, 2006a). It is worthwhile to note that there are several paradigms that have emerged as alternatives for the conventional EAs, such as Particle Swarm Optimization (PSO) (Kennedy & Eberhart, 1995), Ant Colony Optimization (ACO) (Dorigo & Stutzle, 2004), Differential Evolution (DE) (Price, Storn, & Lampinen, 2005), Estimation of Distribution Algorithms (EDA) (Larraanaga & Lozano, 2002), and Artificial Immune Systems (AIS) (Dasgupta, 1998). For them, mutation and crossover operators might be replaced by some specific operator inspired by different phenomena in nature.

This chapter is organized as follows: the second section is for the common concepts and notations in multi-objective optimization using evolutionary algorithms that are used throughout the book. It is followed by descriptions of traditional multi-objective algorithms as well as MOEAs (the third and fourth sections respectively). The fifth and sixth sections are dedicated to the research issues and the performance assessment. The chapter is concluded in the final section.

CONCEPTS AND NOTATIONS

This section will define some common concepts that have been widely used in the literature as well as in this book. Interested readers might refer to Coello, Veldhuizen, and Lamont (2002), Deb (2001), Ehrgott (2005), or Miettinen (1999) for a more detailed description. Note that for evolutionary multi-objective optimization, in addition to the *decision variable space* (phenotype), we have the *decision space* or *search space* (genotype), while also the objectives form another space, called the *objective space*. However, somewhere in this book a continuous representation is used, so there is no distinction between genotype/phenotype. Therefore, the two spaces are identical.

Mathematically, in a k-objective optimization problem, a vector function $\vec{f}(\vec{x})$ of k objectives is defined as:

$$\vec{f}(\vec{x}) = \begin{bmatrix} f_1(\vec{x}) \\ f_2(\vec{x}) \\ \dots \\ f_k(\vec{x}) \end{bmatrix} \quad (1)$$

in which $\vec{x}$ is a vector of decision variables in the n-dimensional space $\mathbf{R}_n$; n and k are not necessarily the same. A solution is assigned a vector $\vec{x}$ and therefore the corresponding objective vector, $\vec{f}$. Therefore, a general MOP is defined as follows:

$$\min f_i(\vec{x}) \Big|_{\vec{x} \in D} \quad (2)$$

where $i = 1, 2, \dots, k$ and $D \in \mathbf{R}_n$, called the *feasible search region*. All solutions (including optimal solutions) that belong to D are called *feasible solutions*.

In general, when dealing with MOPs, a solution x_1 is said to dominate x_2 if x_1 is better than x_2 when measured on all objectives. If x_1 does not dominate x_2 and x_2 also does not dominate x_1, they are said to be nondominated. If we use $\preceq$ between $x1$ and $x2$ as $x_1 \preceq x_2$ to denote that x_1 dominates x_2 and $\triangleleft$ between two scalars a and b, as $a \triangleleft b$ to denote that a is better than b (similarly, $a \triangleright b$ to denote that a is worse than b, and $a \not\triangleright b$ to denote that a is not worse than b), then the dominance concept is formally defined as follows.

Definition 1: $x_1 \preceq x_2$ if the following conditions are held:

1. $f_j(x_1) \not\triangleright f_j(x_2), \forall j \in (1, 2, \dots, k)$
2. $\exists j \in (1, 2, \dots, k)$ in which $f_j(x_1) \triangleleft f_j(x_2)$

The concept defined in Definition 1 is sometimes referred to as *weak dominance*. For the *strict dominance* concept, solution x_1 must be strictly better than x_2 in all objectives. However, this book follows the weak dominance concept as defined in Definition 1. Further, the relation between individuals is called the *dominance relation*.

Generally, there are several properties of binary relations that are related to the dominance relation; and they are listed as follows:

- **Irreflexive:** From Definition 2, clearly a solution does not dominate itself. Therefore, the dominance relation is not reflexive (or is irreflexive).
- **Asymmetric:** The dominance relation is asymmetric since $x1 \preceq x2$ does not imply $x2 \preceq x1$
- **Antisymmetric:** The dominance relation is asymmetric; therefore it is not antisymmetric (recall that this property requires that if $x1 \preceq x2$ and $x2 \preceq x1$ then $x1 = x2$).
- **Transitive:** From Definition 2, we can see that if $x1 \preceq x2$ and $x2 \preceq x3$ then $x1 \preceq x3$. Therefore, the dominance relation is transitive.

Definition 2: A binary relation R is called:

- *Partially ordered* if it is reflexive, antisymmetric and transitive

- *Strictly partially ordered* if it is asymmetric and transitive

Clearly, the dominance relation is a strict partial order relation since it is not reflexive and not antisymmetric. This is an important finding and it has been used in considering theoretical aspects of multi-objective optimization (Ehrgott, 2005).

As stated earlier in the chapter, in dealing with MOPs, EAs use a population of individuals during the optimization process. At the end, we usually have a set of individuals where no one individual dominates any other one in the set. This set is an approximation of the real optimal solutions for the problem.

In general, if an individual in a population is not dominated by any other individual in the population, it is called a nondominated individual. All nondominated individuals in a population form the nondominated set (as formally described in Definition 3). Note that these definitions are equivalent to that from (Deb, 2001).

Definition 3: A set S is said to be the nondominated set of a population P if the following conditions are held:

1. $S \subseteq P$
2. $\forall s \in S, \nexists\, x \in P\; x \prec s$

When the set P represents the entire search space, the set of nondominated solutions S is called the *global Pareto optimal set*. If P represents a subspace, S will be called the *local Pareto optimal set*. There is only one global Pareto optimal set, but there could be multiple local ones. However, in general, we simply refer to the global Pareto optimal set as the Pareto optimal set. Although there are several conditions established in the literature for optimality (Miettinen, 1999; Ehrgott, 2005), however, for practical black-box optimization problems, these conditions generally cannot be verified easily.

Finally, it is worthwhile to mention here two special objective vectors (assuming that the problem is minimization) that are related to the Pareto optimal set (see Ehrgott, 2005, p. 34). For the sake of simplicity, these vectors are also called "solutions."

- **Ideal solution:** This represents the lower bound of each objective in the Pareto optimal set. It can be obtained by optimizing each objective individually in the entire feasible objective space.
- **Nadir solution:** This contains all the upper bound of each objective in the Pareto optimal set. Obtaining the Nadir solution over the Pareto optimal set is not an easy task. One of the common approaches is to estimate the Nadir point by a pay-off table based on the Ideal solution.

TRADITIONAL MULTI-OBJECTIVE ALGORITHMS

This book uses the term "traditional" to differentiate such methods from evolutionary ones. There are many traditional methods, such as the method of global criterion, weighted-sum (Cohon, 1983; Miettinen, 1999), ε-constraint (Haimes, Lasdon, & Wismer, 1971), weighted metric (Miettinen, 1999), and goal programming (Steuer, 1986). This section will only summarize several approaches that represent for different categories.

No-Preference Methods

For methods not using preference, the decision maker will receive the solution of the optimization process. They can make the choice to accept or reject it. For this, the no-preference methods are suitable in the case that the decision maker does not have specific assumptions on the solution. The method of *global criterion* (Miettinen,

1999; Zeleny, 1973) can be used to demonstrate this class of methods.

For this method, the MOPs are transformed into single objective optimization problems by minimizing the distance between some reference points and the feasible objective region. In the simplest form (using Lp-metrics), the reference point is the ideal solution and the problem is represented as follows:

$$\min \left(\sum_{i=1}^{k} |f_i(x) - z_i^*|^p \right)^{\frac{1}{p}} \quad (3)$$

where z^* is the ideal vector, and k is the number of objectives.

When $p = 1$, it is called a Tchebycheff problem with a Tchebycheff metric and is presented as follows:

$$\min \max_{i=1,\ldots,k} |f_i(x) - z_i^*| \quad (4)$$

From the equation, one can see that the obtained solutions depend very much on the choice of the p's value. Also, at the end the method will only give one solution to the decision maker.

Posteriori Methods

For posteriori methods, the decision maker will be given a set of Pareto optimal solutions and the most suitable one will be selected based on the decision maker's preference. Here, the two most popular approaches, weighted sum and ε-constraint, are summarized.

For the weighted-sum method, all the objectives are combined into a single objective by using a weight vector. The problem in equation (2) is now transformed as in equation (5).

$$\min f(\vec{x}) = w_1 f_1(\vec{x}) + w_2 f_2(\vec{x}) + \ldots + w_k f_k(\vec{x}) \mid \vec{x} \in D \quad (5)$$

where $i = 1, 2, \ldots, k$ and $D \in \mathbf{R}_n$.

The weight vector is usually normalized such that $\Sigma w_i = 1$. Figure 2 is used to demonstrate how the method works for problems with a 2D objective space. From equation (5) we can see that:

$$f2 = -\frac{w_1}{w_2} f1 + \frac{f}{w_2}.$$

This equation can be visualized as a straight line in the figure (the left one) with a slop of:

$-\frac{w_1}{w_2}$ and an intercept of $\frac{f}{w_2}$.

Therefore, when the optimization process is progressing, it is equivalent to moving the line towards the origin of the objective space until it reaches point A of the optimal set.

Although the weighted-sum method is simple and easy to use, there are two inherent problems. Firstly, there is the difficulty of selecting the weights in order to deal with scaling problems since the objectives usually have different magnitudes. Therefore, when combining them together, it is easy to cause biases when searching for trade-off solutions. Secondly, the performance of the method is heavily dependent on the shape of the POF. Consequently, it cannot find all the optimal solutions for problems that have a nonconvex POF. We can see this problem from Figure 1b where the optimization process will not reach any of the points of the Pareto set between A and C (such as B).

To overcome the difficulty of nonconvexity, the method of ε-constraint has been introduced, where only one objective is optimized while the others are transformed as constraints. The problem

Figure 2. Demonstration of weighted-sum method in 2D objective space: Problem with convex POF on the left (a), and the one with non-convex POF on the right (b)

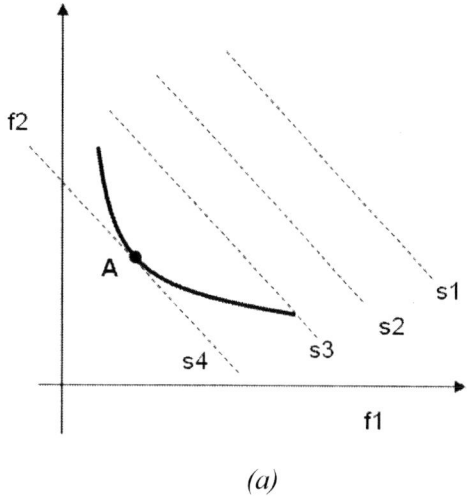

(a)

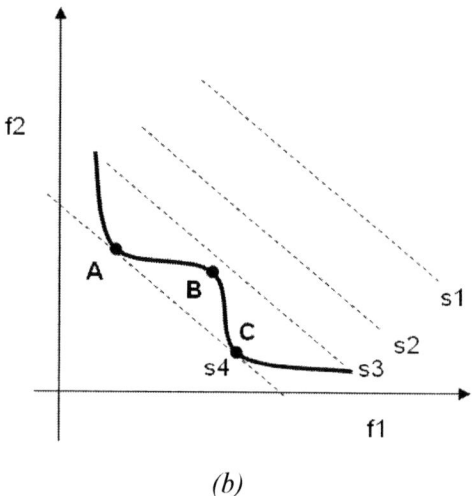

(b)

in equation (2) is now transformed as in equation (6). Again, the problem is now transformed into a single objective one.

$$\min f_j(\vec{x}) \mid \vec{x} \in D \quad (6)$$

subject to $f_i(\vec{x}) \leq \varepsilon_i$ where $i = 1, 2, ..., k, i \neq j$ and $D \in \mathbf{R}_n$.

In this method, the ε vector is determined and uses the boundary (upper bound in the case of minimization) for all objectives i. For a given ε vector, this method will find an optimal solution by optimizing objective j. By changing ε, we will obtain a set of optimal solutions. Although, this method alleviates the difficulty of nonconvexity, it still has to face the problem of selecting appropriate values for the ε vector, since it can happen that for a given ε vector, there does not exist any feasible solution. An example is given in Figure 3 where ε_1 will give an optimal solution, while ε_2 will result in no solution at all.

Priori Methods

For these methods, the decision maker must indicate the assumption about the preferences before the optimization process. Therefore, the issue is how to quantify the preference and incorporate it

Figure 3. Demonstration of the ε-constraint method in 2D objective space.

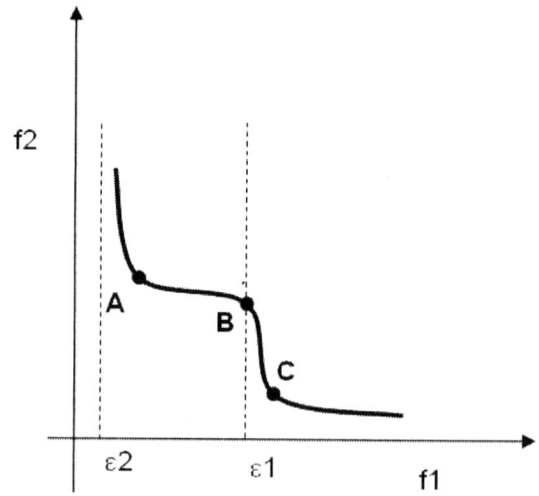

into the problem before the optimization process. Here, one obvious method is the weighted-sum where the weights can be used to represent the decision maker's preference.

However, here the methods of lexicographic ordering and goal programming (Fishburn, 1974; Ignizio, 1974; Miettinen, 1999) are used to demonstrate the use of priori preference. For a lexicographic method, the decision maker is asked to arrange the objective functions by relying on their absolute importance. The optimization process is performed individually on each objective following the order of importance. After optimizing with the most important objective (the first objective), if only one solution is returned, it is the optimal solution. Otherwise, the optimization will continue with the second objective and with a new constraint on the obtained solutions from the first objective. This loop might continue to the last objective.

For the method of goal programming, aspiration levels of the objective functions will be specified by the decision maker. Optimizing the objective function with an aspiration level is seen as a goal to be achieved. In its simplest form, goal programming can be stated as here:

$$\min \sum_{i=1}^{k} |f_i(x) - z_i| \qquad (7)$$

where z is the vector indicating the aspiration levels. A more general formulation of this equation can be derived by replacing $|f_i(x) - z_i|$ by $|f_i(x) - z_i|^p$.

Interactive Methods

The section on traditional methods is concluded by looking at the class of interactive methods, which allows the decision maker to interact with the optimization program (or an analyst). In general, the interaction can be described step-by-step as follows (see Miettinen, 1999):

- **Step 1:** Find an initial feasible solution
- **Step 2:** Interact with the decision maker, and
- **Step 3:** Obtain a new solution (or a set of new solutions). If the new solution (or one of them) or one of the previous solutions is acceptable to the decision maker, stop. Otherwise, go to Step 2.

With the interaction between the program and the decision maker, as indicated in (Miettinen, 1999), many weaknesses from the aforementioned approaches can be alleviated. To date, there are many approaches using an interactive style, namely, GDF (Geoffrion, Dyer, & Feinberg, 1972), Tchebycheff method (Steuer, 1986), Reference point method (Wierzbiki, 1980), NIMBUS (Miettinen, 1994). Recently, interactive methods have also been incorporated with MOEAs (see Abbass, 2006 for an example). Here we use the reference direction approach to demonstrate this class of the methods. The approach is described as follows:

- **Step 1:** Give the decision maker information of the problem such as the ideal solution.
- **Step 2:** Ask the decision maker to specify a reference point z
- **Step 3:** Minimize the achievement function (an example is given in equation (8)) and obtain a Pareto optimal solution x and the corresponding z. Present z to the decision maker.

$$\min \max_{i=1,\ldots,k} [w_i (f_i(x) - z_i)] \qquad (8)$$

- **Step 4:** Calculate a number of k other Pareto optimal solutions by minimizing the achievement function with perturbed reference points:

$$\bar{z}(i) = \bar{z} + de^i,$$

where

$$d = \|\bar{z} - z\|$$

and e^i is the ith unit vector for i=1,...,k

- **Step 5:** Present the alternatives to the decision maker. If the decision maker finds one of the k+1 solutions satisfied, the corresponding x is the final solution. Otherwise, go to Step 3.

From these basic steps, it appears that the approach is very simple and practical. The preference is incorporated into the achievement function and therefore the problem becomes single objective. The perturbation of the reference point gives the decision maker more understanding of the Pareto optimal set.

MULTI-OBJECTIVE EVOLUTIONARY ALGORITHMS

Overview

Multi-objective evolutionary algorithms (MOEAs) are stochastic optimization techniques. Similar to other optimization algorithms, MOEAs are used to find Pareto optimal solutions for a particular problem, but differ by using a population-based approach. The majority of existing MOEAs employ the concept of dominance in their courses of action (however, see VEGA (Schaffer, 1985) for an example of not using a dominance relation); therefore, here the focus is the class of dominance-based MOEAs.

The optimization mechanism of MOEAs is quite similar with that of EAs, except for the use of the dominance relation. In more detail, at each iteration, the objective values are calculated for every individual and are then used to determine the dominance relationships within the population, in order to select potentially better solutions for the production of the offspring population. This population might be combined with the parent population to produce the population for the next generation. Further, the existence of the objective space might give MOEAs the flexibility to apply some conventional supportive techniques such as niching.

Generally, MOEAs have to deal with two major inherent issues (Deb, 2001). The first issue is how to get close to the Pareto optimal front. This is not an easy task, because converging to the POF is a stochastic process. The second is how to keep diversity among the solutions in the obtained set. These two issues have become common criteria for most current algorithmic performance comparisons (Zitzler, Thiele, & Deb, 2000). A diverse set of solutions will give more options for decision makers, designers and so forth. However, working on a set of solutions instead of only one, makes the measurement of the convergence of a MOEA harder, since the closeness of one individual to the optima does not act as a measure for the entire set.

To date, many MOEAs have been developed. Generally speaking, there are several ways to classify MOEAs. However, this chapter follows the one used in Coello (2006b) where they are classified into two broad categories1: Non-elitism and Elitism. Note that in Coello (2006b), the author used the first and second generations of MOEAs. However, the classification actually relied on elitism

Non-Elitism Approach

The non-elitism approach has no concept of explicitly preserving the best solutions when it does selection of individuals for the next generation from the current population (Deb, 2001). Instead, selected individuals from the current generation are used to exclusively generate solutions for the next generation by crossover and mutation operators as in EAs. In Coello (2006b), all algorithms using this approach are listed as instances of the *first generation* of MOEAs which implies simplicity. The only difference from conventional EAs is that they use the dominance relation when assessing solutions. Instances of this category include MOGA (Fonseca & Fleming, 1993), NPGA (Horn, Nafpliotis, & Goldberg, 1994) and NSGA (Deb, 2001).

Although MOEAs are different from each other, the common steps of these algorithms can be summarized as next. Note that Steps 2 and 5 are used for elitism approaches that will be summarized in the next subsection.

- **Step 1:** Initialize a population P
- **Step 2:** (optional): Select elitist solutions from P to create/update an external set FP (For non-elitism algorithms, FP is empty).
- **Step 3:** Create mating pool from one or both of P and FP
- **Step 4:** Perform reproduction based on the pool to create the next generation P
- **Step 5:** Possibly combine FP into P
- **Step 6:** Go to Step 2 if the termination condition is not satisfied.

Elitism Approach

Elitism is a mechanism to preserve the best individuals from generation to generation. By this way, the system never loses the best individuals found during the optimization process. Elitism was used at quite an early stage of evolutionary computing (see DeJong, 1975) for an example); and to date, it has been used widely with EAs. Elitism can be done by placing one or more of the best individuals directly into the population for the next generations, or by comparing the offspring individual with its parents and then the offspring will only be considered if it is better than the parent (Storn & Price, 1995).

In the domain of evolutionary multi-objective optimization, elitist MOEAs usually (but not necessarily) employ an external set (the archive) to store the nondominated solutions after each generation. In general, when using the archive, there are two important aspects as follows:

- **Interaction between the archive and the main population:** This is about how we use the archive during the optimization process; for example, one such way is to combine the archive with the current population to form the population for the next generation as in Zitzler, Laumanns, and Thiele (2001).
- **Updating the archive:** This is about the methodology to build the archive, one such method is by using the neighborhood relationship between individuals using crowded dominance (Deb, Pratap, Agarwal, & Meyarivan, 2002), clustering (Zitzler et al., 2001), or geographical grid (Knowles & Corne, 2000), while another method is by controlling the size of the archive through truncation when the number of nondominated individuals are over a predefined threshold.

Obviously, the current archive might then be a part of the next generation; however, the way to integrate this archive may be different from one algorithm to another. In general, with elitism, the best individuals in each generation are always preserved, and this helps the algorithms to get closer to the POF; a proof of convergence for MOEAs using elitism can be found in (Rudolph & Agapie, 2000). Algorithms such as PAES (Knowles & Corne, 2000), SPEA2 (Zitzler et al., 2001), PDE (Abbass, Sarker, & Newton, 2001), NSGA-II (Deb et al., 2002), and MOPSO (Coello, Pulido, & Lechuga, 2004) are typical examples of this category.

Selected MOEAs

This section will summarize several approaches in the literature.

Nondominated Sorting Genetic Algorithms Version 2: NSGA-II

NSGA-II is an elitism algorithm (Deb, 2001; Deb et al., 2002). The main feature of NSGA-II lies in its elitism-preservation operation. Note that NSGA-II does not use an explicit archive; a population is used to store both elitist and non-elitist solutions for the next generation. However, for consistency, it is still considered as an archive. Firstly, the archive size is set equal to the initial population size. The current archive is then determined based on the combination of the current population and the previous archive. To do this, NSGA-II uses dominance ranking to classify the population into a number of layers, such that the first layer is the nondominated set in the population, the second layer is the nondominated set in the population with the first layer removed, the third layer is the nondominated set in the population with the first and second layers removed and so on. The archive is created based on the order of ranking layers: the best rank being selected first. If the number of individuals in the archive is smaller than the population size, the next layer will be taken into account and so forth. If adding a layer makes the number of individuals in the archive exceed the initial population size, a truncation operator is applied to that layer using *crowding distance*.

The *crowding distance D* of a solution x is calculated as follows: the population is sorted according to each objective to find adjacent solutions to x; boundary solutions are assigned infinite values; the average of the differences between the adjacent solutions in each objective is calculated; the truncation operator removes the individual with the smallest *crowding distance*.

$$D(x) = \sum_{m=1}^{M} \frac{F_m^{I_x^m+1} - F_m^{I_x^m-1}}{F_m^{max} - F_m^{min}} \quad (9)$$

in which F is the vector of objective values, and I_x^m returns the sorted index of solution x, according to objective m^{th}.

An offspring population of the same size as the initial population is then created from the archive, by using crowded tournament selection, crossover, and mutation operators. Crowded tournament selection is a traditional tournament selection method, but when two solutions have the same rank, it uses the crowding distance to break the tie.

A Pareto-Frontier Differential Evolution Algorithm for MOPs: PDE

The algorithm works as follows (Abbass et al., 2001): an initial population is generated at random from a Gaussian distribution with a predefined mean and standard deviation. All dominated solutions are removed from the population. The remaining nondominated solutions are retained for reproduction. If the number of nondominated solutions exceeds some threshold, a distance metric relation is used to remove those parents who are very close to each other. Three parents are selected at random. A child is generated from the three parents as in conventional single-objective Differential Evolution and is placed into the population if it dominates the first selected parent; otherwise a new selection process takes place. This process continues until the population is completed. A maximum number of nondominated solutions in each generation was set to 50. If this maximum is exceeded, the following nearest neighbor distance function is adopted:

$$D(x) = \frac{\min\|x - x_i\| + \min\|x - x_j\|}{2}$$

where $x \ne x_i \ne x_j$. That is, the nearest neighbor distance is the average Euclidean distance between the closest two points. The nondominated solution with the smallest neighbor distance is removed from the population until the total number of nondominated solutions is retained to 50.

Strength Pareto Evolutionary Algorithm 2: SPEA2

SPEA2 is actually an extension of an elitism MOEA called "The Strength Pareto Evolution Algorithm"—SPEA (Zitzler & Thiele, 1999). This section just concentrates on the main points of SPEA2 (Zitzler et al., 2001). The initial population, representation and evolutionary operators are standard: uniform distribution, binary representation, binary tournament selection, single-point crossover, and bit-flip mutation. However, the distinctive feature of SPEA2 lies in the elitism-preserved operation.

An external set (archive) is created for storing primarily nondominated solutions. It is then combined with the current population to form the next archive that is then used to create offspring for the next generation. The size of the archive is fixed. It can be set to be equal to the population size. Therefore, there exist two special situations when filling solutions in the archive. If the number of nondominated solutions is smaller than the archive size, other dominated solutions taken from the remainder part of the population are filled in. This selection is carried out according to a fitness value, specifically defined for SPEA. That is the individual fitness value defined for a solution x, is the total of the SPEA-defined strengths of solutions which dominate x, plus a density value.

The second situation happens when the number of nondominated solutions is over the archive size. In this case, a truncation operator is applied. For that operator, the solution which has the smallest distance to the other solutions will be removed from the set. If solutions have the same minimum distance, the second nearest distance will be considered, and so forth. This is called the *k-th nearest distance rule*.

Pareto Archived Evolutionary Strategy: PAES

This algorithm uses an evolutionary strategy for solving multi-objective problems (Knowles & Corne, 2000). Therefore, it uses the mutation operator only, and the parental solutions are mutated to generate offspring. Similar to evolutionary strategies, it also has different versions such as (1+1), (1+λ), or (μ, λ). The unique property of PAES is the way it uses and maintains elitism. We consider the case (1+1) as an example.

If the newly generated offspring dominates the parent, it replaces its parent. Conversely, if the parent dominates the offspring, it is discarded and new offspring will be generated. However, if both of them are nondominated, there is a further mechanism to compare them (note that PAES also has an archive to store the nondominated solutions over time). To do this, the offspring will be compared against all of the nondominated solutions found so far in the archive. There will be several possible cases as follows:

- **Offspring is dominated by a member of the archive:** It is discarded and the parent is mutated again.
- **Offspring dominates some members of the archive:** These members are deleted from the archive and the offspring is included into the archive. It also will be a parent in the next generation.
- **Offspring is nondominated with all members of the archive:** Offspring will be considered to be included into the archive depending on the current size of the archive. Note that the parent is also a nondominated solution and belongs to the archive. Therefore, it is necessary to calculate the density in the areas of both solutions in order to decide which one will be the parent of the next generation. For this, a hyper-grid is built in the area of the objective occupied by the archive, where all solutions in the archive will belong to different hyper-cells of the grid depending on their locations. Thus, the offspring is selected if its cell is less crowed than that of the parent.

To keep the size of the archive always below its limit, PAES also uses a density measure. The solution associated with the highest-density cell will be replaced by the newcomer (the offspring).

Multi-Objective Particle Swarm Optimizer: MOPSO

This is a MOEA which incorporates Pareto dominance into a particle swarm optimization algorithm in order to allow the PSO algorithm to handle problems with several objective functions (Coello et al., 2004). In PSO, a population of solutions (particles) are used without neither crossover nor mutation operators. Each solution is assigned a velocity and uses this velocity to make a move in the search space. The determination of the velocity of a particle is dependent on both the best position the particle has achieved (the local best) and the best position the population has found so far (the global best). Applying PSO to multi-objective optimization very much relies on how to define the local and global best positions.

MOPSO keeps tracking the local best for every solution over time. In order to find the global best position for each solution, MOPSO uses an external archive (secondary repository) of particles to store all nondominated particles. Each particle will be assigned for a selected one in the archive (as the global best). The selection of a particle in the archive is dependent on the density of the areas surrounding the particle. Further, the archive is updated continuously and its size is controlled by using the grid technique proposed in PAES where a hyper-grid is built in the area of the objective occupied by the archive, and all solutions in the archive will belong to different hyper-cells of the grid depending on their locations.

PROBLEM DIFFICULTIES AND RESEARCH ISSUES

This section introduces a number of possible challenges that MOEAs might face in solving practical problems (note that there are several problem difficulties for conventional optimization that do not matter to MOEAs, such as convexity, concavity, discontinuity, or differentiability). Although they are not always separated, but for the purpose of a clear description, they can be categorized as follows:

- **Multimodality:** This is one of the major hurdles that faces the application of optimization algorithms to many real life problems. Problems with multimodality usually have multiple local optima. This causes the algorithm to become easily attracted to a basin associated with local optima. Solving these problems is the main objective of a class of optimization algorithms called global optimization (Torn & Zilinskas, 1989). In multi-objective optimization, multimodality of a problem is understood in the sense that the problem has many local Pareto optimal fronts and only one global POF.
- **Epitasis among decision variables:** This difficulty introduces interdependency among variables. At the extreme, all of the variables interact with all others. Rotated problems can be seen as examples. Obviously, it is a challenge for optimization algorithms that rely on optimizing along each independent variable, such as dynamic programming. In evolutionary computing, this difficulty is usually referred to as the problem of linkage learning (Goldberg, 2002).
- **Dynamic environments:** The world is dynamic. It is changing from time to time with different levels and at almost all aspects. That is why dynamism happening on many real-world optimization problems, such as timetabling, routing, or path planning. In general, there are several aspects when dealing with dynamic environments including the frequency of change and the severity of change. Further, the performance of algorithms is dependent on their ability to track the optima over time (Branke, 2002; Bui et al., 2005b).
- **Noisy environments:** A noise effect is inevitable in many real-world problems. Sources of noise can vary depending on the way data is obtained such as the sensors,

and actuators, or because of the stochastic elements pertaining in some problems such as multi-agent simulations (Bui et al., 2005a). In the presence of noise, the optimization process might be misled by including inferior solutions. If the distribution of noise is symmetric around zero, such population-based approaches as evolutionary algorithms can maintain well their progress since the population acts as a noise filter (Nissen & Propach, 1998).
- **Scalability:** This matter has a long history associated with optimization. Originally, it was considered in the decision space, where by increasing the number of variables, the search space became larger, more complicated and more vulnerable to the effect of numerical rounding errors. With the development of multi-objective optimization, scalability is also considered in the objective space with more than two objectives (Khare, Yao, & Deb, 2003).
- **Expensive objective-value evaluation:** This difficulty does not cause errors in approaching the optima. However, it sometimes makes the optimization process become impossible, since it has to spend too much time on objective evaluation efforts. In this case, two popular approaches have been using estimated objective functions (Jin, 2005) and employing distributed computation (Cantuz-Paz, 2000; Veldhuizen, Zydallis, & Lamont, 2003; Bui et al., 2007; Bui, 2007).

These aspects pose major challenges to the use of MOEAs (and EAs in general) in solving optimization problems. That is why they are main themes in the research community of evolutionary computation in both theoretical and experimental senses. The consideration of these aspects reveals a key rule that the success of an algorithm is heavily dependent on the study of the search problems with regards to the no-free lunch theorem (Wolpert & Macready, 1997).

Furthermore, for all population-based methods, there is an advantage to model (learn) the fitness landscapes of the testing problems, especially the black-box ones, since the population acts as a sample of the fitness landscape. There is also a possibility to incorporate both evolution and learning during the optimization process.

PERFORMANCE ASSESSMENTS

Performance metrics are usually used to compare algorithms in order to form an understanding of which one is better and in what aspects. However, it is hard to define a concise definition of algorithmic performance. In general, when doing comparisons, a number of criteria are employed (Zitzler et al., 2000):

- Closeness of the obtained nondominated set to the Pareto optimal front.
- A good (in most cases, uniform) distribution of solutions within the set.
- Spread of the obtained nondominated front, that is, for each objective, a wide range of values should be covered by the nondominated solutions.

Based on these criteria, the community of evolutionary multi-objective optimization has developed a number of performance metrics. Recently, there have been a number of works to develop platforms for performance assessments including most popular metrics such as the PISA system (Bleuler, Laumanns, Thiele, & Zitzler, 2003). This section will provide a summary of the most popular ones of these metrics.

Metrics Evaluating Closeness to the POF

The first obvious metric is the error rate, *ER*, introduced by Veldhuizen (Veldhuizen, 1999). It is calculated by the percentage of solutions that are not in the POF:

$$ER = \frac{\sum_{i=1}^{N} e_i}{N} \quad (10)$$

where N is the size of the obtained set and $e_i = 1$ if the solution i is not in the POF, otherwise $e_i = 0$. The smaller the ER, the better the convergence to the POF. However, this metric does not work in the case when all the solutions of two compared sets are not in the POFs. In this case, a threshold is employed, such that if the distance from a solution i to the POF is greater than the threshold, $e_i = 1$, otherwise $e_i = 0$.

The second metric is the generation distance, GD, which is the average distance from the set of solutions found by evolution to the POF (Veldhuizen, 1999)

$$GD = \frac{\sqrt{\sum_{i=1}^{N} d_i^2}}{N} \quad (11)$$

where d_i is the Euclidean distance (in objective space) from solution i to the nearest solution in the POF. If there is a large fluctuation in the distance values, it is also necessary to calculate the variance of the metric. Finally, the objective values should be normalized before calculating the distance.

Metrics Evaluating Diversity Among Obtained Nondominated Solutions

The spread metric is also an important one in performance comparisons. One of its instances is introduced by Schott (1995), called the *spacing* method.

$$S = \frac{\sqrt{\frac{1}{N}\sum_{i=1}^{N}(\overline{d} - d_i)^2}}{\overline{d}} \quad (12)$$

where

$$d_i = \min_{j=1,\dots,N} \sum_{m=1}^{M} |f_m^i - f_m^j|$$

and f_m is the mth objective function. N is the population size and M is the number of objectives. The interpretation of this metric is that the smaller the value of S, the better the distribution in the set. For some problems, this metric might be correlated with the number of obtained solutions. In general, this metric focuses on the distribution of the Pareto optimal set, not the extent of the spread.

In Deb et al. (2002), the authors proposed another method to alleviate the problem of the above spacing method. The spread of a set of nondominated solutions is calculated as follows:

$$\Delta = \frac{\sum_{i=1}^{M} d_i^e + \sum_{i=1}^{N} |d_i - \overline{d}|}{\sum_{i=1}^{M} d_i^e + N\overline{d}} \quad (13)$$

where d_i can be any distance measure between neighboring solutions and $\overline{d}$ is the mean value of these distances. d_i^e is the distance between extreme solutions of the obtained nondominated set and the true Pareto optimal set. Δ ranges from 0 to 1. If it is close to 1, the spread is bad.

Metrics Evaluating Both Closeness and Diversity

Note that all of the metrics in the previous section focus on a single criterion only. This section summarizes the other two that take into account both closeness and diversity. The first one is the hypervolume ratio (Zitzler & Thiele, 1998), one of the most widely accepted by the research community of MOEAs. To calculate the hyper-volume, an area of objective space covered by the obtained POF is measured, called the hyper-area (see Figure 4). Note that calculating the hyper-volume is a time-consuming process (although recently several attempts have been given to speed up this process (While, Bradstreet, Barone, & Hingston, 2005; While, Hingston, Barone, & Huband, 2006). In general, for two sets of solutions, whichever has the greater value of hyper-volume will be the best. However, when using hyper-volume it is sometime difficult to understand the quality of the obtained POF in comparison with the true POF.

As recommended in Coello et al. (2002) and Veldhuizen (1999), it is considered better to use the hyper-volume ratio (HR) that is measured by the ratio between the hyper-volumes of hyperareas covered by the obtained POF and the true POF, called $H1$ and $H2$ respectively. HR is calculated as in equation (14). For this metric, the greater the value of HR, the better the convergence that the algorithm has.

$$HR = \frac{H_1}{H_2} \quad (14)$$

There are some questions on how to determine the reference point for the calculation of the hyper-volume. For example, it can be the origin (Veldhuizen, 1999). However, generally it is dependent on the area of the objective space that is visited by all comparing algorithms. In this revised version, as suggested elsewhere (Deb, 2001), the reference point is the one associated with all the worst values of objectives found by all the algorithms under investigation.

The second metric uses a statistical comparison method. It was first introduced by Fonesca and Fleming (1996). For experiments of MOEAs, which generate a large set of solutions, this metric is often the most suitable, as their data can easily be assessed by statistical methods. Knowles and Corne (2000) modified this metric and instead of drawing parallel lines, all lines originate from the origin. The basic idea is as follows: suppose that two algorithms (A1, A2) result in two non-dominated sets: P1 and P2. The lines that join the solutions in P1 and P2 are called attainment surfaces. The comparison is carried out in the objective space. In order to do the comparison, a number of lines are drawn from the origin (assuming a minimization problem), such that they intersect with the surfaces. The comparison is then individually done for each sampling line to determine which one outperforms the other. Each intersection line will then yield to a number of intersection points. In this case, statistical tests are necessary to determine the percentage an algorithm outperformed the other in each section. For both of these methods, the final results are two numbers that show the percentage of the space where each algorithm outperforms the other.

Statistical Testing

Since MOEAs (and EAs in general) are stochastic, we cannot rely on the results obtained from only

Figure 4. An example of calculating hyper-volume from a Pareto optimal set in 2D objective space

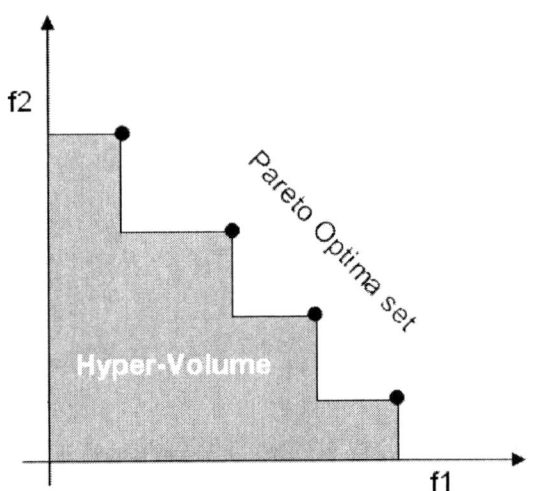

one run tested on a particular problem. Therefore, it is necessary that every algorithm involved in the comparison needs to be tested on the problem for a number of independent runs (equivalent to using different random seeds). In general, all algorithms were usually tested for a number of runs. By applying the aforementioned metrics (except the one using attainment surfaces), at the end, a set of numerical values was obtained for each algorithm. All comparisons will be done on these sets. From the statistical point of view, there are a number of concepts that can be used to compare the sets, including the mean, standard deviation, and median. However, the confidence on using these concepts in comparison is questionable. In general, the final decision on the performance of algorithms will be made after completing a statistical testing.

CONCLUSION

This chapter provided an overview of different aspects of multi-objective optimization. It is important to summarize several implications that emerge from this overview:

- Multi-objectivity naturally adheres to real-world optimization problems.
- MOEAs are practical approaches to solving real-world optimization problems
- Controlling elitism via the use of the archive is the most important issue in developing efficient MOEAs

Lastly, there has been a trend to extend newly introduced paradigms of EAs (rather than the conventional ones), such as the PDE shown in the previous section, to the area of multi-objective optimization. Some of them will be introduced in the next chapters.

REFERENCES

Abbass, H. A. (2006). An economical cognitive approach for bi-objective optimization using bliss points, visualization, and interaction. *Soft Computing, 10*(8), 687-698.

Abbass, H. A., Sarker, R., & Newton, C. (2001). PDE: A Pareto frontier differential evolution approach for multi-objective optimization problems. In *Proceedings of the Congress on Evolutionary Computation* (vol. 2, pp. 971-978), Seoul Korea. IEEE Service Center.

Back, T. (1996). *Evolutionary algorithms in theory and practice*. New York: Oxford University Press.

Bleuler, S., Laumanns, M., Thiele, L., & Zitzler, E. (2003). Pisa: A platform and programming language independent interface for search algorithms. *Evolutionary multi-criterion optimisation. Lecture notes in computer science*, (Vol. 2632, pp. 494-508). Springer.

Branke, J. (2002). *Evolutionary optimization in dynamic environments*. Massachusetts: Kluwer Academic Publishers.

Bui, L. T. (2007). *The role of communication messages and explicit niching in distributed evolutionary multi-objective optimization*. PhD Thesis, University of New South Wales.

Bui, L. T., Abbass, H. A., & Essam, D. (2005a). Fitness inheritance for noisy evolutionary multi-objective optimization. *Proceedings of the Genetic and Evolutionary Computation Conference (GECCO-2005)* (pp. 779-785). Washington, DC: ACM Press.

Bui, L. T., Abbass, H. A., & Essam, D. (2007). Local models. An approach to distributed multi-objective optimization. *Journal of Computational Optimization and Applications*, In press. DOI: 10.1007/s10589-007-9119-8

Bui, L. T., Branke, J., & Abbass, H. A. (2005b). Multi-objective optimization for dynamic environments. *Proceedings of the Congress on Evolutionary Computation (CEC)* (pp. 2349-2356). Edinburgh, UK: IEEE Press.

Cantuz-Paz, E. (2000). *Efficient and accurate parallel genetic algorithms.* Boston, MA: Kluwer Academic Publishers.

Coello, C. (2006a). *EMOO repository.* Retrieved February 5, 2008 from, http://delta.cs.cinvestav.mx/ ccoello/EMOO/

Coello, C. A. C. (2006b). Evolutionary multi-objective optimization: A historical view of the field. *IEEE Computational Intelligence Magazine, 1*(1), 28-36.

Coello, C. A. C., Pulido, G. T., & Lechuga, M. S. (2004). Handling multiple objectives with particle swarm optimization. *IEEE Transactions one Evolutionary Computation, 8*(3), 256-279.

Coello, C. A. C., Veldhuizen, D. A. V., & Lamont, G. B. (2002). *Evolutionary algorithms for solving multi-objective problems.* New York: Kluwer Academic Publishers.

Cohon, J. L. (1983). *Multi-objective programming and planning.* New York: Academic Press.

Dasgupta, D. (1998). *Artificial immune systems and their applications.* Berlin, Germany: Springer.

Deb, K. (2001). *Multi-objective optimization using evolutionary algorithms.* New York: John Wiley and Son Ltd.

Deb, K., Pratap, A., Agarwal, S., & Meyarivan, T. (2002). A fast and elitist multi-objective genetic algorithm: NSGA-II. *IEEE Transactions on Evolutionary Computation, 6*(2), 182-197.

DeJong, K. A. (1975). *An analysis of the behavior of a class of genetic adaptive systems.* Unpublished doctoral thesis, University of Michigan, Ann Arbor.

Dorigo, M. & Stutzle, T. (2004). *Ant colony optimization.* MIT Press.

Ehrgott, M. (2005). *Multicriteria optimisation* (2nd ed.). Berlin, Germany: Springer.

Fishburn, P. C. (1974). Lexicographic orders, utilities, and decision rules: A survey. *Management Science, 20*(11), 1442-1471.

Fonseca, C. & Fleming, P. (1993). Genetic algorithms for multi-objective optimization: Formulation, discussion and generalization. In *Proceedings of the Fifth International Conference on Genetic Algorithms, San Mateo, California* (pp. 416-423). Morgan Kauffman Publishers.

Fonseca, C. & Fleming, P. (1996). On the performance assessement and comparision of stochastic multi-objective optimizers. In H.-M. Voigt, W. Ebeling, I. Rechenberg, and H.-P. Schwefel (Eds.), *Parallel problem solving from nature - PPSN IV, Lecture Notes in Computer Science* (pp. 584-593). Berlin, Germany: Springer Verlag.

Geoffrion, A. M., Dyer, J. S., & Feinberg, A. (1972). An interactive approach for multi-criterion optimization, with an application to the operation of an academic department. *Management Science, 19*(4), 357-368.

Goldberg, D. (2002). *The design of innovation: Lessons from and for competent genetic algorithms.* Massachusetts: Kluwer Academic Publishers.

Goldberg, D. E. (1989). *Genetic algorithms in search, optimization and machine learning.* Boston, MA: Addison-Wesley Longman Publishing Co., Inc.

Haimes, Y. Y., Lasdon, . S., & Wismer, D. A. (1971). On a bicriteriion formulation of the problem of integrated system identification and system optimization. *IEEE Transactions on Systems, Man, and Cybernetics, 1*(3), 296-297.

Horn, J. (1997). Multicriteria decision making. In T. Back, D. B. Gogel, & Z. Michalewicz (Eds.),

Handbook of evolutionary computation. Institute of Physics Publishing.

Horn, J., Nafpliotis, N., & Goldberg, D. (1994). A niched Pareto genetic algorithm for multi-objective optimization. In *Proceedings of the First IEEE Conference on Evolutionary Computation* (Vol. 1, pp. 82-87). IEEE World Congress on Computational Intelligence, Piscataway, New Jersey.

Ignizio, J. P. (1974). Generalized goal programming: An overview. *Computer and Operations Research, 10*(4), 277-289.

Jin, Y. (2005). A comprehensive survey of fitness approximation in evolutionary computation. *Soft Computing, 9*(1), 3-12.

Kennedy, J. & Eberhart, R. C. (1995). Particle swarm optimization. In *Proceedings of IEEE International Conference on Neural Networks* (Vol. 4, pp. 1942-1948).

Khare, V., Yao, X., & Deb, K. (2003). Performance scaling of multi-objective evolutionary algorithms. In *Proceedings of the Evolutionary Multi-Objective Optimization Conference, Lecture notes in computer science* (Vol. 2632, pp. 346-390). Springer.

Knowles, J. & Corne, D. (2000a). Approximating the nondominated front using the pareto archibed evoltion strategy. *Evolutionary Computation, 8*(2), 149-172.

Larraanaga, P. & Lozano, J. A. (2002). *Estimation of distribution algorithms: A new tool for evolutionary computation.* Norwell, MA: Kluwer Academic Publishers.

Michalewicz, Z. (1996). *Genetic algorithms + data structures = evolution programs* (3rd ed.). London: Springer-Verlag..

Miettinen, K. (1994). *On the methodology of multi-objective optimization with applications.* Unpublished doctoral thesis (Rep. No. 60), University of JyvÄaskylÄa, Department of Mathematics.

Miettinen, K. (1999). *Nonlinear multi-objective optimization.* Boston: Kluwer Academic Publishers.

Nissen, V. & Propach, J. (1998). On the robustness of population-based versus point-based optimization in the presence of noise. *IEEE Transactions on Evolutionary Computation, 2*(3), 107-119.

Pareto, V. (1896). *Cours d'e_conomie politique professe_ a_l'universite_ de Lausanne* (Vol. 1,2). F. Rouge, Laussanne.

Price, K., Storn, R., & Lampinen, J. (2005). *Differential evolution - A practical approach to global optimization.* Berlin, Germany: Springer.

Rudolph, G. & Agapie, A. (2000). Convergence properties of some multi-objective evolutionary algorithms. In *Proceedings of the Congress on Evolutionary Computation* (pp. 1010-1016). IEEE Press.

Runyon, R. P., Coleman, K. A., & Pittenger, D. (1996). *Fundamentals of behavioral statistics.* Boston: McGraw-Hill.

Schaffer, J. (1985). Multiple objective optimization with vector evaluated genetic algorithms. *Genetic algorithms and their applications: Proceedings of the first international conference on genetic algorithms* (pp. 93-100). Hillsdale, New Jersey.

Schott, J. (1995). Fault tolerant design using single and multicriteria genetic algorithm optimization. Unpublished master's thesis, Department of Aeronautics and Astronautics, Massachusets Institute of Technology.

Steuer, R. E. (1986). *Multiple criteria optimization: Theory, computation, and applications.* John Wiley & Sons, Inc.

Storn, R. and Price, K. (1995). *Differential evolution—A simple and efficient adaptive scheme for global optimization over continuous spaces* (Tech. Rep. No. tr-95-012). ICSI.

Torn, A. & Zilinskas, A. (1989). *Global optimization*. Springer-Verlag.

Veldhuizen, D. (1999). *Multi-objective evolutionary algorithms: Classifications, analyses, and new innovation*. Unpublished doctoral thesis, Department of Electrical Engineering and Computer Engineering, Air-force Institute of Technology, Ohio.

Veldhuizen, D. A. V., Zydallis, J. B., & Lamont, G. B. (2003). Considerations in engineering parallel multi-objective evolutionary algorithms. *IEEE Transactions on Evolutionary Computation, 7*(2), 144-173.

While, L., Bradstreet, L., Barone, L., & Hingston, P. (2005). Heuristics for optimising the calculation of hypervolume for multi-objective optimization problems. *IEEE congress on evolutionary computation* (Vol. 3, pp. 2225-2232). IEEE Press.

While, R. L., Hingston, P., Barone, L., & Huband, S. (2006). A faster algorithm for calculating hypervolume. *IEEE Transactions on Evolutionary Computation, 10*(1), 29-38.

Wierzbiki, A. P. (1980). Optimization techniques, Part 1. *Metholodlogical guide to multi-objective optimisation, Lecture notes in control and information sciences 22*. (pp. 99-123), Berlin, Germany: Springer-Verlag.

Wolpert, D. H. & Macready, W. G. (1997). No free lunch theorems for optimization. *IEEE Transactions on Evolutionary Computation, 1*(1), 67-82.

Zeleny, M. (1973). Multiple criteria decision making. *Compromise programming* (pp. 262-301). University of South Carolina Press.

Zitzler, E., Laumanns, M., & Thiele, L. (2001). SPEA2: Improving the strength Pareto evolutionary algorithm for multi-objective optimization. In K. C. Giannakoglou, D. T. Tsahalis, J. Periaux, K. D. Papailiou, & T. Fogarty (Eds.), *Evolutionary methods for design optimization and control with applications to industrial problems* (pp. 95-100). International Center for Numerical Methods in Engineering (Cmine).

Zitzler, E. & Thiele, L. (1998). Multi-objective optimization using evolutionary algorithms—A comparative case study. *Parallel problem solving from nature, Lecture notes in computer science* (Vol. 1498, pp. 292-304). Springer.

Zitzler, E. & Thiele, L. (1999). Multi-objective evolutionary algorithms: A comparative case study and the strength Pareto approach. *IEEE Transactions on Evolutionary Computation, 3*(4), 257–271.

Zitzler, E., Thiele, L., & Deb, K. (2000). Comparison of multi-objective evolutionary algorithms: Empirical results. *Evolutionary Computation, 8*(1), 173-195.

Chapter II
Multi-Objective Particles Swarm Optimization Approaches

Konstantinos E. Parsopoulos
University of Patras, Greece

Michael N. Vrahatis
University of Patras, Greece

ABSTRACT

The multiple criteria nature of most real world problems has boosted research on multi-objective algorithms that can tackle such problems effectively, with the smallest possible computational burden. Particle Swarm Optimization has attracted the interest of researchers due to its simplicity, effectiveness and efficiency in solving numerous single-objective optimization problems. Up-to-date, there are a significant number of multi-objective Particle Swarm Optimization approaches and applications reported in the literature. This chapter aims at providing a review and discussion of the most established results on this field, as well as exposing the most active research topics that can give initiative for future research.

INTRODUCTION

Multi-objective optimization problems consist of several objectives that are necessary to be handled simultaneously. Such problems arise in many applications, where two or more, sometimes competing and/or incommensurable, objective functions have to be minimized concurrently. Due to the multicriteria nature of such problems, optimality of a solution has to be redefined, giving rise to the concept of Pareto optimality.

In contrast to the single-objective optimization case, multi-objective problems are characterized by trade-offs and, thus, there is a multitude of Pareto optimal solutions, which correspond to different settings of the investigated multi-objective problem. For example, in shape optimization, different Pareto optimal solutions correspond to different structure configurations of equal fitness but different properties. Thus, the necessity of finding the largest allowed number of such solutions, with adequate variety of their corresponding properties, is highly desirable.

Evolutionary algorithms seem to be particularly suited to multi-objective problems due to their ability to synchronously search for multiple Pareto optimal solutions and perform better global exploration of the search space (Coello, Van Veldhuizen, & Lamont, 2002; Deb, 1999; Schaffer, 1984). Up-to-date, a plethora of evolutionary algorithms have been proposed, implementing different concepts such as fitness sharing and niching (Fonseca & Fleming, 1993; Horn, Nafpliotis, & Goldberg, 1994; Srinivas & Deb, 1994), and elitism (Deb, Pratap, Agarwal, & Meyarivan, 2002; Erickson, Mayer, & Horn, 2001; Zitzler & Thiele, 1999). External archives have also been introduced as a means of memory for retaining Pareto optimal solutions. This addition enhanced significantly the performance of some algorithms, but it has also raised questions regarding the manipulation of the archive and its interaction with the actual population of search points.

Particle Swarm Optimization (PSO) is a swarm intelligence method that roughly models the social behavior of swarms (Kennedy & Eberhart, 2001). PSO shares many features with evolutionary algorithms that rendered its adaptation to the multi-objective context straightforward. Although several ideas can be adopted directly from evolutionary algorithms, the special characteristics that distinguish PSO from them, such as the directed mutation, population representation and operators must be taken into consideration in order to produce schemes that take full advantage of PSO's efficiency.

Up-to-date, several studies of PSO on multi-objective problems have appeared, and new, specialized variants of the method have been developed (Reyes-Sierra & Coello, 2006a). This chapter aims at providing a descriptive review of the state-of-the-art multi-objective PSO variants.

Of course, it is not possible to include in the limited space of a book chapter the whole literature. For this reason, we selected to present the approaches that we considered most important and proper to sketch the most common features considered in the development of algorithms. Thus, we underline to the reader the fundamental issues in PSO-based multi-objective approaches, as well as the most active research directions and future trends. An additional reading section regarding applications and further developments is included at the end of the chapter, in order to provide a useful overview of this blossoming research field.

The rest of the chapter is organized as follows: Section 2 provides concise descriptions of the necessary background material, namely the basic multi-objective concepts and the PSO algorithm. Section 3 is devoted to the discussion of key concepts and issues that arise in the transition from single-objective to multi-objective cases. Section 4 exposes the established PSO approaches reported in the relative literature, and highlights their main features, while Section 5 discusses the most active research directions and future trends. The chapter concludes in Section 6.

BACKGROUND MATERIAL

Although the basic concepts of multi-objective optimization have been analyzed in another chapter of this book, we report the most essential for completeness purposes, along with a presentation of the PSO algorithm.

Basic Multi-Objective Optimization Concepts

Let $S \subset \mathbb{R}^n$ be an n-dimensional search space, and $f_i(x)$, $i=1,\ldots,k$, be k objective functions defined over S. Also, let **f** be a vector function defined as

$$\mathbf{f}(x) = [f_1(x), f_2(x), \ldots, f_k(x)], \quad (1)$$

and

$$g_i(x) \leq 0, \quad i = 1,\ldots, m, \quad (2)$$

be m inequality constraints. Then, we are interested in finding a solution, $x^* = (x_1^*, x_2^*,\ldots, x_n^*)$, that minimizes $\mathbf{f}(x)$. The objective functions $f_i(x)$ may be conflicting with each other, thereby rendering the detection of a single global minimum at the same point in S, impossible. For this purpose, optimality of a solution in multi-objective problems needs to be redefined properly.

Let $u = (u_1,\ldots, u_k)$ and $v = (v_1,\ldots, v_k)$ be two vectors of the search space S. Then, u *dominates* v, if and only if, $u_i \leq v_i$ for all $i=1, 2,\ldots, k$, and $u_i < v_i$ for at least one component. This property is known as *Pareto dominance*. A solution, x, of the multi-objective problem is said to be *Pareto optimal*, if and only if there is no other solution, y, in S such that $\mathbf{f}(y)$ dominates $\mathbf{f}(x)$. In this case, we also say that x is *nondominated* with respect to S. The set of all Pareto optimal solutions of a problem is called the *Pareto optimal set*, and it is usually denoted as $\mathcal{P}^*$. The set

$$\mathcal{PF}^* = \{ \mathbf{f}(x): x \in \mathcal{P}^* \}, \quad (3)$$

is called the *Pareto front*. A Pareto front is *convex* if and only if, for all $u, v \in \mathcal{PF}^*$ and for all $\lambda \in (0, 1)$, there exists a $w \in \mathcal{PF}^*$ such that

$$\lambda \|u\| + (1-\lambda) \|v\| \geq \|w\|,$$

while it is called *concave*, if and only if

$$\lambda \|u\| + (1-\lambda) \|v\| \leq \|w\|.$$

A Pareto front can also be partially convex and/or concave, as well as discontinuous. These cases are considered the most difficult for most multi-objective optimization algorithms.

The special nature of multi-objective problems makes necessary the determination of new goals for the optimization procedure, since the detection of a single solution, which is adequate in the single-objective case, is not valid in cases of many, possibly conflicting objective functions. Based on the definition of Pareto optimality, the detection of all Pareto optimal solutions is the main goal in multi-objective optimization problems. However, since the Pareto optimal set can be infinite and our computations adhere to time and space limitations, we are compelled to set more realistic goals. Thus, we can state as the main goal of the multi-objective optimization procedure, the *detection of the highest possible number of Pareto optimal solutions that correspond to an adequately spread Pareto front, with the smallest possible deviation from the true Pareto front*.

Particle Swarm Optimization

Eberhart and Kennedy (1995) developed PSO as an expansion of an animal social behavior simulation system that incorporated concepts such as nearest-neighbor velocity matching and acceleration by distance (Kennedy & Eberhart, 1995). Similarly to evolutionary algorithms, PSO exploits a population, called a *swarm*, of potential solutions, called *particles*, which are modified stochastically at each iteration of the algorithm. However, the manipulation of swarm differs significantly from that of evolutionary algorithms, promoting a cooperative rather than a competitive model.

More specifically, instead of using explicit mutation and selection operators in order to modify the population and favor the best performing individuals, PSO uses an adaptable velocity vector for each particle, which shifts its position at each iteration of the algorithm. The particles are moving towards promising regions of the search space by exploiting information springing from their own experience during the search, as well as the experience of other particles. For this purpose, a separate memory is used where each particle stores the best position it has ever visited in the search space.

Let us now put PSO more formally in the context of single-objective optimization. Let S be an n-dimensional search space, $f: S \to \mathbb{R}$ be the objective function, and N be the number of particles that comprise the swarm,

$$\mathbb{S} = \{x_1, x_2, \ldots, x_N\}.$$

Then, the i-th particle is a point in the search space,

$$x_i = (x_{i1}, x_{i2}, \ldots, x_{in}) \in S,$$

as well as its best position,

$$p_i = (p_{i1}, p_{i2}, \ldots, p_{in}) \in S,$$

which is the best position ever visited by x_i during the search. The velocity of x_i is also an n-dimensional vector,

$$v_i = (v_{i1}, v_{i2}, \ldots, v_{in}).$$

The particles, their best positions, as well as their velocities, are randomly initialized in the search space.

Let $NG_i \subseteq \mathbb{S}$ be a set of particles that exchange information with x_i. This set is called the *neighborhood* of x_i, and it will be discussed later. Let also, g, be the index of the best particle in NG_i, that is,

$$f(p_g) \leq f(p_l), \quad \text{for all } l \text{ with } x_l \in NG_i,$$

and t denote the iteration counter. Then, the swarm is manipulated according to the equations (Eberhart & Shi, 1998),

$$v_{ij}(t+1) = w\, v_{ij}(t) + c_1\, r_1\, (p_{ij}(t) - x_{ij}(t)) + c_2\, r_2\, (p_{gj}(t) - x_{ij}(t)), \quad (4)$$

$$x_{ij}(t+1) = x_{ij}(t) + v_{ij}(t+1), \quad (5)$$

where $i = 1, 2, \ldots, N; j = 1, 2, \ldots, n$; w is a positive parameter called *inertia weight*; c_1 and c_2 are two positive constants called *cognitive* and *social* parameter, respectively; and r_1, r_2, are realizations of two independent random variables that assume the uniform distribution in the range (0, 1). The best position of each particle is updated at each iteration by setting

$$p_i(t+1) = x_i(t+1), \quad \text{if } f(x_i) < f(p_i),$$

otherwise it remains unchanged. Obviously, an update of the index g is also required at each iteration.

The inertia weight was not used in early PSO versions. However, experiments showed that the lack of mechanism for controlling the velocities could result in *swarm explosion*, that is, an unbounded increase in the magnitude of the velocities, which resulted in swarm divergence. For this purpose, a boundary, v_{max}, was imposed on the absolute value of the velocities, such that, if $v_{ij} > v_{max}$ then $v_{ij} = v_{max}$, and if $v_{ij} < -v_{max}$ then $v_{ij} = -v_{max}$. In later, more sophisticated versions, the new parameter was incorporated in the velocity update equation, in order to control the impact of the previous velocity on the current one, although the use of v_{max} was not abandoned.

Intelligent search algorithms, such as PSO, must demonstrate an ability to combine *exploration*, that is, visiting new regions of the search space, and *exploitation*, that is, performing more refined local search, in a balanced way in order to solve problems effectively (Parsopoulos & Vrahatis, 2004; Parsopoulos & Vrahatis, 2007). Since larger values of w promote exploration, while smaller values promote exploitation, it was proposed and experimentally verified that declining values of the inertia weight can provide better results than fixed values. Thus, an initial value of w around 1.0 and a gradually decline towards 0.0 are considered a good choice. On the other hand, the parameters c_1 and c_2 are usually set to fixed and equal values such that the particle is equally influenced by its own best position, p_i, as well as the best position of its neighborhood, p_g, unless the problem at hand implies the use of a different setting.

An alternative velocity update equation was proposed by Clerc and Kennedy (2002),

$$v_{ij}(t+1) = \chi \left[v_{ij}(t) + c_1 r_1 (p_{ij}(t) - x_{ij}(t)) + c_2 r_2 (p_{gj}(t) - x_{ij}(t)) \right], \quad (6)$$

where χ is a parameter called *constriction factor*. This version is algebraically equivalent with the inertia weight version of equation (4). However, the parameter selection in this case is based on the stability analysis due to Clerc and Kennedy (2002), which expresses χ as a function of c_1 and c_2. Different promising models were derived through the analysis of the algorithm, with the setting $\chi = 0.729$, $c_1 = c_2 = 2.05$, providing the most promising results and robust behavior, rendering it the default PSO parameter setting.

Regardless of the PSO version used, it is clear that its performance is heavily dependent on the information provided by the best positions, p_i and p_g, since they determine the region of the search space that will be visited by the particle.

Therefore, their selection, especially for p_g, which is related to information exchange, plays a central role in the development of effective and efficient PSO variants.

Moreover, the concept of neighborhood mentioned earlier in this section, raises efficiency issues. A neighborhood has been already defined as a subset of the swarm. The most straightforward choice would be to consider as neighbors of the particle x_i, all particles enclosed in a sphere with center x_i and a user-defined radius in the search space. Despite its simplicity, this approach increases significantly the computational burden of the algorithm, since it requires the computation of all distances among particles at each iteration. This deficiency has been addressed by defining neighborhoods in the space of particles' indices instead of the actual search space.

Thus, the neighbors of x_i are determined based solely on the indices of the particles, assuming different *neighborhood topologies*, that is, orderings of the particles' indices. The most common neighborhood is the *ring topology*, depicted in Fig. 1 (left), where the particles are arranged on a ring, with x_{i-1} and x_{i+1} being the immediate neighbors of x_i, and x_1 following immediately after x_N. Based on this topology, a neighborhood of radius r of x_i is defined as

Figure 1. The ring (left) and star (right) neighborhood topologies of PSO

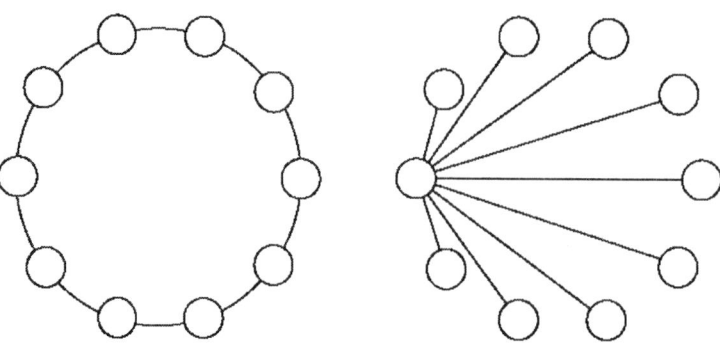

$$NG_i(r) = \{x_{i-r}, x_{i-r+1}, \ldots, x_{i-1}, x_i, x_{i+1}, \ldots, x_{i+r-1}, x_{i+r}\},$$

and the search is influenced by the particle's own best position, p_i, as well as the best position of its neighborhood. This topology promotes exploration, since the information carried by the best positions is communicated slowly through the neighbors of each particle. A different topology is the *star topology*, depicted in Figure 1 (right) where all particles communicate only with a single particle, which is the overall best position, p_g, of the swarm, that is, $NG_i \equiv \mathbb{S}$. This topology promotes exploitation, since all particles share the same information. This is also called the *global variant* of PSO, denoted as *gbest* in the relative literature, while all other topologies with $NG_i \subset \mathbb{S}$, define *local variants*, usually denoted as *lbest*. Different topologies have also been investigated with promising results (Janson & Middendorf, 2004; Kennedy, 1999).

KEY CONCEPTS OF MULTI-OBJECTIVE PSO ALGORITHMS

In the previous section, it was made clear that the search ability of a particle is heavily dependent on the best positions, p_i and p_g, involved in its velocity update equation (equation (4) or (6)). These best positions attract the particle, biasing its movement towards the search space regions they lie, with p_i representing the inherent knowledge accumulated by the particle during its search, while p_g is the socially communicated information of its neighborhood, determined through the adopted neighborhood topology.

In multi-objective problems, we can distinguish two fundamental approaches for designing PSO algorithms (Reyes-Sierra & Coello, 2006a). The first approach consists of algorithms that consider each objective function separately. In these approaches, each particle is evaluated only for one objective function at a time, and the determination of the best positions is performed similarly to the single-objective optimization case. The main challenge in such cases is the proper manipulation of the information coming from each objective function in order to guide the particles towards Pareto optimal solutions.

The second approach consists of algorithms that evaluate all objective functions for each particle, and, based on the concept of Pareto optimality, they produce nondominated best positions (often called *leaders*) that are used to guide the particles. In these approaches, the determination of leaders is not straighforward, since there can be many nondominated solutions in the neighborhood of a particle, but only one is usually selected to participate in the velocity update.

In the aforementioned approaches, the problem of maintaining the detected Pareto optimal solutions must be addressed. The most trivial solution would be to store nondominated solutions as the particles' best positions. However, this choice is not always valid, since the desirable size of the Pareto front may exceed the swarm size. Moreover, two nondominated solutions are equally good, arising questions regarding the selection of the one that will be used as the best position of a particle. The size problem can be addressed by using an additional set, called the *external archive*, for storing the nondominated solutions discovered during search, while the problem of selection of the most proper archive member depends on the approach. Nevertheless, an external archive has also bounded size, thereby making unavoidable the imposition of rules regarding the replacement of existing solutions with new ones.

The general multi-objective PSO scheme can be described with the following pseudocode:

Begin
    Initialize swarm, velocities and best positions
    Initialize external archive (initially empty)

```
    While (stopping criterion not satisfied) Do
        For each particle
            Select a member of the exter-
nal             archive (if needed)
            Update velocity and position
            Evaluate new position
            Update best position and exter-
nal             archive
        End For
    End While
End
```

It is clear that selection of a member of the external archive, as well as the update of archive and best positions, constitute key concepts in the development of multi-objective PSO approaches, albeit not the only ones. Diversity also affects significantly the performance of the algorithm, since its loss can result in convergence of the swarm to a single solution.

The problem of selecting members from the external archive has been addressed through the determination of measures that assess the quality of each archive member, based on *density estimators*. Using such measures, archive members that promote diversity can be selected. The most commonly used density estimators are the *Nearest Neighbor Density Estimator* (Deb et al., 2002) and the *Kernel Density Estimator* (Deb & Goldberg, 1989). Both measures provide estimations regarding the proximity and number of neighbors for a given point.

The problem of updating the archive is more complex. A new solution is included in the archive if it is nondominated by all its members. If some members are dominated by the new solution, then they are usually deleted from the archive. The necessity for a bounded archive size originates from its tendency to increase significantly within a small number of algorithm iterations, rendering domination check computationally expensive.

Also, the user must decide for the action taken in the case of a candidate new solution that is nondominated by all members of a full archive. Obviously, this solution must compete all members of the archive in order to replace an existing member. Diversity is again the fundamental criterion, that is, the decision between an existing and a new solution is taken such that the archive retains the maximum possible diversity. For this purpose, different clustering techniques have been proposed (Knowles & Corne, 2000; Zitzler & Thiele, 1999). A similar approach uses the concept of ε-dominance to separate the Pareto front in boxes and retain one solution for each box. This approach has been shown to be more efficient than simple clustering techniques (Mostaghim & Teich, 2003b).

The update of each particle's own best position, is more straightforward. Thus, in approaches based on distinct evaluation of each objective function, it is performed as in standard PSO for single-objective optimization. On the other hand, in Pareto-based approaches, the best position of a particle is replaced only by a new one that dominates it. If the candidate and the existing best position are nondominated, then the old one is usually replaced in order to promote swarm diversity. At this point, we must also mention the effect of the employed neighborhood topology and PSO variant, on the performance of the algorithm. However, there are no extensive investigations to support the superiority of specific variants and topologies in multi-objective cases.

ESTABLISHED MULTI-OBJECTIVE PSO APPROACHES

In this section we review the state-of-the-art literature on multi-objective PSO algorithms. We will distinguish two fundamental categories of algorithms, based on the two approaches mentioned in the previous section, namely, approaches that exploit each objective function separately, and Pareto-based schemes. The distinction is made mainly for presentation purposes, and it is not strict, since there are algorithms that combine features from both approaches. The exposition of the methods for each category is based on a chronological ordering.

Algorithms that Exploit Each Objective Function Separately

This category consists of approaches that either combine all objective functions to a single one or consider each objective function in turn for the evaluation of the swarm, in an attempt to exploit the efficiency of PSO in solving single-objective problems. This approach has the advantage of straightforward update of the swarm and best positions, with an external archive usually employed for storing nondominated solutions. The main drawback of these methods is the lack of *a priori* information regarding the most proper manipulation of the distinct objective values, in order to converge to the actual Pareto front (Jin, Olhofer, & Sendhoff, 2001).

Objective Function Aggregation Approaches

These approaches aggregate, through a weighted combination, all objective functions in a single one,

$$F(x) = \sum_{i=1}^{k} w_i f_i(x),$$

where w_i are nonnegative weights such that

$$\sum_{i=1}^{k} w_i = 1,$$

and the optimization is performed on $F(x)$, similarly to the single-objective case. If the weights remain fixed during the run of the algorithm, we have the case of *Conventional Weighted Aggregation* (CWA). This approach is characterized by simplicity but it has also some crucial disadvantages. For only a single solution can be attained through the application of PSO for a specific weight setting, the algorithm must be applied repeatedly with different weight settings in order to detect a desirable number of nondominated solutions. Moreover, the CWA approach is unable to detect solutions in concave regions of the Pareto front (Jin et al., 2001).

The aforementioned limitations of CWA were addressed by using dynamically adjusted weights during optimization. Such approaches are the *Bang-Bang Weighted Aggregation* (BWA), which is defined for the case of bi-objective problems as (Jin et al., 2001),

$$w_1(t) = \text{sign}(\sin(2\pi t/a)), \quad w_2(t) = 1 - w_1(t),$$

as well as the *Dynamic Weighted Aggregation* (DWA), which is defined as,

$$w_1(t) = |\sin(2\pi t/a)|, \quad w_2(t) = 1 - w_1(t),$$

where a is a user-defined adaptation frequency and t is the iteration number. The use of the sign function in BWA results in abrupt changes of the weights that force the algorithm to keep moving towards the Pareto front. The same effect is achieved with DWA, although the change in the weights is milder than BWA. Experiments with Genetic Algorithms have shown that DWA approaches perform better than BWA in convex Pareto fronts, while their performance is almost identical in concave Pareto fronts.

Parsopoulos and Vrahatis (2002a, 2002b) proposed the first multi-objective PSO weighted aggregation approach. They considered bi-objective problems with CWA, BWA and DWA approaches. Preliminary results on widely used benchmark problems were promising, and graphical representations showed that the two schemes could provide Pareto fronts with satisfactory spreading. As expected, the dynamically modified scheme outperformed the fixed weights approach. Although the simplicity and straightforward applicability render weighted aggregation schemes very attractive in combination with PSO, their efficiency on problems with more than two objectives has not been investigated extensively.

Baumgartner, Magele and Renhart (2004) considered a similar approach, where subswarms that use a different weight setting each, are used in combination with a gradient-based scheme for the detection of Pareto optimal solutions. More specifically, the swarm is divided in subswarms and each one uses a specific weight setting. The best particle of each subswarm serves as a leader only for itself. Also, a *preliminary pareto decision* is made in order to further investigate points that are candidate Pareto optimal solutions. This decision is made for each particle, x, based on the relation

$$\frac{1}{k}\left|\sum_{j=1}^{k} \text{sgn}\left(f_j(x(t+1)) - f_j(x(t))\right)\right| \neq 1,$$

where t stands for the iteration counter. If it holds, then x could be a Pareto optimal point, and the gradients of the objective functions $f_1,\ldots,f_k$, are computed on a perturbed point $x+\Delta x$. If none objective function improves at the perturbed point, then it is considered as a Pareto optimal point and it is removed from the swarm. Although results on a limited set of test problems are promising, the algorithm has not been fully evaluated and compared with other PSO approaches.

Mahfouf, Chen, and Linkens (2004) proposed a dynamically modified weights approach. However, in this approach, the standard PSO scheme with linearly decreasing inertia weight was modified, by incorporating a mutation operator in order to alleviate swarm stagnation, as well as an acceleration term that accelerates convergence at later stages of the algorithm. More specifically, equation (4) was modified to

$$v_{ij}(t+1) = w\, v_{ij}(t) + a\left(r_1\left(p_{ij}(t) - x_{ij}(t)\right) + r_2\left(p_{gj}(t) - x_{ij}(t)\right)\right),$$

where a is an acceleration factor that depends on the current iteration number,

$$a = a_0 + t/\text{MIT},$$

where MIT is the maximum number of iterations and a_0 lies within the range [0.5, 1]. After the computation of the new positions of the particles, both new and old positions are entered in a list. The *Non-Dominated Sorting* technique (Li, 2003) is applied for this list, and the nondominated particles (that approximate the Pareto front) are selected. These particles suffer a mutation procedure in an attempt to further improve them. The resulting set of particles constitutes the swarm in the next iteration of the algorithm. Results from the application of this scheme on a problem from steel industry are reported with promising results. The algorithm combines characteristics of different approaches that have been shown to enhance the performance of multi-objective methods. Its competitive performance to both PSO and other evolutionary approaches, such as NSGA-II and SPEA2, can be attributed to the mutation operator that preserves swarm diversity, as well as to the Nondominated Sorting technique that allows the direct exploitation and evolution of points approximating the Pareto front, instead of using an external archive.

Objective Function Ordering Approaches

These approaches require the determination of a ranking of the objective functions. Then, minimization is performed for each function independently, starting from the most important one. Hu and Eberhart (2002) proposed a scheme based on such an ordering. Since Pareto front constitutes a boundary of the fitness values space, the algorithm retains the simplest objective function fixed and minimizes the rest of the objective functions. In their scheme, a local PSO variant with dynamic neighborhoods was used, with neighborhoods been defined rather in the fitness values space than the standard index-based scheme described in Section 2.2. Nondominated solutions are stored as particles' best positions and no external archive is used. The approach was applied successfully on problems with two objective functions but the function ordering procedure, which can be crucial for its performance especially in problems with more than two objectives, lacks justification.

An extension of the previous approach was proposed one year later (Hu, Eberhart, & Shi, 2003), incorporating an external archive in the form of external memory for storing nondominated solutions and reducing the computational cost. Albeit the reported preliminary results on problems with two objective functions were promising, further investigation is needed to reveal the algorithm's potential under more demanding situations, as well as its sensitivity to the parameter setting. Also, the authors mentioned the limited applicability of this approach, which was unable to address the binary string problem.

Non-Pareto, Vector Evaluated Approaches

Parsopoulos and Vrahatis (2002a; 2002b) proposed the Vector Evaluated PSO (VEPSO) scheme. This is a multiswarm approach based on the idea of Vector Evaluated Genetic Algorithm (VEGA) (Schaffer, 1985). In VEPSO, there is one swarm devoted to each objective function, and evaluated only for this objective function. However, in the swarm update (the algorithm employed the global variant of PSO), the best positions of one swarm are used for the velocity update of another swarm that corresponds to a different objective function.

Thus, if the problem consists of k objectives, then k swarms are used. If $v_i^{[s]}$ denotes the velocity of the i-th particle in the s-th swarm, $s=1,\ldots, k$, then it is updated based on the relation

$$v_{ij}^{[s]}(t+1) = w\, v_{ij}^{[s]}(t) + c_1\, r_1\, (p_{ij}^{[s]}(t) - x_{ij}^{[s]}(t)) + c_2\, r_2\, (p_{gj}^{[q]}(t) - x_{ij}^{[s]}(t)),$$

where $p_g^{[q]}$ is the best position of the q-th swarm (which is evaluated with the q-th objective function). In this way, the information regarding the promising regions for one objective is inoculated to a swarm that already possesses information for a different objective. Experimental results imply that the algorithm is capable of moving towards the Pareto front, always in combination with the external archive approach of Jin et al. (2001).

A parallel implementation of VEPSO has also been investigated (Parsopoulos, Tasoulis & Vrahatis, 2004) with promising results. In this implementation, each swarm is assigned to a processor and the number of swarms is not necessarily equal to the number of objective functions. The communication among swarms is performed through an island migration scheme, similar to the ring topology used in PSO's ring neighborhood topology. VEPSO has been successfully used in two real-life problems, namely, the optimization of a radiometer array antenna (Gies & Rahmat-Samii, 2004), as well as for determining generator contributions to transmission systems (Vlachogiannis & Lee, 2005).

An approach similar to VEPSO, was proposed by Chow and Tsui (2004). The algorithm, called Multi-Species PSO, was introduced within a generalized autonomous agent response-learning framework, related to robotics. It uses subswarms that form species, one for each objective function. Each subswarm is then evaluated only with its own objective function, and information of best particles is communicated to neighboring subswarms with the form of an extra term in the velocity update of the particles. Thus, the velocity of the i-th particle in the s-th swarm is updated as follows:

$$v_{ij}^{[s]}(t+1) = v_{ij}^{[s]}(t) + a_1\, (p_{ij}^{[s]}(t) - x_{ij}^{[s]}(t)) + a_2\, (p_{gj}^{[s]}(t) - x_{ij}^{[s]}(t))) + A,$$

where

$$A = \sum_{l=1}^{H_s} \left(p_{gj}^{[l]}(t) - x_{ij}^{[s]}(t) \right),$$

with H_s being the number of swarms that communicate with the s-th swarm, and $p_g^{[l]}$ the best position of the l-th swarm, $l = 1,\ldots, H_s$. The algorithm was shown to be competitive to other established multi-objective PSO approaches, although in limited number of experiments. Also, questions arise regarding the velocity update that does not include any constriction factor or inertia weight, as well as on the scheme for defining neighboring swarms, since the schemes employed in the investigated problems are not analyzed.

Algorithms Based on Pareto Dominance

These approaches use the concept of Pareto dominance to determine the best positions (leaders) that will guide the swarm during search. As we mentioned in Section 3, several questions arise regarding the underlying schemes and rules for the selection of these positions among equally good solutions. For the imposition of additional criteria that take into consideration further issues (such as swarm diversity, Pareto front spread, etc.) is inevitable, the development of Pareto-based PSO approaches became a blossoming research area, with a significant number of different approaches reported in the literature. In the following paragraphs we review the most significant developments.

Coello and Salazar Lechuga (2002) proposed the Multi-objective PSO (MOPSO), one of the first Pareto-based PSO approaches (Coello, Toscano Pulido, & Salazar Lechuga, 2004). In MOPSO, the nondominated solutions detected by the particles are stored in a repository. Also, the search space is divided in hypercubes. Each hypercube is assigned a fitness value that is inversely proportional to the number of particles it contains. Then, the classical roulette wheel selection is used to select a hypercube and a leader from it. Thus, the velocity update for the i-th particle becomes

$$v_{ij}(t+1) = w\, v_{ij}(t) + c_1\, r_1\, (p_{ij}(t) - x_{ij}(t)) + c_2\, r_2\, (R_h(t) - x_{ij}(t)),$$

where p_i is its best position and R_h is the selected leader from the repository. The best position p_i is updated at each iteration, based on the domination relation between the existing best position of the particle and its new position.

Also, the repository has limited size and, if it is full, new solutions are inserted based on the *retention* criterion, that is, giving priority to solutions located in less crowded areas of the objective space. MOPSO was competitive against NSGA-II and PAES on typical benchmark problems, under common performance metrics, and it is currently considered one of the most typical multi-objective PSO approaches. A sensitivity analysis on the parameters of the algorithm, including the number of hypercubes used, can provide further useful information on this simple though efficient approach.

Fieldsend and Singh (2002) proposed a multi-objective PSO scheme that addresses the inefficiencies caused by the truncation of limited archives of nondominated solutions. For this purpose, a complex tree-like structure for unconstrained archiving maintenance, called the *dominated tree*, is used (Fieldsend, Everson, & Singh, 2003). The algorithm works similarly to MOPSO, except the repository, which is maintained through the aforementioned structures. An additional feature that works beneficially is the use of mutation, called *craziness*, on the particle velocity, in order to preserve diversity. The algorithm has shown to be competitive with PAES, although the authors underline the general deficiency of such approaches in cases where closeness in the objective space is loosely related to closeness in the parameter space.

Ray and Liew (2002) proposed an approach that employs the nearest neighbor density estimator in combination with a roulette wheel scheme for the selection of leaders. More specifically, leaders are generated through a multilevel sieve procedure that ranks individuals. Initially, all nondominated particles are assigned a rank of 1 and removed from swarm. The nondominated solutions from the remaining particles are assigned a rank of 2, and the procedure continues until all particles have been assigned a rank. If at most half of the swarm has been assigned a rank of 1, then all particles with rank smaller than the average rank are assigned to the set of leaders. Otherwise, only particles with a rank of 1 are assigned to the set of leaders. For the rest of the particles, a leader is selected and used for updating their position.

The selection of leader is based on the computation of the crowding radius for each leader and a roulette wheel selection mechanism that uses these values. Leaders with higher crowding radius have higher selection probability and, therefore, promote the uniform spread of solutions on the Pareto front. Special care is taken in constrained problems, where ranking takes into consideration both the objective and constraint values. The algorithm was tested on benchmark as well as engineering design problems and results were represented graphically. However, neither numerical results nor comparisons with any other multi-objective algorithm are reported to convince the reader regarding its efficiency.

Bartz-Beielstein, Limbourg, Mehnen, Schmitt, Parsopoulos, & Vrahatis (2003) proposed DOPS, a method based on an elitist archiving scheme. Their analysis considered different schemes for updating the archive and selecting the most proper solutions for the particles' update, using functions that assess the performance and contribution of each particle to the Pareto front spreading. More specifically, two functions, F_{sel} and F_{del}, are used to assign a *selection* and a *deletion* fitness value to each particle, respectively. The selection fitness value is a measure of the particle's influence to the spreading of the Pareto front, and increases with its distance to its nearest neighbors. Thus, every time a personal or a globally best position is needed, a member is chosen from the archive based on a roulette wheel selection over F_{sel}. If the number of available nondominated solutions surpasses the archive size, then a member of the archive is selected for deletion based on F_{del}. Different selection and deletion functions are proposed and evaluated. The method was supported by sensitivity analysis on its parameters, providing useful hints on the effect of archiving on the performance of multi-objective PSO.

Srinivasan and Seow (2003) introduced the Particle Swarm inspired Evolutionary Algorithm (PS-EA). This algorithm can only roughly be characterized as a PSO-based approach, since the update of particles is completely different than any PSO algorithm. More specifically, the particle update equations (equations (4) and (5)) are substituted by a *probability inheritance tree*. Thus, instead of moving in the search space with an adaptable velocity, the particle rather inherits the parameters of its new position. Therefore, it can inherit parameters from an *elite particle*, that is, its own or the overall best position, or inherit parameters from a randomly selected neighboring particle. Further choices are pure mutation and the retainment of the existing parameter in the new position.

All these choices are made probabilistically, based on a *dynamic inheritance probability adjuster* (DIPA). This mechanism controls the probabilities based on feedback from the convergence status of the algorithm, and more specifically on the fitness of the overall best particle. If the overall best seems to stagnate or does not change positions frequently, DIPA adjusts the probabilities. Unfortunately, the authors do not provide details regarding the exact operation of DIPA even in their experiments. Thus, although the algorithm is shown to be competitive with a GA approach, there are no indications regarding the complexity of setting the DIPA mechanism properly in order to achieve acceptable performance.

Mostaghim and Teich proposed several algorithms based on MOPSO, incorporating special schemes for the selection of archive members that participate in the update of the particles' velocity. In Mostaghim and Teich (2003a), a MOPSO approach is proposed in combination with the *sigma method* that assigns a numerical value to each particle and member of the archive. For example, in a bi-objective problem, if the i-th particle has objective values (f_1, f_2), then it is assigned a sigma value,

$$\sigma = \frac{(K_2 f_1)^2 - (K_1 f_2)^2}{(K_2 f_1)^2 + (K_1 f_2)^2},$$

where K_1, K_2, are the maximum objective values of the particles for f_1 and f_2, respectively. Then, a particle uses as leader the archive member with the closest sigma value to its own. Also, a turbulence (mutation) factor is used for the position update of the particle, to maintain swarm diversity. The algorithm outperformed SPEA2 in typical bi-objective problems but the opposite happened for problems with three objectives. Also, the authors underline the necessity for large swarm sizes, since an adequate number of distributed solutions are required in the objective space.

Mostaghim and Teich (2003b) studied further the performance of MOPSO using also the concept of ε-dominance, and compared it to clustering-based approaches, with promising results. The investigation in this work focused mostly on the archiving methodology rather than the search algorithm itself, indicating the superiority of the ε-dominance approach with respect to the quality of the obtained Pareto fronts through MOPSO, in terms of convergence speed and diversity.

Furthermore, an algorithm for covering the Pareto front by using subswarms and an unbounded external archive, after the detection of an initial approximation of the Pareto front through MOPSO, was proposed by Mostaghim and Teich (2004). In this approach, an initial approximation of the Pareto front is detected through MOPSO, and subswarms are initialized around each nondominated solution in order to search the neighborhood around it. The algorithm outperformed an evolutionary approach (Hybrid MOEA) that incorporates a space subdivision scheme, on an antenna design problem. The applicability of the proposed MOPSO scheme on problems of any dimension and number of objectives, constitutes an additional advantage of the algorithm, as claimed by the authors.

Li (2004) proposed an approach called the MaximinPSO that exploits the maximin fitness function (Balling, 2003). For a given decision vector x, this fitness function is defined as,

$$\max_{j=1,\ldots,N; x \neq y} \min_{i=1,\ldots,k} \{f_i(x) - f_i(y)\},$$

where k is the number of objective functions and N is the swarm size. Obviously, only decision vectors with a maximin function value less than zero can be nondominated solutions with respect to the current population. The maximin function promotes diversity of the swarm, since it penalizes particles that cluster in groups. Also, it has been argued that it favors the middle solutions in convex fronts and the extreme solutions in concave fronts (Balling, 2003). However, Li (2004) has shown that this effect can be addressed through the use of adequately large swarms. The particles in the proposed algorithm are evaluated with the maximin function and nondominated solutions are stored in an archive to serve as leaders (randomly selected by the particles). MaximinPSO outperformed NSGA-II on typical benchmark problems. However, experiments were restricted in bi-objective unconstrained problems, thus, no sound conclusions can be derived regarding its efficiency in more demanding cases.

Toscano Pulido and Coello (2004) proposed Another MOPSO (AMOPSO), an approach similar to VEPSO, where subswarms are used to probe different regions of the search space. Each subswarm has its own group of leaders. These groups are formed from a large set of nondominated solutions through a clustering technique. Then, each subswarm is assigned a group of leaders and select randomly those that will serve as its guides towards the Pareto front. This approach can alleviate problems related to disconnected search spaces, where a particle may be assigned a leader that lies in a disconnected region, wasting a lot of search effort. However, at some points, information exchange is allowed among subswarms. The authors show that AMOPSO is competitive to NSGA-II, and could be considered as a viable alternative.

AMOPSO does not use an external archive (nondominated solutions are stored as best positions of the particles), in contrast to OMOPSO, the approach of Reyes-Sierra and Coello (2005), which employs two external archives. This approach uses the nearest neighbor estimator and stores the selected best positions for the current iteration of PSO in the one archive and the overall nondominated solutions (final solutions) in the other archive. Established concepts such as turbulence (mutation) and ε-dominance are also used for diversity and archive maintenance purposes, respectively, increasing the complexity of the algorithm significantly, when compared to AMOPSO. The special feature of the algorithm is the incorporation of a mechanism for removing leaders, when their number exceeds a threshold. The aforementioned features result in an increased efficiency and effectiveness of the OMOPSO, which is shown to outperform previously presented MOPSO approaches as well as NSGA-II and SPEA2, rendering it a highly efficient method.

A different idea has been introduced in (Villalobos-Arias et al., 2005), where stripes are used on the search space and they are assigned particles that can exploit a unique leader that corresponds to a specific stripe. The core of this work is the stripes-based technique and its ability to maintain diversity in the employed optimizer. Its combination with MOPSO exhibits promising results, although it is not clear if this is independent of the search algorithm or the specific technique is beneficial specifically for MOPSO (the authors mention it as a future work direction).

Ho, Yang, Ni, Lo & Wong (2005) proposed a multi-objective PSO-based algorithm for design optimization. However, they introduced a plethora of unjustified modifications to the PSO algorithm regarding its parameter configuration and velocity update. Similarly to AMOPSO, the resulting scheme uses several external archives, one for the overall solutions and one for each particle, where it stores the most recent Pareto optimal solutions it has discovered. For the velocity update of the particle x_i, its best position, p_i, is selected from the latter archive, while p_g is selected from the overall archive, through a roulette wheel selection procedure. Aging of the leaders in the repositories is also introduced, as a means of biasing the selection scheme towards these leaders that have not been selected frequently. The algorithm is tested only on two problems and no comparisons with other methods are provided (the authors just mention its superiority against a simulated annealing approach), thus, no clear conclusions can be derived regarding its usefulness.

Raquel and Naval (2005) proposed MOPSO-CD, an approach that incorporates a *crowding distance* mechanism for the selection of the global best particle, as well as for the deletion of nondominated solutions from the external archive. Mutation is also employed to maintain diversity of the nondominated solutions in the external archive. Crowding distance is computed for each nondominated solution separately. If $f_1,...,f_k$ are the objective functions and R is the external archive, then for the computation of the crowding distance of p in R, with respect to f_j, $j=1,..., k$, we sort all points in R with respect to their f_j objective value and take

$$CD\_f_j = f_j(q) - f_j(r),$$

where q is the point of R that follows immediately after p in the sorting with respect to the f_j objective values, and r is the point that precedes p in the same ordering. Thus, the total crowding distance of p is given by

$$\sum_{j=1}^{k} CD\_f_j.$$

A proportion of the nondominated points of R with the highest crowding distances serve as leaders of the swarm (selected randomly). Also, mutation applied on the particles at randomly selected iterations promotes swarm diversity. Typical constraint-handling techniques adopted from the NSGA-II algorithm (Deb et al., 2002) are incorporated for addressing constrained problems. MOPSO-CD was compared to MOPSO, with results implying its viability as an alternative.

Alvarez-Benitez, Everson & Fieldsend (2005) proposed the *Rounds*, *Random*, and *Prob* techniques, which are based solely on the concept of Pareto dominance, for selecting leaders from the external archive. Each technique promotes different features in the algorithm. Rounds promotes as global guide of a particle x_i the nondominated solution that dominates the fewest particles of the swarm, including x_i. This solution is then excluded from selection for the rest of the particles. The procedure can be computationally expensive for large archives, however it is shown that promotes diversity. On the other hand, Random uses as global guide of a particle x_i a probabilistically selected nondominated solution that dominates x_i, with each nondominated solution having the same probability of selection. Prob constitutes an extension of Random that favors the archive members that dominate the smallest number of points. Mutation is also employed, while constraint-handling techniques are proposed and discussed, deriving the conclusion that careful handling of exploration near the boundaries of the search space can be beneficial for all multi-objective optimization approaches. However, this concept needs further experimentation to be confirmed.

As described earlier, MOPSO has an implicit fitness sharing mechanism for the selection of hypercubes. Salazar Lechuga and Rowe (2005) introduced MOPSO-*fs*, a MOPSO variant with explicit fitness sharing. According to this approach, each particle p_i in the repository of nondominated solutions, is assigned a fitness

$$F\_sh_i = 10 \bigg/ \sum_{j=1}^{n} s_i^j,$$

where

$$s_i^j = \begin{cases} 1 - \left(\dfrac{d_i^j}{\sigma_{share}}\right)^2, & \text{if } d_i^j < \sigma_{share}, \\ 0, & \text{otherwise}, \end{cases}$$

with σ_{share} being a user-defined distance and d_i^j be a distance measure between nondominated solutions p_i and p_j. This fitness-sharing scheme assigns higher fitness values to solutions with small number of other solutions around them. Then, the leaders of the swarm are selected through a roulette wheel selection technique that uses the assigned fitness values. MOPSO-*fs* has shown to be competitive with MOPSO, as well as with NSGA-II and PAES, although the analysis of choosing the fitness sharing parameters is under further investigation.

Mostaghim and Teich (2006) proposed recently a new idea, similar to that of Ho *et al.* (2005) described above. More specifically, each particle retains all nondominated solutions it has encountered in a personal archive. Naturally, a question arises regarding the final selection of the leader from the personal archive. The authors propose different techniques, ranging from pure random selection to the use of weights and diversity-preserving techniques. Experiments with the sigma-MOPSO (Mostaghim & Teich, 2003a) provided promising results on typical benchmark problems.

Huo, Shen Zhu (2006) proposed an interesting idea for the selection of leaders. More specifically, they evaluated each particle according to each objective function separately, and then, they assumed the mean of the best particles per function, as the global best position for the swarm update. Diversity of the swarm is preserved through a distance measure that biases the leader selection towards nondominated solutions that promote the alleviation of particle gathering in clusters. The resulting SMOPSO algorithm was tested on a limited number of test problems, and no comparisons were provided with other methods, to fully evaluate its efficiency.

Reyes-Sierra and Coello (2006b) conducted an interesting investigation on a hot research topic of both single- and multi-objective optimization, namely the on-line parameter adaptation of multi-objective algorithms. More specifically, the inertia weight, w, acceleration coefficients, c_1 and c_2, and selection method (dominance or crowding values) probability, P_s, of the MOPSO approach described earlier, were investigated using Analysis of Variance (ANOVA). The analysis has shown that large values of P_s, w, and c_2 provide better results, while c_1 seems to have a mild effect on MOPSO's performance. After identifying the most crucial parameters, different adaptation techniques, based on a reward system, were proposed. Thus, the parameter level selection could be *proportional*, *greedy*, or based on the *soft max strategy* that employs Gibbs distribution. The results are very promising, opening the way towards more efficient self-adaptive multi-objective approaches.

FUTURE RESEARCH DIRECTIONS

The non-Pareto algorithms describe above, share some characteristics that have concentrated the interest of the research community. With simplicity and straightforward applicability being their main advantage, while increased computational cost being their common drawback in some cases, these algorithms can be considered as significant alternatives that provide satisfactory solutions without complex implementation requirements.

However, there are still fundamental questions unanswered. More specifically, for the weighted aggregation approaches, the most efficient schedule for changing weights remains an open question. In most cases, the problem is addressed on a problem-dependent base, since there are no extensive investigations that can imply specific choices based on possible special characteristics of the problem at hand.

The same holds for the function ordering approaches. If the problem at hand implies a specific significance ordering for the objective functions, then these algorithms can be proved valuable. On the other hand, if there are no such indications, it is very difficult to make proper orderings and hold the overall computational cost at an acceptable level.

The non-Pareto vector evaluated approaches are the most popular in this category of algorithms, due to their straightforward applicability and use of the fundamental element of swarm intelligence, that is, the exchange of information among swarms. Still, there are features of these algorithms that need further investigation, such as the frequency and direction of information exchange among swarms. The size and number of swarms used, as well as the incorporation of external archives, constitute further interesting research issues.

It has been made obvious that the category of Pareto-based approaches is significantly wider than that of non-Pareto approaches. This can be partially attributed to the direct attack to the multi-objective problem through algorithms that incorporate in their criteria the key-property of Pareto dominance. In this manner, many non-dominated solutions are considered in a single run of the algorithm, and stored as the resulting approximation of the Pareto front.

Naturally, there are crucial issues that need to be addressed prior to the design of efficient Pareto-based algorithms. In PSO Pareto-based approaches, we can distinguish three fundamental issues:

1. Selection of leaders,
2. Promotion of diversity, and
3. Archive maintenance.

The first two issues depend only on the swarm dynamics, while the latter can be considered as a more general issue that arises in all multi-objective algorithms that use archives. However, since the specific workings of an algorithm can mutually interact with the archiving procedures, it is possible that some archiving schemes fit better the multi-objective PSO approaches, resulting in more efficient algorithms.

Unfortunately, although there is a plethora of approaches for tackling the aforementioned issues, most of them are based on recombinations of established ideas from the field of evolutionary multi-objective algorithms. Also, the vast majority of experiments is conducted on a narrow set of test problems of small dimensionality, and perhaps this is the most proper point for underlining the necessity for extensive investigations of the algorithms, since this is the only way to reveal their advantages and deficiencies. The assumption of widely acceptable performance metrics from the multi-objective optimization community would also help towards this direction. It is not rare for two algorithms to compete completely different under two different metrics, but only favorable metrics are reported in most papers, hindering the user from detecting and interfering to the weak aspects of the algorithms.

Parallel implementations of multi-objective PSO approaches constitute also an active research area. Although PSO fits perfectly the framework for parallel implementations that can save significant computational effort in demanding problems, the development of such schemes as well as the interaction of the algorithms' modules (multiple swarms, archives, etc.) under this framework has not been studied extensively.

Furthermore, self-adaptation is considered a very challenging topic in almost all application areas where evolutionary algorithms are involved. The development of self-adaptive PSO schemes that can tackle multiple objectives will disengage the user from the necessity of providing proper parameter values, and it will render the algorithm applicable to any environment and problem, since it will be able to adapt its dynamic in order to fit the problem at hand.

The aforementioned topics can be extended to the field of dynamic multi-objective optimization, where the problem changes over time, along with its constraints. The dynamic case is far harder than the static one, since the algorithm shall be able to both approximate the Pareto front and track it through time. The literature in this field is limited and the development of PSO-based approaches for such problems is an open (although not very active yet) research area.

Finally, as time passes, the necessity for novel ideas that can tackle the aforementioned issues, while retaining the highest possible simplicity and efficiency for the algorithms, becomes more vivid. It is the authors' opinion that, besides the aforementioned topics, special emphasis should be given to it in future research.

CONCLUSION

This chapter provided a descriptive review of the state-of-the-art multi-objective PSO variants. Issues related to the operation of PSO in multi-objective environments have been pointed out and a plethora of approaches with various characteristics have been exposed. Naturally, the collection of algorithms described in the previous sections is far from complete, since the number of research works published on the field has been significantly increased in the late years. However, we provided the most significant results from our perspective, in order to sketch the up-to-date state of research in multi-objective PSO algorithms.

Since multi-objective optimization is intimately related to real-life applications, efficiency must be the key issue in the development of new multi-objective PSO approaches. The plethora of established approaches provides a wide variety of ideas and combinations of existing techniques for better manipulation of the algorithms, but only a minority of the existing methods have shown their potential in real-life problems. Thus, further work is needed to verify the nice properties of existing approaches in practice. Also, theoretical analyses that will provide further information on multi-objective PSO dynamics are expected to encourage the development of less complex and easily parametrized algorithms. Nevertheless, the development of multi-objective PSO approaches is currently and will remain a very active and exciting research field.

REFERENCES

Alvarez-Benitez, J. E., Everson, R. M., & Fieldsend, J. E. (2005). A MOPSO algorithm based exclusively on Pareto dominance concepts. *Lecture notes in computer science* (Vol. 3410, pp. 459-473). Springer-Verlag.

Balling, R. (2003). The maximin fitness function; Multi-objective city and regional planning. *Lecture notes in computer science* (Vol. 2632, pp. 1-15). Springer-Verlag.

Bartz-Beielstein, T., Limbourg, P., Mehnen, J., Schmitt, K., Parsopoulos, K. E., & Vrahatis, M. N. (2003). Particle swarm optimizers for Pareto optimization with enhanced archiving techniques. In *Proceedings of the IEEE 2003 Congress on Evolutionary Computation* (pp. 1780-1787). IEEE Press.

Baumgartner, U., Magele, C., & Renhart, W. (2004). Pareto optimality and particle swarm optimization. *IEEE Transactions on Magnetics, 40*(2), 1172-1175.

Chow, C.-K. & Tsui, H.-T. (2004). Autonomous agent response learning by a multi-species particle swarm optimization. In *Proceedings of the 2004 IEEE Congress on Evolutionary Computation* (pp. 778-785). IEEE Service Center.

Clerc, M. & Kennedy, J. (2002). The particle swarm-explosion, stability, and convergence in a multidimensional complex space. *IEEE Trans. Evol. Comput., 6*(1), 58-73.

Coello, C. A. & Salazar Lechuga, M. (2002). MOPSO: A proposal for multiple objective particle swarm optimization. In *Proceedings of the 2002 IEEE Congress of Evolutionary Compututation* (pp. 1051-1056). IEEE Service Center.

Coello, C. A., Toscano Pulido, G., & Salazar Lechuga, M. (2004). Handling multiple objectives with particle swarm optimization. *IEEE Trans. Evol. Comput., 8*(3), 256-279.

Coello, C. A., Van Veldhuizen, D. A., & Lamont, G. B. (2002). *Evolutionary algorithms for solving multi-objective problems.* New York: Kluwer.

Deb, K. (1999). Multi-objective genetic algorithms: Problem difficulties and construction of test problems. *Evolutionary Computation, 7*(3), 205-230.

Deb, K., & Goldberg, D. E. (1989). An investigation of niche and species formation in genetic function optimization. In *Proceedings of the 3rd International Conference on Genetic Algorithms* (pp. 42-50). Morgan Kaufmann Publishing.

Deb, K., Pratap, A., Agarwal, S., & Meyarivan, T. (2002). A fast and elitist multi-objective genetic algorithm: NSGA-II. *IEEE Trans. Evol. Comput., 6*(2), 182-197.

Eberhart, R. C. & Kennedy, J. (1995). A new optimizer using particle swarm theory. In *Proceedings of the Sixth Symposium on Micro Machine and Human Science* (pp. 39-43). Piscataway, NJ: IEEE Service Center.

Eberhart, R. C. & Shi, Y. (1998). Comparison between genetic algorithms and particle swarm optimization. In V. W. Porto et al. (Eds.), *Evolutionary programming: Vol. VII* (pp. 611-616). Springer.

Erickson, M., Mayer, A., & Horn, J. (2001). The niched Pareto genetic algorithm 2 applied to the design of groundwater remediation systems. *Lecture notes in computer science* (Vol. 1993, pp. 681-695). Springer-Verlag.

Fieldsend, J. E., Everson, R. M., & Singh, S. (2003). Using unconstrained elite archives for multi-objective optimization. *IEEE Trans. Evol. Comp., 7*(3), 305-323.

Fieldsend, J. E. & Singh, S. (2002). A multi-objective algorithm based upon particle swarm optimisation, An efficient data structure and turbulence. In *Proceedings of the 2002 UK Workshop on Computational Intelligence* (pp. 34-44). Birmingham, UK.

Fonseca, C. M. & Fleming, P. J. (1993). Genetic algorithms for multi-objective optimization: Formulation, discussion and generalization. In *Proceedings of the 5th International Conference on Genetic Algorithms* (pp. 416-423).

Gies, D. & Rahmat-Samii, Y. (2004). Vector evaluated particle swarm optimization (VEPSO): Optimization of a radiometer array antenna. In *Proceedings of the AP-S IEEE International Symposium (Digest) of Antennas and Propagation Society, Vol. 3* (pp. 2297-2300).

Ho, S. L., Yang, S., Ni, G., Lo, E. W. C., & Wong, H. C. (2005). A particle swarm optimization-based method for multi-objective design optimizations. *IEEE Trans. Magnetics, 41*(5), 1756-1759.

Horn, J., Nafpliotis, N., & Goldberg, D. E. (1994). A niched Pareto genetic algorithm for multi-objective optimization. In *Proceedings of the 1st IEEE Conference on Evolutionary Computation* (pp. 82-87).

Hu, X. & Eberhart, R. (2002). Multi-objective optimization using dynamic neighborhood particle swarm optimization. In *Proceedings of the 2002 IEEE Congress Evolutionary Compututation* (pp. 1677-1681). IEEE Service Center.

Hu, X., Eberhart, R. C., & Shi, Y. (2003). Particle swarm with extended memory for multi-objective optimization. In *Proceedings of the 2003 IEEE Swarm Intelligence Symposium* (pp. 193-197). IEEE Service Center.

Huo, X. H., Shen, L. C., Zhu, H. Y. (2006). A smart particle swarm optimization algorithm for multi-objective problems. *Lecture notes in computer science* (Vol. 4115, pp. 72-80). Springer-Verlag.

Janson, S. & Middendorf, M. (2004). A hierarchical particle swarm optimizer for dynamic optimization problems. *Lecture notes in computer science* (Vol. 3005, pp. 513-524). Springer-Verlag.

Jin, Y., Olhofer, M., & Sendhoff, B. (2001). Evolutionary dynamic weighted aggregation for multi-objective optimization: Why does it work and how? In *Proceedings of the GECCO 2001 Conference* (pp. 1042-1049), San Francisco, CA.

Kennedy, J. (1999). Small worlds and mega-minds: effects of neighborhood topology on particle swarm performance. In *Proceedings of the IEEE Congress Evolutionary Computation* (pp. 1931-1938). IEEE Press.

Kennedy, J. & Eberhart, R. C. (1995). Particle swarm optimization. In *Proceedings of the IEEE International Conference Neural Networks, Vol. IV* (pp. 1942-1948). Piscataway, NJ: IEEE Service Center.

Kennedy, J. & Eberhart, R. C. (2001). *Swarm intelligence*. Morgan Kaufmann Publishers.

Knowles, J D. & Corne, D. W. (2000). Approximating the nondominated front using the Pareto archived evolution strategy. *Evolutionary computation, 8*(2), 149-172.

Li, X. (2003). A non-dominated sorting particle swarm optimizer for multi-objective optimization. *Lecture notes in computer science, Vol. 2723* (pp. 37-48). Springer-Verlag.

Li, X. (2004). Better spread and convergence: Particle swarm multi-objective optimization using the maximin fitness function. *Lecture notes in computer science, Vol. 3102* (pp. 117-128). Springer-Verlag.

Mahfouf, M., Chen, M.-Y., & Linkens, D. A. (2004). Adaptive weighted particle swarm optimisation for multi-objective optimal design of alloy steels. *Lecture notes in computer science* (Vol. 3242, pp. 762-771). Springer.

Mostaghim, S. & Teich, J. (2003a). Strategies for finding good local guides in multi-objective particle swarm optimization (MOPSO). In *Proceedings of the 2003 IEEE Swarm Intelligence Symposium* (pp. 26-33). IEEE Service Center.

Mostaghim, S. & Teich, J. (2003b). The role of ε-dominance in multi objective particle swarm optimization methods. In *Proceedings of the IEEE 2003 Congress on Evolutionary Computation* (pp. 1764-1771). IEEE Press.

Mostaghim, S. & Teich, J. (2004). Covering Pareto-optimal fronts by subswarms in multi-objective particle swarm optimization. In *Proceedings of the IEEE 2004 Congress on Evolutionary Computation* (pp. 1404-1411). IEEE Press.

Mostaghim, S. & Teich, J. (2006). About selecting the personal best in multi-objective particle swarm optimization. *Lecture notes in computer science* (Vol. 4193, pp. 523-532). Springer.

Parsopoulos, K. E., Tasoulis, D. K., & Vrahatis, M. N. (2004). Multi-objective optimization using parallel vector evaluated particle swarm optimization. In *Proceedings of the IASTED 2004 International Conference on Artificial Intelligence and Applications* (pp. 823-828). IASTED/ACTA Press.

Parsopoulos, K. E. & Vrahatis, M. N. (2002a). Recent approaches to global optimization problems through particle swarm optimization. *Natural Computing, 1*(2-3), 235-306.

Parsopoulos, K. E. & Vrahatis, M. N. (2002b). Particle swarm optimization method in multi-objective problems. In *Proceedings of the ACM 2002 Symposium on Applied Computing* (pp. 603-607). ACM Press.

Parsopoulos, K. E. & Vrahatis, M. N. (2004). On the computation of all global minimizers through particle swarm optimization. *IEEE Transactions on Evolutionary Computation, 8*(3), 211-224.

Parsopoulos, K. E. & Vrahatis, M. N. (2007). Parameter selection and adaptation in unified particle swarm optimization. *Mathematical and Computer Modelling, 46*(1-2), 198-213.

Raquel, C. R. & Naval, P. C., Jr. (2005). An effecive use of crowding distance in multi-objective particle swarm optimization. In *Proceedings of the GECCO 2005* (pp. 257-264). ACM Press.

Ray, T. & Liew, K. M. (2002). A swarm metaphor for multi-objective design optimization. *Engineering Optimization, 34*(2), 141-153.

Reyes-Sierra, M. & Coello, C. A. (2005). Improving PSO-based multi-objective optimisation using crowding, mutation and ε-dominance. *Lecture notes in computer science* (Vol. 3410, pp. 505-519). Springer-Verlag.

Reyes-Sierra, M. & Coello, C. A. (2006a). Multi-objective particle swarm optimizers: A survey of the state-of-the-art. *International Journal of Computational Intelligence Research, 2*(3), 287-308.

Reyes-Sierra, M. & Coello, C. A. (2006b). On-line adaptation in multi-objective particle swarm optimization. In *Proceedings of the 2006 IEEE Swarm Intelligence Symposium* (pp. 61-68). IEEE Press.

Salazar Lechuga, M. & Rowe, J. E. (2005). Particle swarm optimization and fitness sharing to solve multi-objective optimization problems. In *Proceedings of the 2005 IEEE Congress on Evolutionary Computation* (pp. 1204-1211). IEEE Service Center.

Schaffer, J. D. (1984). *Multiple objective optimization with vector evaluated genetic algorithms.* Unpublished doctoral thesis, Vanderbilt University, Nashville, TN.

Schaffer, J. D. (1985). Multiple objective optimisation with vector evaluated genetic algorithm. In *Proceedings of the 1st International Conference on Genetic Algorithms* (pp. 93-100). Morgan Kaufmann Publishers.

Srinivas, N. & Deb, K. (1994). Multi-objective optimization using nondominated sorting in genetic algorithms. *Evolutionary Computation, 2*(3), 221-248.

Srinivasan, D. & Seow, T. H. (2003). Particle swarm inspired evolutionary algorithm (PS-EA) for multi-objective optimization problem. In *Proceedings of the IEEE 2003 Congress on Evolutionary Computation* (pp. 2292-2297). IEEE Press.

Toscano Pulido, G., & Coello, C. A. (2004). Using clustering techniques to improve the performance of a particle swarm optimizer. *Lecture notes in computer science* (Vol. 3102, pp. 225-237). Springer.

Villalobos-Aria, M. A., Toscano Pulido, G., & Coello, C. A. (2005). A proposal to use stripes to maintain diversity in a multi-objective particle swarm optimizer. In *Proceedings of the 2005 IEEE Swarm Intelligence Symposium* (pp. 22-29). IEEE Service Center.

Vlachogiannis, J. G. & Lee, K. Y. (2005). Determining generator contributions to transmission system using parallel vector evaluated particle swarm optimization. *IEEE Transactions on Power Systems, 20*(4), 1765-1774.

Zitzler, E. & Thiele, L. (1999). Multi-objective evolutionary algorithms: A comparative case study and the strength Pareto approach. *IEEE Trans. Evol. Comput., 3*(4), 257-271.

ADDITIONAL READING

The reader is strongly encouraged to visit the *Evolutionary Multi-objective Optimization Repository*, which is maintained by Carlos A. Coello Coello at the Web address:

http://delta.cs.cinvestav.mx/~ccoello/EMOO/

This excellent and up-to-date source of literature and software provides links and online copies of a plethora of papers published in the field. We selected some papers for the interested reader, with an emphasis in further developments and applications that were not discussed in the chapter due to space limitations:

Book Chapters

Hernandez Luna, E. & Coello Coello, C. A. (2004). Using a particle swarm optimizer with a multi-objective selection scheme to design combinational logic circuits. In Carlos A. Coello Coello & Gary B. Lamont (Eds.), *Applications of multi-objective evolutionary algorithms* (pp. 101-124). Singapore: World Scientific.

Reyes-Sierra, M. & Coello Coello, C. A. (2007). A study of techniques to improve the efficiency of a multi-objective particle swarm optimiser. In Shengxiang Yang, Yew Soon Ong, & Yaochu Jin (Eds.), *Evolutionary computation in dynamic and uncertain environments* (pp. 269-296). Springer.

Santana-Quintero, L. V., Ramirez-Santiago, N., Coello Coello, C. A., Molina Luque, J., & Hernandez-Diaz, A. G. (2006). A new proposal for multi-objective optimization using particle swarm optimization and rough sets theory. *Lecture notes in computer science* (Vol. 4193, pp. 483-492). Springer.

Santana-Quintero, L. V., Ramirez-Santiago, N., & Coello Coello, C. A. (2006). A multi-objective particle swarm optimizer hybridized with scatter search. *Lecture notes in artificial intelligence* (Vol. 4293, pp. 294-304). Springer.

Journal Papers

Gill, M. K., Kaheil, Y. H., Khalil, A., Mckee, M., & Bastidas, L. (2006). Multi-objective particle swarm optimization for parameter estimation in hydrology. *Water Resources Research, 42*(7), 2006.

Goudos, S. K. & Sahalos, J. N. (2006). Microwave absorber optimal design using Multi-objective particle swarm optimization. *Microwave and Optical Technology Letters, 48*(8), 1553-1558.

Huang, V. L., Suganthan, P. N., & Liang, J. J. (2006). Comprehensive learning particle swarm optimizer for solving multi-objective optimization problems. *International Journal of Intelligent Systems, 21*(2), 209-226.

Rahimi-Vahed, A. R. & Mirghorbani, S. M. (2007). A multi-objective particle swarm for a flow shop scheduling problem. *Journal of Combinatorial Optimization, 13*(1), 79-102.

Zhao, B. & Cao, Y.-J. (2005). Multiple objective particle swarm optimization technique for economic load dispatch. *Journal of Zhejiang University SCIENCE, 6A*(5), 420-427.

Conference Papers

Baltar, A. M. & Fontane, D. G. (2006, March). A generalized multi-objective particle swarm optimization solver for spreadsheet models: Application to water quality. In *Proceedings of Hydrology Days 2006*, Fort Collins, Colorado.

Brits, R., Engelbrecht, A. P., & van den Bergh, F. (2002). A niching particle swarm optimizer. In *Proceedings of the 4th Asia-Pacific Conference on Simulated Evolution and Learning (SEAL'02)* (pp. 692-696).

Goldbarg, E. F. G., de Souza, G. R., & Goldbarg, M. C. (2006). Particle swarm optimization for the bi-objective degree-constrained minimum spanning tree. In *Proceedings of the 2006 IEEE Congress on Evolutionary Computation (CEC'2006)* (pp. 1527-1534). IEEE.

Gong, D. W., Zhang, Y., & Zhang, J. H. (2005). Multi-objective particle swarm optimization based on minimal particle angle. *Lecture notes in computer science* (Vol. 3644, pp. 571-580). Springer-Verlag.

Halter, W. & Mostaghim, S. (2006). Bilevel optimization of multi-component chemical systems using particle swarm optimization. In *Proceedings of the 2006 IEEE Congress on Evolutionary Computation (CEC'2006)* (pp. 4383-4390). IEEE.

Hendtlass, T. (2005). WoSP: A multi-optima particle swarm algorithm. In *Proceedings of the 2005 IEEE Congress on Evolutionary Computation (CEC'2005)* (pp. 727-734). IEEE Service Center.

Ma, M., Zhang, L. B., Ma, J., & Zhou, C. G. (2006). Fuzzy neural network optimization by a particle swarm optimization algorithm. *Lecture notes in computer science* (Vol. 3971, pp. 752-761). Springer.

Meng, H. Y., Zhang, X. H., & Liu, S. Y. (2005). Intelligent multi-objective particle swarm optimization based on AER model. *Lecture notes in artificial intelligence* (Vol. 3808, pp. 178-189). Springer.

Salazar-Lechugam, M. & Rowe, J. E. (2006). Particle swarm optimization and auto-fitness sharing to solve multi-objective optimization problems. In *Proceedings of the 2006 Swarm Intelligence Symposium (SIS'06)* (pp. 90-97). IEEE Press.

Wang, L. & Singh, C. (2006). Multi-objective stochastic power dispatch through a modified particle swarm optimization algorithm. In *Proceedings of the 2006 Swarm Intelligence Symposium (SIS'06)* (pp. 128-135). IEEE Press.

Yapicioglu, H., Dozier, G., & Smith, A. E. (2004). Bi-criteria model for locating a semi-desirable facility on a plane using particle swarm optimization. In *Proceedings of the 2004 Congress on Evolutionary Computation (CEC'2004)* (pp. 2328-2334). IEEE Service Center.

Munoz Zavala, A. E., Villa Diharce, E. R., & Hernandez Aguirre, A. (2005). Particle evolutionary swarm for design reliability optimization. *Lecture notes in computer science* (Vol. 3410, pp. 856-869). Springer.

Theses

Reyes-Sierra, M. (2006). *Use of coevolution and fitness inheritance for multi-objective particle swarm optimization.* Unpublished doctoral Thesis, Computer Science Section, Department of Electrical Engineering, CINVESTAV-IPN, Mexico.

Toscano Pulido, G. (2005). *On the use of self-adaptation and elitism for multi-objective particle swarm optimization.* Unpublished doctoral thesis, Computer Science Section, Department of Electrical Engineering, CINVESTAV-IPN, Mexico.

Tayal, M. (2003). *Particle swarm optimization for mechanical design.* Unpublished master's thesis, The University of Texas at Arlington, Arlington, Texas.

Chapter III
Generalized Differential Evolution for Constrained Multi-Objective Optimization

Saku Kukkonen
Lappeenranta University of Technology, Finland

Jouni Lampinen
University of Vaasa, Finland

ABSTRACT

Multi-objective optimization with Evolutionary Algorithms has been gaining popularity recently because its applicability in practical problems. Many practical problems contain also constraints, which must be taken care of during optimization process. This chapter is about Generalized Differential Evolution, which is a general-purpose optimizer. It is based on a relatively recent Evolutionary Algorithm, Differential Evolution, which has been gaining popularity because of its simplicity and good observed performance. Generalized Differential Evolution extends Differential Evolution for problems with several objectives and constraints. The chapter concentrates on describing different development phases and performance of Generalized Differential Evolution but it also contains a brief review of other multi-objective DE approaches. Ability to solve multi-objective problems is mainly discussed, but constraint handling and the effect of control parameters are also covered. It is found that GDE versions, in particular the latest version, are effective and efficient for solving constrained multi-objective problems.

INTRODUCTION

During the last two decades, Evolutionary Algorithms (EAs) have gained popularity since EAs are capable of dealing with difficult objective functions, which are, for example, discontinuous, non-convex, multimodal, and nondifferentiable. Multi-objective EAs (MOEAs) have also gained popularity since they are capable of providing multiple solution candidates in a single run that is desirable with multi-objective optimization problems (MOPs).

Differential Evolution (DE) is a relatively new EA and it has been gaining popularity during previous years. Several extensions of DE for multi-objective optimization have already been proposed. The simplest approaches just convert MOPs to single-objective forms and use DE to solve these (Babu & Jehan, 2003; Chang & Xu, 2000; Wang & Sheu, 2000), whereas more recent ones use the concept of Pareto-dominance. The chapter contains a brief review of multi-objective DE approaches as well as constraint handling techniques used with DE.

This chapter concentrates on describing a DE extension called Generalized Differential Evolution (GDE), its development phases, and performance. GDE is a general-purpose optimizer for problems with constraints and objectives. Since different GDE versions differ in their ability to handle multiple objectives, the chapter mainly concentrates on this aspect but it also deals with constraint handling and the effect of control parameters. It is found that GDE versions, in particular the latest version, are effective and efficient for solving constrained multi-objective problems.

The rest of the chapter is organized as follows: In Section BACKGROUND, the concept of multi-objective optimization with constraints is handled briefly. Also, basic DE and its extensions for multi-objective and constrained optimization have been described. Section GENERALIZED DIFFERENTIAL EVOLUTION describes different development phases of GDE with experimental illustrations. Subjects of future work are given in Section FUTURE RESEARCH DIRECTIONS, and finally conclusions are drawn in Section CONCLUSION.

BACKGROUND

Multi-Objective Optimization with Constraints

Many practical problems have multiple objectives and several aspects cause multiple constraints to problems. For example, mechanical design problems have several objectives such as obtained performance and manufacturing costs, and available resources may cause limitations. Constraints can be divided into boundary constraints and constraint functions. Boundary constraints are used when the value of a decision variable is limited to some range, and constraint functions represent more complicated constraints, which are expressed as functions. A term *multi-objective* is used when the number of objectives is more than one. A term *many-objective* is used when the number of objectives is more than two or three (the term is not settled yet).

A constrained multi-objective optimization problem (MOP) can be presented in the form (Miettinen, 1998, p. 37):

minimize $\{f_1(\vec{x}), f_2(\vec{x}), \ldots, f_M(\vec{x})\}$

subject to $\left(g_1(\vec{x}), g_2(\vec{x}), \ldots, g_K(\vec{x})\right)^T \leq 0^T$

Thus, there are M functions to be optimized and K constraint functions. Maximization problems can be easily transformed to minimization problems and constraint functions can be converted to form $g_j(\vec{x}) \leq 0$, thereby the formulation above is without loss of generality.

Typically, MOPs are often converted to single-objective optimization problems by predefining weighting factors for different objectives, expressing the relative importance of each objective. Optimizing several objectives simultaneously without articulating the relative importance of each objective *a priori* is often called Pareto-optimization (Pareto, 1896). An obtained solution is *Pareto-optimal* if none of the objectives can be improved without impairing at least one other objective (Miettinen, 1998, p. 11). If the obtained solution can be improved in such a way that at least one objective improves and the other objectives do not decline, then the new solution (Pareto-) dominates the original solution. The objective of Pareto-optimization is to find a set of solutions that are not dominated by any other solution.

A set of Pareto-optimal solutions form a Pareto front, and an approximation of the Pareto front is called a set of nondominated solutions, because the solutions in this set are not dominating each other in the space of objective functions. From the set of nondominated solutions the decision-maker may pick a solution, which provides a suitable compromise between the objectives. This can be viewed as *a posteriori* articulation of the decision-makers preferences concerning the relative importance of each objective. Besides *a priori* and *a posteriori* methods, also no-preference and interactive methods exist (Miettinen, 1998). The first ones do not take any preference information and the second ones have the decision-maker interacting/guiding the solution process. In a way interactive methods are the most developed and provide the most satisfactory results (Miettinen, 1998, p. 131).

Weak dominance relation $\preceq$ between two vectors is defined such that $\vec{x}_1$ weakly dominates $\vec{x}_2$, that is, $\vec{x}_1 \preceq \vec{x}_2$ iff $\forall i : f_i(\vec{x}_1) \leq f_i(\vec{x}_2)$. Dominance relation $\prec$ between two vectors is defined such a way that $\vec{x}_1$ dominates $\vec{x}_2$, i.e., $\vec{x}_1 \prec \vec{x}_2$ iff $\vec{x}_1 \preceq \vec{x}_2 \wedge \exists i : f_i(\vec{x}_1) < f_i(\vec{x}_2)$. The dominance relationship can be extended to take into consideration constraint values besides objective values. *Constraint-domination* $\prec_c$ is defined here such a way that $\vec{x}_1$ constraint-dominates $\vec{x}_2$, i.e., $\vec{x}_1 \prec_c \vec{x}_2$ iff any of the following conditions is true (Lampinen, 2001):

1. $\vec{x}_1$ and $\vec{x}_2$ are infeasible and $\vec{x}_1$ dominates $\vec{x}_2$ in the constraint function violation space.
2. $\vec{x}_1$ is feasible and $\vec{x}_2$ is not.
3. $\vec{x}_1$ and $\vec{x}_2$ are feasible and $\vec{x}_1$ dominates $\vec{x}_2$ in the objective function space.

The definition for weak constraint-domination $\preceq_c$ is analogous when the dominance relation is changed to weak dominance in the above definition. The weak constraint-domination relation can be formally defined as, (see Box 1), where $g'_k(\vec{x}) = \max(g_k(\vec{x}), 0)$ represents a constraint violation. In the case of no constraints and a single objective $\vec{x}_1 \preceq_c \vec{x}_2$ iff $f(\vec{x}_1) \leq f(\vec{x}_2)$. This con-

Box 1.

$$\vec{x}_1 \preceq_c \vec{x}_2 \text{ iff } \begin{cases} \begin{cases} \exists k \in \{1,\ldots,K\} : g_k(\vec{x}_1) > 0 \\ \wedge \\ \forall k \in \{1,\ldots,K\} : g'_k(\vec{x}_1) \leq g'_k(\vec{x}_2) \end{cases} \\ \vee \\ \begin{cases} \forall k \in \{1,\ldots,K\} : g_k(\vec{x}_1) \leq 0 \\ \wedge \\ \exists k \in \{1,\ldots,K\} : g_k(\vec{x}_2) > 0 \end{cases} \\ \vee \\ \begin{cases} \forall k \in \{1,\ldots,K\} : g_k(\vec{x}_1) \leq 0 \wedge g_k(\vec{x}_2) \leq 0 \\ \wedge \\ \forall m \in \{1,\cdots,M\} : f_m(\vec{x}_1) \leq f_m(\vec{x}_2) \end{cases} \end{cases},$$

straint-domination is a special case of more general concept of having goals and priorities that is presented in (Fonseca & Fleming, 1998). A slightly different definition for constraint-domination also exists (Deb, 2001, pp. 301-302; Deb, 2000). It makes selection based on a sum of constraint violations instead of domination principle in the case of two infeasible vectors.

Only the convergence aspect of multi-objective optimization has been considered above. MOEAs are able to provide several solution candidates in a single run and besides of convergence, also a good diversity is desired. Diversity is usually considered in the objective space (instead of decision variable space) and a good diversity means that the spread of extreme solutions is as high as possible, and the relative distance between solutions is as equal as possible. This kind of set would provide an ideal presentation about existing solutions to choose from.

Differential Evolution

The Differential Evolution (DE) algorithm (Price, Storn, & Lampinen, 2005) belongs to the family of EAs and the concept was introduced by Storn and Price (1995). Design principles in DE are simplicity, efficiency, and use of floating-point encoding instead of binary numbers, which is a usual way of coding in Genetic Algorithms (GA) (Goldberg, 1989). The name of the method is referring to the idea of using differences of individuals to mutate an individual.

DE has been gaining popularity during previous years because of its good performance in practical problems. It has also performed well with number of test problems (Price & Storn, 1996; Rönkkönen, Kukkonen, & Lampinen, 2005a; Rönkkönen, Kukkonen, & Price, 2005b). The 2006 Congress on Evolutionary Computation (CEC 2006) was the first major conference to arrange a special session dedicated solely to DE.

There exist several variations of the idea and these are referred as DE strategies in the literature (Price et al., 2005). In the following section, probably the most popular DE strategy is described in detail.

Basic Differential Evolution, DE/rand/1/bin

Basic DE is meant for unconstrained single-objective optimization and therefore notations in this section are for single-objective optimization. Like in a typical EA, the idea in DE is to have some random initial population, which is then improved using selection, mutation, and crossover operations. Several ways exist to determine a stopping criterion for EAs but usually a predefined upper limit G_{max} for the number of generations to be computed provides appropriate stopping condition.

Initialization of Population

Values for the initial population in DE are typically drawn from uniform distribution. Formally this can be presented as (Price, 1999):

$$P_G = \{\vec{x}_{1,G}, \vec{x}_{2,G}, \ldots, \vec{x}_{NP,G}\}, \quad \vec{x}_{i,G} = x_{j,i,G}$$
$$x_{j,i,G=0} = x_j^{(lo)} + rand_j[0,1] \cdot (x_j^{(hi)} - x_j^{(lo)})$$
$$i = 1, 2, \ldots, NP, \quad NP \geq 4, \quad j = 1, 2, \ldots, D$$

In this representation P_G denotes a population after G generations (0 is an initial generation), $\vec{x}_{i,G}$ denotes a decision vector (or individual) of the population, and $rand_j[0,1]$ denotes a uniformly distributed random variable in the range [0, 1]. Terms $x_j^{(lo)}$ and $x_j^{(hi)}$ denote lower and upper parameter bounds, respectively. The size of the population is denoted by NP and the dimension of decision vectors is denoted by D.

Other ways of initialization also exist, for example, if some knowledge exists about the position of the optimum, part of the initial population may be initialized around the possible position of the optimum using normal distribution.

Mutation and Crossover

DE goes through each decision vector $\vec{x}_{i,G}$ of the population and creates a corresponding trial vector $\vec{u}_{i,G}$ as follows (Price, 1999), (see Box 2).

Indices r_1, r_2, and r_3 are mutually different and drawn from the set of the population indices. Both CR and F are user defined control parameters for the DE algorithm and they remain fixed during the whole execution of the algorithm. Parameter CR, controlling the crossover operation, represents the probability that an element for the trial vector is chosen from a linear combination of three randomly chosen vectors and not from the old decision vector $\vec{x}_{i,G}$. The condition $j == j_{rand}$ ensures that at least one element of the trial vector is different compared to the elements of the old vector. Parameter F is a scaling factor for mutation and its value is typically (0, 1+] (i.e., larger than 0 and upper limit is in practice around 1 although there is no hard upper limit). In practice, CR controls the rotational invariance of the search, and its small value (e.g., 0.1) is practicable with separable problems while larger values (e.g., 0.9) are for non-separable problems. Control parameter F controls the speed and robustness of the search, that is, a lower value for F increases the convergence rate but also the risk of getting stuck into a local optimum. Parameters CR and NP have the similar effect on the convergence rate as F has.

The difference between two randomly chosen vectors $(x_{j,r_1,G} - x_{j,r_2,G})$ defines magnitude and direction of mutation. When the difference is added to a third randomly chosen vector $x_{j,r_3,G}$, this corresponds mutation of this third vector. The basic idea of DE is that mutation is self-adaptive to the objective function space and to the current population in the same way as in Covariance Matrix Adaptation Evolutionary Strategy (CMA-ES) (Hansen & Ostermeier, 1996) but without the computational burden of covariance matrix calculations that are scaling unfavorably with the dimensionality of the problem. At the beginning of generations the magnitude of mutation is large because vectors in the population are far away from each other in the search space. When the evolution proceeds and the population converges, the magnitude of mutation gets smaller. The self-adaptive mutation of DE permits to balance between global and local search. Other strengths are simplicity and ability to perform a rotationally invariant search.

Box 2.

$r_1, r_2, r_3 \in \{1, 2, \ldots, NP\}$,
(randomly selected, except mutually different and different from i)
$j_{rand} = \text{int}(rand_i[0,1) \cdot D) + 1$
for $(j = 1; j \leq D; j = j + 1)$
{
    if $(rand_j[0,1) < CR \lor j == j_{rand})$
        $u_{j,i,G} = x_{j,r_3,G} + F \cdot (x_{j,r_1,G} - x_{j,r_2,G})$
    else
        $u_{j,i,G} = x_{j,i,G}$
}

Selection

After each mutation and crossover operation the trial vector $\vec{u}_{i,G}$ is compared to the old decision vector $\vec{x}_{i,G}$. If the trial vector has equal or lower objective value, then it replaces the old vector. This can be presented as follows (Price, 1999):

$$\vec{x}_{i,G+1} = \begin{cases} \vec{u}_{i,G} & \text{if } f(\vec{u}_{i,G}) \leq f(\vec{x}_{i,G}) \\ \vec{x}_{i,G} & \text{otherwise} \end{cases}$$

The average objective value of the population will never deteriorate, because the trial vector replaces the old vector only if it has equal or lower objective value. Therefore, DE is an elitist search method.

Overall Algorithm

The overall presentation of basic DE (sometimes also referred as "classic DE") is presented below (Price, 1999). This DE strategy is identified with a notation *DE/rand/1/bin* in the DE literature. In this notation, *rand* indicates how the mutated vector is selected (it could be also the *best* among the current population). The number of vector differences used in the mutation is indicated next, and *bin* indicates the way the old vector and the trial vector are combined (an alternative exponential recombination procedure also exists). (See Box 3).

Differential Evolution for Multiple Objectives and Constraints

The first method extending DE for multi-objective optimization using the Pareto approach was Pareto-based DE approach (Chang, Xu, & Quek, 1999). It used separated set for obtained nondominated solutions and fitness sharing (Deb, 2001, pp. 149-160) to achieve diversity in the population.

Box 3.

Input: D, G_{max}, $NP \geq 4$, $F \in (0, 1+]$, $CR \in [0,1]$, and initial bounds: $\vec{x}^{(lo)}, \vec{x}^{(hi)}$

Initialize:
$$\begin{cases} \forall i \leq NP \wedge \forall j \leq D : x_{j,i,G=0} = x_j^{(lo)} + rand_j[0,1] \cdot \left(x_j^{(hi)} - x_j^{(lo)}\right) \\ i = \{1, 2, \ldots, NP\}, j = \{1, 2, \ldots, D\}, G = 0, rand_j[0,1] \in [0,1] \end{cases}$$

While $G < G_{max}$

    Mutate and recombine:

    $r_1, r_2, r_3 \in \{1, 2, \ldots, NP\}$, randomly selected,

        except mutually different and different from i

    $j_{rand} \in \{1, 2, \ldots, D\}$, randomly selected for each i

$$\forall i \leq NP \; \forall j \leq D, \; u_{j,i,G} = \begin{cases} x_{j,r_3,G} + F \cdot \left(x_{j,r_1,G} - x_{j,r_2,G}\right) \\ \quad \text{if } rand_j[0,1) < CR \vee j == j_{rand} \\ x_{j,i,G} \quad \text{otherwise} \end{cases}$$

    Select:

$$\vec{x}_{i,G+1} = \begin{cases} \vec{u}_{i,G} & \text{if } f(\vec{u}_{i,G}) \leq f(\vec{x}_{i,G}) \\ \vec{x}_{i,G} & \text{otherwise} \end{cases}$$

$G = G + 1$

Pareto Differential Evolution (Bergey, 1999) was also mentioned about the same time, unfortunately without an explicit description of the method. After these, the Pareto(-frontier) Differential Evolution (PDE) algorithm (Abbass & Sarker, 2002; Abbass, Sarker, & Newton, 2001) and the first version of Generalized Differential Evolution (GDE) (Lampinen, 2001) were introduced. PDE algorithm modified basic DE in several ways and used variable size population containing only nondominated individuals. If the size of the population increased above allowed maximum, the most crowded members were removed according to distance to the nearest neighbors.

Then, Self-adaptive PDE (SPDE) (Abbass, 2002), the Pareto DE Approach (PDEA) (Madavan, 2002), Adaptive Pareto DE (APDE) (Zaharie, 2003b), Multi-objective DE (MODE) (Xue, Sanderson, & Graves, 2003), Vector Evaluated DE (VEDE) (Parsopoulos, Tasoulis, Pavlidis, Plagianakos, & Vrahatis, 2004), and the second version of GDE (Kukkonen & Lampinen, 2004c) have been proposed. SPDE is an extension of PDE to have the adaptation of control parameters along the optimization process (the control parameters evolve similarly to decision variables to be optimized). PDEA is basically the same as the elitist Non-Dominated Sorting Genetic Algorithm (NSGA-II) (Deb, Pratap, Agarwal, & Meyarivan, 2002) except GA replaced with DE. Research demonstrating the performance of PDEA over NSGA-II with rotated MOPs has also been reported (Iorio & Li, 2004). APDE is the same as PDEA except DE replaced with earlier proposed Adaptive Differential Evolution (Zaharie, 2003a), which has a parameter adaptation guided by a theoretical rule about the population variance evolution. MODE is another approach combining ideas of DE and NSGA-II. In MODE, basic DE is modified and also an extra crowding parameter is introduced to prevent similar individuals entering the next generation. VEDE is inspired by the classical Vector Evaluated GA (VEGA) and is based on subpopulations optimizing individual objectives separately. VEDE does not have any diversity maintenance technique.

Later, DE for Multi-objective Optimization (DEMO) (Robič & Filipič, 2005) and the third version of GDE (Kukkonen & Lampinen, 2005b) were introduced. DEMO is a slight modification of PDEA and will be discussed later. Some of the latest proposals are Differential Evolution for Multi-objective Optimization with Random Sets (DEMORS) (Hernández-Diaz et al., 2006), Multi-objective Differential Evolution based Decomposition (MODE/D) (Li & Zhang, 2006), and DE algorithm based on ε-dominance and an orthogonal design method (ε -ODEMO) (Cai, Gong, & Huang, 2007). DEMORS has a relatively complicate two-phase approach combining a global search using Pareto-adaptive ε-dominance and a local search using rough sets. MODE/D decomposes a MOP into the number of different scalar optimization problems and solves these simultaneously using DE. ε -ODEMO uses the orthogonal design method to generate an initial population and then the ε -dominance concept to maintain archive of nondominated solutions. Use of ε -dominance maintains distribution of solutions automatically.

There exist also some other relevant studies. Iorio & Li (2006) examined incorporating directional information in selection of vectors for the mutation step of DE. Comparison between GA and DE in multi-objective optimization has been done by Tušar & Filipič (2007) and it has been concluded that DE explores the decision variable space better than GA. A comparison between four different multi-objective DE variants is in (Zielinski & Laur, 2007). The variants differ in their selection scheme and based on experimental results it is found that a selection mechanism that is used, for example, in DEMO and the third version of GDE is better than the one used, for example, in PDEA.

Besides solving problems with multiple objectives, DE has also been modified for handling problems with constraints (Chang & Chang, 1998;

Lampinen & Zelinka, 1999; Lin, Hwang, & Wang, 2002; Storn, 1999; Wang & Chiou, 1997). Many of these approaches are based on applying penalty functions, which have a problem of selecting penalty parameters. To overcome this problem, following selection rules has been used:

1. Between two feasible solutions, the one with a better fitness value is selected.
2. If one solution is feasible and the other one is infeasible, the feasible is selected.
3. Between two infeasible solutions, the one with less constraint violation is selected.

For measuring constraint violation in the third rule, the Pareto-dominance relation between constraint violations (Lampinen, 2002) and the sum of constraint violations (Mezura-Montes, Coello Coello, & Tun-Morales, 2004) have been used with DE. The first one has the scale of individual constraint functions and it is used in Generalized Differential Evolution.

GENERALIZED DIFFERENTIAL EVOLUTION

Generalized Differential Evolution (GDE) is an extension of DE for optimization with an arbitrary number of objectives and constraints. Leading idea and justification for the name has been that the extension falls back to basic DE in the case of unconstrained single-objective problem. This property is contrary to the other multi-objective DE approaches described in the previous section. The property makes it possible to change *DE/rand/1/bin* strategy to any other DE strategy such as presented in (Feoktistov & Janaqi, 2004; Price et al., 2005; Zaharie, 2003b) or, generally, to any method where a child vector is compared against a parent vector and the better one is preserved.

Several GDE development versions exist and they can be implemented in such a way that the number of function evaluations is reduced. The reason for this is that in the case of infeasible solutions, the old vector is preferred unless the trial vector weakly dominates it in the space of constraint violations. Already comparison between single constraint values can reveal that both solutions are infeasible and the trial vector does not dominate the old vector. This reduces number of needed constraint function evaluations that is helpful in the case of many and/or computationally heavy constraint functions.

In the following, different development versions of GDE are described. Performance is demonstrated with two sets of well known test problems. The first set consist of five bi-objective benchmark problems, which are described in (Deb, 2001, pp. 356-360; Zitzler, Deb, & Thiele, 2000) and known as ZDT1, ZDT2, ZDT3, ZDT4, & ZDT6 (ZDT5 is commonly left out since it has binary-coded variables whereas other ZDT problems have real-coded variables). They are designed to test the ability of a multi-objective optimization method to handle convexity (ZDT1), non-convexity (ZDT2), discontinuity (ZDT3), multimodality (ZDT4), and non-uniformity (ZDT6) of the Pareto front. With these problems population size of 100 and 250 generations are used. The second set consist of five tri-objective benchmark problems, which are described in (Deb, Thiele, Laumanns, & Zitzler, 2005) and known as DTLZ1, DTLZ2, DTLZ4, DTLZ5, and DTLZ7. These problems are solved using population size 200 and 250 generations. The control parameter values are $CR = 0.2$ and $F = 0.2$ for all the problems except values $CR = 0.0$ and $F = 0.5$ are used with ZDT4 (ZDT4 has multiple equally spaced local Pareto fronts and $F = 0.5$ advances moving from one local front to another). Since the objectives of the ZDT problems, especially ZDT4, are in different order of difficulty, using a large CR value would lead to convergence along the first objective far before the second objective. Therefore a small CR value is used. More about the issue is given in (Kukkonen & Lampinen, 2005a; Kukkonen

Figure 1. Results for the ZDT problems using GDE1

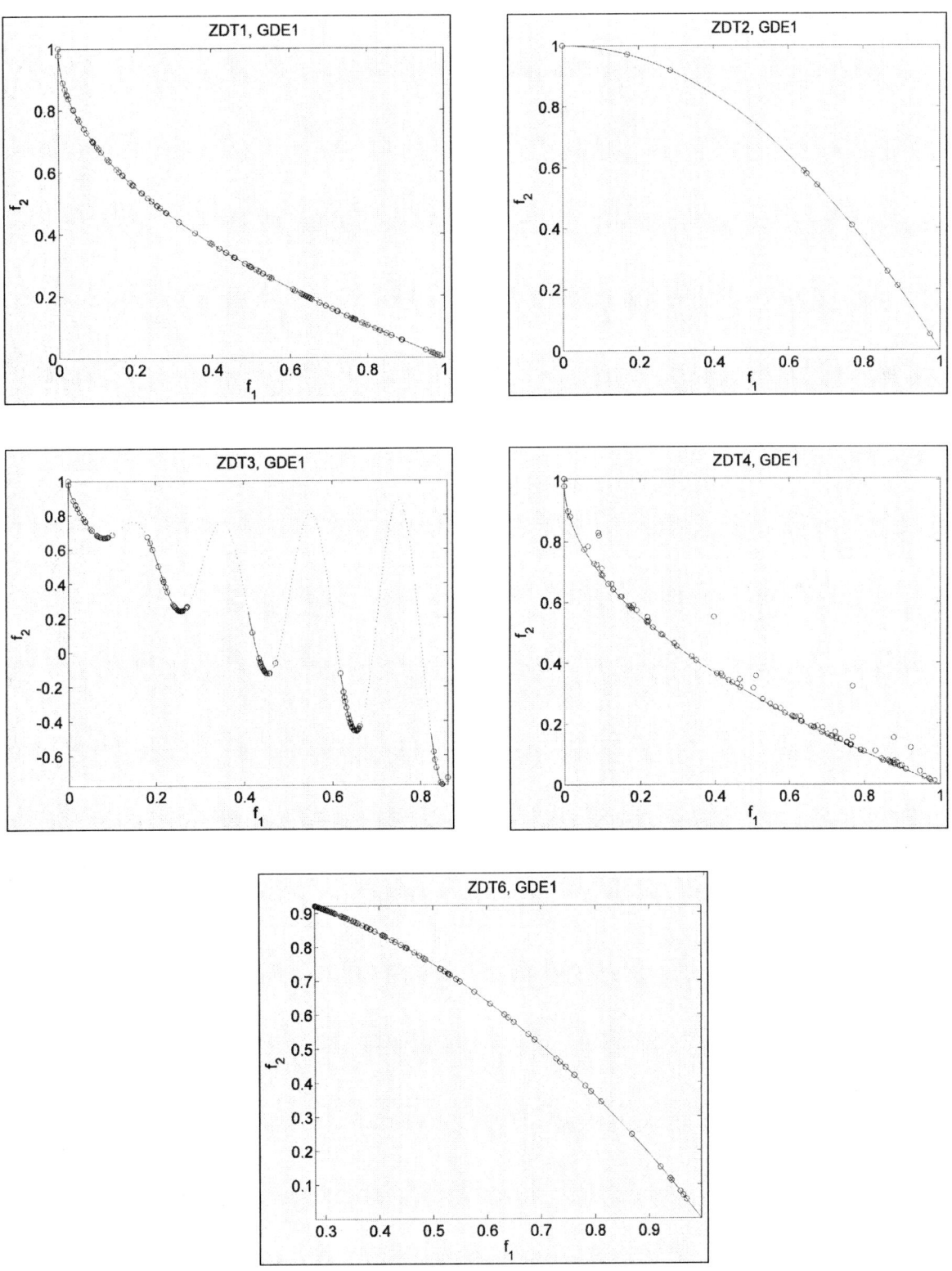

Figure 2. Results for the DTLZ problems using GDE1

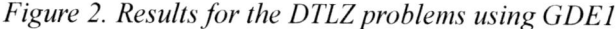

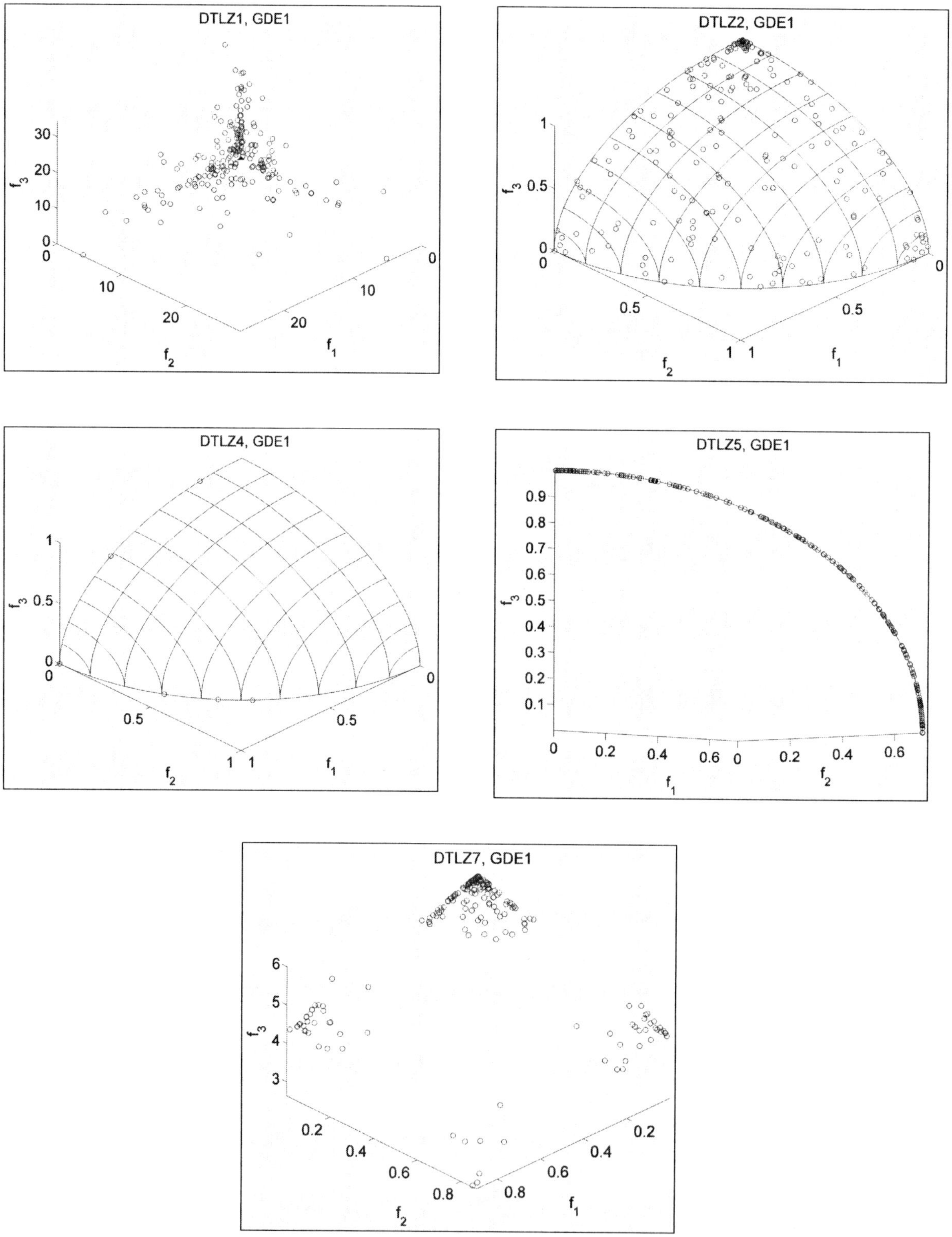

& Lampinen, 2006b). Results for the problems solved with different GDE versions are shown in Figure 1 – Figure 8.

In all the experiments in this chapter, possible boundary constraint violations have been handled by reflecting violating variable values back from the violated boundary using the following rule before the selection operation of GDE:

$$u_{j,i,G} = \begin{cases} 2x_j^{(lo)} - u_{j,i,G} & \text{if } u_{j,i,G} < x_j^{(lo)} \\ 2x_j^{(hi)} - u_{j,i,G} & \text{if } u_{j,i,G} > x_j^{(hi)} \end{cases}$$

The First Version, GDE1

The first version, GDE1, was proposed by Lampinen (2001) as a further development from the constraint handling approach based on dominance relation (Lampinen, 2002), and name Generalized Differential Evolution appeared first time in (Kukkonen & Lampinen, 2004b). GDE1 extends basic DE for constrained multi-objective optimization simply by modifying the selection operation of DE. In GDE1, the selection operation is based on constraint-domination and can be simply defined as:

$$\vec{x}_{i,G+1} = \begin{cases} \vec{u}_{i,G} & \text{if } \vec{u}_{i,G} \prec=_c \vec{x}_{i,G} \\ \vec{x}_{i,G} & \text{otherwise} \end{cases}$$

The weak constraint-domination relation is used to have a congruity with the selection operation of DE. Thus, in the case of equality, the trial vector is preferred.

As mentioned earlier, a major benefit of using the dominance relation in the selection is that it can be implemented in a way that the number of function evaluations is reduced because not always all the constraints and objectives need to be evaluated, for example, inspecting constraint violations (even one constraint) is often enough to determine, which vector to select for the next generation (Lampinen, 2002; Price et al., 2005). Dependent on a problem, the reduction can be truly remarkable as noted in (Kukkonen & Lampinen, 2006a). In practice, it is wise to evaluate computationally expensive functions last, since the later a function is in evaluation order, the fewer times it gets evaluated. Order of functions has also an effect on the search process since the search is directed at the beginning according to the first functions. This property may be either useful or harmful.

GDE1 does not have any kind of diversity maintenance that is rare compared to the present MOEAs. Still, GDE1 has been able to provide surprisingly good results with some problems (Kukkonen & Lampinen, 2004a; Kukkonen & Lampinen, 2004d) but has been found too sensitive to the selection of the control parameters values as noted in (Kukkonen & Lampinen, 2005a).

A final population for the ZDT and DTLZ problems is shown in Figure 1 and Figure 2. The members of the final population are shown instead of just the nondominated members to have a better idea about the behavior of a search method in hand. Difficulty to find the concave Pareto-front of ZDT2 is observable in Figure 1. Also, only edges of Pareto-front of DTLZ4 are found. DTLZ4 is similar to DTLZ2 except DTLZ4 posses more difficulty for diversity maintenance.

The Second Version, GDE2

The second version, GDE2, introduced a diversity maintenance operation to GDE. Again, only the selection operation of basic DE was modified. The selection is done based on crowding in the objective space when the trial and old vector are feasible and nondominating each other in the objective function space (Kukkonen & Lampinen, 2004c). More formally, the selection operation is now, (see Box 4), where d_i is a distance measure for measuring the distance from a particular solution i to its neighbor solutions. Implementation was done using *crowding distance* (Deb,

Box 4.

$$\vec{x}_{i,G+1} = \begin{cases} \vec{u}_{i,G} & \text{if } \begin{cases} \vec{u}_{i,G} \prec=_c \vec{x}_{i,G} \\ \vee \\ \begin{cases} \forall j \in \{1,\ldots,K\}: g_j(\vec{u}_{i,G}) \leq 0 \\ \wedge \\ \neg[\vec{x}_{i,G} \prec \vec{u}_{i,G}] \\ \wedge \\ d_{\vec{u}_{i,G}} \geq d_{\vec{x}_{i,G}} \end{cases} \end{cases} \\ \vec{x}_{i,G} & \text{otherwise} \end{cases}$$

2001, pp. 248-249), which is a distance measure used in NSGA-II. However, any other distance measure could be used instead that is advisable if the number of objectives is more than two, since crowding distance does not estimate true crowding anymore in a such case (Kukkonen & Deb, 2006b).

Since there is no nondominated sorting (Deb, 2001, pp. 33-44), crowding is measured among the whole population. This improves the extent and distribution of the obtained set of solutions but slows down the convergence of the overall population because it favors isolated solutions far from the Pareto-front until all the solutions are converged near the Pareto-front. GDE2 is also too sensitive to the selection of the control parameter values.

A final population for the ZDT and DTLZ problems is shown in Figure 3 and Figure 4. Better obtained diversity for ZDT2 and DTLZ4 compared to GDE1 can be observed by comparing Figure 3 and Figure 4 to Figure 1 and Figure 2.

Also, a slower convergence compared to GDE1 can be observed with ZDT3 and DTLZ1.

The Third Version, GDE3

The third and currently the latest enumerated version is GDE3 (Kukkonen & Lampinen, 2005b; Kukkonen & Deb, 2006b). Besides the selection, another part of basic DE has also been modified. Now, in the case of comparing feasible and non-dominating solutions, both vectors are saved. Therefore, at the end of a generation the population might be larger than originally. Before continuing to the next generation, the size of the population is reduced using nondominated sorting and pruning based on diversity preservation to select the best solution candidates to survive.

Whole GDE3 is presented below. Notation CD is referring to crowding distance, but some other distance measure for crowding could be used. GDE3 can be seen as a combination of GDE2 and PDEA. A similar approach was also proposed in

Figure 3. Results for the ZDT problems using GDE2

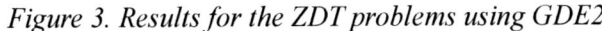

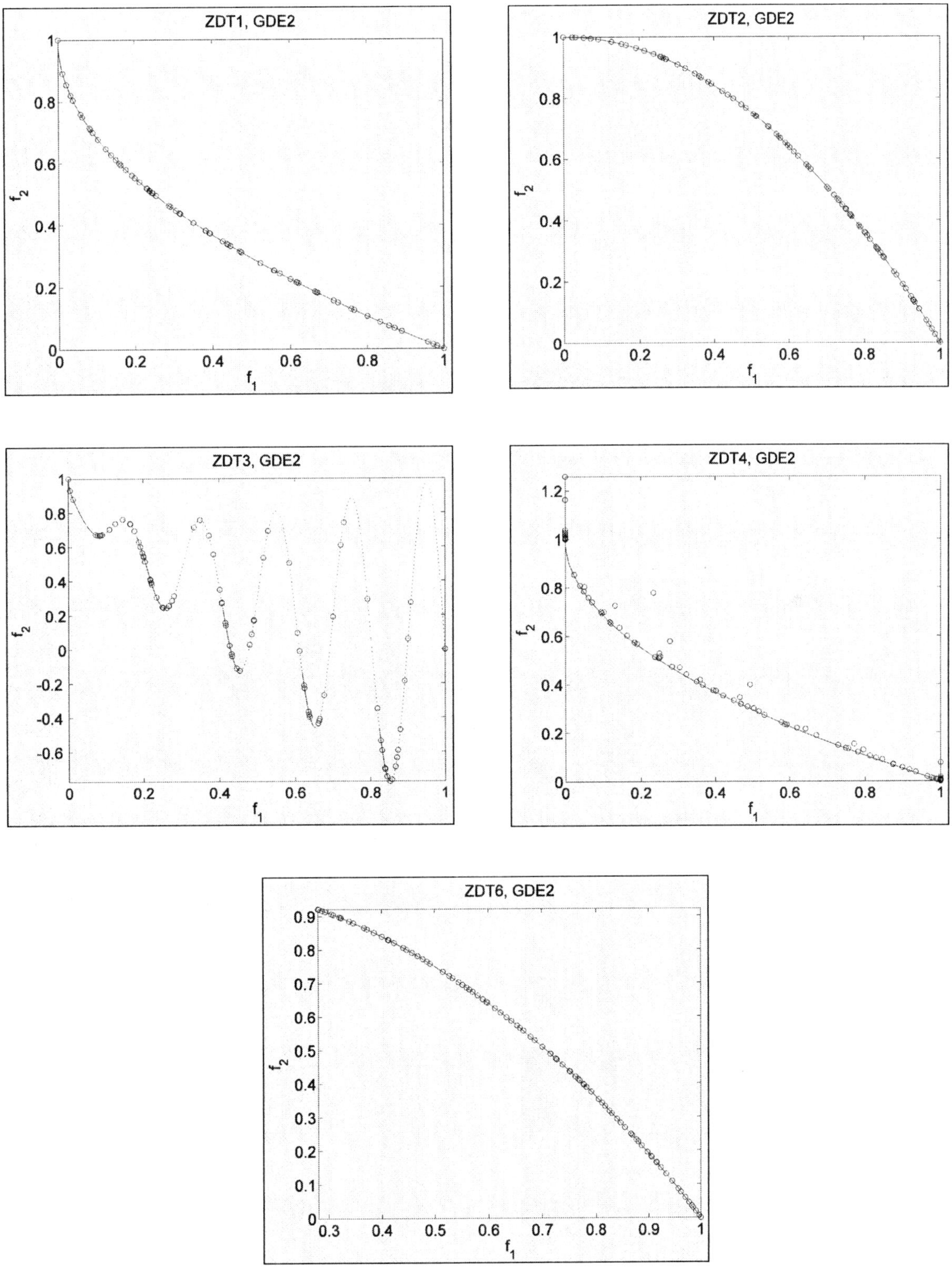

Figure 4. Results for the DTLZ problems using GDE2

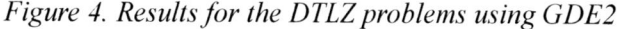

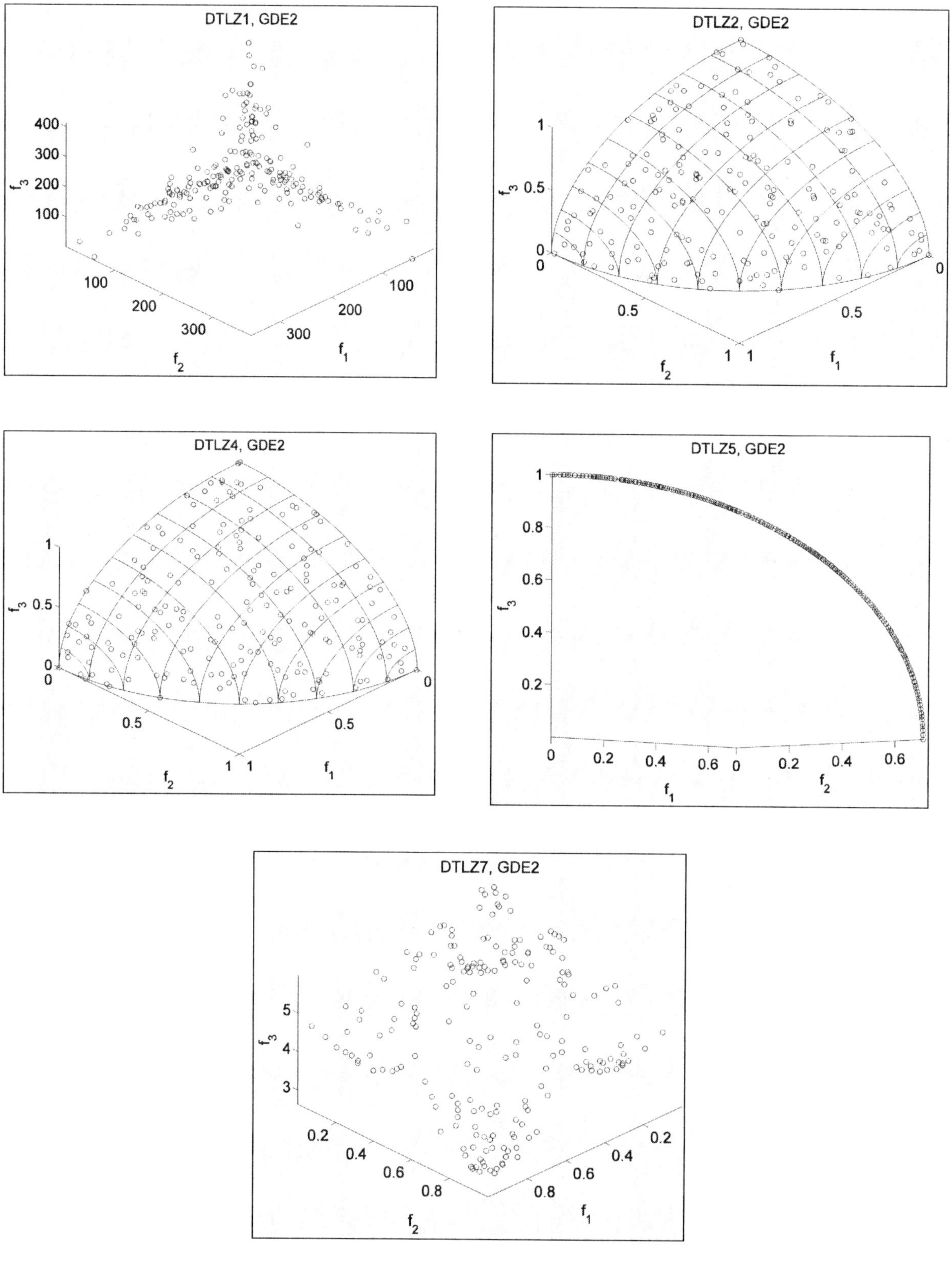

DEMO (Robič & Filipič, 2005) without constraint handling, and DEMO does not fall back to basic DE in the case of a single objective as GDE3 does. (See Box 5).

After a generation, the size of the population may be larger than originally. If this is the case, the population is then decreased back to the original size based on a similar selection approach used in

Box 5.

$$\text{Input: } D, G_{max}, NP \geq 4, F \in (0, 1+], CR \in [0,1], \text{ and initial bounds: } \vec{x}^{(lo)}, \vec{x}^{(hi)}$$

$$\text{Initialize: } \begin{cases} \forall i \leq NP \land \forall j \leq D : x_{j,i,G=0} = x_j^{(lo)} + rand_j[0,1] \cdot \left(x_j^{(hi)} - x_j^{(lo)}\right) \\ i = \{1,2,\ldots,NP\}, j = \{1,2,\ldots,D\}, G = 0, n = 0, rand_j[0,1] \in [0,1] \end{cases}$$

While $G < G_{max}$

  Mutate and recombine:

  $r_1, r_2, r_3 \in \{1,2,\ldots,NP\}$, randomly selected, except mutually different and different from i

  $j_{rand} \in \{1,2,\ldots,D\}$, randomly selected for each i

  $$\forall j \leq D, u_{j,i,G} = \begin{cases} x_{j,r_3,G} + F \cdot \left(x_{j,r_1,G} - x_{j,r_2,G}\right) \\ \quad \text{if } rand_j[0,1) < CR \lor j == j_{rand} \\ x_{j,i,G} \quad \text{otherwise} \end{cases}$$

$\forall i \leq NP$

  Select:

  $$\vec{x}_{i,G+1} = \begin{cases} \vec{u}_{i,G} & \text{if } \vec{u}_{i,G} \prec=_c \vec{x}_{i,G} \\ \vec{x}_{i,G} & \text{otherwise} \end{cases}$$

  Set:

  $$\begin{aligned} n &= n+1 \\ \vec{x}_{NP+n,G+1} &= \vec{u}_{i,G} \end{aligned} \quad \text{if } \begin{cases} \forall j \in \{1,\ldots,K\}: g_j(\vec{u}_{i,G}) \leq 0 \\ \land \\ \vec{x}_{i,G+1} == \vec{x}_{i,G} \\ \land \\ \neg\left[\vec{x}_{i,G} \prec \vec{u}_{i,G}\right] \end{cases}$$

While $n > 0$

  Select $\vec{x} \in \{\vec{x}_{1,G+1}, \vec{x}_{2,G+1},\ldots,\vec{x}_{NP+n,G+1}\}$:

  $$\begin{cases} \forall i \in \{1,\ldots,NP+n\}: \neg\left[\vec{x} \prec_c \vec{x}_{i,G+1}\right] \\ \land \\ \forall \left(\vec{x}_{i,G+1} : \neg\left[\vec{x}_{i,G+1} \prec_c \vec{x}\right]\right) CD(\vec{x}) \leq CD(\vec{x}_{i,G+1}) \end{cases}$$

  Remove $\vec{x}$

  $n = n - 1$

$G = G + 1$

NSGA-II. Population members are sorted based on nondominance and crowding. The worst population members according to these measurements are removed to decrease the size of the population to the original size. Nondominated sorting is modified to take into consideration also constraints. The selection based on crowding distance is improved over the original method of NSGA-II to provide a better distributed set of vectors (Kukkonen & Deb, 2006b). This improvement is described in following section.

When $M = 1$ and $K = 0$, there are no constraints to be evaluated and the selection is simply

$$\vec{x}_{i,G+1} = \begin{cases} \vec{u}_{i,G} & \text{if } f(\vec{u}_{i,G}) \leq f(\vec{x}_{i,G}) \\ \vec{x}_{i,G} & \text{otherwise} \end{cases},$$

which is the same as for basic DE. The population size does not increase because this requires that $\vec{x}_{i,G}$ and $\vec{u}_{i,G}$ do not weakly dominate each other that cannot be true in the case of a single objective. Since the population size does not increase, there is no need to remove elements. Therefore, GDE3 is identical to basic DE in this case.

In NSGA-II and PDEA, the size of the population after a generation is $2\,NP$, which is then decreased to NP. In GDE3 and DEMO, the size of the population after a generation is between NP and $2\,NP$ because the size of the population is increased only if the trial and the old vector are feasible and do not dominate each other.

Decreasing the size of the population at the end of a generation is the most complex operation in the algorithm. The reduction is done using nondominated sorting and pruning based on crowding. The run-time complexity of nondominated sorting is $O(N \log^{M-1} N)$ (Jensen, 2003). The pruning of population members based on crowding is also a complex operation if clustering techniques are applied. Instead of clustering, the operation is performed using an approximate distance measure, crowding distance, which can be calculated in time $O(M N \log N)$ for whole population (Jensen, 2003). The overall run-time complexity of GDE3 is $O(G_{max} N \log^{M-1} N)$ for large N.

Compared to the earlier GDE versions GDE3 improves the ability to handle MOPs by giving a better distributed set of solutions and being less sensitive to the selection of control parameter values. GDE3 has been compared to NSGA-II and found at least comparable according to experimental results (Kukkonen & Lampinen, 2005b).

Diversity Maintenance for Bi-Objective Problems

Diversity preservation of originally introduced GDE3 is based on crowding distance but it is a modified version from the approach used in NSGA-II. In NSGA-II crowding distance values are calculated once for all the members of a nondominated set. Then members having the smallest crowding distance values are removed without taking account that removal of a member will affect to the crowding distance value of its neighbors. Outcome is that the diversity of the remaining members is nonoptimal. Therefore, the diversity maintenance operation in GDE3 removes the most crowded members from a nondominated set one by one and updates the crowding distance value of the remaining members after each removal. Straightforward approach for this would have a time complexity class $O(M N^2)$ but a more sophisticated algorithm exists and it has a time complexity class $O(M N \log N)$, which is the same as for the approach used with NSGA-II (Kukkonen & Deb, 2006b).

A final population for the ZDT and DTLZ problems is shown in Figure 5 and Figure 6. Obtained distributions are almost optimal for the ZDT problems but less optimal for DTLZ problems (except for DTLZ5, which has a curved shape Pareto-front). In (Kukkonen & Deb, 2006b) it was shown that diversity maintenance based on crowding distance does not estimate crowding properly when the number of objectives is more than two. It should be noted that several multi-objective DE approaches mentioned in Section Differential Evolution for Multiple Objectives and

Figure 5. Results for the ZDT problems using GDE3

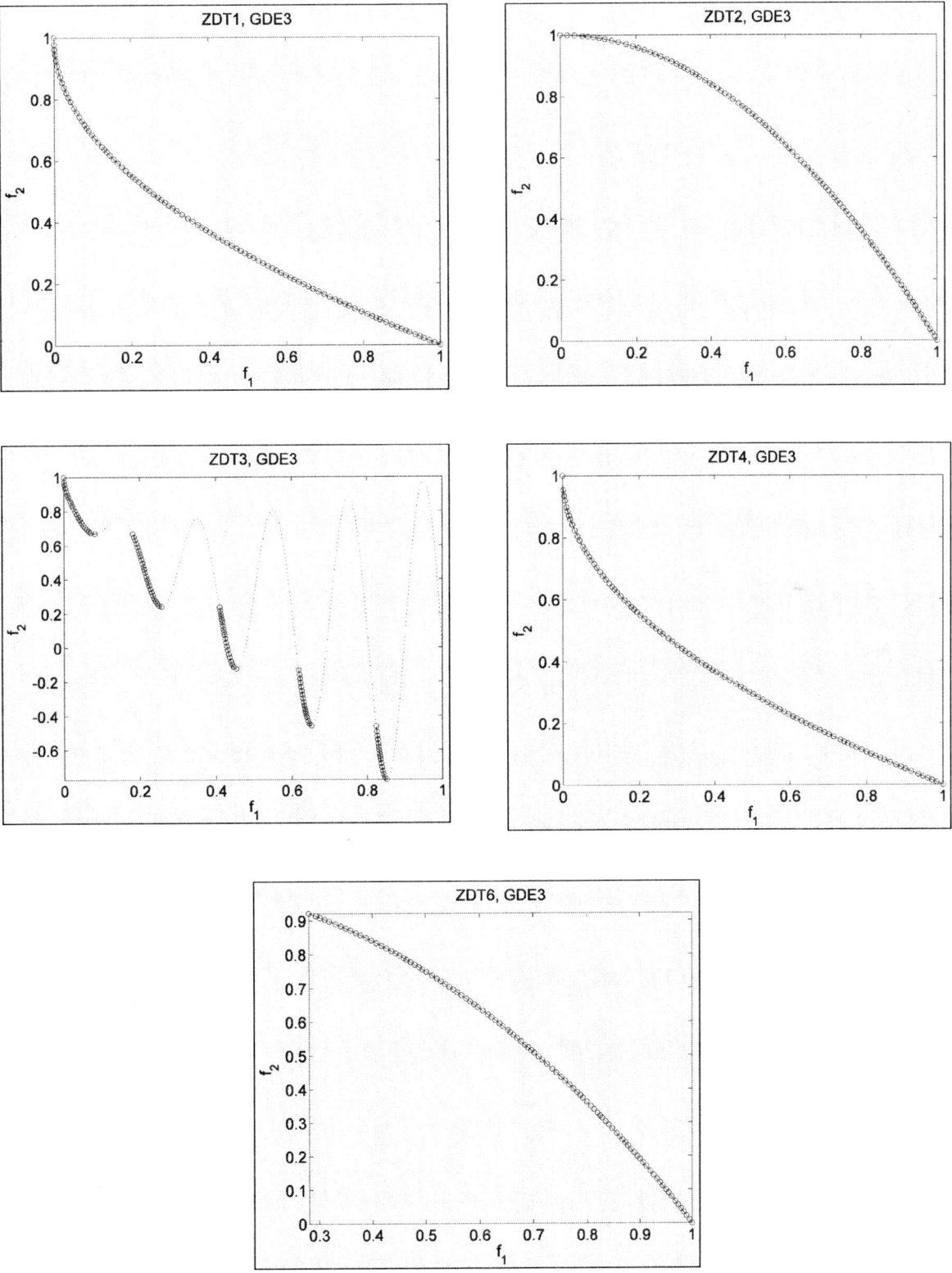

Figure 6. Results for the DTLZ problems using GDE3

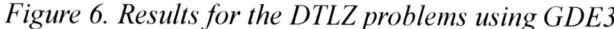

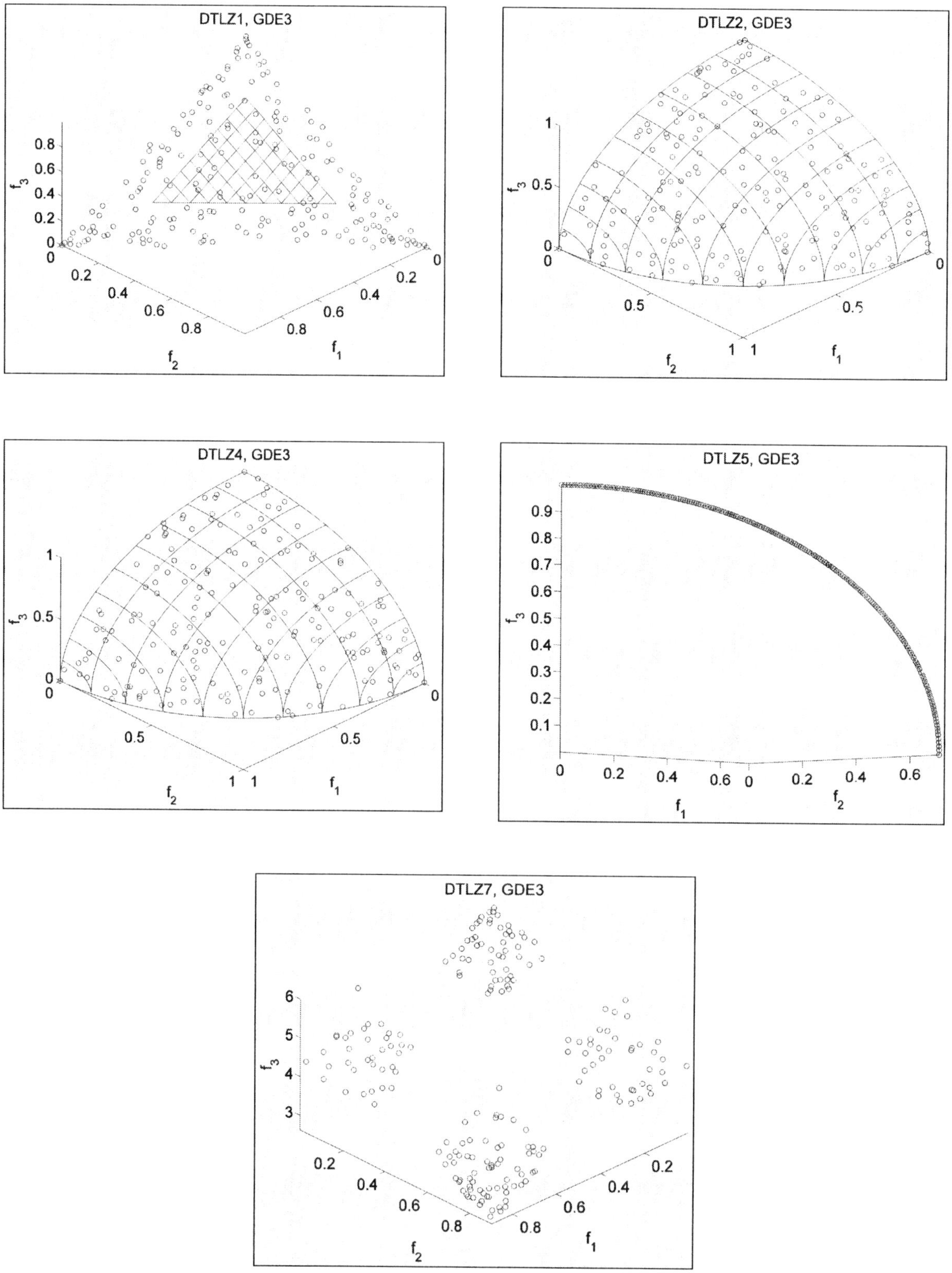

Figure 7. Results for the ZDT problems using GDE3 with the 2-NN diversity maintenance technique

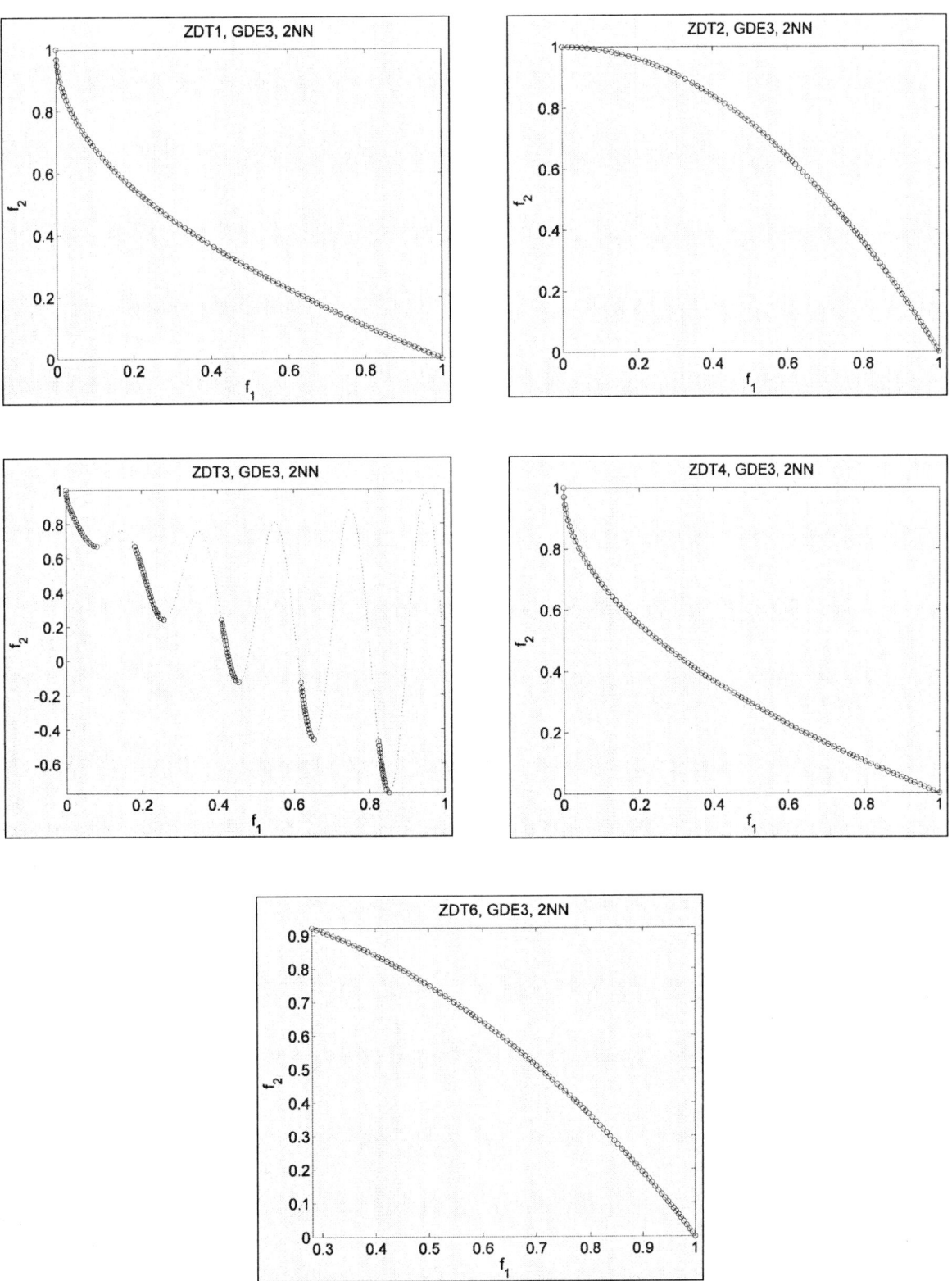

Figure 8. Results for the DTLZ problems using GDE3 with the 2-NN diversity maintenance technique

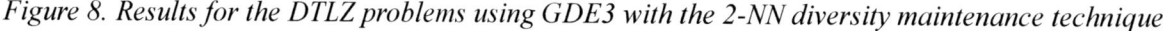

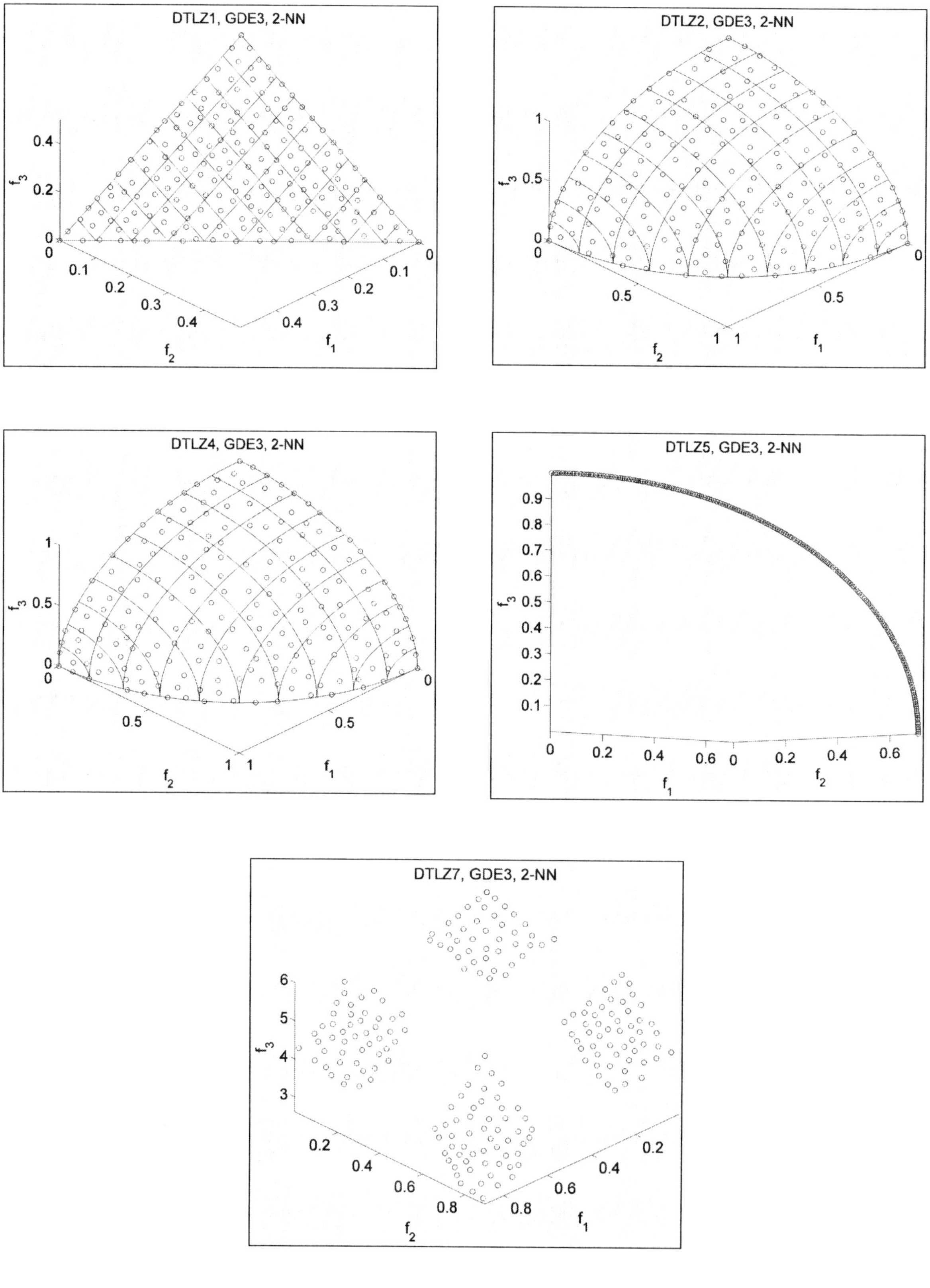

Constraints use crowding distance and therefore do not provide good diversity when the number of objectives is three or more.

Diversity Maintenance for Many-Objective Problems

As noted in the previous section, the original diversity maintenance technique in GDE3 does not provide good diversity in many-objective cases. Therefore, a new efficient diversity maintenance technique was needed. A pruning method intended to be effective and relatively fast at the same time was proposed by Kukkonen and Deb (2006a). The basic idea of the method is to eliminate the most crowded members of a nondominated set one by one, and update the crowding information of the remaining members after each removal. Crowding estimation was done based on the nearest neighbors of solution candidates, and the nearest neighbors were found using an efficient search method. Two crowding estimation techniques were proposed: one that always uses two nearest neighbors for the crowding estimation (2-NN) and one that uses as many neighbors as there are objectives (M-NN). The efficient exact k-NN search technique used was the *equal-average nearest neighbor search (ENNS) algorithm* (Guan & Kamel, 1992; Ra & Kim, 1993). ENNS projects data to a projection axis and uses an inequality between the projected values and corresponding Euclidean distance to reduce the number of actual distance calculations. The quickness of the proposed method was further improved by using a priority queue to store elements. Details of the algorithm can be found from (Kukkonen & Deb, 2006a).

The diversity maintenance technique used in GDE3 can be directly replaced with the technique intended for many-objective problems. A final population for the ZDT and DTLZ problems is shown in Figure 7 and Figure 8. Now, distribution can be observed to be near optimal for all the problems.

Study of Control Parameter Values for GDE

The effect of control parameters CR and F has been studied with GDE1 and GDE3 (Kukkonen & Lampinen, 2005a; Kukkonen & Lampinen, 2006b). Different control parameter values were tested using common bi-objective test problems and performance metrics measuring the convergence and diversity of solutions. It was interesting to know how the control parameter values affect to results when there is no diversity maintenance (Kukkonen & Lampinen, 2005a) and when diversity maintenance is used (Kukkonen & Lampinen, 2006b).

According to experimental results, GDE3 provides a better distribution than GDE1. GDE3 is also able to produce a good Pareto-front approximation with a larger amount of points, when the control parameter values are varied. Therefore, GDE3 seems to be more robust in terms of the control parameter values selection, and GDE3 provides better results than GDE1 in general.

Based on the empirical results, suitable control parameter value ranges for multi-objective optimization are the same as for single-objective optimization, that is, $CR \in [0,1]$ and $F \in (0,1+]$. The results also proposed that a larger F value than usually used in the case of single-objective optimization, does not give any extra benefit in the case of multi-objective optimization. It seems that in some cases it is better to use a smaller CR value to prevent the population from converging to a single point of the Pareto-front.

From the results in (Kukkonen & Lampinen, 2005a; Kukkonen & Lampinen, 2006b), a nonlinear relationship between the CR and F values was observed, that is, a larger F value can be used with a small CR value than with a large CR value, and this relationship is nonlinear. An

Figure 9. Curves c = 1.0 and c = 1.5 for NP = 100 in the CR-F control parameter space

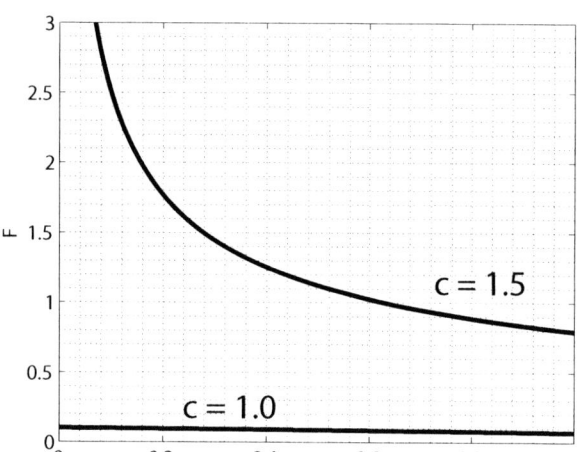
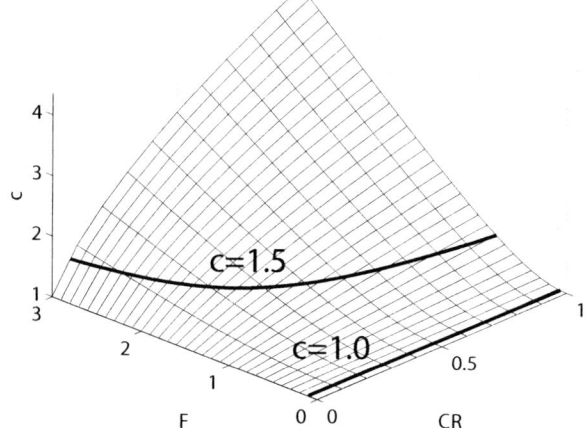

explanation for this was found from a theory for the single-objective DE algorithm. A formula for the relationship between the control parameters of DE and the evolution/development of the population variance has been conducted by Zaharie (2002). The change in the standard deviation (i.e., square root of variance) of the population between successive generations due to the crossover and mutation operations is denoted with c and its value is calculated as:

$$c = \sqrt{2F^2 CR - 2CR/NP + CR^2/NP + 1}$$

When $c < 1$, the crossover and mutation operations decrease the population variance. When $c = 1$, the variance do not change, and when $c > 1$, the variance increases. Since the selection operation of an EA usually decreases the population variance, $c > 1$ is recommended to prevent too high convergence rate and a poor search coverage, which typically results in a premature convergence. On the other hand, if c is too large, the search process proceeds reliably, but too slowly. In practice it has been observed that $c < 1.5$ is suitable upper limitation for most of the cases (Price et al., 2005).

When the size of the population is relatively large (e.g., $NP > 50$), the value of c depends mainly on the values of CR and F. Curves $c = 1.0$ and $c = 1.5$ for $NP = 100$ are shown in Figure 9.

Observations in (Kukkonen & Lampinen, 2005a; Kukkonen & Lampinen, 2006b) proposed that the theory for the population variance between successive generations is applicable also in the case of multi-objective DE and provides

Figure 10. The spring design problem solved with GDE1, GDE2, and GDE3

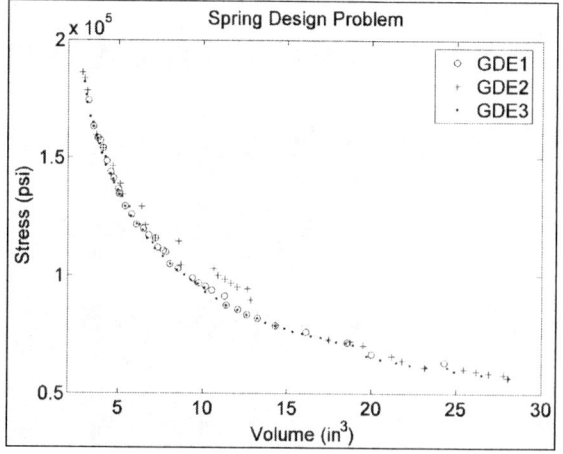

a way to select good control parameter value combinations. This is natural, since single-objective optimization can be seen as a special case of multi-objective optimization, and a large c means a slow but reliable search while a small c means opposite. According to results, it is advisable to select values for CR and F satisfying the condition $1.0 < c < 1.5$.

The observed results were good with small CR and F values that also means a low c value (close to 1.0). One reason for the good performance with small control parameter values is that the test problems had conflicting objectives, which reduced overall selection pressure and prevented the premature convergence. Another reason is that most of the problems had relatively easy objective functions to solve, leading to a faster convergence with a small F, while a bigger F might be needed for harder functions with several local optima and/or if NP is smaller.

Constrained Optimization with the GDE Versions

Above the performance of GDE versions has been described only with unconstrained problems. However, the GDE versions include in their definition also constraint handling approach, which is identical in all the versions. This constraint handling approach was first introduced and evaluated for single-objective optimization with DE by Lampinen (2002) and later extended into multi-objective optimization with the GDE versions.

In Kukkonen and Lampinen (2004d) a small set of mechanical design problems including several constraints was solved using GDE1. Surprisingly good estimations of the Pareto-front were obtained. The extend of approximation sets was measured and found comparable to results with NSGA-II.

GDE1 has been used also to solve a given set of constrained single-objective optimization problems in the CEC 2006 Special Session on Constrained Real-Parameter Optimization (Kukkonen & Lampinen, 2006a). GDE1 was able to solve almost all the problems in a given maximum number of solution candidate evaluations. A better solution than previously known was found for some problems. It was also demonstrated that GDE actually needs lower number of function evaluations than usually required.

In (Kukkonen & Lampinen, 2005b) the ability of GDE versions to handle several constraints and different types of decision variables has been demonstrated using a bi-objective spring design problem (Deb, 2001, pp. 453-455). GDE versions use real-coded variables as genotypes, which are converted to corresponding phenotypes before evaluation of the objective and constraint functions (Price et al., 2005).

In the spring design problem, the problem is to design a helical compression spring, which has a minimum volume and minimal stress. Objective functions are nonlinear and the problem has three variables: the number of spring coils x_1 (integer), the wire diameter x_2 (discrete having 42 non-equispaced values), and the mean coil diameter x_3 (real). Besides the boundary constraints, the

Table 1. Number of needed constraint (g) and objective (f) function evaluations by GDE1, GDE2, and GDE3 for the spring design problem

	g_1	g_2	g_3	g_4	g_5	g_6	g_7	g_8	f_1	f_2
GDE1	10100	8665	8571	8389	7764	7764	4669	4143	4136	2045
GDE2	10100	8304	8210	8050	7562	7562	5297	4792	4777	4777
GDE3	10100	8974	8905	8763	8351	8350	4744	4275	4261	4261

problem has eight inequality constraint functions from which most are nonlinear. Formal description of the problem is (Deb, Pratap, & Moitra, 2000), (see Box 6).

The parameters used are as follows, (see Box 7).

Nondominated points extracted from the final population of the different GDE versions after a single run are shown in Figure 10. The size of the population and the number of generations were 100. The control parameter values for the GDE versions were $CR = 0.5$ and $F = 0.3$, and the number of function evaluations needed for the GDE versions are reported in Table 1. It can be observed that the constraint handling approach used in the GDE versions reduce the actual number of function evaluations.

The performance of GDE3 is compared with NSGA-II in Figure 11 – Figure 14 using a set of common bi-objective test problems given in (Deb, 2001, pp. 362-367). The constraint handling technique in NSGA-II is the same as in GDE3 except in the case of infeasible solution candidates, NSGA-II makes selection based on sums

Box 6.

$$\begin{aligned}
\text{Minimize} \quad & f_1(\vec{x}) = 0.25\pi^2 x_2^2 x_3 (x_1 + 2) \\
\text{Minimize} \quad & f_2(\vec{x}) = \frac{8KP_{max} x_3}{\pi x_2^3} \\
\text{Subject to} \quad & g_1(\vec{x}) = l_{max} - \frac{P_{max}}{k} - 1.05(x_1 + 2)x_2 \geq 0 \\
& g_2(\vec{x}) = x_2 - d_{min} \geq 0 \\
& g_3(\vec{x}) = D_{max} - (x_2 + x_3) \geq 0 \\
& g_4(\vec{x}) = C - 3 \geq 0 \\
& g_5(\vec{x}) = \delta_{pm} - \delta_p \geq 0 \\
& g_6(\vec{x}) = \frac{P_{max} - P}{k} - \delta_w \geq 0 \\
& g_7(\vec{x}) = S - \frac{8KP_{max} x_3}{\pi x_2^3} \geq 0 \\
& g_8(\vec{x}) = V_{max} - 0.25\pi^2 x_2^2 x_3 (x_1 + 2) \geq 0 \\
& x_1 \text{ is integer, } x_2 \text{ is discrete, and } x_3 \text{ is continuous.}
\end{aligned}$$

Box 7.

$$K = \frac{4C-1}{4C-4} + \frac{0.615 x_2}{x_3}, \quad P = 300 \text{ lb}, \quad D_{max} = 3 \text{ in}, \quad k = \frac{G x_2^4}{8 x_1 x_3^3},$$

$$P_{max} = 1000 \text{ lb}, \quad \delta_w = 1.25 \text{ in}, \quad \delta_p = \frac{P}{k}, \quad l_{max} = 14 \text{ in},$$

$$\delta_{pm} = 6 \text{ in}, \quad S = 189 \text{ kpsi}, \quad d_{min} = 0.12 \text{ in}, \quad C = D/d,$$

$$G = 11500000, \quad V_{max} = 30 \text{ in}^3.$$

of constraint violations whereas GDE3 makes selection based on Pareto-dominance relations in the space of constraint violations.

The first problem is known as BNH and it has two variables and constraints. Results for this problem are shown in Figure 11. The population size of 100 and 150 generations were used. The control parameter values for GDE3 were $CR = 0.4$ and $F = 0.3$, and for NSGA-II $p_c = 0.9$, $p_m = 1/D$, $\eta_c = 10$, and $\eta_m = 20$ (the control parameter values of NSGA-II for the problems were obtained with the program code from the Web site http://www.iitk.ac.in/kangal/codes.shtml). The second problem, OSY, has six variables and constraints. Results for this problem are shown in Figure 12. The population size of 200 and 250 generations were used. The control parameter values for GDE3 were $CR = 0.4$ and $F = 0.3$, and for NSGA-II $p_c = 0.9$, $p_m = 1/D$, $\eta_c = 5$, and $\eta_m = 5$. The third problem, SRN, has two variables and constraints. Results for this

Figure 11. Solutions for BNH using GDE3 and NSGA-II

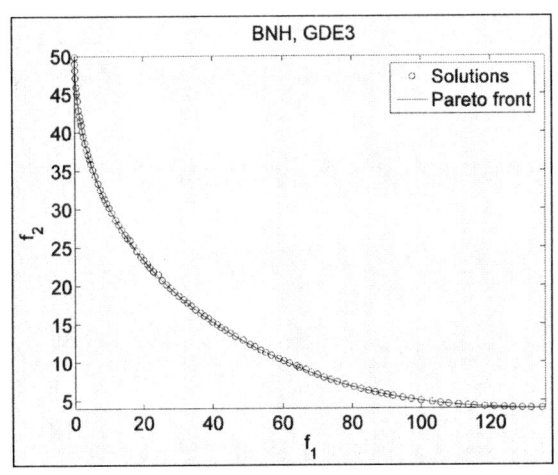
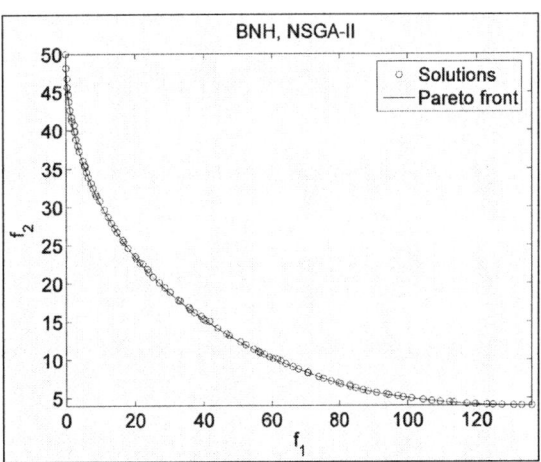

Figure 12. Solutions for OSY using GDE3 and NSGA-II

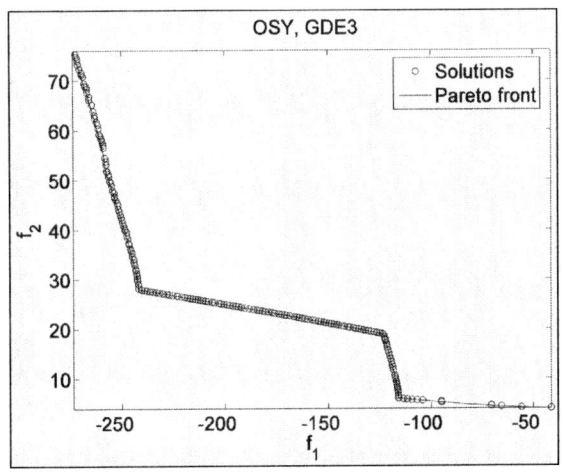
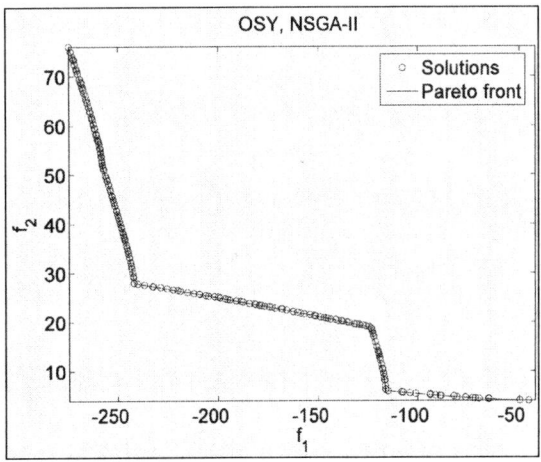

problem are shown in Figure 13. The population size of 100 and 100 generations were used. The control parameter values for GDE3 were $CR = 0.4$ and $F = 0.3$, and for NSGA-II $p_c = 0.9$, $p_m = 1/D$, $\eta_c = 5$, and $\eta_m = 5$. The last problem, TNK, also has two variables and constraints. Results for this problem are shown in Figure 14. The population size of 200 and 300 generations were used. The control parameter values for GDE3 were $CR = 0.4$ and $F = 0.3$, and for NSGA-II $p_c = 0.9$, $p_m = 1/D$, $\eta_c = 5$, and $\eta_m = 5$. From the results, a similar performance between the methods can be observed. GDE3 provides a better diversity in general but NSGA-II is slightly better in the case of OSY.

Figure 13. Solutions for SRN using GDE3 and NSGA-II

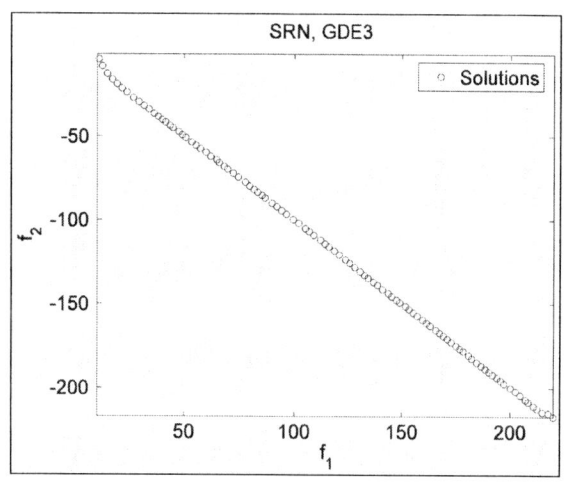
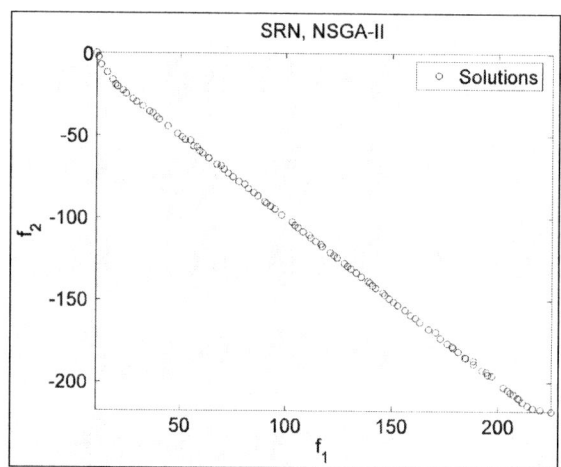

Figure 14. Solutions for TNK using GDE3 and NSGA-II

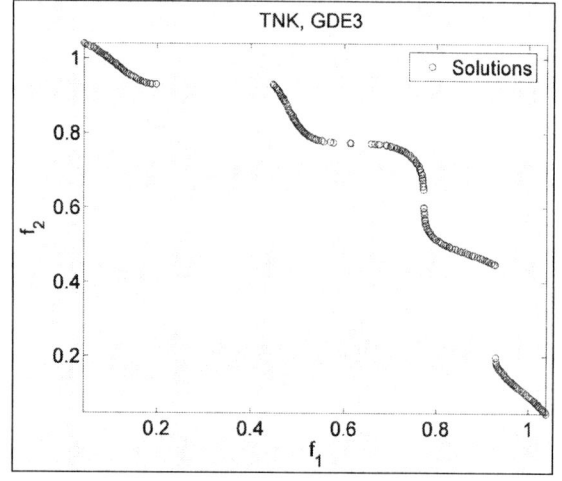
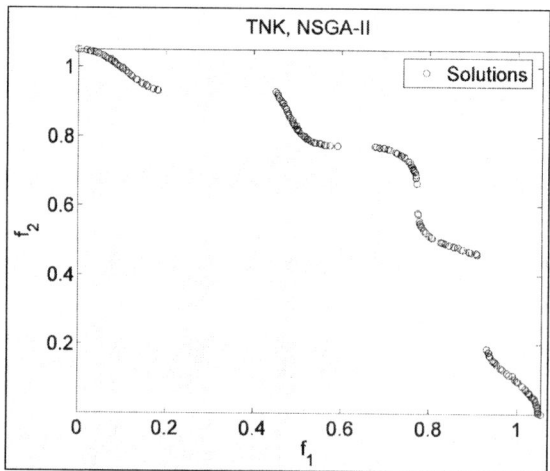

The GDE versions have been successfully applied also for more challenging constrained multi-objective optimization problems such as a scaling filter design (Kukkonen, Sampo, & Lampinen, 2004), a multi-objective scheduling for NASA's future deep space network array (Johnston, 2006), and a molecular sequence alignment problem (Kukkonen, Jangam, & Chakraborti, 2007). The last problem is interesting because it is a nonlinear problem with thousands of integer variables.

FUTURE RESEARCH DIRECTIONS

Currently GDE is a potential general purpose optimizer for problems with constraints and relatively low (e.g., 1-5) number of objectives. However, when the number of objectives increases, the speed of the search will rapidly slow down. The reason for this is that GDE (as many other MOEAs) applies the Pareto-dominance relation in its selection. When the number of objectives increases, the proportion of non-dominating members in the population will also increase rapidly and the selection based on Pareto-dominance is not able to sort members. Often already ten objectives are too much and cause stagnation of the search. This phenomenon is referred as a *curse of dimensionality* (Deb & Saxena, 2006). Increase of objectives cause also other problems, that is, visualization of the obtained optimization result becomes harder when the number of objectives increases. Probably for these reasons the most of the research has dealt with problems, which have only a couple of objectives (Coello Coello, Van Veldhuizen, & Lamont, 2002) although there are many problems with more objectives. It seems that solving problems with a large number of objectives is one direction of future research.

In the control parameter study, a further investigation of the theory about the development of the population variance with multi-objective problems is necessary. Also, extending studies for problems with more than two objectives remains to be studied. Special cases, as multi-objective problems without conflicting objectives and single-objective problems transformed into multi-objective forms, might be interesting to investigate.

There exists already some research on an automatic control parameter adaptation (Abbass, 2002; Huang, Qin, & Suganthan, 2006; Zaharie, 2003a). This is an interesting and important topic of research in order to increase the usability of DE.

In general, the intention of authors is to continue the development of GDE towards a widely applicable, effective, and efficient general purpose optimizer. This work will probably include parallelization the algorithm and extending it to use metamodels (Jin, 2005) to approximate functions.

CONCLUSION

Development history of Generalized Differential Evolution (GDE) has been described with a brief review of other multi-objective approaches based on Differential Evolution (DE). GDE is a real-coded general purpose EA extended from DE to handle multiple objectives and constraints. Each GDE version falls back to DE in the case of an unconstrained single-objective problem. DE has been found as an effective and widely applicable evolutionary search "engine" because of its simplicity, linear scalability, and ability for a rotational invariant search.

The first version, GDE1, extends DE for constrained multi-objective optimization in a simple way and was obtained by modifying the selection rule of basic DE. The basic idea in the selection rule is that the trial vector is selected to replace the old vector in the next generation if the trial vector weakly constraint-dominates the old vector. There is neither explicit nondominated sorting during the optimization process nor any mechanism for maintaining diversity. Also, there is no extra repository for nondominated vectors. Still, GDE1 has been observed to provide surprisingly good results but has been found rather sensitive to the selection of the control parameter values.

The second version, GDE2, makes a decision based on crowding when the trial and the old vector are feasible and nondominating each other in the objective function space. This improves the extent and distribution of an obtained set of solutions but slows down the convergence of the population because it favors isolated solutions far from the Pareto-front until all the solutions are converged near the Pareto-front. Also this version has been observed to be rather sensitive to the selection of the control parameters values.

The third and latest enumerated version is GDE3. Besides the selection, another part of basic DE has also been modified. Now, in the case of feasible and nondominating solutions, both vectors are saved for the population of the next generation. Before starting the next generation, the size of the population is reduced using nondominated sorting and pruning based on diversity preservation. The diversity maintenance technique is an improvement from the technique used in NSGA-II but it has been noticed to provide a good diversity only in the case of two objectives because of properties of the crowding distance metric. Therefore, later on GDE3 has been further developed with the diversity maintenance technique designed for many-objective problems. The latest version of GDE3 provides better distribution than the earlier GDE versions, and it seems to be also more robust in terms of the selection of the control parameter values.

The experimental results demonstrate how the performance of the method has improved over the development steps. The GDE versions have performed well with a number of problems having a different number of objectives and constraints. However, some limitations exist. Because of the Pareto-dominance relation used in the GDE versions (as well as in many other MOEAs), the search slows down when the number of objectives increases.

The influence of the control parameters has been also discussed. It has been found that suitable control parameter ranges for multi-objective optimization are the same as for single-objective optimization, i.e., $CR \in [0,1]$ and $F \in (0,1 +]$. It also seems that in some cases it is better to use a smaller CR value to prevent the population from converging to a single point of the Pareto-front. The nonlinear relationship between CR and F was observed according to the theory of basic single-objective DE, concerning the relationship between the control parameters and the development in the standard deviation of the population. It is advisable to select the values for CR and F satisfying the condition $1.0 < c < 1.5$, where c denotes the change of the population variance between successive generations due to the crossover and mutation operations.

In the end, it can be concluded that GDE3 with the diversity maintenance technique for many-objective problems is a good choice for constrained multi-objective optimization with different types of variables and a few objectives.

REFERENCES

Abbass, H. A. (2002). The self-adaptive Pareto differential evolution algorithm. In *Proceedings of the 2002 Congress on Evolutionary Computation (CEC 2002)* (pp. 831-836). Honolulu, HI: IEEE Service Center.

Abbass, H. A. & Sarker, R. (2002). The Pareto differential evolution algorithm. *International Journal on Artificial Intelligence Tools, 11*(4), 531-552.

Abbass, H. A., Sarker, R., & Newton, C. (2001). PDE: A Pareto-frontier differential evolution approach for multi-objective optimization problems.

In *Proceedings of the 2001 Congress on Evolutionary Computation (CEC 2001)* (pp. 971-978). Seoul, South Korea: IEEE Service Center.

Babu, B. V. & Jehan, M. M. L. (2003). Differential evolution for multi-objective optimization. In *Proceedings of the 2003 Congress on Evolutionary Computation (CEC 2003)* (pp. 2696-2703), Canberra, Australia: IEEE Service Center.

Bergey, P. K. (1999). An agent enhanced intelligent spreadsheet solver for multi-criteria decision making. In *Proceedings of the Fifth Americas Conference on Information Systems (AMCIS 1999)* (pp. 966-968), Milwaukee, WI.

Cai, Z., Gong, W., & Huang, Y. (2007). A novel differential evolution algorithm based on ε-domination and orthogonal design method for multi-objective optimization. In *Proceedings of the 4th International Congress on Evolutionary Multi-Criterion Optimization (EMO 2007)* (pp. 286-301). Matsushima, Japan: Springer.

Chang, C. S. & Xu, D. Y. (2000). Differential evolution based tuning of fuzzy automatic train operation for mass rapid transit system. *IEE Proceedings on Electric Power Applications, 147*(3), 206-212.

Chang, C. S., Xu, D. Y., & Quek, H. B. (1999). Pareto-optimal set based multi-objective tuning of fuzzy automatic train operation for mass transit system. *IEE Proceedings on Electric Power Applications,* 146(5), 577-583.

Chang, T.-T. & Chang, H.-C. (1998). Application of differential evolution to passive shunt harmonic filter planning. In *8th International Conference on Harmonics and Quality of Power* (pp. 149-153). Athens, Greece.

Coello Coello, C. A., Van Veldhuizen, D. A., & Lamont, G. B. (2002). *Evolutionary algorithms for solving multi-objective problems.* New York: Kluwer Academic.

Deb, K. (2000). An efficient constraint handling method for genetic algorithms. *Computer Methods in Applied Mechanics and Engineering, 186*(2-3), 311-338.

Deb, K. (2001). *Multi-objective optimization using evolutionary algorithms.* Chichester, England: John Wiley & Sons.

Deb, K., Pratap, A., Agarwal, S., & Meyarivan, T. (2002). A fast and elitist multi-objective genetic algorithm: NSGA-II. *IEEE Transactions on Evolutionary Computation, 6*(2), 182-197.

Deb, K., Pratap, A., & Moitra, S. (2000). Mechanical component design for multiple objectives using elitist non-dominated sorting GA. In *Proceedings of the Parallel Problem Solving from Nature VI (PPSN-VI)* (pp. 859-868), Paris, France: Springer.

Deb, K. & Saxena, D. K. (2006). Searching for Pareto-optimal solutions through dimensionality reduction for certain large-dimensional multi-objective optimization problems. In *Proceedings of the 2006 Congress on Evolutionary Computation (CEC 2006)* (pp. 3353-3360), Vancouver, BC, Canada: IEEE Service Center.

Deb, K., Thiele, L., Laumanns, M., & Zitzler, E. (2005). Scalable test problems for evolutionary multi-objective optimization. *Evolutionary multi-objective optimization* (pp. 105-145). London: Springer-Verlag.

Feoktistov, V. & Janaqi, S. (2004). New strategies in differential evolution. In *Proceedings of the 6th International Conference on Adaptive Computing in Design and Manufacture (ACDM 2004)* (pp. 335-346), Bristol, United Kingdom: Springer.

Fonseca, C. M. & Fleming, P. J. (1998). Multi-objective optimization and multiple constraint handling with evolutionary algorithms-Part I: A unified formulation. *IEEE Transactions on Systems, Man, and Cybernetics-Part A: Systems and Humans, 28*(1), 26-37.

Goldberg, D. E. (1989). *Genetic algorithms in search, optimization & machine learning.* Addison-Wesley.

Guan, L. & Kamel, M. (1992). Equal-average hyperplane portioning method for vector quantization of image data. *Pattern Recognition Letters, 13*(10), 693-699.

Hansen, N. & Ostermeier, A. (1996). Adapting arbitrary normal mutation distributions in evolutionary strategies: the covariance matrix adaptation. In *Proceedings of the 1996 IEEE International Conference on Evolutionary Computation (ICEC '96)* (pp. 312-317), Nayoya, Japan: IEEE Service Center.

Hernández-Diaz, A. G., Santana-Quintero, L. V., Coello Coello, C. A., Caballero, R., & Molina, J. (2006). A new proposal for multi-objective optimization using Differential Evolution and rough sets theory. In *Proceedings of the Genetic and Evolutionary Computation Conference (GECCO 2006)* (pp. 675-682). Seattle, WA: ACM Press.

Huang, V. L., Qin, A. K., & Suganthan, P. N. (2006). Self-adaptive differential evolution algorithm for constrained real-parameter optimization. In *Proceedings of the 2006 Congress on Evolutionary Computation (CEC 2006)* (pp. 324-331). Vancouver, BC, Canada: IEEE Service Center.

Iorio, A. & Li, X. (2004). Solving rotated multi-objective optimization problems using differential evolution. In *Proceedings of the 17th Australian Joint Conference on Artificial Intelligence (AI 2004)* (pp. 861-872). Cairns, Australia.

Iorio, A. & Li, X. (2006). Incorporating directional information within a differential evolution for multi-objective optimization. In *Proceedings of the Genetic and Evolutionary Computing Conference (GECCO 2006)* (pp. 691-697). Seattle, WA: ACM Press.

Jensen, M. T. (2003). Reducing the run-time complexity of multi-objective EAs: the NSGA-II and other algorithms. *IEEE Transactions on Evolutionary Computation, 7*(5), 503-515.

Jin, Y. (2005). A comprehensive survey of fitness approximation in evolutionary computation. *Soft Computing, 9*(1), 3-12.

Johnston, M. D. (2006). Multi-objective scheduling for NASA's future deep space network array. In *Proceedings of the 5th International Workshop on Planning and Scheduling for Space (IWPSS 2006)* (pp. 27-35). Baltimore, MD.

Kukkonen, S. & Deb, K. (2006a). A fast and effective method for pruning of non-dominated solutions in many-objective problems. In *Proceedings of the 9th International Conference on Parallel Problem Solving from Nature (PPSN IX)* (pp. 553-562). Reykjavik, Iceland: Springer.

Kukkonen, S. & Deb, K. (2006b). Improved pruning of non-dominated solutions based on crowding distance for bi-objective optimization problems. In *Proceedings of the 2006 Congress on Evolutionary Computation (CEC 2006)* (pp. 3995-4002). Vancouver, BC, Canada: IEEE Service Center.

Kukkonen, S., Jangam, S. R., & Chakraborti, N. (2007). Solving the molecular sequence alignment problem with generalized differential evolution 3 (GDE3). In *Proceedings of the 2007 IEEE Symposium on Computational Intelligence in Multi-Criteria Decision-Making (MCDM 2007)* (pp. 302-309). Honolulu, HI: IEEE Service Center.

Kukkonen, S. & Lampinen, J. (2004a). Comparison of generalized differential evolution algorithm to other multi-objective evolutionary algorithms. In *Proceedings of the 4th European Congress on Computational Methods in Applied Sciences and Engineering (ECCOMAS 2004).* Jyväskylä, Finland.

Kukkonen, S. & Lampinen, J. (2004b). A differential evolution algorithm for constrained multi-objective optimization: Initial assessment.

In *Proceedings of the IASTED International Conference on Artificial Intelligence and Applications (AIA 2004)* (pp. 96-102). Innsbruck, Austria: ACTA Press.

Kukkonen, S. & Lampinen, J. (2004c). An extension of generalized differential evolution for multi-objective optimization with constraints. In *Proceedings of the 8th International Conference on Parallel Problem Solving from Nature (PPSN VIII)* (pp. 752-761). Birmingham, England: Springer.

Kukkonen, S. & Lampinen, J. (2004d). Mechanical component design for multiple objectives using generalized differential evolution. In *Proceedings of the 6th International Conference on Adaptive Computing in Design and Manufacture (ACDM 2004)* (pp. 261-272). Bristol, United Kingdom: Springer.

Kukkonen, S. & Lampinen, J. (2005a). An empirical study of control parameters for generalized differential evolution. In *Proceedings of the Sixth Conference on Evolutionary and Deterministic Methods for Design, Optimization and Control with Applications to Industrial and Societal Problems (EUROGEN 2005)*. Munich, Germany.

Kukkonen, S. & Lampinen, J. (2005b). GDE3: The third evolution step of generalized differential evolution. In *Proceedings of the 2005 Congress on Evolutionary Computation (CEC 2005)* (pp. 443-450). Edinburgh, Scotland: IEEE Service Center.

Kukkonen, S. & Lampinen, J. (2006a). Constrained real-parameter optimization with generalized differential evolution. In *Proceedings of the 2006 Congress on Evolutionary Computation (CEC 2006)* (pp. 911-918). Vancouver, BC, Canada: IEEE Service Center.

Kukkonen, S. & Lampinen, J. (2006b). An empirical study of control parameters for the third version of generalized differential evolution (GDE3). In *Proceedings of the 2006 Congress on Evolutionary Computation (CEC 2006)* (pp. 7355-7362). Vancouver, BC, Canada: IEEE Service Center.

Kukkonen, S., Sampo, J., & Lampinen, J. (2004). Applying generalized differential evolution for scaling filter design. In *Proceedings of Mendel 2004, 10th International Conference on Soft Computing* (pp. 28-33). Brno, Czech Republic.

Lampinen, J. (2001). *DE's selection rule for multi-objective optimization* (Tech. Rep.). Lappeenranta University of Technology, Department of Information Technology.

Lampinen, J. (2002). A constraint handling approach for the differential evolution algorithm. In *Proceedings of the 2002 Congress on Evolutionary Computation (CEC 2002)* (pp. 1468-1473). Honolulu, HI: IEEE Service Center.

Lampinen, J. & Zelinka, I. (1999). Mechanical engineering design optimization by Differential Evolution. *New ideas in optimization* (pp. 128-146). London: McGraw-Hill.

Li, H. & Zhang, Q. (2006). A multi-objective differential evolution based on decomposition for multi-objective optimization with variable linkages. In *Proceedings of the 9th International Conference on Parallel Problem Solving from Nature (PPSN IX)* (pp. 583-592). Reykjavik, Iceland: Springer.

Lin, Y.-C., Hwang, K.-S., & Wang, F.-S. (2002). Hybrid differential evolution with multiplier updating method for nonlinear constrained optimization problems. In *Proceedings of the 2002 Congress on Evolutionary Computation (CEC 2002)* (pp. 872-877). Honolulu, HI: IEEE Service Center.

Madavan, N. K. (2002). Multi-objective optimization using a Pareto differential evolution approach. In *Proceedings of the 2002 Congress on Evolutionary Computation (CEC 2002)* (pp. 1145-1150). Honolulu, HI: IEEE Service Center.

Mezura-Montes, E., Coello Coello, C. A., & Tun-Morales, E. I. (2004). Simple feasibility rules and differential evolution for constrained optimization. In *Proceedings of the 3rd Mexican International Conference on Artificial Intelligence (MICAI 2004)* (pp. 707-716). Mexico City, Mexico.

Miettinen, K. (1998). *Nonlinear multiobjective optimization*. Boston: Kluwer Academic Publishers.

Pareto, V. (1896). *Cours d'economie politique*. Geneve: Libraire Droz.

Parsopoulos, K. E., Tasoulis, D. K., Pavlidis, N. G., Plagianakos, V. P., & Vrahatis, M. N. (2004). Vector evaluated differential evolution for multi-objective optimization. In *Proceedings of the 2004 Congress on Evolutionary Computation (CEC 2004)* (pp. 204-211). Portland, OR: IEEE Service Center.

Price, K. & Storn, R. (1996). Minimizing the real functions of the ICEC'96 contest by differential evolution. In *Proceedings of the 1996 IEEE International Conference on Evolutionary Computation (ICEC '96)* (pp. 842-844). Nagoya, Japan: IEEE Service Center.

Price, K. V. (1999). An introduction to differential evolution. *New ideas in optimization* (pp. 79-108). London: McGraw-Hill.

Price, K. V., Storn, R. M., & Lampinen, J. A. (2005). *Differential evolution: A practical approach to global optimization*. Berlin: Springer-Verlag.

Ra, S.-W. & Kim, J.-K. (1993). A fast mean-distance-ordered partial codebook search algorithm for image vector quantization. *IEEE Transactions on Circuits and Systems-II, 40*(9), 576-579.

Robič, T. & Filipič, B. (2005). DEMO: Differential evolution for multi-objective optimization. In *Proceedings of the 3rd International Conference on Evolutionary Multi-Criterion Optimization (EMO 2005)* (pp. 520-533). Guanajuato, Mexico: Springer.

Rönkkönen, J., Kukkonen, S., & Lampinen, J. (2005a). A comparison of differential evolution and generalized generation gap model. *Journal of Advanced Computational Intelligence and Intelligent Informatics, 9*(5), 549-555.

Rönkkönen, J., Kukkonen, S., & Price, K. V. (2005b). Real-parameter optimization with differential evolution. In *Proceedings of the 2005 Congress on Evolutionary Computation (CEC 2005)* (pp. 506-513). Edinburgh, Scotland: IEEE Service Center.

Storn, R. (1999). System design by constraint adaptation and Differential Evolution. *IEEE Transactions on Evolutionary Computation, 3*(1), 22-34.

Storn, R. & Price, K. V. (1995). *Differential evolution—A simple and efficient adaptive scheme for global optimization over continuous spaces* (Tech. Rep.). ICSI, University of California, Berkeley.

Tušar, T. & Filipič, B. (2007). Differential evolution versus genetic algorithms in multi-objective optimization. In *Proceedings of the 4th International Conference on Evolutionary Multi-Criterion Optimization (EMO 2007)* (pp. 257-271). Matsushima, Japan: Springer.

Wang, F.-S. & Chiou, J.-P. (1997). Differential evolution for dynamic optimization of differential-algebraic systems. In *Proceedings of the 1997 IEEE International Conference on Evolutionary Computation (ICEC 1997)* (pp. 531-536). Indianapolis, IN: IEEE Service Center.

Wang, F.-S. & Sheu, J.-W. (2000). Multi-objective parameter estimation problems of fermentation processes using a high ethanol tolerance yeast. *Chemical Engineering Science, 55*(18), 3685-3695.

Xue, F., Sanderson, A. C., & Graves, R. J. (2003). Pareto-based multi-objective differential evolution. In *Proceedings of the 2003 Congress on Evolutionary Computation (CEC 2003)* (pp. 862-869). Canberra, Australia: IEEE Service Center.

Zaharie, D. (2002). Critical values for the control parameters of differential evolution algorithms. In *Proceedings of Mendel 2002, 8th International Conference on Soft Computing* (pp. 62-67). Brno, Czech Republic.

Zaharie, D. (2003a). Control of population diversity and adaptation in differential evolution algorithms. In *Proceedings of Mendel 2003, 9th International Conference on Soft Computing* (pp. 41-46). Brno, Czech Republic.

Zaharie, D. (2003b). Multi-objective optimization with adaptive Pareto differential evolution. In *Proceedings of Symposium on Intelligent Systems and Applications (SIA 2003)*. Iasi, Romania.

Zielinski, K. & Laur, R. (2007). Variants of differential evolution for multi-objective optimization. In *Proceedings of the 2007 Symposium on Computational Intelligence in Multi-Criteria Decision-Making (MCDM 2007)* (pp. 91-98). Honolulu, HI: IEEE Service Center.

Zitzler, E., Deb, K., & Thiele, L. (2000). Comparison of multi-objective evolutionary algorithms: empirical results. *Evolutionary Computation, 8*(2), 173-195.

ADDITIONAL READING

Feoktistov, V. (2006). *Differential evolution: In search of solutions*. Springer.

Mezura-Montes, E., Velázquez-Reyes, J., & Coello Coello, C. A. (2006). Comparative study of differential evolution variants for global optimization. In *Proceedings of the Genetic and Evolutionary Computation Conference (GECCO 2006)* (pp. 485-492). Seattle, WA: ACM Press.

Mezura-Montes, E., Velázquez-Reyes, J., & Coello Coello, C. A. (2005). Promising infeasibility and multiple offspring incorporated to differential evolution for constrained optimization. In *Proceedings of the Genetic and Evolutionary Computation Conference (GECCO 2005)* (pp. 225-232). New York: ACM Press.

Robič, T. (2005). Performance of DEMO on new test problems: A comparison study. In *Proceedings of the 14th International Electrotechnical and Computer Science Conference (ERK 2005)* (pp. 121-124). Partaraž, Slovenia.

Wolpert, D. H. & Macready, W. G. (1997). No free lunch theorems for optimization. *IEEE Transactions on Evolutionary Computation, 1*(1), 67-82.

Chapter IV
Towards a More Efficient Multi-Objective Particle Swarm Optimizer

Luis V. Santana-Quintero
CINVESTAV-IPN, Evolutionary Computation Group (EVOCINV), Mexico

Noel Ramírez-Santiago
CINVESTAV-IPN, Evolutionary Computation Group (EVOCINV), Mexico

Carlos A. Coello Coello[*]
CINVESTAV-IPN, Evolutionary Computation Group (EVOCINV), Mexico

ABSTRACT

This chapter presents a hybrid between a particle swarm optimization (PSO) approach and scatter search. The main motivation for developing this approach is to combine the high convergence rate of the PSO algorithm with a local search approach based on scatter search, in order to have the main advantages of these two types of techniques. We propose a new leader selection scheme for PSO, which aims to accelerate convergence by increasing the selection pressure. However, this higher selection pressure reduces diversity. To alleviate that, scatter search is adopted after applying PSO, in order to spread the solutions previously obtained, so that a better distribution along the Pareto front is achieved. The proposed approach can produce reasonably good approximations of multi-objective problems of high dimensionality, performing only 4,000 fitness function evaluations. Test problems taken from the specialized literature are adopted to validate the proposed hybrid approach. Results are compared with respect to the NSGA-II, which is an approach representative of the state-of-the-art in the area.

INTRODUCTION

Despite the considerable volume of research developed on evolutionary multi-objective optimization during the last 20 years, certain topics such as algorithmic design emphasizing efficiency have become popular only within the last few years (Coello Coello, Van Veldhuizen, & Lamont, 2002).

In this chapter, we propose a new hybrid multi-objective evolutionary algorithm (MOEA) based on particle swarm optimization (PSO) and scatter search (SS). The main motivation of this work was to design a MOEA that could produce a reasonably good approximation of the true Pareto front of a problem with a relatively low number of fitness function evaluations. The core idea of our proposal is to combine the high convergence rate of PSO with the use of SS as a local search mechanism that compensates for the diversity lost during the search (due to the high selection pressure generated by the leader selection scheme that we propose for our PSO). As we show later, our proposed hybrid scheme constitutes an efficient MOEA, which can produce reasonably good approximations of the Pareto fronts of both constrained and unconstrained multi-objective problems of high dimensionality, performing a relatively low number of fitness function evaluations. Our results are compared with respect to a MOEA that is representative of the state-of-the-art in the area: the NSGA-II (Deb, Pratap, Agarwal, & Meyarivan, 2002).

The remainder of this chapter is organized as follows. First, we provide some basic concepts from multi-objective optimization required to make the chapter self-contained. This includes an introduction to the PSO strategy and to SS. We also present a brief review of several multi-objective particle swarm optimizers previously proposed in the specialized literature. Then, we provide the details of our proposed approach and the mechanism adopted to maintain diversity. Our comparison of results is provided in a further section. Our conclusions are presented after that, and some promising paths for future research are then briefly described. Finally, for those interested in gaining more in-depth knowledge about the topics covered in this chapter, a list of additional readings is provided at the end of the chapter.

BASIC CONCEPTS

In this section, we introduce some basic definitions which aim to make the paper self-contained. We introduce some basic terminology from the multi-objective optimization literature (assuming minimization) and we provide an introduction to both particle swarm optimization and scatter search.

Multi-Objective Optimization

The multi-objective optimization problem can be formally defined as the problem of finding:

$$\vec{x}^* = [x_1^*, x_2^*, ..., x_n^*]^T$$

which satisfies the m inequality constraints:

$$g_i(\vec{x}) \leq 0; i = 1,...,m$$

the p equality constraints:

$$h_i(\vec{x}) = 0; i = 1,...,p$$

and optimizes the vector function:

$$\vec{f}(\vec{x}) = f_1(\vec{x}), f_2(\vec{x}),..., f_k(\vec{x})$$

In other words, we aim to determine from among the set F of all vectors (points) which satisfy the constraints those that yield the optimum values for all the k-objective functions simultaneously. The constraints define the feasible region F and any point $\vec{x}$ in the feasible region is called a feasible point.

Pareto Dominance

Pareto dominance is formally defined as follows:

A vector $\bar{u} = (u_1,...,u_k)$ is said to dominate $\bar{v} = (v_1,...,v_k)$ if and only if $\bar{u}$ is partially less than $\bar{v}$, i.e.,

$$\forall i \in (1,...,k), u_i \leq v_i \wedge \exists i \in (1,...,k) : u_i < v_i.$$

In words, this definition says that a solution dominates another one, only if it's strictly better in at least one objective, and not worse in any of them. So, when we are comparing two different solutions A and B, there are 3 possibilities:

- A dominates B
- A is dominated by B
- A and B are nondominated

Pareto Optimality. The formal definition of *Pareto optimality* is provided next:

A solution $\bar{x}_u \in F$ (where F is the feasible region) is said to be Pareto optimal if and only if there is no $\bar{x}_v \in F$ for which $v = f(x_v) = (v_1, v_2,...,v_k)$ dominates $u = f(x_u) = (u_1, u_2,...,u_k)$, where k is the number of objectives.

In words, this definition says that $\bar{x}_u$ is Pareto optimal if there exists no feasible vector $\bar{x}_v$ which would decrease some objective without causing a simultaneous increase in at least one other objective.

This does not provide us a single solution (in decision variable space), but a set of solutions which form the so-called *Pareto Optimal Set*. The vectors that correspond to the solutions included in the Pareto optimal set are *nondominated*.

Pareto Front

When all nondominated solutions are plotted in objective space, the nondominated vectors are collectively known as the *Pareto Front*. Formally:

For a given MOP $\vec{f}(x)$ and Pareto optimal set P^*, the Pareto front (PF^*) is defined as:

$$PF^* = \{\vec{f} = [f_1(x),...,f_k(x)] \mid x \in P^*\}$$

Figure 1. Multi-objective optimization problem

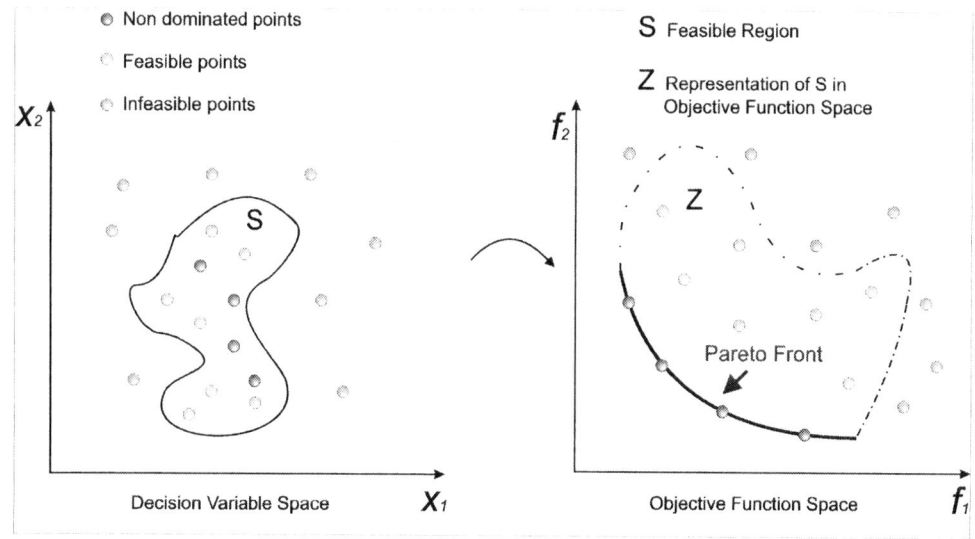

The previous definitions are graphically depicted in Figure 1, showing the *Pareto front*, the *Pareto Optimal Set* and *dominance* relations among solutions.

Particle Swarm Optimization (PSO)

PSO is a bio-inspired optimization algorithm that was proposed by James Kennedy and Russell Eberhart in the mid-1990's (Kennedy & Eberhart, 2001), and which is inspired on the choreography of a bird flock. PSO has been found to be a very successful optimization approach both in single-objective and in multi-objective problems (Kennedy & Eberhart, 2001; Reyes-Sierra & Coello Coello, 2006).

In PSO, each solution is represented by a particle. Particles group in "swarms" (there can be either one swarm or several in one population) and the evolution of the swarm to the optimal solutions is achieved by a velocity equation. This equation is composed of three elements: a velocity inertia, a cognitive component "*pbest*" and a social component "*gbest*". Depending on the topology adopted, each particle can be affected by either the best local and/or the best global particle in its swarm. In some of our previous work, we noticed that PSO normally has difficulties to achieve a good distribution of solutions with a low number of fitness function evaluations (Coello Coello, Toscano Pulido, & Salazar Lechuga, 2004). That is why we adopted scatter search (which can be useful at finding solutions within the neighborhood of a reference set) in this work in order to have a local optimizer whose computational cost is low.

In the PSO algorithm, the particles (including the *pbest*) are randomly initialized at the beginning of the search process. Next, the fittest particle from the swarm is identified and assigned to the *gbest* solution (i.e., the global best, or best particle found so far). After that, the swarm flies through the search space (in k dimensions, in the general case). The flight function adopted by PSO is determined by equation (1), which updates the position and fitness of the particle (see equation (2)). The new fitness is compared with respect to the particle's *pbest* position. If it is better, then it replaces the *pbest* (i.e., the personal best, or the best value that has been found for this particle so far). This procedure is repeated for every particle in the swarm until the termination criterion is reached.

$$v_{i,j} = w \cdot v_{i,j} + c_1 \cdot U(0,1)(pbest_{i,j} - x_{i,j}) \\ + c_2 \cdot U(0,1)(gbest_j - x_{i,j}) \quad (1)$$

$$x_{i,j} = x_{i,j} + v_{i,j} \quad (2)$$

where c_1 and c_2 are constants that indicate the attraction from the *pbest* or *gbest* position, respectively; w refers to the inertia of the previous movement; $x_i = (x_{i1}, x_{i2}, ..., x_{i,j})$ represents the $i-th$ particle; $j = 1, 2, ..., k$ and k represents the dimension; $U(0,1)$ denotes a uniformly random number generated within the range $(0,1)$; $v_i = (v_{i1}, v_{i2}, ..., v_{i,D})$ represents the rate change (velocity) of particle i. Equation (1) describes the velocity that is constantly updated by each particle and equation (2) updates the position of the particle in each decision variable.

Multi-Objective Algorithms Based on PSO

There are plenty of proposals to extend PSO for dealing with multiple objectives (see for example Alvarez-Benitez, Everson, & Fieldsend, 2005; Bartz-Beielstein, Limbourg, Parsopoulos, Vrahatis, Mehnen, & Schmitt, 2003; Baumgartner, Magele, & Renhart, 2004; Coello Coello & Salazar Lechuga, 2002; Mahfouf, Chen, & Linkens, 2004) and the survey by Reyes-Sierra and Coello Coello (2006). A brief description of the most representative proposals is provided next and a summary of their features is presented in Table 1:

Table 1. Characteristics of different multi-objective particle swarm optimizers

Author(s) / (reference)	Selection	Elitism	Mutation	Constraint-Handling
Alvarez-Benitez et al. (2005)	Pareto Ranking	Yes	No	No
Bartz-Beilstein et al. (2003)	Population-based	Yes	No	No
Baumgartner et al. (2004)	Linear Aggregation	No	No	No
Coello et al. (2004)	Pareto Ranking	Yes	Yes	Yes
Fieldsend and Singh (2002)	Dominated Tree based	Yes	Yes	No
Mahfouf et al. (2004)	Population-based	No	Yes	No
Moore and Chapman (1999)	Population-based	No	No	No
Parsopoulos et al. (2004)	Population-based	No	Yes	No
Reyes and Coello (2005)	Pareto Ranking	Yes	Yes	No

- **Alvarez-Benitez et al. (2005):** The authors propose methods based exclusively on Pareto dominance for selecting leaders from an unconstrained nondominated (external) archive. The authors propose and evaluate four mechanisms for confining particles to the feasible region, that is, constraint-handling methods. The authors show that a probabilistic selection favoring archival particles that dominate few particles provides good convergence towards the Pareto front while properly covering it at the same time. Also, they conclude that allowing particles to explore regions close to the constraint boundaries is important to ensure convergence to the Pareto front. This approach uses a turbulence factor that is added to the position of the particles with certain probability.

- **Bartz-Beielstein et al. (2003):** This approach starts from the idea of introducing elitism (through the use of an external archive) into PSO. Different methods for selecting and deleting particles (leaders) from the archive are analyzed to generate a satisfactory approximation of the Pareto front. Selecting methods are either inversely related to the fitness value or based on the previous success of each particle. The authors provide some statistical analysis in order to assess the impact of each of the parameters used by their approach.

- **Baumgartner et al. (2004):** This approach, based on the *fully connected* topology, uses linear aggregating functions. In this case, the swarm is equally partitioned into n sub-swarms, each of which uses a different set of weights and evolves into the direction of its own swarm leader. The approach adopts a gradient technique to identify the Pareto optimal solutions.

- **Coello Coello et al.(2004):** This proposal is based on the idea of having an external archive in which every particle deposits its flight experiences after each flight cycle. The search space explored is divided in hypercubes. Each hypercube receives a fitness value based on the number of particles it contains. Once a hypercube has been selected, the leader is randomly chosen. This approach also uses a mutation operator that acts both on the particles of the swarm, and on the range of each design variable of the problem to be solved.

- **Fieldsend and Singh (2002):** This approach uses an unconstrained elite external archive (in which a special data structure called "dominated tree" is adopted) to store the nondominated individuals. The archive interacts with the primary population in order to define leaders. The selection of the *gbest* for a particle in the swarm is based on the structure defined by the dominated tree. First, a composite point of the tree is located based on dominance relations, and then the closest member (in objective function space) of the composite point is chosen as the leader. On the other hand, a set of personal best particles found (nondominated) is also maintained for each swarm member, and the selection is performed uniformly. This approach also uses a "turbulence" operator that is basically a mutation operator that acts on the velocity value used by the PSO algorithm.

- **Mahfouf et al. (2004):** The authors propose an Adaptive Weighted PSO (AWPSO) algorithm, in which the velocity is modified by including an acceleration term that increases as the number of iterations increases. This aims to enhance the global search ability at the end of the run and to help the algorithm to jump out of local optima. The authors use dynamic weights to generate Pareto optimal solutions. When the population is losing diversity, a mutation operator is applied to the positions of certain particles and the best of them are retained. Finally, the authors include a nondominated sorting algorithm to select the particles from one iteration to the next.

- **Moore and Chapman (1999):** This was the first attempt to produce a multi-objective particle swarm optimizer. In this approach, the personal best (*pbest*) of a particle is a list of all the nondominated solutions it has found in its trajectory. When selecting a *pbest*, a particle from the list is randomly chosen. Since the ring topology is used, when selecting the best particle of the neighborhood, the solutions contained in the *pbest* lists are compared, and a nondominated solution with respect to the neighborhood is chosen. The authors do not indicate how they choose the *lbest* particle when more than one nondominated solution is found in the neighborhood.

- **Parsopoulos Tasoulis, and Vrahatis (2004):** studied a parallel version of the Vector Evaluated Particle Swarm (VEPSO) method for multi-objective problems. VEPSO is a multi-swarm variant of PSO, which is inspired on the Vector Evaluated Genetic Algorithm (VEGA) (Schaffer, 1985). In VEPSO, each swarm is evaluated using only one of the objective functions of the problem under consideration, and the information it possesses for this objective function is communicated to the other swarms through the exchange of their best experience (*gbest* particle). The authors argue that this process can lead to Pareto optimal solutions.

- **Reyes-Sierra and Coello Coello (2005):** This approach is based on Pareto dominance and the use of a nearest neighbor density estimator for the selection of leaders (by means of a binary tournament). This proposal uses two external archives: one for storing the leaders currently used for performing the flight and another for storing the final solutions. On the other hand, the concept of ε-dominance is used to select the particles that remain in the archive of final solutions. Additionally, the authors propose a scheme in which they subdivide the population (or swarm) into three different subsets. A different mutation operator is applied to each subset. Finally, this approach incorporates fitness inheritance (Smith, Dike, & Stegmann, 1995) in order to reduce the total number of fitness function evaluations performed. However, this approach performs 20,000 fitness function evaluations, which is considerably higher than the number of evaluations performed by the algorithm proposed in this chapter.

Scatter Search

Scatter search (SS) is an evolutionary method that was originally proposed in the 1970's by Fred Glover (1977) for combining decision rules and problem constraints. This method uses strategies for combining solution vectors that have been found effective during the search (the so called "reference set") (Laguna & Martí, 2003). SS has been successfully applied to hard optimization problems, and it constitutes a very flexible heuristic, since it can be implemented in a variety of ways, offering numerous alternatives for exploiting its fundamental ideas.

In 1994 (Glover, 1994), the range of applications of SS was expanded to nonlinear optimization problems, binary and permutation problems. Finally, in 1998 a new publication on scatter search (Glover, 1998) triggered the interest of researchers and practitioners, who translated these ideas into different computer implementations to solve a variety of problems.

Scatter search operates on a set of solutions (the reference set) by combining these solutions to create new ones. When the main mechanism for combining solutions is such that a new solution is created from the linear combination of two other solutions, the reference starts to evolve and the new solutions generated become part of the reference set.

Unlike a population in genetic algorithms, the reference set of solutions in scatter search is relatively small. In genetic algorithms, two solutions are randomly chosen from the population and a crossover or combination mechanism is applied to generate one or more offspring. A typical population size in a genetic algorithm consists of 100 elements, which are randomly sampled to create combinations. In contrast, scatter search chooses two or more elements of the reference set in a systematic way with the purpose of creating new solutions. Typically, the reference set in scatter search has 20 solutions or less. The scatter search algorithm contains five

Figure 2. Scatter search scheme

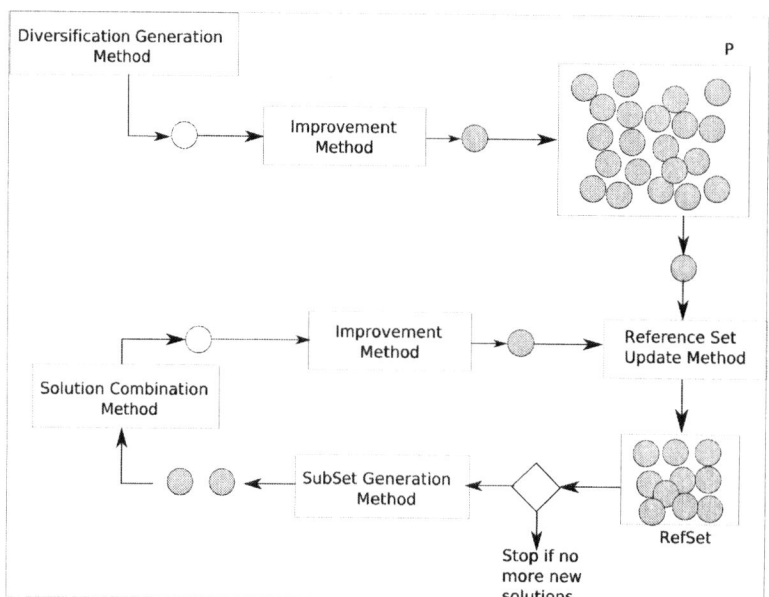

different methods, that are illustrated in Figure 2 and are briefly explained next:

The *Diversification Generation Method* (generates a scatter solutions set) and *Improvement Method* (makes a local search, and aims to improve the solutions) are initially applied to all the solutions in the *P* set. A *RefSet* set is generated based on the *P* set. *RefSet* contains the best solutions in terms of quality and diversity found so far. The *Subset Generation Method* takes the reference solutions as its input to produce solution subsets to be combined; the solution subsets contain two or more solutions from *RefSet*. Then, the *Combination Method* is applied to the solution subsets to get new solutions. We try to improve the generated solutions with the *Improvement Method* and the result of the improvement is handled by the *Reference Set Update Method*. This method applies rules regarding the admission of solutions to the reference set *RefSet*.

Handling Well-Distributed Solutions

Researchers have proposed several mechanisms to reduce the number of nondominated solutions generated by a MOEA (most of them applicable to external archives): clusters (Zitzler & Thiele, 1999), adaptive grids (Knowles & Corne, 2000), crowding (Deb et al. 2002) and relaxed forms of Pareto dominance (Laumanns, Thiele, Deb, & Zitzler, 2002). However, we only mention those that need an external archive to store nondominated solutions, such as:

- **Adaptive Grid**: Proposed by Knowles and Corne (2000), the adaptive grid is really a space formed by hypercubes. Such hypercubes have as many components as objective functions has the problem to be solved. Each hypercube can be interpreted as a geographical region that contains an *n* number of individuals. The adaptive grid allows us to store nondominated solutions and to redistribute them when its maximum capacity is reached.

- **ε-dominance**: This is a relaxed form of dominance proposed by Laumanns et al. (2002). The so-called ε-Pareto set is an archiving strategy that maintains a subset of generated solutions. It guarantees convergence and diversity according to well-defined criteria, namely the value of the ε parameter, which defines the resolution of the grid to be adopted for the secondary population. The general idea of this mechanism is to divide objective function space into boxes of size ε. In Figure 3 it is shown an ε-dominance example in which it can be seen the main difference between Pareto dominance and ε-dominance. Each box can be interpreted as a geographical region that contains a single solution. This algorithm is very attractive both from a theoretical and from a practical point of view. However, in order to achieve the best performance, it is necessary to provide the size of the box (the ε parameter) which is problem-dependent, and it's normally not known before executing a MOEA.

OUR PROPOSED APPROACH

Our proposed approach, called **Constrained Multi-objective Optimization using Particle Swarm Optimization with Scatter Search (C-MOPSOSS)**, is divided in two phases, and each of them consumes a fixed number of fitness function evaluations. During Phase I, our PSO-based MOEA is applied for 2000 fitness function evaluations for unconstrained problems and 2500 evaluations for constrained problems. During Phase II, a local search procedure based on scatter search is applied (for the same number of fitness function evaluations as in Phase I), in order to improve the solutions (i.e., spread them

Figure 3. ε-dominance relation example

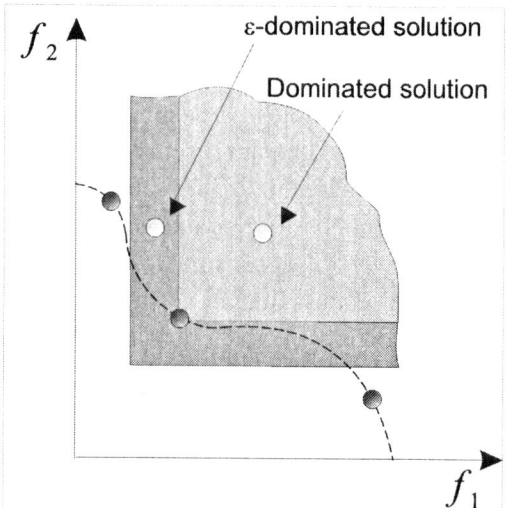

along the Pareto front) produced at the previous phase. Each of these two phases is described next in more detail.

Phase I: Particle Swarm Optimization

Our proposed PSO-based approach adopts a very small population size ($P = 5$ particles). The leader is determined using a simple criterion: the first N particles (N is the number of objectives of the problem) are guided by the best particle in each objective, considered separately. The remainder $P - N$ particles are adopted to build an approximation of the ideal vector. The ideal

Algorithm 1

Algorithm 1: Phase I - PSO Algorithm
1 **begin**
2   *Initialize Population (P) with randomly generated solutions*
3   *getLeaders()*
4   **repeat**
5   **for** $i = 1$ *to* P **do**
6       $g = GetLeader(i)$
7   **for** $d = 1$ *to* $nVariables$ **do**
8   /*$L_{g,d}$ is the leader of particle i*/
9         $v_{i,d} = w \cdot v_{i,d} + c_1 \cdot U(0,1)(p_{i,d} - x_{i,d}) + c_2 \cdot U(0,1)(L_{g,d} - x_{i,d})$
10         $x_{i,d} = x_{i,d} + v_{i,d}$
11   **end**
12   **if** $x_i \notin search\ space$ **then**
13         $x_i = BLX - \alpha(L_g, p_i)$
14   **end**
15   **if** $U(0,1) < p_m$ **then**
16         $x_i = Mutate(x_i)$
17   **end**
18   **if** x_i *is nondominated and* x_i *is feasible* **then**
19   **for** $d=1$ *to* $nVariables$ **do**
20           $p_{i,d} = x_{i,d}$
21   **end**
22   **end**
23   **end**
24   *getLeaders()*
25   **until** *MaxIter*
26 **end**

vector is formed with $(f_1^*, f_2^*, ..., f_N^*)$ where f_i^* is the best solution found so far for the *i-th* objective function. Then, we identify the individual which is closest to this ideal vector (using an euclidian distance) and such individual becomes the leader for the remainder *P-N* particles. The purpose of these selection criteria is twofold: first, we aim to approximate the optimum for each separate objective, by exploiting the high convergence rate of PSO in single-objective optimization. The second purpose of our selection rules is to encourage convergence towards the "knee" of the Pareto front (considering the bi-objective case).

Algorithm 1 shows the pseudocode of Phase I from our proposed approach. First, we randomly generate the initial population, but in the population we need at least the same number of individuals as the number of objectives plus one. This last individual is needed to form the ideal vector; for this purpose, we chose 5 individuals to perform the experiments reported in this work. In the *getLeaders($\bar{x}$)* function, we identify the best particles in each objective and the closest particle to the ideal vector. Those particles (the leaders) are stored in the set *L*. Then the *getLeaders($\bar{x}$)* function returns the position of the leader from the set *L* for a particle *x*. Then, we perform the flight in order to obtain a new particle. If this solution is beyond the allowable bounds for a decision variable, then we adopt the *BLX-α*[a] recombination operator (Eshelmann & Schaffer, 1993), and a new vector solution $Z = (z_1, z_2, ..., z_d)$ is generated, where $z_i \in [c_{min} - I \cdot \alpha, c_{max} + I \cdot \alpha]$; $c_{max} = \max(a_i, b_i)$, $c_{min} = \min(a_i, b_i)$, $I = c_{max} - c_{min}$, $\alpha = 0.5$, $a = L_g$ (the leader of the particle) and $b = pbest$ (i.e., the personal best of the particle). Note that the use of a recombination operator is not a common practice in PSO, and some people may consider our approach as a PSO-variant because of that. PSO does not use a specific mutation operator either (the variation of the factors of the flight equation may compensate for that). However, it has become common practice in MOPSOs to adopt some sort of mutation (or turbulence) operator that improves the exploration capabilities of PSO (Mostaghim & Teich, 2003; Reyes-Sierra & Coello Coello, 2006). The use of a mutation operator is normally simpler (and easier) than varying the factors of the flight equation and therefore its extended use. We adopted Parameter-Based Mutation (Deb et al., 2002) in our approach with

$$p_m = \frac{1}{nVariables}.$$

Our proposed approach uses an external archive (also called secondary population) and a selection procedure which is described in detail in a further section.

The second phase of our algorithm is based on Scatter Search, and it requires a set of dominated points to work properly. For this purpose, we decided to include a third population that stores the dominated points that are being removed constantly from the secondary population as the search progresses. Thus, this third population contains solutions that are (globally) dominated, but that are close from being nondominated (as shown in Figure 4).

Phase II: Scatter Search

Phase II departs from the nondominated set generated in Phase I. This set is contained within the secondary population. We also have the dominated set, which is contained within the third population. From the nondominated set we choose *MaxScatterSolutions* points. These particles have to be scattered in the nondominated set, so we choose them based on a distance L_α which is determined by equation (3):

$$L_\alpha(x) = \max_{i=1,...,k} \left\{ \frac{f_i^{max(x)} - f_i(x)}{f_i^{max(x)} - f_i^{min(x)}} \right\} \quad (3)$$

Figure 4. Secondary and third population

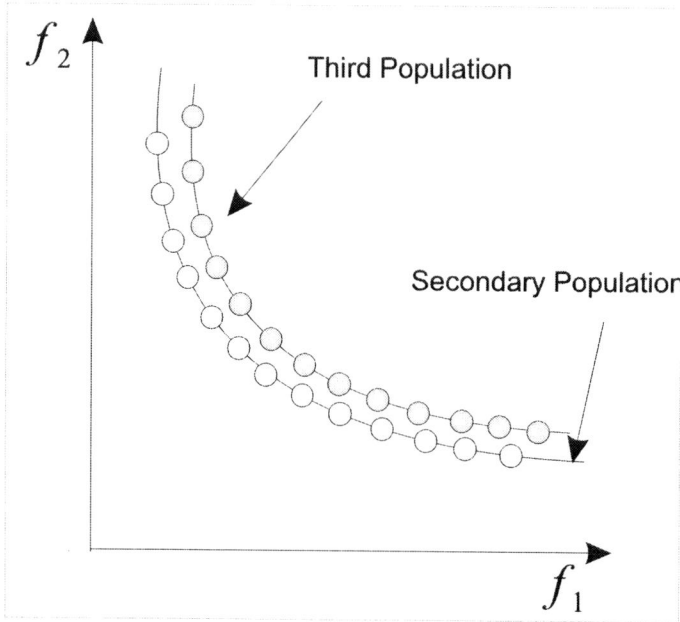

Generalizing, to obtain the scatter solutions set among the nondominated set, we use equation (4):

$$L_{set}(x) = \max_{\forall u \in U}\left\{\min_{\forall v \in V}\left\{\max_{i=1,\ldots,k}\left\{\frac{|f_{vi}(x) - f_{ui}(x)|}{f_i^{\max(x)} - f_i^{\min(x)}}\right\}\right\}\right\} \quad (4)$$

where L_{set} is the Leaders set, U is the nondominated set and V contains the scatter solutions set, $f_i^{\max}$ and $f_i^{\min}$ are the upper and lower bound of the i-th objective function in the secondary population.

This selection process is shown in Figure 5, where the black points are the scatter particles that we use to obtain the reference set. Algorithm 2 describes the scatter search process used in the second phase of our approach. This process is graphically depicted in Figure 6. The **getScatterSolution()** function returns the scatter solutions set in the nondominated set V. The **getScatterSolution(n)** function returns the n-th scatter solution and stores it in pl. **CreateRefSet(pl)** creates the reference set of the pl scatter solution. This function returns a set of solutions C_n as it is shown in Figure 5 (those which are enclosed by the continuous black line). Regarding the Solution Combination Method required by SS, we used the *BLX-α* recombination operator (Eshelmann & Schaffer, 1993) with α = 0.5. This operator combines the i-th particle with the j-th particle from the C_n set. Finally, we used a Parameter-Based mutation as the Improvement Method with

$$p_m = \frac{1}{nVariables}.$$

Use of ε-Dominance

As indicated before, our proposed approach uses an external archive (also called secondary population) together with the ε-dominance concept

Figure 5. Solutions selected to create the reference set used in scatter search

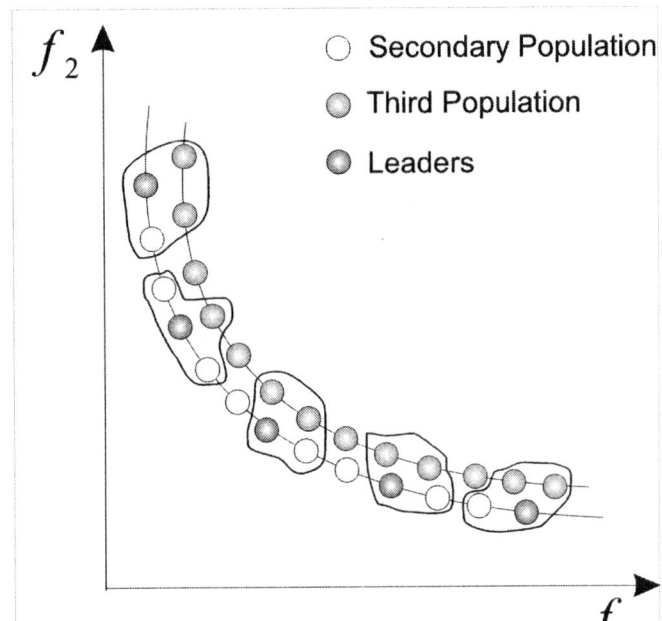

Figure 6. Multi-objective optimization problem

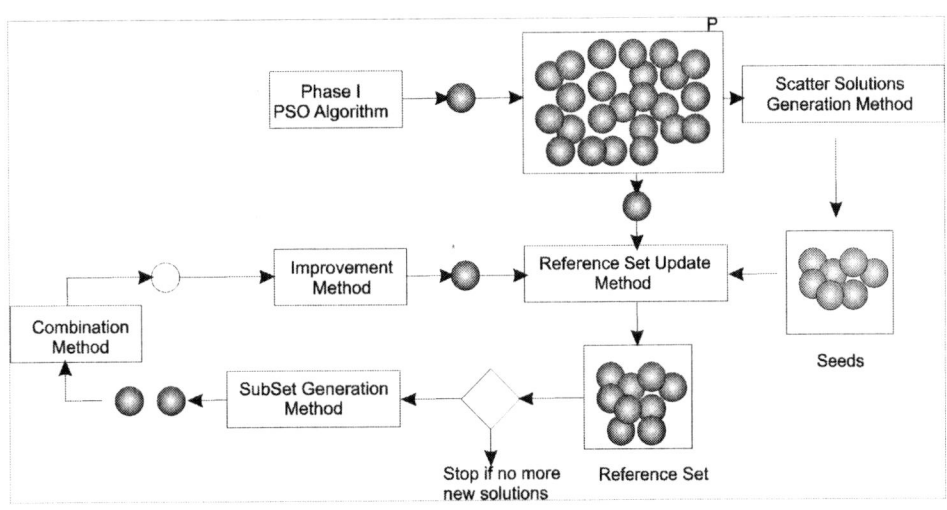

Algorithm 2

Algorithm 2: Phase II - Scatter Search Algorithm
1 **begin**
2   **repeat**
3   *getScatterSolutions()*
4   **for** $n = 0$ *to MaxScatterSolutions* **do**
5          $pl = getScatterSolution(n)$
6   //Reference Set Update and Create Method
7   *CreateRefSet(pl)*
8   **for** $i = 0$ *to SizeRefSet* **do**
9   **for** $j = i + 1$ *to RefSetSize* **do**
10   //Solution Combination Method
11               $x = BLX - \alpha(popRefSet(i), popRefSet(j))$
12   //Improvement Method
13               $x = Mutate(x)$
14   **if** *x is nondominated and x is feasible* **then**
15   *Add Particle x into secondary population*
16   **end**
17   **end**
18   **end**
19   **end**
20   **until** *MaxIter*
21 **end**

proposed by Laumanns et al. (2002). In order to include a solution into this archive, it is compared with respect to each member already contained in the archive using ε-dominance. The procedure is described next.

Every solution in the archive is assigned an identification array $B = (B_1, B_2, ..., B_k)^T$, where k is the total number of objectives) as follows:

$$B_j(f) = \begin{cases} \left\lfloor \dfrac{f_j - f_j^{min}}{\varepsilon_j} \right\rfloor, \text{ for minimizing} \cdot (f_j) \\ \left\lceil \dfrac{f_j - f_j^{min}}{\varepsilon_j} \right\rceil, \text{ for maximizing} \cdot (f_j) \end{cases}$$

where: f_j^{min} is the minimum possible value of the j-th objective $\lfloor \rfloor \lceil \rceil$ are the ceiling and floor functions, respectively, and ε_j is the allowable tolerance in the j-th objective (Laumanns et al., 2002). The identification array divides the whole objective space into hyper-boxes, each having ε_j size in the j-th objective. With the identification arrays calculated for the offspring c_i and each archive member a, we use the procedure illustrated in Figure 7 and described next:

- If the identification array B_a of any archive member a dominates that of the offspring c_i, then it means that the offspring is ε-dominated by this archive member and so the offspring *is not accepted*. This is case (A) in Figure 7.
- If B_{ci} of the offspring dominates the B_a of any archive member a, the archive member is deleted and the offspring *is accepted*. This is case (B) in Figure 7.

If neither of the two cases occur, then it means that the offspring is ε-nondominated with respect to the archive contents. There are two further possibilities in this case:

Figure 7. Four cases of inserting a child into the external archive

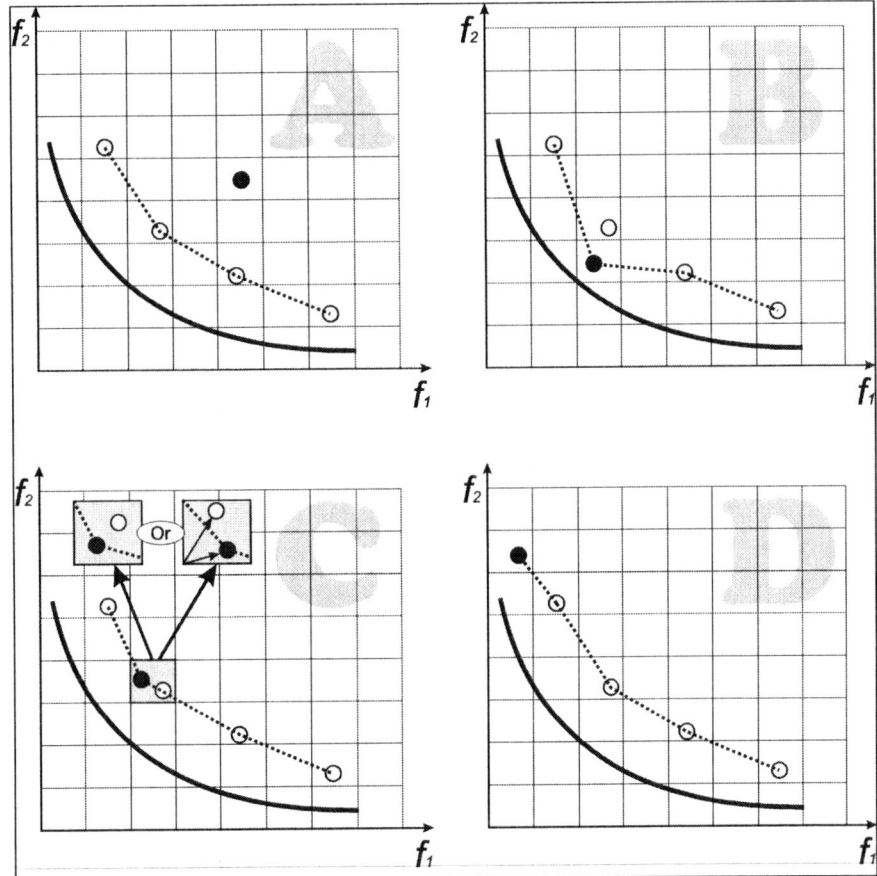

- If the offspring shares the same **B** vector with an archive member (meaning that they belong to the same hyper-box), then they are first checked for the usual nondomination. If the offspring dominates the archive member or the offspring is nondominated with respect to the archive member but is closer to the **B** vector (in terms of the Euclidian distance) than the archive member, then the offspring *is retained*. This is case (C) in Figure 7.
- In the event of an offspring not sharing the same **B** vector with any archive member, the offspring *is accepted*. This is case (D) in Figure 7.

Using this procedure, we can guarantee the generation of a well-distributed set of nondominated solutions. Also, the value of ε adopted (defined by the user) regulates the size of the external archive. Thus, there is no need to pre-fix an upper limit on the size of the archive as done in most traditional multi-objective evolutionary algorithms.

COMPARISON OF RESULTS

We chose 14 test problems with different geometrical characteristics for our experimental study (10 of them are unconstrained and 3 with constraints). The problems selected are the following: **Kursawe**'s problem (Kursawe, 1991) (the Pareto front is disconnected); 5 problems from the **ZDT** set (multimodal problems) (Zitzler, Deb, & Thiele, 2000); 4 from the **DTLZ** set (Deb, Thiele, Laumanns, & Zitzler, 2005) (three-objective problems); and 4 more functions have constraints: **Osyczka** (Osyczka & Kundu, 1995)**, Kita** (Kita, Yabumoto, Y., Mori, & Nishikawa, 1996)**, Welded Beam** (Ragsdell & Phillips, 1975) and **Speed Reducer** (Golinski, 1970). The full description of **Welded Beam** and **Speed Reducer** is presented in Table 6. The description of the other test functions is available from their original sources, and was omitted due to space limitations.

In order to allow a quantitative comparison of results, we adopted two performance measures that are used to determine if our approach has converged to the true Pareto front (Two Set Coverage and Inverted Generational Distance) and a third one was adopted to determine if the solutions are uniformly distributed along the Pareto front (Spread). A brief description of each of them is provided next:

Two Set coverage (SC) Zitzler et al. (2000) proposed this metric that can be termed relative coverage comparison of two sets. SC is defined as the mapping of the order pair (X', X'') to the interval [0,1] as follows:

$$SC(X',X'') = \frac{|\{a'' \in X''; \exists a' \in X': a' \succ a''\}|}{|X''|}$$

Consider $X', X'' \subseteq X'$ as two sets of decision vectors. If all points in X' dominate or are equal to all points in X'', then by definition SC = 1. SC = 0 implies the opposite. Observe that this is not a distance measure that allows to determine how close these sets are from each other.

Inverted Generational Distance (IGD): Van Veldhuizen and Lamont (1998; 2000) proposed the Generational Distance (GD) metric as a way of estimating how far are the elements in the Pareto front produced by an algorithm from those in the true Pareto front of the problem. Mathematically:

$$IGD = \frac{\sqrt{\sum_{i=1}^{n} d_i^2}}{n}$$

where n is the number of nondominated solutions found by the algorithm being analyzed and d_i is the Euclidean distance between each of these and the nearest member of the true Pareto front. A value of zero for this metric indicates that our algorithm has converged to the true Pareto front. Therefore, any other value indicates how "far" we are from the true Pareto front. We adopted a variation of this metric, called Inverted Generational Distance (IGD) in which we use as a reference the true Pareto front, and we compare each of its elements with respect to the approximation produced by an algorithm. This provides a better estimate and avoids some of the pathological cases of poor convergence that could arise (see Coello Coello & Cruz Cortés (2005) for a more extended discussion on this metric).

Spread metric (S) Deb (2001) proposed the metric Δ with the idea of measuring both progress towards the Pareto-optimal front and the extent of spread. To this end, if P is a subset of the Pareto-optimal front, Δ is defined as follows

$$\Delta = \frac{\sum_{i=1}^{m} d_i^e + \sum_{i=1}^{|F|} |d_i - \bar{d}|}{\sum_{i=1}^{m} d_i^e + |F|\bar{d}}$$

where d_i^e denotes the distance between the i-th coordinate for both extreme points in P and F, and d_i measures the distance of each point in F to its closer point in F.

From this definition, it is easy to conclude that $0 \leq \Delta \leq 1$ and the lower the Δ value, the better the distribution of solutions. A perfect distribution, that is $\Delta = 0$, means that the extreme points of the Pareto-optimal front have been found and d_i is constant for all i.

Discussion of Results

This section is divided in four parts: (1) in the first one, we compare our approach with respect to the NSGA-II, which is a MOEA representative of the state-of-the-art in the area. (2) In the second part we compare our proposed approach against the MOPSO proposed by Coello Coello et al. (2004). (3) In the third part we compare our approach without scatter search (i.e., using only the first phase) with respect to the full approach (i.e., using the two phases) in order to assess the usefulness of the scatter search algorithm. Finally, (4) the fourth part is dedicated to show that the C-MOPSOSS is capable of converging to the true Pareto front of all the test functions adopted in our study, if allowed a sufficiently large number of fitness function evaluations.

It is important to mention the parameters that we use for all the different test functions in order to make all the comparisons in this section. The first phase of our approach uses four parameters: population size (P), leaders number (N), mutation probability (P_m), recombination parameter α, plus the traditional PSO parameters (w, c_1, c_2). On the other hand, the second phase uses two more parameters: reference set size (*RefSetSize*) and number of scatter search solutions (*MaxScatterSolutions*). Finally, the ε-vector used to generate the ε-dominance grid was set to 0.05 in Kursawe's function, 0.02 in the ZDT and the DTLZ test functions, and to 0.1 for the constrained functions. In all cases, the parameters of our approach were set as follows: $P=5$, $N = k+1$ (k = number of objective functions), $P_m=1/n$, w = 0.3, $c_1= 0.1$, $c_2 =1.4$, *RefSetSize* = 4, *MaxScatterSolutions*=7 and α=0.5. These values were empirically derived after numerous experiments.

C-MOPSOSS vs NSGA-II Comparison

In order to validate our proposed approach, we compare results with respect to the NSGA-II (Deb et al., 2002), which is a MOEA representative of the state-of-the-art in the area.

The NSGA-II was used with the following parameters[b]: crossover rate = 0.9, mutation rate = $1/n$ (n = number of decision variables), $\eta_c=15$, $\eta_m = 20$ (as suggested in (Deb et al., 2002)), population size = 100 and maximum number of generations = 40 or 50 for constrained problems. The population size of the NSGA-II is the same as the size of the grid of our approach. In order to allow a fair comparison of results, both approaches adopted real-numbers encoding and performed the same number of fitness function evaluations per run because with our approach we only need 4,000 (and 5,000 for constrained problems) fitness function evaluations to produce a reasonably good approximation of the true Pareto front in most of the test problems adopted in our study. For each test problem, 30 independent runs were performed. Our results reported in Table 2 correspond to the mean and standard deviation of the performance metrics (SC, IGD and S). We show in boldface the best mean values for each test function.

In Table 2, it can be observed that in the ZDT test problems, our approach produced the best results with respect to the SC, IGD and S metrics, in all cases. Our approach also outperformed the NSGA-II with respect to the SC metric in the DTLZ1, DTLZ2 and DTLZ3 test problems. The NSGA-II found better results in three cases with respect to the IGD, and S metrics. In constrained problems, our C-MOPSOSS obtained better results with respect to the SC and Spread metrics in all three cases, and the NSGA-II outperformed it with respect to the IGD metric for Osyczka's and the Welded beam problems. Based on these results, we can conclude that our approach obtained better solutions than the NSGA-II with the same number of function evaluations in almost all the problems except for DTLZ4. With respect to the IGD metric, we obtained better results than the NSGA-II in 10 of the 14 test functions adopted. We also concluded that the use of ε-dominance helped our approach to maintain a well-distributed set of nondominated solutions because we were able to outperform the NSGA-II with respect to

Table 2. Comparison of results between our hybrid (called C-MOPSOSS) and the NSGA-II with 4000 (and 5000 for constrained problems) fitness function evaluations

Function	SC				IGD				Spread			
	C-MOPSOSS		NSGA-II		C-MOPSOSS		NSGA-II		C-MOPSOSS		NSGA-II	
	Mean	σ	Mean	σ	Mean	σ	Mean	σ	Mean	σ	Mean	σ
KURSAWE	**0.1738**	0.0635	0.2166	0.0664	**0.0005**	0.0004	0.0036	0.0002	**0.3978**	0.0257	0.4383	0.0370
ZDT1	**0.0000**	0.0000	0.8662	0.0418	**0.0018**	0.0011	0.0097	0.0019	**0.3190**	0.0634	0.5444	0.0380
ZDT2	**0.0000**	0.0000	0.8894	0.1718	**0.0052**	0.0064	0.0223	0.0064	**0.3984**	0.1108	0.7213	0.1102
ZDT3	**0.0117**	0.0391	0.9011	0.0483	**0.0047**	0.0033	0.0155	0.0020	**0.6462**	0.0635	0.7492	0.0353
ZDT4	**0.0000**	0.0000	0.2415	0.1316	**0.1065**	0.0421	0.4297	0.1304	**0.6992**	0.0771	0.9840	0.0193
ZDT6	**0.0000**	0.0000	0.5375	0.1426	**0.0011**	0.0006	0.0420	0.0041	**0.4261**	0.1557	0.8747	0.0778
DTLZ1	**0.0551**	0.0993	0.6826	0.1502	**0.3942**	0.1181	0.7318	0.2062	**0.9939**	0.0040	0.9981	0.0008
DTLZ2	**0.0656**	0.0800	0.1806	0.0800	**0.0006**	0.0001	0.0004	0.0000	0.7600	0.0686	**0.2155**	0.0202
DTLZ3	**0.0036**	0.0140	0.5165	0.2214	**0.8367**	0.2348	1.4228	0.2690	**0.9963**	0.0029	0.9992	0.0002
DTLZ4	0.4329	0.3815	**0.0815**	0.1760	0.0222	0.0043	**0.0096**	0.0025	0.7345	0.1168	**0.7251**	0.0898
OSYCZKA	**0.1613**	0.2248	0.6233	0.2363	0.0020	0.0011	**0.0012**	0.0006	**0.9667**	0.0173	0.9848	0.0251
KITA	**0.2663**	0.0696	0.4033	0.0675	**0.0009**	0.0001	**0.0009**	0.0001	**0.5620**	0.0964	0.6400	0.1861
WELBEAM	**0.3694**	0.3399	0.3812	0.2049	0.0047	0.0059	**0.0024**	0.0019	**0.7050**	0.0992	0.8601	0.0998
SPD RED	**0.2247**	0.1139	0.4430	0.1006	0.0027	0.0002	**0.0026**	0.0001	**0.9996**	0.0001	0.9990	0.0001

the S metric in 12 of the 14 test functions, in spite of the fact that the NSGA-II uses a very powerful density estimator (the crowded-comparison operator).

Figures 8 and 9 show the graphical results produced by our C-MOPSOSS and the NSGA-II for all the test problems adopted. The solutions displayed correspond to the median result with respect to the IGD metric. The true Pareto front (obtained by enumeration or using the corresponding analytical expressions, where applicable) is shown with a continuous line and the approximation produced by each algorithm is shown with circles. In Figures 8 and 9, we can clearly see that in problems Kursawe, ZDT1, ZDT2, ZDT3, ZDT4 and ZDT6, the NSGA-II is very far from the true Pareto front, whereas our C-MOPSOSS is very close to the true Pareto front after only 4,000 fitness function evaluations (except for ZDT4). Graphically, the results are not entirely clear for the DTLZ test problems. However, if we pay attention to the scale, its evident that, in most cases, our approach has several points closer to the true Pareto front than the NSGA-II. In constrained problems, we can see that the performance of both approaches is very similar in Kita's problem, but in Osyczka's problem our approach gets closer to the true Pareto front with a good spread of solutions. In the Welded beam problem, the NSGA-II gets a well-distributed set of solutions along the Pareto front.

Our results indicate that the NSGA-II, despite being a highly competitive MOEA, is not able to converge to the true Pareto front in most of the test problems adopted when performing a low number of fitness function evaluations. Note however that if we perform a higher number of evaluations, the NSGA-II would certainly produce a very good (and well-distributed) approximation of the Pareto front. However, our aim was precisely to provide an alternative approach that requires a lower number of evaluations than a state-of-the-art MOEA while still providing a highly competitive performance. Such an approach could be useful in real-world applications having objective functions that require a very high computational cost.

Towards a More Efficient Multi-Objective Particle Swarm Optimizer

Figure 8. Pareto fronts generated by C-MOPSOSS and NSGA-II for Kursawe's, ZDT1, ZDT2, ZDT3, ZDT4, ZDT6 and DTLZ1 test functions

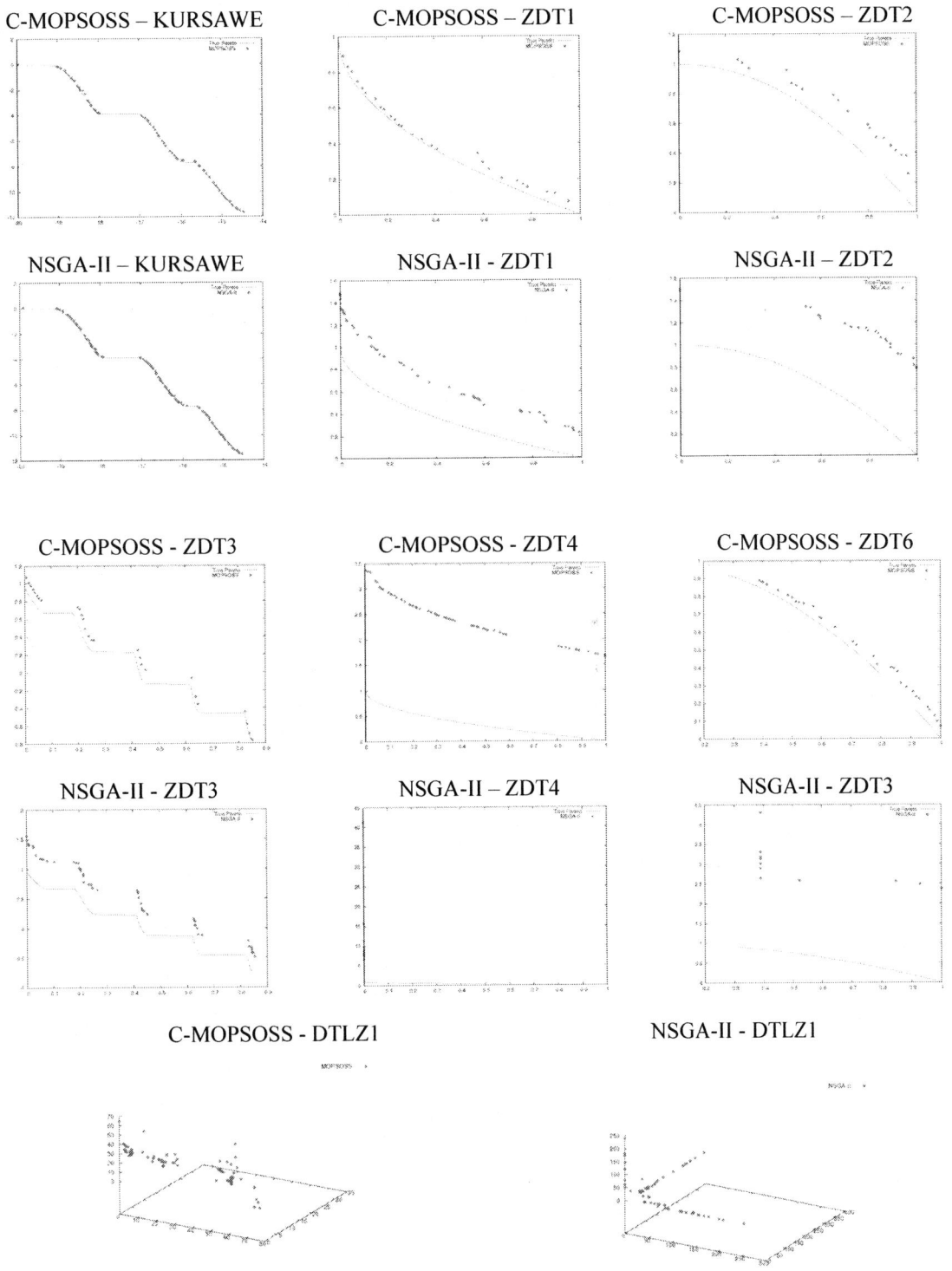

Figure 9. Pareto fronts generated by our C-MOPSOSS and the NSGA-II for the DTLZ2, DTLZ3, DTLZ4, Osyczka, Kita, Welded Beam and Speed Reducer test functions

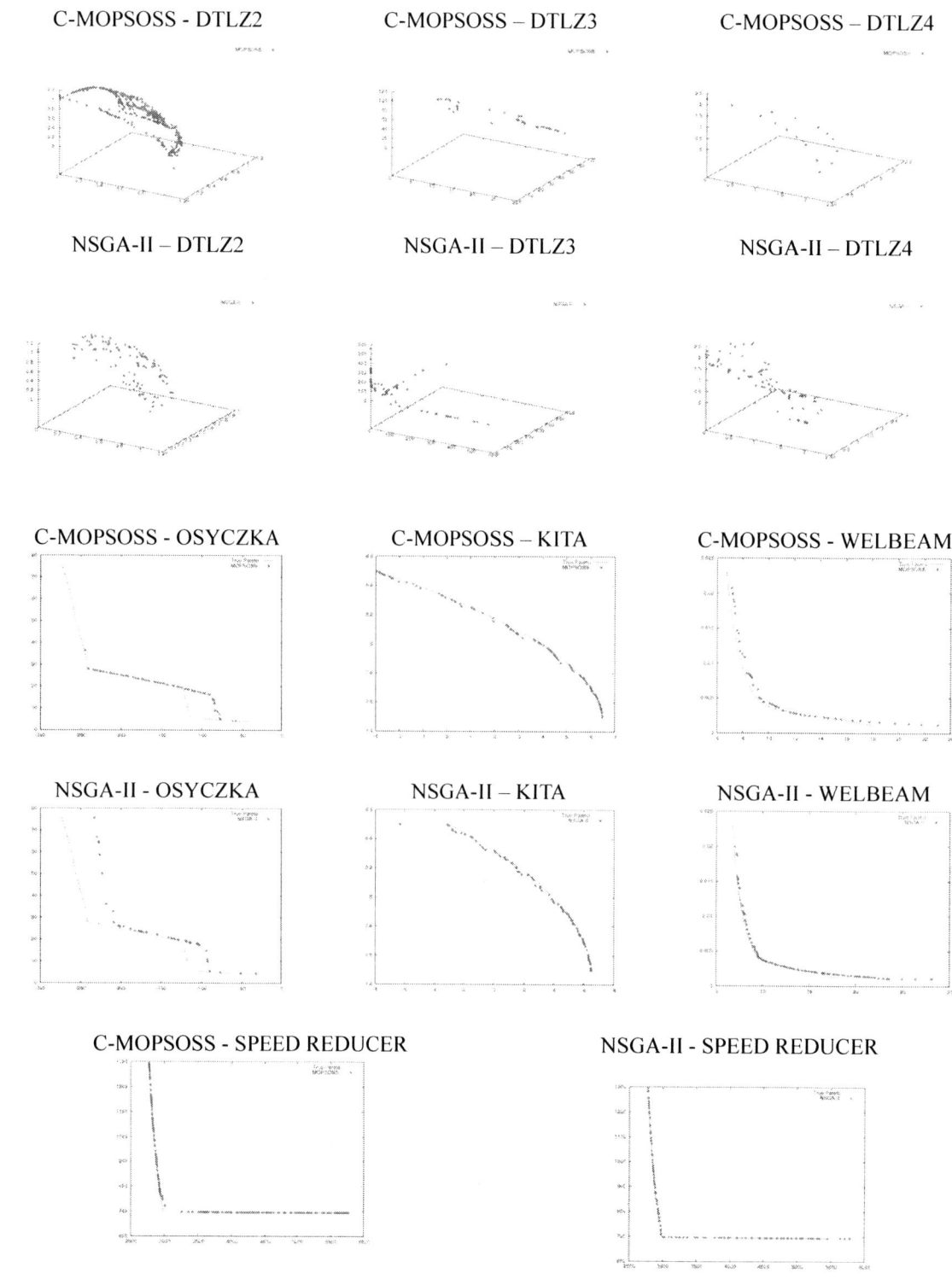

Comparison Between Our C-MOPSOSS and MOPSO

We now compare the results produced by our C-MOPSOSS with respect to the MOPSO proposed in (Coello Coello et al., 2004)[c]: number of Particles = 50, number of cycles = 80, mutation rate = 0.05, w = 0.4, c_1 = 2.0, c_2 =2.0,. For each test problem, 30 independent runs were performed. The results obtained are shown in Table 3 and correspond to the mean and standard deviation of the performance metrics (SC, IGD and S). We show in boldface the best mean values for each test function. Due to space limitations, we do not include any graphical comparison of results, and we only limited our comparison to the unconstrained test problems.

In Table 3, it can be observed that in all the test problems, our C-MOPSOSS obtained the best results with respect to the SC and IGD metrics, except for ZDT4, in which there was a tie (both obtain a zero value).[d] With respect to the S metric, we obtained the best results in all the test problems, except for DTLZ2.

From these results, we can conclude that our approach clearly outperforms MOPSO (Coello Coello et al., 2004), which is one of the few multi-objective particle swarm optimizers published in a specialized journal.

Comparing the Two Stages of Our Approach

The intention of this subsection is to illustrate the effect of the second phase of our approach. For that sake, we adopted a version of our algorithm that only uses the first phase (i.e., without scatter search) and which we call C-MOPSO. This approach is compared to C-MOPSOSS (i.e., the version with the two phases) performing the same number of fitness function evaluations as before (4000 for unconstrained and 5000 for constrained problems) and using the same test functions. The parameters used for C-MOPSO are exactly the same as the ones described before: $P = 5$, $N = k+1$ (k = number of objective functions), $P_m = 1/n$, $w = 0.3$, $c_1 = 0.1$, $c_2 = 1.4$. For each test problem, 30 independent runs were performed. Our results are reported in Table 4. Such results correspond to the mean and standard deviation of the performance metrics (SC, IGD and S); we show in boldface the best mean values for each test function. Figure 10 shows the graphical results produced by C-MOPSO for all the test problems adopted. The

Table 3. Comparison of results between our hybrid (called C-MOPSOSS) and MOPSO with 4000 (and 5000 for constrained problems) fitness function evaluations

Function	SC				IGD				Spread			
	C-MOPSOSS		MOPSO		C-MOPSOSS		MOPSO		C-MOPSOSS		MOPSO	
	Mean	σ	Mean	σ	Mean	σ	Mean	σ	Mean	σ	Mean	σ
KURSAWE	0.1421	0.3083	0.0852	0.0664	**0.0005**	0.0004	0.0014	0.0027	**0.3978**	0.0257	0.5715	0.0766
ZDT1	**0.0000**	0.0000	0.9374	0.0149	**0.0018**	0.0011	0.0507	0.0043	**0.3190**	0.0634	0.6362	0.0211
ZDT2	**0.0000**	0.0000	0.4662	0.4984	**0.0052**	0.0064	0.1162	0.0203	**0.3984**	0.1108	0.9287	0.0749
ZDT3	**0.0000**	0.0000	0.9530	0.0159	**0.0047**	0.0033	0.0580	0.0045	**0.6462**	0.0635	0.8396	0.0221
ZDT4	**0.0000**	0.0000	**0.0000**	0.0000	**0.1065**	0.0421	0.8777	0.6170	**0.6992**	0.0771	0.9698	0.0327
ZDT6	**0.0000**	0.0000	0.0150	0.0584	**0.0011**	0.0006	0.4041	0.0115	**0.4261**	0.1557	0.9878	0.0109
DTLZ1	**0.1680**	0.3386	0.7300	0.3157	**0.3942**	0.1181	2.6280	1.3218	**0.9939**	0.0040	0.9960	0.0038
DTLZ2	**0.0000**	0.0000	0.9730	0.0586	**0.0006**	0.0001	0.0079	0.0006	0.7600	0.0686	**0.6609**	0.0398
DTLZ3	**0.0000**	0.0000	0.7321	0.2087	**0.8367**	0.2348	3.5866	0.0699	**0.9963**	0.0029	0.9983	0.0009
DTLZ4	**0.0000**	0.0000	0.6893	0.4189	**0.0222**	0.0043	0.0431	0.0009	**0.7345**	0.1168	0.7699	0.0255

solutions displayed correspond to the median result with respect to the IGD metric.

In Table 4, it can be observed that, with respect to the SC metric, our C-MOPSOSS obtains better results only in 8 from the 14 test functions. This result was anticipated, since allowing that the search engine performs more evaluations should produce a better approximation of the Pareto front. With respect to the IGD metric, we obtained better results with our C-MOPSOSS in all, but two cases, because this metric penalizes a poor spread of solutions, even when an algorithm has converged to the true Pareto front. With respect to the S metric, we obtained better results with our C-MOPSOSS in 13 of the 14 test functions (except for DTLZ2). In Figure 10, we can observe the Pareto fronts obtained by our C-MOPSO algorithm. In this figure, it can be observed that very few solutions are obtained in each case, and that they present a poor distribution along the Pareto front.

Based on these results, we conclude that the use of the second phase of our approach is beneficial to improve the spread of solutions along the Pareto front. It is worth noting, however, that such an improvement in spread is obtained by sacrificing a slight improvement in terms of convergence.

Convergence Capability of Our C-MOPSOSS

Here, we show that our proposed hybrid approach, C-MOPSOSS, is capable of converging to the true Pareto front of all the test functions adopted in our study, if allowed a sufficiently large number of fitness function evaluations. Table 5 shows the total number of fitness function evaluations required to reach the true Pareto front for each test function. Figure 11 shows these results in graphical form. No metrics are adopted in this case, since we only aimed to illustrate the convergence capabilities of our proposed approach.

Table 4. Comparison of results between our hybrid (called C-MOPSOSS) and a version that only uses the first phase (called C-MOPSO) with 4000 (and 5000 for constrained problems) fitness function evaluations

Function	SC				IGD				Spread			
	C-MOPSOSS		C-MOPSO		C-MOPSOSS		C-MOPSO		C-MOPSOSS		C-MOPSO	
	Mean	σ	Mean	σ	Mean	σ	Mean	σ	Mean	σ	Mean	σ
KURSAWE	0.0719	0.0319	0.3745	0.0685	**0.0005**	0.0000	0.0009	0.0001	**0.3978**	0.0257	0.6830	0.0652
ZDT1	0.4155	0.1699	**0.1071**	0.0737	**0.0018**	0.0011	**0.0018**	0.0006	**0.3190**	0.0634	0.7102	0.0841
ZDT2	0.3049	0.2377	**0.1197**	0.1704	0.0052	0.0064	**0.0037**	0.0048	**0.3984**	0.1108	0.5374	0.0795
ZDT3	0.3043	0.1511	**0.1404**	0.0839	**0.0047**	0.0033	0.0110	0.0045	**0.6462**	0.0635	1.1051	0.1057
ZDT4	**0.0000**	0.0000	0.7444	0.2291	**0.1065**	0.0421	0.8452	0.4025	**0.6992**	0.0771	0.9741	0.0201
ZDT6	0.7702	0.2254	**0.0465**	0.0894	0.0011	0.0006	**0.0007**	0.0007	**0.4261**	0.1557	0.6280	0.2688
DTLZ1	**0.1299**	0.1699	0.4067	0.2445	**0.3942**	0.2432	0.9439	0.2790	**0.9930**	0.0040	0.9939	0.0050
DTLZ2	0.1391	0.0947	**0.0627**	0.0672	**0.0006**	0.0001	0.0008	0.0003	0.7600	0.0686	**0.4643**	0.0688
DTLZ3	**0.0735**	0.1139	0.3521	0.2449	**0.8367**	0.2348	1.0328	0.3063	**0.9963**	0.0029	0.9967	0.0025
DTLZ4	**0.1604**	0.2792	0.1843	0.3085	**0.0222**	0.0043	0.0246	0.0033	**0.7345**	0.1168	0.7517	0.1175
OSYCZKA	**0.2077**	0.2261	0.4020	0.2560	**0.0020**	0.0011	0.0026	0.0013	**0.9667**	0.0173	0.9793	0.0156
KITA	0.3857	0.1014	**0.2055**	0.0512	**0.0009**	0.0001	0.0029	0.0015	**0.5620**	0.0964	0.8585	0.1252
WELBEAM	**0.2131**	0.2377	0.5533	0.2366	**0.0047**	0.0059	0.0085	0.0048	**0.7050**	0.0992	0.7226	0.0969
SPD RED	**0.0203**	0.0970	0.3297	0.1459	**0.0027**	0.0002	0.0034	0.0013	**0.9996**	0.0000	0.9999	0.0001

Figure 10. Pareto fronts generated by C-MOPSO for all the 14 test functions adopted

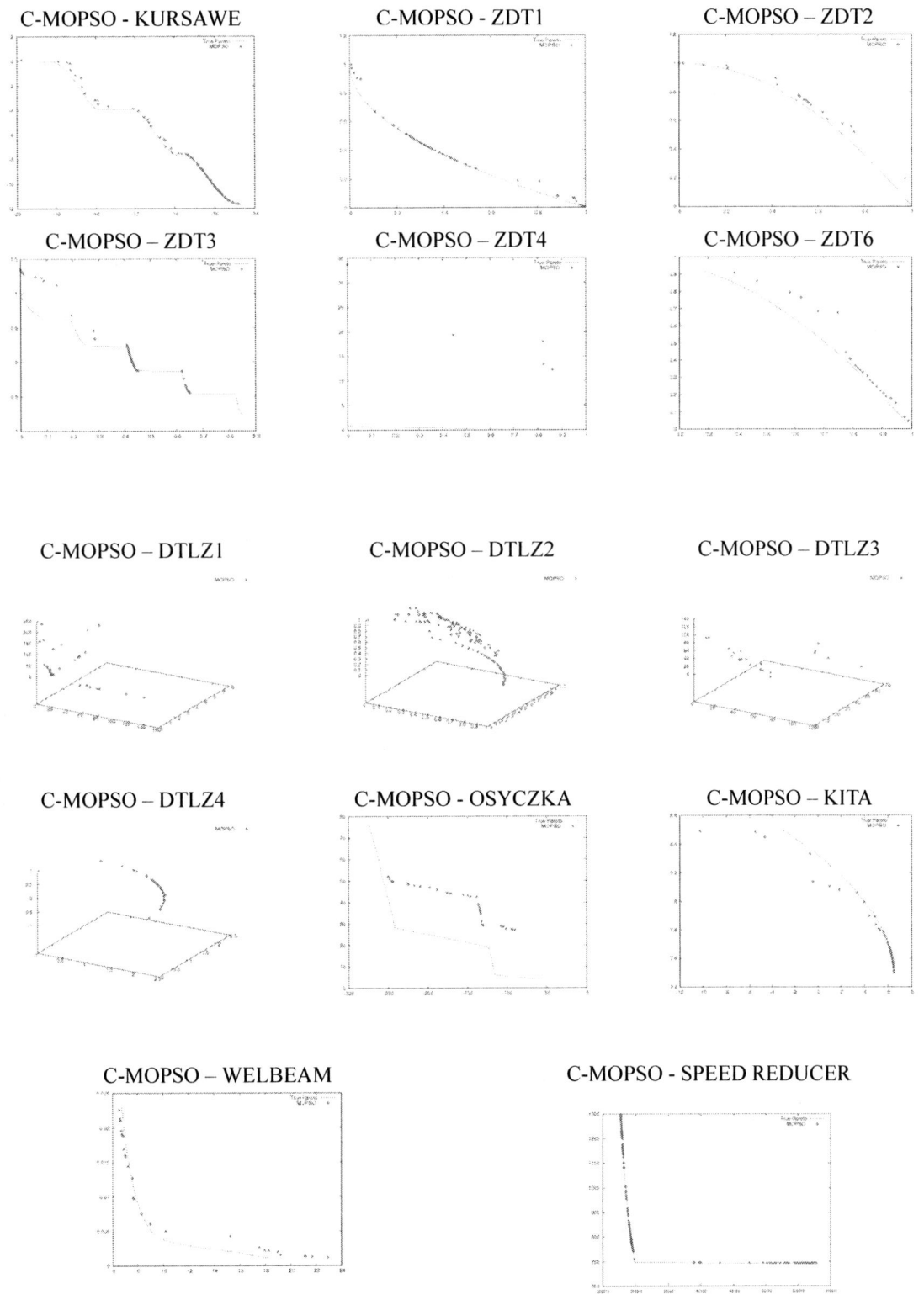

Figure 11. Pareto fronts generated by C-MOPSOSS for all the 14 test functions adopted

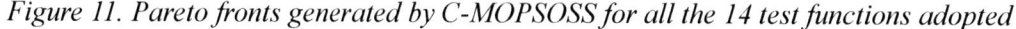

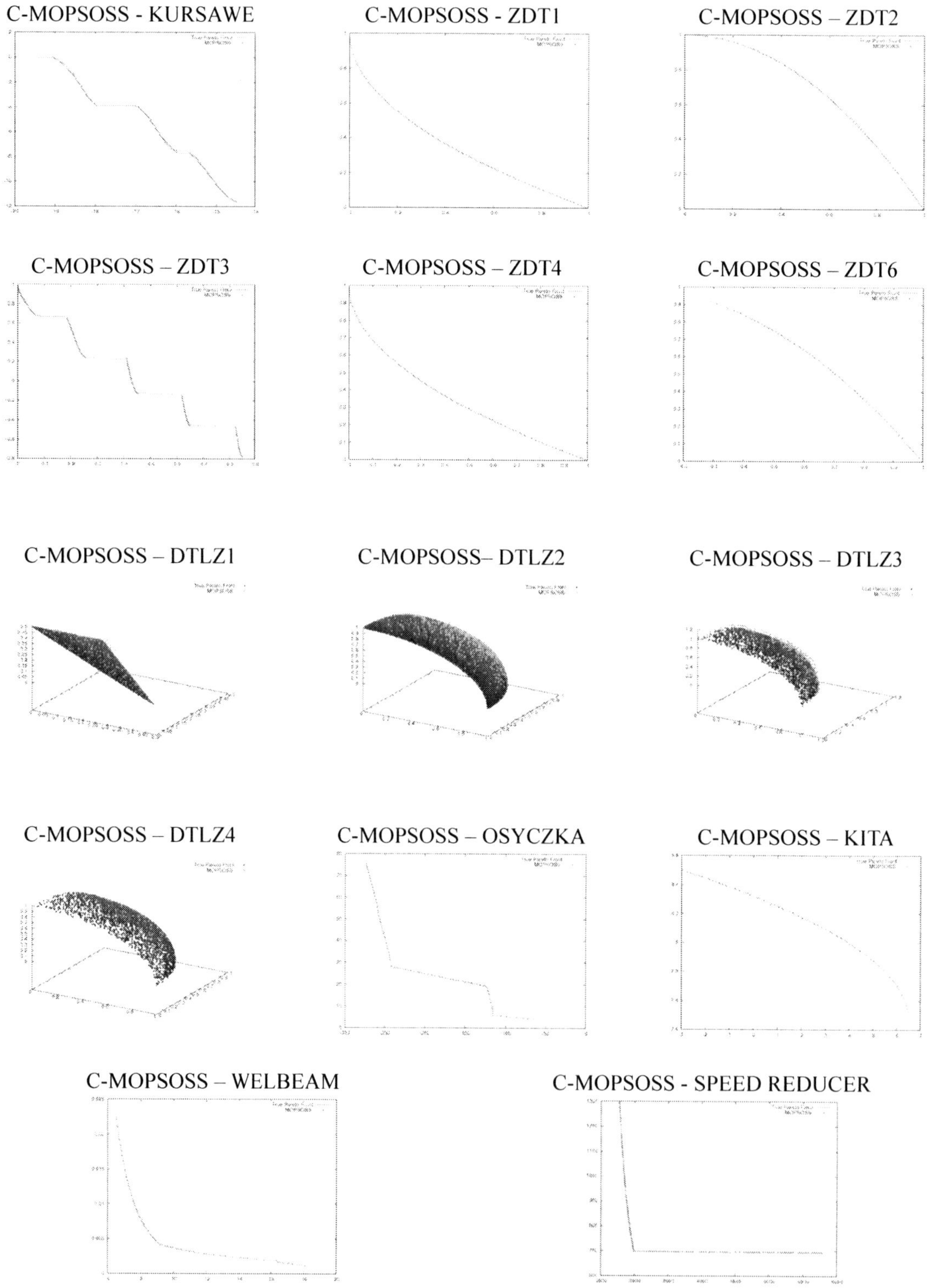

Table 5. Number of Fitness Function Evaluations required to reach the true Pareto front in all the test problems adopted

Function	# eval	Function	# eval
Kursawe	7,000	DTLZ2	7,000
ZDT1	7,000	DTLZ3	150,000
ZDT2	7,000	DTLZ4	150,000
ZDT3	7,000	OSYCZKA	30,000
ZDT4	30,000	KITA	10,000
ZDT6	7,000	WELDED BEAM	10,000
DTLZ1	150,000	SPEED REDUCER	7,000

CONCLUSION

We have presented a hybrid between a MOEA based on PSO and a local search mechanism based on scatter search to solve both unconstrained and constrained multi-objective optimization problems. This hybrid combines the high convergence rate of PSO with the good neighborhood exploration capabilities of the scatter search algorithm. We have also found out that the leader selection scheme adopted in PSO is a key element of our algorithm, since it is responsible of the high convergence that our approach requires. With SS we observe that the selection of solutions closer to the Pareto front generates smooth moves that give us more solutions closer to the true Pareto front of the problem being solved. Our approach also adopts the concept of ε-dominance to produce well-distributed sets of nondominated solutions. The results obtained are very competitive with respect to the NSGA-II in problems whose dimensionality goes from 3 up to 30 decision variables.

The main aim of this chapter has been to present practitioners a tool that they can use in applications in which each fitness function evaluation consumes a considerable amount of CPU time (such applications are common in areas such as aeronautical engineering). In those cases, the approach proposed in this chapter may provide reasonably good approximations of the true Pareto front at an affordable computational cost.

FUTURE RESEARCH DIRECTIONS

The design of highly efficient multi-objective particle swarm optimizers is an area that certainly deserves more research. Next, some of the most promising future research directions within this topic are briefly described.

One interesting path for future work is to improve the performance of the PSO approach proposed in this chapter. The leader selection mechanism is of particular interest, since it is known to be a critical element in any multi-objective particle swarm optimizer (Branke & Mostaghim, 2006). Additionally, the implementation adopted for the ε-dominance mechanism needs to be improved, since it currently loses the extremes of the Pareto front when dealing with segments that are almost horizontal or vertical. A variation of ε-dominance such as the one proposed in (Hernández-Díaz, Santana-Quintero, Coello Coello, & Molina, 2006) could be adopted to deal with this problem. Additionally, the ideas presented in this chapter may also serve as a basis to design entirely new multi-objective particle swarm optimizers whose main design emphasis is efficiency.

Another interesting path for future research is the exploration of self-adaptation and online adaptation schemes that allow the design of parameter-less multi-objective particle swarm optimizers. In order to reach this goal, it is necessary to have an in-depth knowledge of the behavior of multi-objective particle swarm optimizers when dealing with a wide variety of different test problems (see for example: Toscano Pulido, 2005). However, a proper setting of the parameters of a multi-objective particle swarm optimizer is not an easy task, and a lot of research is still needed in this direction. Nevertheless, progress in this research area would allow the design of mechanisms to properly deal with the (potentially wide) variety of situations that could arise in practice.

Although we propose in this chapter the use of scatter search as a diversification mechanism, other techniques are also possible (see for example: Hernández-Díaz, Santana-Quintero, Coello Coello, Caballero, & Molina, 2006, in which

Table 6. MOP test functions

WELDED BEAM (Ragsdell & Phillips, 1975)	
Definition	**Bounds**
$F = (f_1(\vec{x}), f_2(\vec{x}))$ where: $f_1(\vec{x}) = 1.1047 \cdot h^2 \cdot l + 0.04811 \cdot t \cdot b \cdot (14.0 + l)$ $f_2(\vec{x}) = \delta(\vec{x})$ subject to: $$g_1(\vec{x}) \equiv 13600 - \tau(\vec{x}) \geq 0,$$ $$g_2(\vec{x}) \equiv 30000 - \sigma(\vec{x}) \geq 0,$$ $$g_3(\vec{x}) \equiv b - h \geq 0,$$ $$g_4(\vec{x}) \equiv P_c - 6000 \geq 0.$$ where: $$\tau(\vec{x}) = \sqrt{\frac{(\tau')^2 + (\tau'')^2 + (l \cdot \tau' \cdot \tau'')}{\sqrt{0.25(l^2 + (h+t)^2)}}},$$ $$\tau' = \frac{6000}{\sqrt{2}hl},$$ $$\tau'' = \frac{6000(14 + 0.5l)\sqrt{0.25(l^2 + (h+t)^2)}}{2\{0.707hl(l^2/12 + 0.25(h+t)^2)\}},$$ $$\sigma(\vec{x}) = \frac{504000}{t^2 b},$$ $$P_c(\vec{x}) = 64746.022(1 - 0.0282346t)tb^3.$$	$0.125 \leq h, b \leq 5$ $0.1 \leq l, t \leq 10.0$
SPEED REDUCER (Golinski, 1970)	

Table 6. continued

$F = (f_1(\vec{x}), f_2(\vec{x}))$ where: $$f_1(\vec{x}) = \begin{array}{c} 0.7854 x_1 \cdot x_2^2 (3.3333 x_3^2 + 14.9334 x_3 - 43.0934) - \\ 1.5079(x_6^2 + x_7^2)x_1 + 7.477(x_6^3 + x_7^3) + \\ 0.7854(x_4 \cdot x_6^2 + x_5 \cdot x_7^2) \end{array}$$ $$f_2(\vec{x}) = \frac{\sqrt{\left(\frac{745 \cdot x_4}{x_2 x_3}\right)^2 + 1.69 e^7}}{0.1 x_6^3}$$ subject to: $$g_1(\vec{x}) \equiv \frac{1}{x_1 \cdot x_2^2 \cdot x_3} - \frac{1}{27} \leq 0,$$ $$g_2(\vec{x}) \equiv \frac{1}{x_1 \cdot x_2^2 \cdot x_3^2} - \frac{1}{397.5} \leq 0,$$ $$g_3(\vec{x}) \equiv \frac{x_3^3}{x_2 \cdot x_3 \cdot x_6^4} - \frac{1}{1.93} \leq 0,$$ $$g_4(\vec{x}) \equiv \frac{x_5^3}{x_2 \cdot x_3 \cdot x_7^4} - \frac{1}{1.93} \leq 0,$$ $$g_5(\vec{x}) \equiv x_2 \cdot x_3 - 40 \leq 0,$$ $$g_6(\vec{x}) \equiv \frac{x_1}{x_2} - 12 \leq 0,$$ $$g_7(\vec{x}) \equiv 5 - \frac{x_1}{x_2} \leq 0,$$ $$g_8(\vec{x}) \equiv 1.9 - x_4 + 1.5 \cdot x_6 \leq 0,$$ $$g_9(\vec{x}) \equiv 1.9 - x_5 + 1.1 \cdot x_7 \leq 0,$$ $$g_{10}(\vec{x}) \equiv f_2 - 1300 \leq 0,$$ $$g_{11}(\vec{x}) \equiv \frac{\sqrt{\left(\frac{745 \cdot x_5}{x_1 \cdot x_2}\right)^2 + 1.575 e^8}}{0.1 \cdot x_6^3} - 1100 \leq 0.$$	$2.6 \leq x_1 \leq 3.6$ $0.7 \leq x_2 \leq 0.$ $17 \leq x_3 \leq 28$ $7.3 \leq x_4, x_5 \leq 8.3$ $2.9 \leq x_6 \leq 3.9$ $5.0 \leq x_7 \leq 5.5$

rough sets are adopted for this sake). It is worth noting, however, that attention must be paid to the computational cost of the diversification technique adopted, since such cost must be as low as possible in order to be of practical use.

A more extended use of multi-objective particle swarm optimizers in real-world applications is expected to happen within the next few years. The relative simplicity of implementation and ease of use of multi-objective particle swarm optimizers makes them a suitable candidate for practitioners to use. Thus, an important number of real-world applications of this sort of heuristic are expected to appear in the next few years.

REFERENCES

Alvarez-Benitez, J. E., Everson, R. M., & Fieldsend, J. E. (2005, March). A MOPSO algorithm based exclusively on Pareto dominance concepts. In C. A. C. Coello, A. H. Aguirre, & E. Zitzler

(Eds.), *Evolutionary multi-criterion optimization*. In *Proceedings of the Third International Conference, EMO 2005* (pp. 459–473), Guanajuato, México: Springer.

Bartz-Beielstein, T., Limbourg, P., Parsopoulos, K. E., Vrahatis, M. N., Mehnen, J., & Schmitt, K. (2003, December). Particle swarm optimizers for Pareto optimization with enhanced archiving techniques. In *Proceedings of the 2003 Congress on Evolutionary Computation (CEC'2003)* (Vol. 3, pp. 1780–1787), Canberra, Australia: IEEE Press.

Baumgartner, U., Magele, C., & Renhart, W. (2004, March). Pareto optimality and particle swarm optimization. *IEEE Transactions on Magnetics, 40*(2), 1172–1175.

Branke, J., & Mostaghim, S. (2006, September). About selecting the personal best in multi-objective particle swarm optimization. In T. P. Runarsson, H-G. Beyer, E. Burke, J. J. Merelo-Guervós, L. D. Whitley, & X. Yao (Eds.), *Parallel problem solving from nature—PPSN IX*, In *Proceedings of the 9th International Conference* (pp. 523–532). Reykjavik, Iceland: Springer. *Lecture notes in computer science* (Vol. 4193).

Coello Coello, C. A., & Cruz Cortés, N. (2005, June). Solving multi-objective optimization problems using an artificial immune system. *Genetic Programming and Evolvable machines, 6*(2), 163–190.

Coello Coello, C. A., & Salazar Lechuga, M. (2002, May). MOPSO: A proposal for multiple objective particle swarm optimization. In *Proceedings of the Congress on Evolutionary Computation (CEC'2002)* (Vol. 2, pp. 1051–1056), Piscataway, New Jersey: IEEE Service Center.

Coello Coello, C. A., Toscano Pulido, G., & Salazar Lechuga, M. (2004, June). Handling multiple objectives with particle swarm optimization. *IEEE Transactions on Evolutionary Computation, 8*(3), 256–279.

Coello Coello, C. A., Van Veldhuizen, D. A., & Lamont, G. B. (2002). *Evolutionary algorithms for solving multi-objective problems*. New York: Kluwer Academic Publishers.

Deb, K. (2001). *Multi-objective optimization using evolutionary algorithms*. John Wiley & Sons.

Deb, K. & Agrawal, R. B. (1995). Simulated binary crossover for continuous search space. *Complex Systems, 9*, 115–148.

Deb, K., Pratap, A., Agarwal, S., & Meyarivan, T. (2002, April). A fast and elitist multi-objective genetic algorithm: NSGA–II. *IEEE Transactions on Evolutionary Computation, 6*(2), 182–197.

Deb, K., Thiele, L., Laumanns, M., & Zitzler, E. (2005). Scalable test problems for evolutionary multi-objective optimization. In A. Abraham, L. Jain, & R. Goldberg (Eds.), *Evolutionary multi-objective optimization. Theoretical advances and applications*, (pp. 105–145). Springer.

Eshelman, L. J. & Schaffer, J. D. (1993). Real-coded genetic algorithms and interval-schemata. In L. D. Whitley, (Ed.), *Foundations of genetic algorithms 2*, (pp. 187–202). California: Morgan Kaufmann Publishers.

Fieldsend, J. E. & Singh, S. (2002, September). A multi-objective algorithm based upon particle swarm optimisation, An efficient data structure and turbulence. In *Proceedings of the 2002 U.K. Workshop on Computational Intelligence* (pp. 37–44), Birmingham, UK.

Glover, F. (1977). Heuristic for integer programming using surrogate constraints. *Decision Sciences, 8*, 156–166.

Glover, F. (1994). Tabu search for nonlinear and parametric optimization (with links to genetic algorithms). *Discrete Applied Mathematics, 49*(1-3), 231–255.

Glover, F. (1998). A template for scatter search and path relinking. In *AE '97: Selected papers from the third European conference on artificial evolution*, (pp. 13–54). London, UK: Springer-Verlag.

Golinski J. (1970). Optimal synthesis problems solved by means of nonlinear programming and random methods. *Journal of Mechanisms, 5,* 287 – 309.

Hernández-Díaz, A. G., Santana-Quintero, L. V., Coello Coello, C., & Molina, J. (2006, March). *Pareto-adaptive ε-dominance* (Tech. Rep. No. EVOCINV-02-2006). México: Evolutionary computation group at CINVESTAV, Sección de Computación, Departamento de Ingeniería Eléctrica, CINVESTAV-IPN.

Hernández-Díaz, A. G., Santana-Quintero, L. V., Coello Coello, C., Caballero, R., & Molina, J. (2006, July). A new proposal for multi-objective optimization using differential evolution and rough sets theory. In M. K. et al., (Eds.), *2006 genetic and evolutionary computation conference (GECCO'2006),* (Vol. 1, pp. 675–682). Seattle, Washington: ACM Press.

Kennedy, J. & Eberhart, R. C. (2001). *Swarm intelligence.* California: Morgan Kaufmann Publishers.

Kita, H., Yabumoto, Y., Mori, N., & Nishikawa, Y. (1996, September). Multi-objective optimization by means of the thermodynamical genetic algorithm. In H-M. Voigt, W. Ebeling, I. Rechenberg, & H-P. Schwefel, (Eds.), *Parallel problem solving from nature—PPSN IV (*pp. 504–512*),* Berlin, Germany: Springer-Verlag.

Knowles, J. D. & Corne, D. W. (2000). Approximating the nondominated front using the Pareto archived evolution strategy. *Evolutionary Computation, 8*(2), 149–172.

Kursawe, F. (1991, October). A variant of evolution strategies for vector optimization. In H. P. Schwefel & R. Männer, (Eds.), *Parallel problem solving from nature.* In *Proceedings of the 1st Workshop, PPSN I,* (Vol. 496, pp. 193–197), Berlin, Germany: Springer-Verlag.

Laguna, M. & Martí, R. (2003). *Scatter search: Methodology and implementations in C.* Kluwer Academic Publishers.

Laumanns, M., Thiele, L., Deb, K., & Zitzler, E. (2002, Fall). Combining convergence and diversity in evolutionary multi-objective optimization. *Evolutionary Computation, 10*(3), 263–282.

Mahfouf, M., Chen, M-Y., & Linkens, D. A. (2004, September). Adaptive weighted particle swarm optimisation for multi-objective optimal design of alloy steels. *Parallel problem solving from nature - PPSN VIII,* (pp. 762–771). Birmingham, UK: Springer-Verlag.

Moore, J. & Chapman, R. (1999). *Application of particle swarm to multi-objective optimization.* Unpublished manuscript, Department of Computer Science and Software Engineering, Auburn University.

Mostaghim, S. & Teich, J. (2003, April). Strategies for finding good local guides in multi-objective particle swarm optimization (MOPSO). In *2003 IEEE SIS Proceedings,* (pp. 26–33). Indianapolis, IN: IEEE Service Center.

Osyczka, A. & Kundu, S. (1995). A new method to solve generalized multicriteria optimization problems using the simple genetic algorithm. *Structural Optimization, 10,* 94–99.

Parsopoulos, K. E., Tasoulis, K. E., & Vrahatis, K. E. (2004, February). Multi-objective optimization using parallel vector evaluated particle swarm optimization. In *Proceedings of the IASTED International Conference on Artificial Intelligence and Applications (AIA 2004),* (Vol. 2, pp. 823–828). Innsbruck, Austria: ACTA Press.

Ragsdell, K. E. & Phillips, D. T. (1975). Optimal design of a class of welded structures using geometric programming. *Journal of Engineering for Industry Series B, B*(98), 1021–1025.

Reyes Sierra, M. & Coello Coello, C. A. (2005, June). Fitness inheritance in multi-objective particle swarm optimization. In *2005 IEEE Swarm Intelligence Symposium (SIS'05)* (pp. 116–123). Pasadena, California: IEEE Press.

Reyes-Sierra, M. & Coello Coello, C. A. (2006). Multi-objective particle swarm optimizers: A survey of the state-of-the-Art. *International Journal of Computational Intelligence Research, 2*(3), 287–308.

Schaffer, J. D. (1985). Multiple objective optimization with vector evaluated genetic algorithms. *Genetic algorithms and their applications: Proceedings of the first international conference on genetic algorithms* (pp. 93–100). Lawrence Erlbaum.

Smith, R. E., Dike, B. A., & Stegmann, S. A. (1995). Fitness inheritance in genetic algorithms. *SAC '95: Proceedings of the 1995 ACM symposium on applied computing* (pp. 345–350). Nashville, Tennessee: ACM Press.

Toscano Pulido, G. (2005). *On the use of self-adaptation and elitism for multi-objective particle swarm optimization.* Unpublished doctoral dissertation, Computer Science Section, Department of Electrical Engineering, CINVESTAV-IPN, Mexico.

Veldhuizen, D. A. V. & Lamont, G. B. (1998). *Multi-objective evolutionary algorithm research: A history and analysis* (Tech. Rep. No. TR-98-03), Wright-Patterson AFB, Ohio: Department of Electrical and Computer Engineering, Graduate School of Engineering, Air Force Institute of Technology.

Veldhuizen, D. A. V. & Lamont, G. B. (2000, July). On measuring multi-objective evolutionary algorithm performance. *2000 congress on evolutionary computation* (Vol. 1, pp. 204–211). Piscataway, New Jersey: IEEE Service Center.

Zitzler, E., Deb, K., & Thiele, L. (2000, Summer). Comparison of multi-objective evolutionary algorithms: Empirical results. *Evolutionary Computation, 8*(2), 173–195.

Zitzler, E. & Thiele, L. (1999, November). Multi-objective evolutionary algorithms: A comparative case study and the strength Pareto approach. *IEEE Transactions on Evolutionary Computation, 3*(4), 257–271.

ADDITIONAL READING

There are several good (general) references on particle swarm optimization. The following are suggested as additional readings:

1. Engelbrecht, A. P. (2005). *Fundamentals of computational swarm intelligence.* John Wiley & Sons, Ltd.
2. Kennedy, J. & Eberhart, R. C. (2001). *Swarm intelligence.* San Francisco, California: Morgan Kaufmann Publishers.

There are also several references that focus on evolutionary multi-objective optimization and others that specifically deal with multi-objective particle swarm optimizers. See for example:

1. Coello Coello, C. A., Van Veldhuizen, D. A., & Lamont, G. B. (2002). *Evolutionary algorithms for solving multi-objective problems.* New York: Kluwer Academic Publishers.
2. Coello Coello, C. A., Toscano Pulido, G. & Salazar Lechuga, M. (2004, June). Handling multiple objectives with particle swarm optimization. *IEEE Transactions on Evolutionary Computation, 8*(3), 256-279.
3. Deb, K. (2001). *Multi-objective optimization using evolutionary algorithms.* Chichester, UK: John Wiley & Sons.
4. Reyes-Sierra, M. & Coello Coello, C. A. (2006). Multi-objective particle swarm optimizers: A survey of the state-of-the-art. *International Journal of Computational Intelligence Research, 2*(3), 287-308.

5. Tan, K. C., Khor, E. F., & Lee, T.H. (2005). *Multi-objective evolutionary algorithms and applications*. London: Springer-Verlag.
6. Toscano-Pulido, G., Coello Coello, C. A., & Santana-Quintero, L. V. (2007). EMOPSO: A multi-objective particle swarm optimizer with emphasis on efficiency. In S. Obayashi, K. Deb, C. Poloni, T. Hiroyasu, & T. Murata (Eds.), *Evolutionary multi-criterion optimization, 4th International Conference, EMO 2007* (pp. 272-285). *Lecture notes in computer science* (Vol. 4403). Matshushima, Japan: Springer.

Finally, there are also several papers dealing with real-world applications of multi-objective particle swarm optimizers that are worth reading. See for example:

1. Baltar, A. M. & Fontane, D. G. (2006, March). A generalized multi-objective particle swarm optimization solver for spreadsheet models: Application to water quality. In *Proceedings of Hydrology Days 2006*, Fort Collins, Colorado.
2. Gill, M. K., Kaheil, Y. H., Khalil, A., Mckee, M., & Bastidas, L. (2006, July 22). Multi-objective particle swarm optimization for parameter estimation in hydrology. *Water Resources Research, 42*(7).
3. Reddy, M. J. & Kumar, D. N. (2007, January). An efficient multi-objective optimization algorithm based on swarm intelligence for engineering design. *Engineering Optimization, 39*(1), 49-68.

ENDNOTES

[*] Carlos A. Coello Coello acknowledges support from CONACyT project No 45683-Y.

[a] *BLX-α* crossover is commonly used for real numbers encoding. This operator generates an offspring between two real numbers *a* and *b*, randomly selected from an interval of width $2 \cdot |a-b|$ centered on the mean of the *a* and *b* values.

[b] The NSGA-II used in this work was obtained from http://www.iitk.ac.in/kangal/codes.shtml using the parameters suggested by its authors (Deb et al., 2002).

[c] The MOPSO used was obtained from http://www.cs.cinvestav.mx/~EVOCINV/software.html using the parameters suggested by its authors in (Coello Coello et. al, 2004)

[d] In ZDT4, MOPSO only generates a few solutions, but since they lie on the true Pareto front, the solutions produced by our C-MOPSOSS cannot dominate them, and vice versa. This explains the zero value obtained.

Chapter V
Multi-Objective Optimization Using Artificial Immune Systems

Licheng Jiao
Xidian University, P.R. China

Maoguo Gong
Xidian University, P.R. China

Wenping Ma
Xidian University, P.R. China

Ronghua Shang
Xidian University, P.R. China

ABSTRACT

The human immune system (HIS) is a highly evolved, parallel and distributed adaptive system. The information processing abilities of HIS provide important aspects in the field of computation. This emerging field is referring to as the Artificial Immune Systems (AIS). In recent years, AIS have received significant amount of interest from researchers and industrial sponsors. Applications of AIS include such areas as machine learning, fault diagnosis, computer security and optimization. In this chapter, after surveying the AIS for multi-objective optimization, we will describe two multi-objective optimization algorithms using AIS, the Immune Dominance Clonal Multi-objective Algorithm (IDCMA), and the Nondominated Neighbor Immune Algorithm (NNIA). IDCMA is unique in that its fitness values of current dominated individuals are assigned as the values of a custom distance measure, termed as Ab-Ab affinity, between the dominated individuals and one of the nondominated individuals found so far. According to the values of Ab-Ab affinity, all dominated individuals (antibodies) are divided into two kinds, subdominant antibodies and cryptic antibodies. And local search only applies to the subdominant antibodies while the cryptic antibodies are redundant and have no function during local search, but they can become subdominant (active) antibodies during the subsequent evolution. Furthermore, a new immune operation, Clonal Proliferation is provided to enhance local search. Using the Clonal Proliferation operation, IDCMA reproduces individuals and selects their improved maturated progenies after local search, so single individuals can exploit their surrounding space effectively and the newcomers yield a broader exploration of the search space. The performance comparison of IDCMA with MISA, NSGA-II, SPEA, PAES, NSGA, VEGA, NPGA and HLGA in solving six well-known multi-objective function optimization problems and nine multi-objective 0/1 knapsack problems shows that IDCMA has a good performance in converging to approximate Pareto-optimal fronts with a good distribution. NNIA solves multi-objective optimization problems by using a nondominated neighbor-based selection technique, an immune inspired operator, two heuristic search operators and elitism. The unique selection technique of NNIA only selects minority isolated nondominated individuals in population. The selected individuals are then cloned proportionally to their crowding-distance values before heuristic search. By using the nondominated neighbor-based selection and proportional cloning, NNIA pays more attention to the less-crowded regions of the current trade-off front. We compare NNIA with NSGA-II, SPEA2, PESA-II, and MISA in solving five DTLZ problems, five ZDT problems and three low-dimensional problems. The statistical analysis based on three performance metrics including the Coverage of two sets, the Convergence metric, and the Spacing, show that the unique selection method is effective, and NNIA is an effective algorithm for solving multi-objective optimization problems.

INTRODUCTION

The human immune system (HIS) is a highly evolved, parallel and distributed adaptive system. The information processing abilities of HIS provide important aspects in the field of computation. This emerging field is referring to as the Immunological Computation, Immunocomputing or Artificial Immune Systems (AIS) (Tarakanov & Dasgupta, 2000) which can be defined as computational systems inspired by theoretical immunology and observed immune functions, principles and models, which are applied to problem solving (de Castro & Timmis, 2002a). In recent years, AIS have received a significant amount of interest from researchers and industrial sponsors. Some of the first work in applying HIS metaphors was undertaken in the area of fault diagnosis (Ishida, 1990). Later work applied HIS metaphors to the field of computer security (Forrest, Perelson, Allen, & Cherukuri, 1994), which seemed to act as a catalyst for further investigation of HIS as a metaphor in such areas as Anomaly Detection (Gonzalez, Dasgupta, & Kozma, 2002), Pattern Recognition (Carter, 2000; Timmis, Neal, & Hunt, 2000; White, & Garrett, 2003), Job Shop Scheduling (Hart & Ross, 1999; Coello Coello, Rivera, & Cortes, 2003), Optimization (de Castro & Von Zuben, 2002; Jiao &Wang, 2000) and Engineering Design Optimization (Gong, Jiao, Du, & Wang, 2005; Hajela, Yoo, & Lee, 1997).

In this chapter, after surveying the AIS for optimization, we will describe two multi-objective optimization algorithms using AIS, the Immune Dominance Clonal Multi-objective Algorithm (IDCMA) and the Nondominated Neighbor Immune Algorithm (NNIA). IDCMA is unique in that its fitness values of current dominated individuals are assigned as the values of a custom distance measure, termed as Ab-Ab affinity, between the dominated individuals and one of the nondominated individuals found so far. According to the values of Ab-Ab affinity, all dominated individuals (antibodies) are divided into two kinds, subdominant antibodies and cryptic antibodies. And local search only applies to the subdominant antibodies while the cryptic antibodies are redundant and have no function during local search, but they can become subdominant (active) antibodies during the subsequent evolution. Furthermore, an immune operation, Cloning is provided to enhance local search. Using the Cloning operation, IDCMA reproduces individuals and selects their improved maturated progenies after local search. NNIA solves multi-objective optimization problems by using a nondominated neighbor-based selection technique, an immune inspired operator, two heuristic search operators and elitism. The nondominated neighbor-based selection technique selects partial less-crowded nondominated individuals to perform cloning, recombination and hypermutation. The selection only performs on nondominated individuals, so we do not assign fitness to dominated individuals, and the fitness value of each current nondominated individual is the average distance of two nondominated individuals on either side of this individual along each of the objectives, which is called crowding-distance and proposed in NSGA-II (Deb, Pratap, Agarwal, & Meyarivan, 2002). The cloning operator clones each selected individual proportionally to its fitness value, viz. the individuals with larger crowding-distance values are reproduced more times. Then, recombination and static hypermutation are performed on each clone.

The remainder of this chapter is organized as follows: Section 2 describes related background including immune system inspired optimization algorithms and five terms used in this chapter. Section 3 describes the Immune Dominance Clonal Multi-objective Algorithm and experimental study on combinatorial MO problems. Section 4 describes the Nondominated Neighbor Immune Algorithm and experimental study on five DTLZ problems (Deb, Thiele, Laumanns, & Zitzler, 2002), five ZDT problems (Zitzler, Deb, & Thiele, 2000) and three low-dimensional problems. In Section 5, concluding remarks are presented. Finally, the future research directions are given.

RELATED BACKGROUND

The ability of the immune system to respond to an antigen relies on the prior formation of an incredibly diverse population of B cells and T cells. The specificity of both the B-cell receptors (BCRs) and T-cell receptors (TCRs), that is the epitope, is created by a remarkable genetic mechanism. Each receptor is created even though the epitope it recognizes may never have been present in the body. If an antigen with that epitope should enter the body, those few lymphocytes able to bind to it will do so. If they also receive a second costimulatory signal, they may begin repeated rounds of mitosis. In this way, clones of antigen-specific lymphocytes (B and T) develop providing the basis of the immune response. This phenomenon is called clonal selection (Abbas, Lichtman, & Pober, 2000).

The majority of immune system inspired optimization algorithms are based on the applications of the clonal selection and hypermutation (Hart & Timmis, 2005). The first immune optimization algorithm proposed by Fukuda, Mori, and Tsukiyama (1993) that included an abstraction of clonal selection to solve computational problems. But the clonal selection algorithm for optimization has been popularized mainly by de Castro and Von Zuben's CLONALG (de Castro, & Von Zuben, 2002). CLONALG selects part fittest antibodies to clone proportionally to their antigenic affinities. The hypermutation operator performs an affinity maturation process inversely proportional to the fitness values generating the matured clone population. After computing the antigenic affinity of the matured clone population, CLONALG creates randomly part new antibodies to replace the lowest fitness antibodies in current population and retain best antibodies to recycle. de Castro and Timmis (2002) proposed an artificial immune network called opt-aiNet for multimodal optimization. In opt-aiNet, antibodies are part of an immune network and the decision about the individual which will be cloned, suppressed or maintained depends on the interaction established by the immune network. Garrett has presented an attempt to remove all the parameters from clonal selection algorithm (Garrett, 2004). This method attempts to self-evolve various parameters during a single run. Cutello and Nicosia proposed an immune algorithm for optimization called opt-IA (Cutello, Nicosia, & Pavone, 2004; Cutello, Narzisi, Nicosia, & Pavone, 2005). Opt-IA solves optimization problems by using three immune operators, cloning, hypermutation and aging, and a standard evolutionary operator, $(\mu + \lambda)$-selection operator. As far as multi-objective optimization is concerned, MISA (Coello Coello, & Cortes, 2002; Coello Coello, & Cortes, 2005) may be the first attempt to solve general multi-objective optimization problems using AIS. MISA encodes the decision variables of the problem to be solved by binary strings, clones the Nondominated and feasible solutions, and applies two types of mutation to the clones and other individuals, respectively. Luh, Chueh, and Liu (2003) proposed a multi-objective Immune Algorithm (MOIA) and then adapted it to deal with constrained multi-objective problems (Luh, Chueh, & Liu, 2003). MOIA uses binary representation with each variable of the candidate solutions represented by a heavy chain part (the most significant bits) and a light chain (less significant bits), and implements a local search procedure around the most promising solutions of the population. Campelo, Guimaraes, Saldanha, Igarashi, Noguchi, Lowther, and Ramirez (2004) proposed the Multi-Objective Clonal Selection Algorithm (MOCSA) by combining ideas from CLONALG and opt-AINet in a MO-AIS algorithm for real-valued optimization. In MOCSA, the quality values are calculated using nondominated sorting. The population is sorted based on these values, and good solutions are selected for cloning. MOCSA uses real-coding and Gaussian mutation similarly to opt-AINet. The number of clones in the proliferation phase depends on the ranking of the individual in the nondominated fronts. More recently, Freschi and Repetto (2005) proposed a vector Artificial Immune System (VAIS) for solving multi-objective optimization problems based on the opt-aiNet. VAIS adopted the flowchart of opt-aiNet and the fitness assignment method in SPEA2 with some simplification that for Nondominated individuals the fitness is the strength defined in SPEA2 and for dominated individuals the fitness is the number of individuals which dominate them. Cutello, Narzisi, and Nicosia (2005) modified the (1+1)-PAES using two immune inspired operators, cloning and hypermutation, and applied the improved PAES for solving the protein structure prediction problem. Campelo, Guimaraes, and Igarashi (2007) have made a recent survey of artificial immune systems for multi-objective optimization, which covers most of the references referred to this topic.

Most of the immune system inspired optimization algorithms essentially evolve solutions to problems via repeated application of a cloning, mutation and selection cycle to a population of candidate solutions and remaining good solutions in the population. Just as Hart and Timmis (2005) said, anyone familiar with the EA literatures will recognize all of these features as equally applicable to an EA. It may be due to the striking similarity between the functioning of immune system and the adaptive biological evolution. In particularly, the central processes involved in the production of antibodies, genetic recombination and mutation, are the same ones responsible for the biological evolution of species (de Castro & Von Zuben, 2002).

In order to describe the algorithm well, we define the terms used in this chapter as follows.

Antigen Ψ

In immunology, an antigen is any substance that causes immune system to produce antibodies against it. In this chapter, for multi-objective optimization problem,

$$(P) \begin{cases} \max F(x) = (f_1(x), f_2(x), ... f_p(x))^T \\ \text{subject to} \quad g_i(x) \leq 0 \quad i=1,2,\cdots m \end{cases} \quad (1)$$

where $x = (x_1, x_2, ... x_d)$ is called the decision vector, d is the variable dimension, $p \geq 2$ is the number of objective functions, and m is the number of constraints, the antigen Ψ is defined as the objective vector $F(x)$.

Antibody and Antibody Population

In this chapter, B cells, T cells and antigen-specific lymphocytes are generally called antibodies. An antibody is a representation of a candidate solution of an antigen. The antibody $b = b_1 b_2 ... b_l$ with coding length l, is the coding of variable x, denoted by $b = e(x)$, and x is called the decoding of antibody b, expressed as $x = e^{-1}(b)$.

Set I is called antibody space, namely $b \in I$. An antibody population,

$$B = (b_1, b_2, \cdots, b_n), \quad b_k \in I, \quad 1 \leq k \leq n \quad (2)$$

is an n-dimensional group of antibody b, where the positive integer n is the antibody population size.

Ab-Ag Affinity ∂

Ab-Ag Affinity is the affinity between an antibody and an antigen. The Ab-Ag Affinity between antibody $b = e(x)$ and the antigen Ψ in equation (1) is defined as,

$$\partial(b, \Psi) \triangleq F\left(e^{-1}(b)\right) = \left(f_1\left(e^{-1}(b)\right), f_2\left(e^{-1}(b)\right), ... f_p\left(e^{-1}(b)\right)\right)^T \quad (3)$$

Ab-Ab Affinity Ω

Ab-Ab Affinity is the affinity between two antibodies. The Ab-Ab Affinity between binary coding antibodies $b_1 = b_{1,1} b_{1,2} ... b_{1,l}$ and $b_2 = b_{2,1} b_{2,2} ... b_{2,l}$ is defined as, (see equation (4)).

Where $|\cdot|$ denotes the cardinality of a set and $b_{1,0} \neq b_{2,0}$, $b_{1,l+1} \neq b_{2,l+1}$. If the coding of antibodies is not the binary string, it should be converted to binary string in advance.

For example, if $b_1 = 11000010001$ and $b_2 = 11010110101$, then the number of genes matched between the two antibodies is $\left|\{b_i^1 | b_{1,i} = b_{2,i}, i=1,2,3,\cdots,l\}\right| = 8$, the matched gene segments whose length are greater than 2 are '110', '10' and '01', and the corresponding lengths are 3, 2 and 2, so $\Omega(b_1, b_2) = 8 + 3^2 \times 1 + 2^2 \times 2 = 25$.

Dominant Antibody

For the antigen Ψ shown in equation (1), the antibody b_i is a dominant antibody in antibody population $B = \{b_1, b_2, ..., b_n\}$, if and only if there is no antibody $b_j (j=1,2,...n \wedge j \neq i)$ in antibody population B satisfied the equation (5),

Equation (4).

$$\Omega(b_1, b_2) \triangleq \left|\{b_i^1 | b_{1,i} = b_{2,i}, i=1,2,3,\cdots,l\}\right| + \sum_{j=2}^{l}\left(j^2 \times \left|\begin{matrix}\{b_i^j | b_{1,i}b_{1,i+1}\cdots b_{1,i+m} = b_{2,i}b_{2,i+1}\cdots b_{2,i+j} \\ \cap b_{1,i-1} \neq b_{2,i-1} \cap b_{1,i+j+1} \neq b_{2,i+j+1}, i=1,2,3,\cdots,l-j\}\end{matrix}\right|\right)$$

$$\left(\forall k \in \{1,2,\cdots p\}, f_k\left(e^{-1}(b_j)\right) \leq f_k\left(e^{-1}(b_i)\right)\right)$$
$$\wedge \left(\exists l \in \{1,2,\cdots p\}, f_l\left(e^{-1}(b_j)\right) < f_l\left(e^{-1}(b_i)\right)\right) \quad (5)$$

So the dominant antibodies are the nondominated individuals in current population B.

IMMUNE DOMINANCE CLONAL MULTI-OBJECTIVE ALGORITHM

Description of the Algorithm

In this section, we describe a novel artificial immune system algorithm for multi-objective optimization, termed as Immune Dominance Clonal Multi-objective Algorithm (IDCMA). IDCMA is composed of three operations which are the Immune Dominance Recognizing Operation (IDRO), the Immune Dominance Clone Operation (IDCO) and the Dominance Clonal Selection Operation (DCSO). Antibody populations at time k are represented by time-dependent variable matrices.

Immune Dominance Recognizing Operation

IDRO is the process of constructing the initial dominant antibody population, the initial subdominant antibody population and the initial cryptic antibody population.

Algorithm 1: Immune Dominance Recognizing Operation

- **Step 1:** Randomly generate the initial antibody population $A(0)$, and compute the Ab-Ag affinities of the antibodies of $A(0)$.
- **Step 2:** Copy all the dominant antibodies in $A(0)$ to form the initial dominant antibody population $D(0)$.
- **Step 3:** Replace the dominant antibodies in $A(0)$ by new antibodies generated randomly.
- **Step 4:** Randomly Select a dominant antibody d_s from $D(0)$ and compute the values of Ab-Ab affinity between the antibodies of $A(0)$ and the antibody d_s.
- **Step 5:** Select n_s antibodies with the largest Ab-Ab affinities from $A(0)$ to form the initial subdominant antibody population $S(0)$, and other antibodies constitute the initial cryptic antibody population $C(0)$.

Immune Dominance Clone Operation

IDCO includes the cloning operation, recombination operation and mutation operation on the subdominant antibody population. Here, we denote the population after cloning by $CS(k)$, and denote the populations before mutation and after mutation by $CRS(k)$ and $CRMS(k)$, respectively.

Algorithm 2: Immune Dominance Clone Operation

- **Step 1:** Get the antibody population $CS(k)$ by applying the cloning operation T^P to $S(k)$.
- **Step 2:** Get the antibody population $CRS(k)$ by replacing a random gene segment of each antibody in $CS(k)$ with the corresponding gene segment of the dominant antibody d_s.
- **Step 3:** Get the antibody population $CRMS(k)$ by applying a conventional mutation operation to the antibodies of $CRS(k)$ with probability p_m.

The cloning T^P on antibody population $S = \{s_1, s_2, s_3, ..., s_n\}$ is defined as:

$$T^P(s_1 + s_2 + \cdots + s_n) = T^P(s_1) + T^P(s_2) + \cdots + T^P(s_n)$$
$$= \{s_1^1 + s_1^2 + \cdots + s_1^{q_1}\} + \{s_2^1 + s_2^2 + \cdots + s_2^{q_2}\}$$
$$+ \cdots + \{s_n^1 + s_n^2 + \cdots + s_n^{q_n}\} \quad (6)$$

where $T_C^P(s_i) = \{s_i^1 + s_i^2 + ... + s_i^{q_i}\}$; $s_i^j = s_i$, $i = 1,2,...n$; $j = 1,2,...q_i$. $q_i \in [1, n_c]$, termed as clone scale, is a self-adaptive parameter, or set as an constant; n_c is a given value related to the upper limit of clone scale. The representation '+' is not the arithmetical operator, but only separates the antibodies here. $q_i = 1$ represents that there is no cloning on antibody s_i. It is obvious that cloning operation is similar to that of immunology, which is a simple process of asexual propagation. All the antibodies in subpopulation $\{s_i^1, s_i^2, ..., s_i^{q_i}\}$ result from the cloning on the same antibody s_i, and have the same property as antibody s_i.

Dominance Clonal Selection Operation

DCSO includes the update of dominant antibody population, the update of subdominant antibody population and the update of cryptic antibody population.

Algorithm 3: Dominance Clonal Selection Operation

- **Step 1:** Compute the Ab-Ag affinities of the antibodies in $CRMS(k)$.
- **Step 2:** Get the antibody population $A(k+1)$ by uniting the three antibody populations $CRMS(k)$, $D(k)$ and $C(k)$.
- **Step 3:** Copy all the dominant antibodies in $A(k+1)$ to form the temporary dominant antibody population $DT(k+1)$.
- **Step 4:** If the size of $DT(k+1)$ is no larger than a given parameter n_d, let $D(k+1)=DT(k+1)$, go to Step 6; Otherwise, go to Step 5.
- **Step 5:** Prune $DT(k+1)$ by means of clustering until the size of $DT(k+1)$ is n_d, let $D(k+1)=DT(k+1)$.
- **Step 6:** Replace the dominant antibodies in $A(k+1)$ by new antibodies generated randomly.
- **Step 7:** Randomly Select a dominant antibody d_s from $D(k+1)$; Compute the Ab-Ab affinities between the antibodies of $A(k+1)$ and the antibody d_s.
- **Step 8:** Select n_s antibodies with the largest Ab-Ab affinities from $A(k+1)$ to form the subdominant antibody population $S(k+1)$, and randomly select n_n antibodies from $A(k+1)$ to constitute the cryptic antibody population $C(k+1)$.

DCSO applies different update strategies to the three populations. At the beginning of DCSO, the combination of $CRMS(k)$, $D(k)$ and $C(k)$ is propitious to increase the global search ability. The update of dominant antibody population remains the diversity of nondominated individuals. The update of subdominant antibody population can select the dominant niche and assure the validity of the local search in the next generation. The existence of the cryptic antibody population preserves the population diversity.

The Main Loop

In this section, the Immune Dominance Clonal Multi-objective Algorithm (IDCMA) is put forward by integrating IDRO, IDCO and DCSO.

Algorithm 4: Immune Dominance Clonal Multi-objective Algorithm, IDCMA

- **Step 1:** Set the maximum number of iterations G_{max}, the size of Dominant antibody population n_d, the size of Subdominant antibody population n_s, the size of Cryptic antibody population n_n, and the upper limit of clone scale n_c. Set the mutation probability p_m, recombination probability p_c and coding length c. Randomly generate the antibody population $A(0)$ whose population size is $n_s + n_n$.
- **Step 2:** Get $D(0)$, $S(0)$ and $C(0)$ by applying IDRO to $A(0)$; $k=0$.
- **Step 3:** Get $CRMS(k)$ by applying IDCO to $S(k)$.
- **Step 4:** Get $D(k+1)$, $S(k+1)$ and $C(k+1)$ by applying DCSO to $CRMS(k)$, $D(k)$ and $C(k)$.

- **Step 5:** If $k<G_{max}$ is satisfied, $k=k+1$, go to Step 3; Otherwise, export $D(k+1)$ as the output of the algorithm, Stop.

Analysis of the Algorithm

It can be seen that IDCMA uses some well-known techniques such as storing the nondominated solutions previously found externally and performing clustering to reduce the number of nondominated solutions stored without destroying the characteristics of the trade-off front. But IDCMA is unique in its fitness assignment strategy and local search strategy.

Fitness Assignment and Population Evolution

In general, one can distinguish MOEAs where the objectives are considered separately, approaches that are based on the classical aggregation techniques and methods which make direct use of the concept of Pareto dominance (Zitzler, 1999). But in this chapter, we provide a novel fitness assignment method based on the Ab-Ab affinity which is a custom distance measure. In IDCMA, the fitness values of current dominated individuals are assigned as the values of Ab-Ab affinity between the dominated individuals and one of the nondominated individuals found so far. According to the values of Ab-Ab affinity, all dominated antibodies are divided into two kinds, subdominant antibodies and cryptic antibodies. And local search only applies to the subdominant antibodies while the cryptic antibodies are redundant and have no function during local search, but they can become subdominant antibodies during the subsequent evolution.

To make the process of population evolution in IDCMA clearly, we take a simple example in Figure 1. As can be seen in Figure 1(a), the objective space is covered by three nondominated individuals d_1, d_2, and d_3 found so far, hereinto d_2 is selected for calculating Ab-Ab affinities of all dominated individuals which are divided into two kinds, the subdominant antibodies r_1, r_2, r_3 and the cryptic antibodies n_1, n_2, n_3, n_4. Figure 1(b) shows the distribution of all the individuals in Ω space, namely, the distance between two antibodies denotes their Ab-Ab affinity. Because d_2 is the selected antibody for calculating Ab-Ab affinities, so the niche circled by the broken line around d_2 in Figure 1(b) is the local search region (in Ω space) in this generation. Figure 1(c) and (d) show the distribution of all individuals in objective space and Ω space after IDCO. Cloning copies the subdominant antibodies multiple times (double in this example). After recombination and mutation operation, these cloned antibodies distribute broad in the niche though few of them can beyond the niche such as p_{32} in Figure 1(d). Above niching search generates some new non-dominated individuals (as p_{12} in Figure 1(c) and (d)). After DCSO, the distribution of all antibodies in objective space and Ω space are shown in Figure 1(e) and (f). The new target niche becomes around another nondominated individual d_3', and the new subdominant antibodies ($r_1'=n_2, r_2'=n_3, r_3'=p_{11}$) and cryptic antibodies ($n_1'=n_1, n_2'=p_{32}, n_3'=r_3, n_4'=n_4$) are obvious different to those in the previous generation shown in Figure 1(a) and (b). IDCMA will do new local search in the niche circled by the broken line around d_3' in Figure 1(f) by the following IDCO.

Population Diversity

In order to approximate the Pareto-optimal set in a single run, MOEAs have to perform a multimodal search where multiple, widely different solutions should be found. Therefore, maintaining a diverse population is crucial for the efficacy of an MOEA (Zitzler, 1999).

IDCMA adopts three strategies to preserve the population diversity, that is, storing dominated individuals with less fitness externally, reducing the dominance antibody population by clustering and reinitialization.

Figure 1. Population evolution in IDCMA

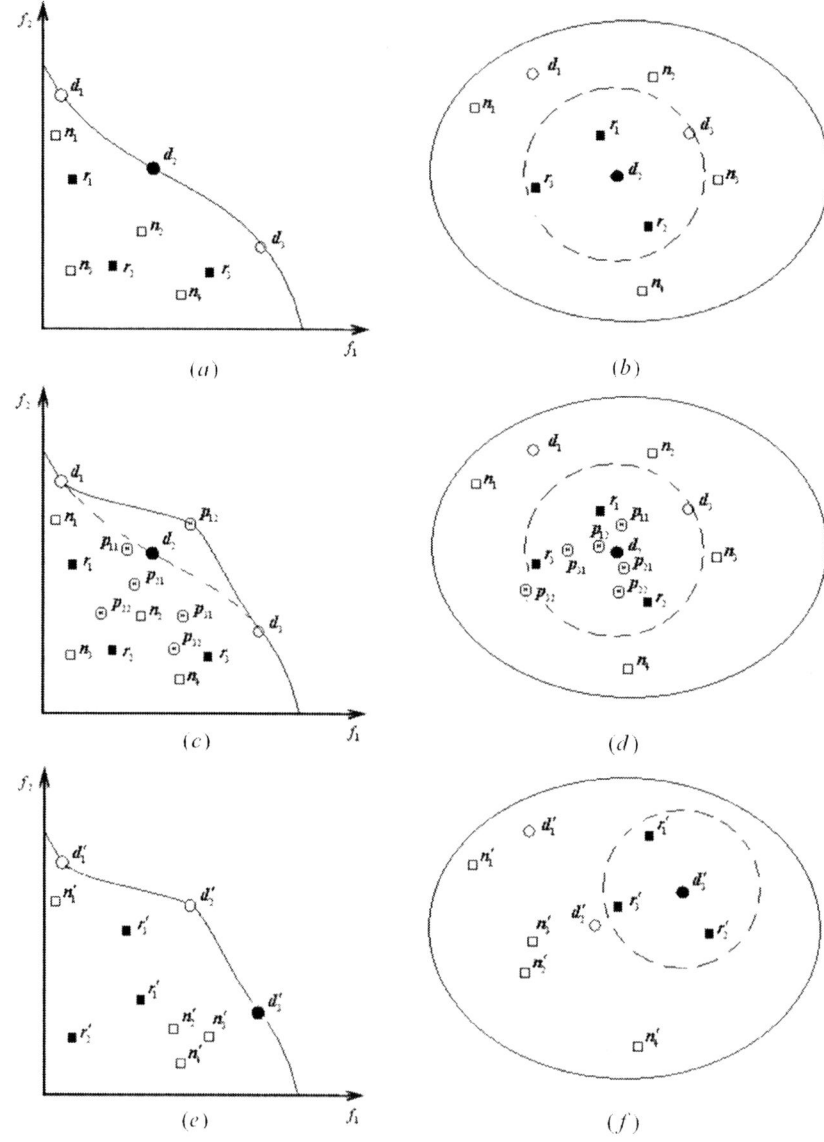

In IDCMA, the cryptic antibody population is set for storing dominated individuals with less Ab-Ab Affinity per generation. With this method, the individuals in cryptic antibody population are redundant and have no function during local search, but they can become subdominant antibodies during the subsequent evolution. So information can be hidden in an individual. A similar technique proposed by Goldberg (1989) can be found in some MOEAs.

Another technique to prevent premature convergence is to reinitialize the parts of the population at each generation, that is, a small number of new individuals generated randomly are introduced in DCSO.

A method that has been applied to prune the dominant antibody population while maintaining its characteristics is cluster analysis, which is widely used in MOEAs. We chose the average linkage method, which is also adopted in SPEA (Zitzler &Thiele, 1999).

Computational Complexity

Analyzing IDCMA's computational complexity is revealing. In this section, we only consider population size in computational complexity. Assuming that the size of dominant antibody population size is n_d, the subdominant antibody population size is n_s, the cryptic antibody population size is n_n, and the clone scale is n_c, then the time complexity of one iteration for the algorithm can be calculated as follows:

The time complexity for calculating Ab-Ag Affinities in IDRO is $O(n_s + n_n)$; The worst time complexity for update the dominant antibody population is $O((n_d + n_s \times n_c)^2)$; The time complexity for calculating the Ab-Ab Affinities of all dominated antibodies is $O(n_n + n_s \times n_c)$; The worst time complexity for update the subdominant antibody population and cryptic antibody population is $O((n_d + n_n + n_s \times n_c)\log(n_d + n_n + n_s \times n_c))$; The time complexity for Cloning is $O(n_s \times n_c)$; And the time complexity for recombination and mutation operation is $O(n_s \times n_c)$; The time complexity for calculating Ab-Ag Affinities in DCSO is $O(n_s \times n_c)$. So the worst total time complexity is

$$O((n_s + n_n)) + O((n_d + n_s \times n_c)^2) + O(n_n + n_s \times n_c) + O(n_s \times n_c)$$
$$+ O((n_d + n_n + n_s \times n_c)\log(n_d + n_n + n_s \times n_c)) + O(n_s \times n_c) + O(n_s \times n_c)$$
(7)

According to the operational rules of the symbol O, the worst time complexity of one generation for IDCMA can be simplified as follow:

$$O((n_d + n_s \times n_c)^2) + O((n_d + n_n + n_s \times n_c)\log(n_d + n_n + n_s \times n_c))$$
(8)

If we denote the total size of all populations as N, namely, $N = n_d + n_n + n_s \times n_c$, then the computational complexity of IDCMA is

$$O((n_d + n_s \times n_c)^2) + O((n_d + n_n + n_s \times n_c)\log(n_d + n_n + n_s \times n_c)) < O(N^2)$$
(9)

NSGA-II (Deb, Pratap, Agarwal, & Meyarivan, 2002) and SPEA2 (Zitzler, Laumanns, & Thiele, 2002) are two representative of the state-of-the-art in multi-objective optimization. As their authors' analysis, the worst computational complexities of NSGA-II and SPEA2 are $O(N^2)$ and $O((N + \bar{N})^3)$, respectively, where N is the size of population and $\bar{N}$ is the size of archive. Therefore, the computational complexities of IDCMA and NSGA-II are no worse than $O(N^2)$ which are much smaller than that of SPEA2. In fact, the cost of determining the Pareto optimal individuals in population dominates the computational complexity of IDCMA and NSGA-II while environmental selection dominates the computational complexity of SPEA2.

Experimental Study on Combinatorial MO Problems

The knapsack problem is an abstract of restricted resource problems with some purposes, which has broad projective background. A 0/1 knapsack problem is a typical combinatorial optimization problem with NP-hard (Zitzler &Thiele, 1999). In order to validate the algorithm, we compare IDCMA with another five MOEAs in solving nine multi-objective 0/1 knapsack problems. The five selected algorithms are SPEA (Zitzler & Thiele, 1999), VEGA (Schaffer, 1984), HLGA (Hajela & Lin, 1992), NPGA (Horn & Nafpliotis, 1993) and NSGA (Srinivas & Deb, 1994). The teat data sets are available from Zitzler's homepages (http://www.tik.ee.ethz.ch/~zitzler/testdata.html/), where two, three and four knapsacks with 250, 500, 750 items are taken under consideration.

The parameter settings of IDCMA are the same as that in Section V except the binary coding length *l* is equal to the number of items. A greedy repair method adopted in Zitzler and Thiele (1999) is also applied in IDCMA that the repair method removes items from the infeasible solutions step by step until all capacity constraints are fulfilled. The order in which the items are deleted is determined by the maximum profit/weight ratio per item. Thirty independent runs of IDCMA are performed per test problem. The reported results of SPEA, HLGA, NPGA, NSGA and VEGA are directly gleaned from Zitzler's website.

The direct comparisons of IDCMA with the other algorithms based on the coverage of two sets measure (Zitzler, 1999) are shown in Figure 2. For each ordered pair of algorithms, there is a sample of 30 values of the coverage of two sets measure per test problem according to the 30 runs performed.

Here, box plots are used to illustrate the distribution of these samples. The upper and lower ends of the box are the upper and lower quartiles, while a thick line within the box denotes the median and thin appendages summarize the spread and shape of the distribution. Each rectangle contains nine box plots representing the distribution of the measure values for a certain ordered pair of algorithms. The third box to the left relate to 2 knapsacks and (from left to right) 250,500,750 items. Correspondingly, the three middle box plots relate to 3 knapsacks and the three to the right relate to 4 knapsacks. The scale is 0 at the bottom and 1 at the top per rectangle.

Figure 2. Box plots based on the coverage of two sets measure

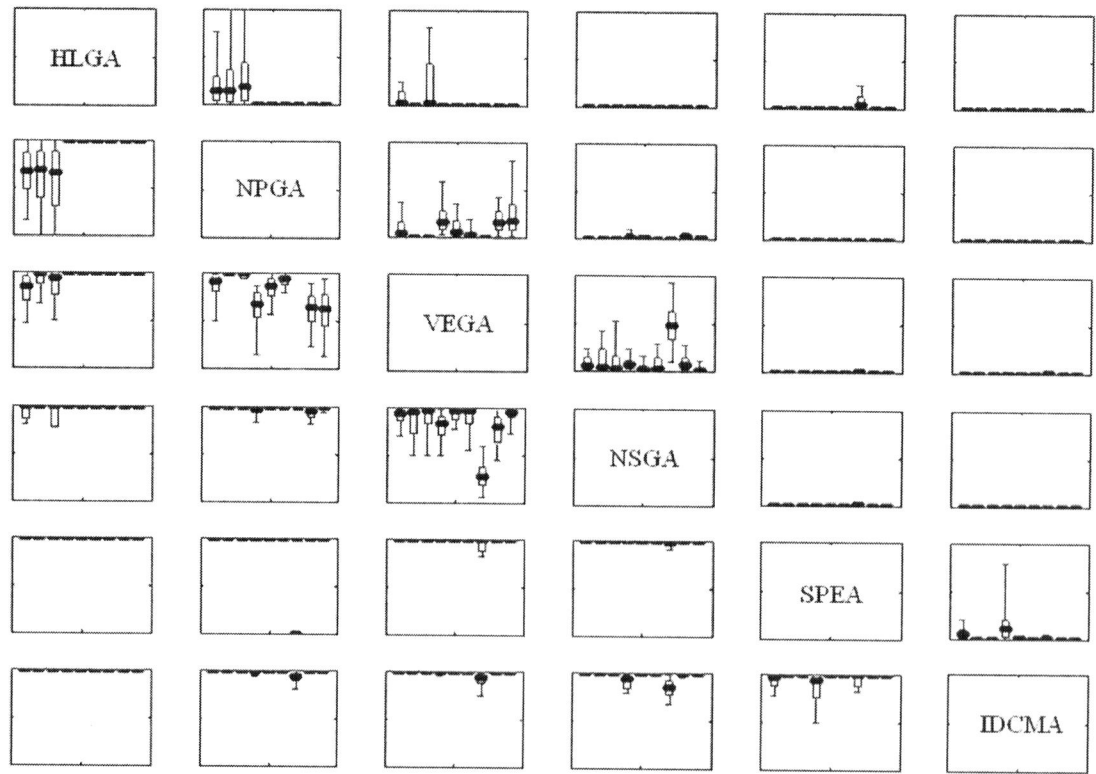

As Figure 2 shows, IDCMA achieves the best performance among these MOEAs in terms of the coverage metric. In detail, the solution sets obtained by IDCMA cover 100% of the nondominated solutions found by HLGA for all the nine test problems, and covers 100% of the nondominated solutions found by NPGA and NSGA for seven of the nine test problems, and covers 100% of the nondominated solutions found by VEGA for eight of the nine test problems, and covers 100% of the nondominated solutions found by SPEA for six of the nine test problems. In contrast, those algorithms except SPEA cover IDCMA less than 2% in all the 270 runs while SPEA covers IDCMA less than 15% on average.

For a typical example, the Pareto fronts of the problems with two knapsacks and 250, 500 and 750 items obtained by IDCMA, SPEA, NSGA, VEGA, NPGA and HLGA are shown in Figure 3. Here, the nondominated individuals regarding the first 5 runs are plotted. For better visualization, the points obtained by a particular method are connected by real lines.

Figure 3 illustrates that for the problems with two knapsacks, the Pareto fronts obtained by IDCMA dominate obviously the Pareto fronts

Figure 3. Pareto fronts for 2 knapsacks problems obtained by IDCMA, SPEA, NSGA, VEGA, NPGA, and HLGA

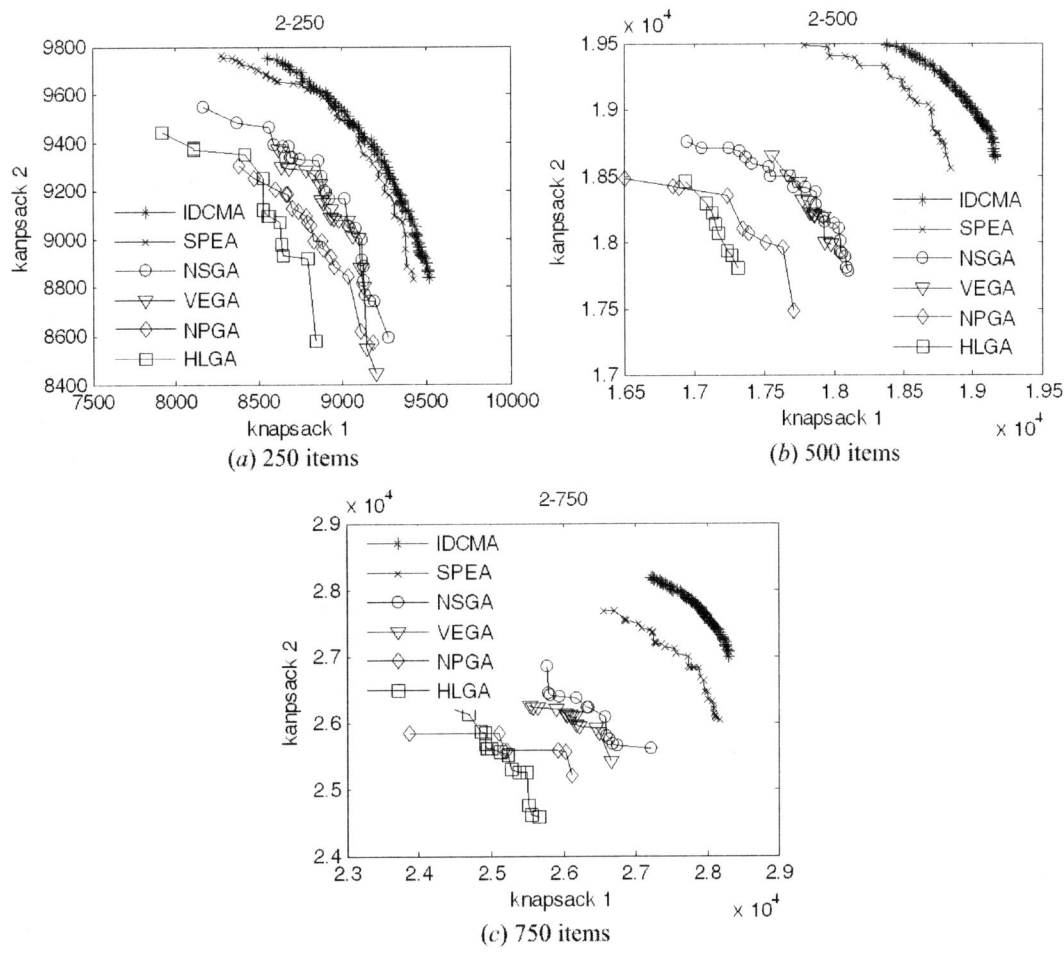

obtained by SPEA, NSGA, VEGA, NPGA and HLGA. Furthermore, IDMCA does much better than the other MOEAs in keeping the distribution of solutions uniformly. But the spread of the Pareto fronts obtained by IDCMA is narrower than those of SPEA and NSGA especially for the problem with 2 knapsacks and 750 items due to the fitness assignment method based on the Ab-Ab affinity did not guarantees the preservation of boundary solutions.

The experimental results reveal that IDCMA outperforms SPEA, HLGA, NPGA, NSGA and VEGA in solving the nine multi-objective combinatorial optimization problems in terms of the coverage metric. But IDCMA does a little worse than SPEA and NSGA in terms of the spread of the Pareto fronts due to the Ab-Ab affinity did not guaratees the preservation of boundary solutions. This disadvantage will be modified in the following algorithm, NNIA.

NONDOMINATED NEIGHBOR IMMUNE ALGORITHM

Description of the Algorithm

In this section, we describe a novel multi-objective optimization algorithm, termed as Nondominated Neighbor Immune Algorithm (NNIA). NNIA stores nondominated solutions found so far in an external population, called Dominant Population. Only partial less-crowded nondominated individuals, called active antibodies are selected to do proportional cloning, recombination, and static hypermutation (Cutello, Nicosia & Pavone, 2004). Furthermore, the population storing clones is called Clone Population. Dominant Population, Active Population and Clone Population at time t are represented by time-dependent variable matrices D_t, A_t and C_t respectively. The main loop of NNIA is as follows.

Algorithm 5: Nondominated Neighbor Immune Algorithm

Input: *Gmax* (maximum number of generations)
n_D (maximum size of Dominant Population)
n_A (maximum size of Active Population)
n_C (size of Clone Population)
Output: D_{Gmax+1} (final Pareto-optimal set)

- **Step 1—Initialization:** Generate an initial antibody population B_0 with the size n_D. Create the initial $D_0= \varphi$, $A_0 = \varphi$, and $C_0 = \varphi$. Set $t=0$.
- **Step 2—Update Dominant Population:** Identify dominant antibodies in B_t; Copy all the dominant antibodies to form the temporary *dominant population* DT_{t+1}; If the size of DT_{t+1} is no larger than n_D, let $D_{t+1}=DT_{t+1}$. Otherwise, calculate the crowding-distance values of all individuals in DT_{t+1}, sort them in descending order of crowding-distance, choose the first n_D individuals to form D_{t+1}.
- **Step 3—Termination:** If $t \geq Gmax$ is satisfied, export D_{t+1} as the output of the algorithm, Stop; Otherwise, $t=t+1$.
- **Step 4—Nondominated Neighbor-based Selection:** If the size of D_t is no larger than n_A, let $A_t=D_t$. Otherwise, calculate the crowding-distance values of all individuals in D_t, sort them in descending order of crowding-distance, choose the first n_A individuals to form A_t.
- **Step 5—Proportional Cloning Operator:** Get the clone population C_t by applying the proportional cloning T^C to A_t.
- **Step 6—Recombination and Hypermutation:** Perform recombination and hypermutation on C_t and set C'_t to the resulting population.
- **Step 7:** Get the antibody population B_t by combining the C'_t and D_t; go to Step 2.

When the number of dominant antibodies is larger than the maximum limitation and the size of dominant population is larger than the maximum size of active population, both the reduction of dominant population and the selection of active antibodies use the crowding-distance based truncation selection. The value of crowding-distance serves as an estimate of the perimeter of the cuboid formed by the nearest neighbors as the vertices in objective space. The crowding-distance assignment is described in full in Deb, Pratap, Agarwal, and Meyarivan (2002). The proportional cloning operation, recombination operation and hypermutation operation are described as follows.

Proportional Cloning

In immunology, Cloning means asexual propagation so that a group of identical cells can be descended from a single common ancestor, such as a bacterial colony whose members arise from a single original cell as the result of mitosis. In this study, the proportional cloning T^C on active population $A = (a_1, a_2, a_3, ..., a_{|A|})$ is defined as

$$T^C(a_1 + a_2 + \cdots + a_{|A|}) = T^C(a_1) + T^C(a_2) + \cdots + T^C(a_{|A|})$$
$$= \{a_1^1 + a_1^2 + \cdots + a_1^{q_1}\} + \{a_2^1 + a_2^2 + \cdots + a_2^{q_2}\} + \cdots + \{a_{|A|}^1 + a_{|A|}^2 + \cdots + a_{|A|}^{q_{|A|}}\} \quad (10)$$

where $T^C(a_i) = \{a_i^1 + a_i^2 + ... + a_i^{q_i}\}$; $a_i^j = a_i$, $i = 1, 2, ..., |A|$, $j = 1, 2, ... q_i$. q_i is a self-adaptive parameter, and $\sum_{i=1}^{|A|} q_i = n_C$, n_C is a given value of the size of the clone population. The representation + is not the arithmetical operator, but only separates the antibodies here. $q_i = 1$ denotes that there is no cloning on antibody a_i. In this study, the individual with larger crowding-distance value is reproduced more times, viz. the individual with larger crowding-distance value has a larger q_i. Because the crowding-distance values of boundary solutions are positive infinity, before computing the value of q_i for each active antibody, we set the crowding-distance values of the boundary individuals be equal to the double values of the maximum value of active antibodies except the boundary individuals. Then the values of q_i are calculated as

$$q_i = \left\lceil n_C \times \frac{i_{\text{distance}}}{\sum_{i=1}^{n_A} i_{\text{distance}}} \right\rceil, \quad (11)$$

where i_{distance} denotes the crowding-distance values of the i-th active antibodies. All the antibodies in sub-population $\{a_i^1 + a_i^2 + \cdots + a_i^{q_i}\}$ are resulted from the cloning on antibody a_i, and have the same property as a_i. In fact, cloning on antibody a_i is to make multiple identical copies of a_i. The aim is that the larger the crowding-distance value of an individual, the more times the individual will be reproduced. So more chances exist to do search in less-crowded regions of the trade-off fronts.

Recombination and Hypermutation

If $C = (c_1, c_2, c_3, ..., c_{|C|})$ is the resulting population from applying the proportional cloning to $A = (a_1, a_2, a_3, ..., a_{|A|})$, then the recombination T^R on clone population C is defined as

$$T^R(c_1 + c_2 + \cdots + c_{|C|}) = T^R(c_1) + T^R(c_2) + \cdots + T^R(c_{|C|})$$
$$= crossover(c_1, A) + crossover(c_2, A) + \cdots + crossover(c_{|C|}, A) \quad (12)$$

where $crossover(c_i, A)$, $i = 1, 2, ..., |C|$ denotes selecting equiprobably one individual from the two offsprings generated by a general crossover operator on clone c_i and an active antibody selected randomly from A.

In this study, we use static hypermutation operator (Cutello, Nicosia, & Pavone, 2004) on the clone population after recombination. Cutello, Nicosia, and Pavone (2004) designed three hypermutation methods, namely, static hypermutation (the number of mutations is independent from the fitness values), proportional hypermutation (the number of mutations is proportional to the fitness value), and inversely proportional hypermutation (the number of mutations is inversely proportional to the fitness value). We chose the static hypermutation in our algorithm for the following reasons:

1. The hypermutation operator is implemented on the clone population after recombination. If we chose the proportional hypermutation or the inversely proportional hypermutation, we have to calculate the fitness values for all the individuals of the clone population. However, in other phases of NNIA, the dominated individuals are not assigned fitness. Therefore we have to define a fitness assignment strategy to dominated individuals only for the hypermuation operator unless we use a mutation operator independent from the fitness values.
2. In order to reducing complexity, the fitness evaluation is as less as possible. Suppose we define a fitness assignment strategy suitable for the proportional hypermutation or the inversely proportional hypermutation, we have to calculate the fitness values of all recombined clones before mutation.
3. The experimental study in Cutello, Nicosia, and Pavone (2004) showed that the inversely proportional hypermutation did only slightly better than static and proportional hypermutation in solving the Trap function problems. But if the combination of multiple operators was not considered, the static hypermutation achieved the best results among the three hypermutation operators in solving the protein structure prediction problems.

Depending on the above reasons, we design the hypermutation operator as the static hypermutation operator. If $R = (r_1, r_2, r_3, \cdots, r_{|R|})$ is the clone population after recombination, then the static hypermutation operator T^H on clone population R is defined as

$$T^H(r_1 + r_2 + \cdots + r_{|R|}) = T^H(r_1) + T^H(r_2) + \cdots + T^H(r_{|R|})$$
$$= mutate(r_1) + mutate(r_2) + \cdots + mutate(r_{|R|})$$
(13)

where $mutate(r_i)$, $i = 1, 2, \cdots, |R|$ denotes changing each element of the variable vector r_i by a general mutation operator with probability p_m, so each

Figure 4. Population evolution of NNIA

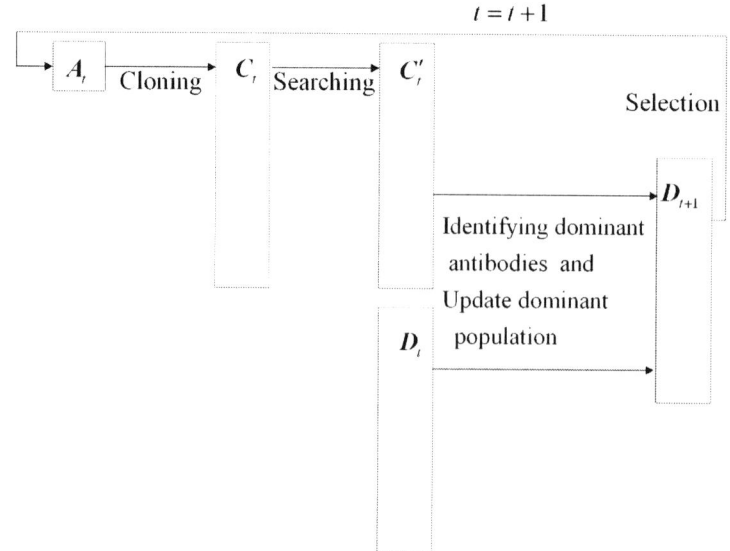

individual in the clone population R at each time step will undergo about $m \times p_m$ mutations, where m is the dimension of variable vector.

Fitness Assignment and Population Evolution

It can be seen that NNIA uses some well-known techniques such as storing the nondominated solutions previously found externally and reducing the number of nondominated solutions stored without destroying the characteristics of the trade-off front. Furthermore, NNIA adopts the nondominated neighbor-based selection. It is the same as NSGA-II in computing the crowding-distance; selection is therefore biased towards individuals with a high isolation value. NSGA-II needs to classify all individuals into several layers, and selection is performed on layer by layer until the population size is achieved. In NNIA, the dominant population is set as an external population for elitism. Nondominated neighbor-based selection only performs on the external population based on the crowding-distance. Only partial nondominated individuals (much less than nondominated individuals found so far) with high crowding-distance values are selected. And cloning, recombination and mutation only apply to the selected individuals (active antibodies). So in a single generation, only less-crowded individuals perform heuristic search in order to obtain more solutions in the less-crowded regions of the trade-off fronts. In contrast to NSGA-II, proportional cloning makes the less-crowded individuals have more chances to do recombination and mutation. The population evolution in a single generation at time t is shown in Figure 4.

Computational Complexity

Analyzing NNIA's computational complexity is revealing. In this section, we only consider population size in computational complexity. Assuming that the maximum size of dominant population is n_D, the maximum size of active population is n_A, the clone population size is n_C, then the time complexity of one generation for the algorithm can be calculated as follows:

The time complexity for identifying nondominated solutions in population is $O((n_D + n_C)^2)$; the worst time complexity for updating the dominant population is $O((n_D + n_C)\log(n_D + n_C))$; the worst time complexity for Nondominated neighbor-based selection is $O(n_D \log(n_D))$; the time complexity for cloning is $O(n_C)$; and the time complexity for recombination and mutation operation is $O(n_C)$. So the worst total time complexity is,

$$O((n_D + n_C)^2) + O((n_D + n_C)\log(n_D + n_C)) + O(n_D \log(n_D)) + O(n_C) + O(n_C) \quad (14)$$

According to the operational rules of the symbol O, the worst time complexity of one generation for NNIA can be simplified as

$$O((n_D + n_C)^2). \quad (15)$$

So the cost of identifying the Pareto optimal individuals in population dominates the computational complexity of NNIA.

Evaluation of NNIA'S Effectiveness

In this section, we compare PESA-II (Corne, Jerram, Knowles, & Oates, 2001), NSGA-II (Deb, Pratap, Agarwal & Meyarivan, 2002), SPEA2 (Zitzler, Laumanns, & Thiele, 2002), and MISA (Coello Coello & Cortes, 2005) with NNIA in solving 13 well-known multi-objective function optimization problems including three low-dimensional bi-objective problems, five ZDT problems (Zitzler, Deb, & Thiele, 2000) and five DTLZ problems (Deb, Thiele, Laumanns & Zitzler, 2002). The MOEA toolbox for Matlab 7.0 designed by the authors including NNIA, MISA, SPEA2, NSGA-II and PESA-II for solving the 13 problems and 20 other problems is available at the first author's homepage (http://see.xidian.

Table 1. Test problems used in this study

Problem	n	Variable bounds	Objective functions (minimize)
SCH	1	[-5,10]	$f_1(x) = \begin{cases} -x & \text{if } x \leq 1 \\ -2+x & \text{if } 1 < x < 3 \\ 4-x & \text{if } 3 < x \leq 4 \\ -4+x & \text{if } x > 4 \end{cases}$ $f_2(x) = (x-5)^2$
DEB	2	[0,1]	$f_1(x) = x_1$ $f_2(x) = (1+10x_2) \times [1 - (\frac{x_1}{1+10x_2})^2 - \frac{x_1}{1+10x_2}\sin(8\pi x_1)]$
KUR	3	[-5,5]	$f_1(x) = \sum_{i=1}^{n-1}\left(-10e^{(-0.2)\sqrt{x_i^2+x_{i+1}^2}}\right)$ $f_2(x) = \sum_{i=1}^{n}\left(\|x_i\|^{0.8} + 5\sin(x_i)^3\right)$
ZDT1	30	[0,1]	$f_1(x) = x_1$ $f_2(x) = g(x)\left[1 - \sqrt{x_1/g(x)}\right]$ $g(x) = 1 + 9\left(\sum_{i=2}^{n} x_i\right)/(n-1)$
ZDT2	30	[0,1]	$f_1(x) = x_1$ $f_2(x) = g(x)\left[1 - (x_1/g(x))^2\right]$ $g(x) = 1 + 9\left(\sum_{i=2}^{n} x_i\right)/(n-1)$
ZDT3	30	[0,1]	$f_1(x) = x_1$ $f_2(x) = g(x)\left[1 - \sqrt{x_1/g(x)} - \frac{x_1}{g(x)}\sin(10\pi x_1)\right]$ $g(x) = 1 + 9\left(\sum_{i=2}^{n} x_i\right)/(n-1)$
ZDT4	10	$x_1 \in [0,1]$ $x_i \in [-5,5]$ $i = 2,\cdots,n$	$f_1(x) = x_1$ $f_2(x) = g(x)\left[1 - \sqrt{x_1/g(x)}\right]$ $g(x) = 1 + 10(n-1) + \sum_{i=2}^{n}[x_i^2 - 10\cos(4\pi x_i)]$
ZDT6	10	[0,1]	$f_1(x) = 1 - \exp(-4x_1)\sin^6(4\pi x_1)$ $f_2(x) = g(x)\left[1 - (f_1(x)/g(x))^2\right]$ $g(x) = 1 + 9\left[\left(\sum_{i=2}^{n} x_i\right)/(n-1)\right]^{0.25}$
DTLZ1	$M+\|x_M\|-1$	[0,1]	$f_1(x) = \frac{1}{2}x_1 x_2 \cdots x_{M-1}(1+g(x_M))$ $f_2(x) = \frac{1}{2}x_1 x_2 \cdots (1-x_{M-1})(1+g(x_M))$ $\vdots$ $f_{M-1}(x) = \frac{1}{2}x_1(1-x_2)(1+g(x_M))$ $f_M(x) = \frac{1}{2}(1-x_1)(1+g(x_M))$ where $g(x_M) = 100\left[\|x_M\| + \sum_{x_i \in x_M}\left((x_i - 0.5)^2 - \cos(20\pi(x_i - 0.5))\right)\right]$

Table 1. continued

Problem	n	Variable bounds	Objective functions (minimize)
DTLZ2	$M+\|x_M\|-1$	[0,1]	$f_1(x) = (1+g(x_M))\cos(x_1\pi/2)\cos(x_2\pi/2)\cdots\cos(x_{M-2}\pi/2)\cos(x_{M-1}\pi/2)$ $f_2(x) = (1+g(x_M))\cos(x_1\pi/2)\cos(x_2\pi/2)\cdots\cos(x_{M-2}\pi/2)\sin(x_{M-1}\pi/2)$ $\vdots$ $f_{M-1}(x) = (1+g(x_M))\cos(x_1\pi/2)\sin(x_2\pi/2)$ $f_M(x) = (1+g(x_M))\sin(x_1\pi/2)$ where $g(x_M) = \sum_{x_i \in x_M}(x_i - 0.5)^2$
DTLZ3	$M+\|x_M\|-1$	[0,1]	$f_1(x) = (1+g(x_M))\cos(x_1\pi/2)\cos(x_2\pi/2)\cdots\cos(x_{M-2}\pi/2)\cos(x_{M-1}\pi/2)$ $f_2(x) = (1+g(x_M))\cos(x_1\pi/2)\cos(x_2\pi/2)\cdots\cos(x_{M-2}\pi/2)\sin(x_{M-1}\pi/2)$ $\vdots$ $f_{M-1}(x) = (1+g(x_M))\cos(x_1\pi/2)\sin(x_2\pi/2)$ $f_M(x) = (1+g(x_M))\sin(x_1\pi/2)$ where $g(x_M) = 100\left[\|x_M\| + \sum_{x_i \in x_M}\left((x_i - 0.5)^2 - \cos(20\pi(x_i - 0.5))\right)\right]$
DTLZ4	$M+\|x_M\|-1$	[0,1]	$f_1(x) = (1+g(x_M))\cos(x_1^\alpha\pi/2)\cos(x_2^\alpha\pi/2)\cdots\cos(x_{M-2}^\alpha\pi/2)\cos(x_{M-1}^\alpha\pi/2)$ $f_2(x) = (1+g(x_M))\cos(x_1^\alpha\pi/2)\cos(x_2^\alpha\pi/2)\cdots\cos(x_{M-2}^\alpha\pi/2)\sin(x_{M-1}^\alpha\pi/2)$ $\vdots$ $f_{M-1}(x) = (1+g(x_M))\cos(x_1^\alpha\pi/2)\sin(x_2^\alpha\pi/2)$ $f_M(x) = (1+g(x_M))\sin(x_1^\alpha\pi/2)$ where $g(x_M) = \sum_{x_i \in x_M}(x_i - 0.5)^2$, $\alpha = 100$
DTLZ6	$M+\|x_M\|-1$	[0,1]	$f_1(x) = x_1$ $f_2(x) = x_2$ $\vdots$ $f_{M-1}(x) = x_{M-1}$ $f_M(x) = (1+g(x_M))h(f_1,f_2,\cdots,f_{M-1},g)$ where $g(x_M) = 1 + \frac{9}{\|x_M\|}\sum_{x_i \in x_M} x_i$, $h(f_1,f_2,\cdots,f_{M-1},g) = M - \sum_{i=1}^{M}\left[\frac{f_i}{1+g}(1+\sin(3\pi f_i))\right]$

edu.cn/graduate/mggong). All the simulations run at a personal computer with P-*IV* 3.2G CPU and 2G RAM.

Experimental Setup

First, we describe the 13 test problems used in this study. The first three low-dimensional bi-objective problems were defined by (Deb, 1999; Schaffer, 1984) and (Kursawe, 1991), respectively. The next five ZDT problems were developed by (Zitzler, Deb & Thiele, 2000). The last five DTLZ problems were developed by (Deb, Thiele, Laumanns & Zitzler, 2002). We describe these problems in Table 1, where *n* denotes the number of variables. More details of them can be found in (Deb, 2001), (Zitzler, Deb & Thiele, 2000) and (Deb, Thiele, Laumanns & Zitzler, 2002). It is necessary to note that the performance of an MOEA in tackling multi-objective constrained optimization problems maybe largely depend on the constraint-handling technique used (Van Veldhuizen, 1999), so we do not mentioned side-constrained problems in this study. For DTLZ problems, in Section 4.2.2, we set the values of M and $|x_M|$ be the values suggested by Deb, Thiele, Laumanns, and Zitzler (2002) and Deb, Thiele, Laumanns, and Zitzler (2001), that is, $M=3$ and $|x_M|=5$ for DTLZ1, $M=3$ and $|x_M|=10$ for DTLZ2, DTLZ3 and DTLZ4, $M=3$ and $|x_M|=20$ for DTLZ6.

Zitzler, Thiele, Laumanns, Fonseca, and da Fonseca (2003) suggested that for an M-objective optimization problem, at least M performances are needed to compare two or more solutions and an infinite number of metrics to compare two or more set of solutions. Deb and Jain (2002) suggested a running performance metrics for measuring the convergence to the reference set at each generation of an MOEA run. As the reference (Khare, Yao, & Deb, 2003), in Section 4.2, we apply this metric only to the final Pareto-optimal set obtained by an MOEA to evaluate its performance. Zitzler, Thiele, Laumanns, Fonseca, and da Fonseca (2003) and Knowles, Thiele, and Zitzler (2006) have suggested that the power of unary quality indicators was restricted. So we choose a binary quality metric, coverage of two sets (Zitzler & Thiele, 1998). We also adopt the Spacing (Schott, 1995) metric to measure the diversity in population individuals. The three metrics are summarized as follows.

Coverage of Two Sets: Let A, B be two Pareto-optimal sets. The function I_C maps the ordered pair (A, B) to the interval [0, 1]:

$$I_C(A, B) \triangleq \frac{|\{b \in B; \exists a \in A : a \succeq b\}|}{|B|} \quad (16)$$

where $\succeq$ means dominate or equal (also called weakly dominate). The value $I_C(A, B)=1$ means that all decision vectors in B are weakly dominated by A. $I_C(A, B)=0$ implies no decision vector in B is weakly dominated by A. Note that always both directions have to be considered because $I_C(A, B)$ is not necessarily equal to $1 - I_C(A, B)$.

Convergence Metric: Let $P^* = (p_1, p_2, p_3, ..., p_{|P^*|})$ be the reference or target set of points on the true Pareto-optimal front and let $A = (a_1, a_2, a_3, ..., a_{|A|})$ be the final Pareto-optimal set obtained by an MOEA. Then for each point a_i in A the smallest normalized Euclidean distance to P^* will be:

$$d_i = \min_{j=1}^{|P^*|} \sqrt{\sum_{k=1}^{M} \left(\frac{f_k(a_i) - f_k(p_j)}{f_k^{max} - f_k^{min}} \right)^2} \quad (17)$$

Here, f_k^{max} and f_k^{min} are the maximum and minimum values of k-th objective function in P^*. The convergence metric is the average value of the normalized distance for all points in A.

$$C(A) \triangleq \frac{\sum_{i=1}^{|A|} d_i}{|A|} \quad (18)$$

The convergence metric represents the distance between the set of converged Pareto-optimal solutions and the true Pareto-optimal fronts. Hence lower values of the convergence metric represent good convergence ability. Similar metrics were proposed by Schott (1995), Rudolph (1998), Zitzler, Deb, & Thiele (2000) and Van Veldhuizen and Lamont (2000b) et al.

Spacing: Let A be the final Pareto-optimal set obtained by an MOEA. The function S,

$$S \triangleq \sqrt{\frac{1}{|A|-1} \sum_{i=1}^{|A|} (\bar{d} - d_i)^2} \quad (19)$$

Where,

$$d_i = \min_j \left\{ \sum_{k=1}^{M} |f_k(\boldsymbol{a}_i) - f_k(\boldsymbol{a}_j)| \right\}$$
$$\boldsymbol{a}_i, \boldsymbol{a}_j \in A \quad i, j = 1, 2, \cdots, |A| \quad (20)$$

$\bar{d}$ is the average value of all d_i, and M is the number of objective functions. A value of zero for this metric indicates all the Pareto-optimal solutions found are equidistantly spaced in objective space.

Comparison of NNIA with PESA-II, SPEA2, NSGA-II and MISA

In this Section, NNIA was compared with PESA-II, NSGA-II, SPEA2 and MISA. NSGA-II was proposed by Deb, Pratap, Agarwal, and Meyarivan (2002) as an improvement of NSGA by using a more efficient nondominated sorting method, elitism and a crowded comparison operator without specifying any additional parameters for diversity maintaining. SPEA2 was proposed by Zitzler, Laumanns, and Thiele (2002) as a revised version of SPEA by incorporating a revised fitness assignment strategy, a nearest neighbor density estimation technique and an enhanced archive truncation method. The revised fitness assignment strategy takes for each individual into account the number of individuals it dominates and it is dominated by. PESA-II was proposed by Corne, Jerram, Knowles, & Oates (2001) as a revised version of PESA by introducing a new selection technique, region-based selection. In region-based selection technique, selective fitness is assigned to the hyperboxes (Corne, Jerram, Knowles & Oates, 2001) in objective space instead of the Pareto-optimal individuals. Its update of auxiliary population (external population) also used the hyperboxes division. MISA (Coello Coello & Cortes, 2002; Coello Coello & Cortes, 2005) may be the first attempt to solve general multi-objective optimization problems using artificial immune systems. MISA encodes the decision variables of the problem to be solved by binary strings, clones the Pareto-optimal and feasible solutions, and applies two types of mutation to the clones and other individuals, respectively. MISA updates its external population by using the grid based techniques used in PAES (Knowles & Corne, 2000).

We use the simulated binary crossover (SBX) operator and polynomial mutation (Deb & Beyer, 2001) for NNIA, PESA-II, NSGA-II and SPEA2. The SBX and polynomial mutation has been adopted in many MOEA literatures (Deb, Pratap, Agarwal & Meyarivan, 2002; Deb & Jain, 2002; Igel, Hansen & Roth, 2007; Khare, Yao & Deb, 2003; Zitzler, Laumanns, & Thiele, 2002). Before the actual experimentation, some tuning of the parameters involved was required. Finding the values of parameters for which an MOEA works best is a difficult MOP in itself. We tuned the parameter values on DTLZ2 and DTLZ3 as (Khare, Yao, & Deb, 2003) when obtained the best value of the Convergence metric. The tuned parameter values are listed in Table 2. Because MISA is a binary-coded algorithm, the mutation is bit-flip with the probability described in Coello Coello and Cortes (2005). For SPEA2, we use a population of size 100 and an external population of size 100. For NSGA-II, the population size is

Table 2. Tuned parameter values

Parameter	PESA-II	SPEA2	NSGA-II	NNIA
Crossover probability p_c	0.8	0.8	0.8	1
Distribution index for SBX	15	15	15	15
Mutation probability p_m	1/n	1/n	1/n	1/n
Distribution index for polynomial mutation	20	20	20	20

Figure 5. Statistical Values of the Coverage of the two sets obtained by NNIA and PESA-II in solving the 13 problems. Here, box plots are used to illustrate the distribution of these samples. In a notched box plot the notches represent a robust estimate of the uncertainty about the medians for box-to-box comparison. Symbol '+' denote for outliers. The 13 plots denote the results of the 13 problems respectively. In each plot, the left box represents the distribution of $I_C(I,P)$ and the right box represents the distribution of $I_C(P,I)$.

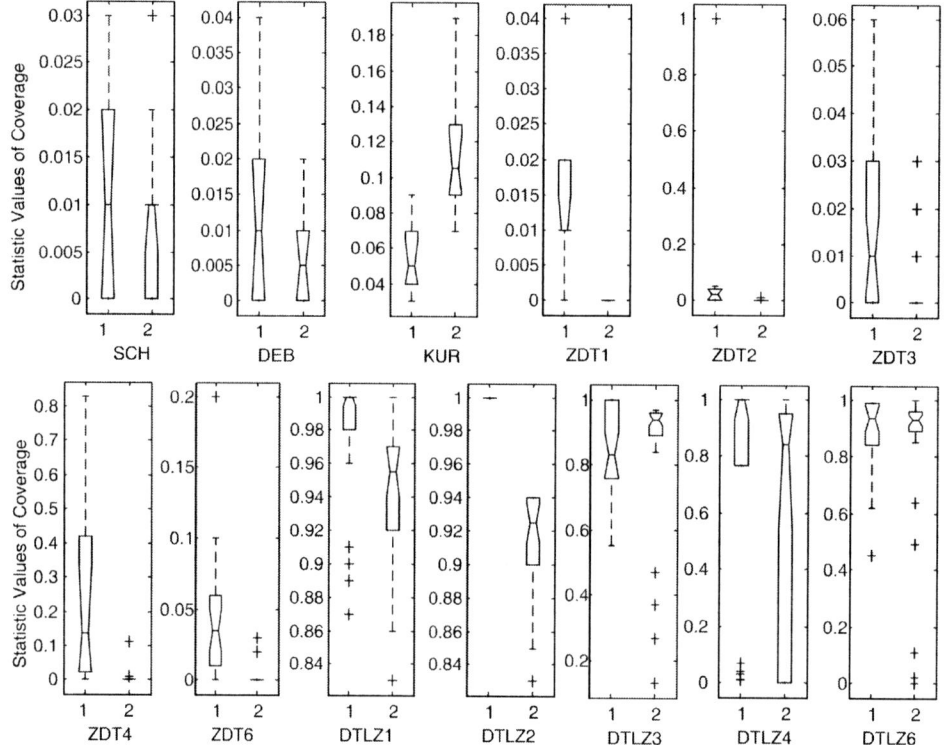

100. For PESA-II, the internal population size is 100, the archive size is 100, and the number of hyper-grid cells per dimension is 10. For NNIA, the maximum size of dominant population n_D = 100, the maximum size of active population n_A = 20, and the size of clone population n_C = 100. For MISA, the population size is 100, the size of the external population is 100, the total number of clones is 600, the number of grid subdivisions is 25, the four values are suggested by Coello Coello and Cortes (2005), and the coding length for each decision variable is 30. It is difficult to formulate the optimal and evidential stop criterion (Coello Coello, 2004) for an MOEA. Researchers usually stop the algorithm when the algorithm reaches a given number of iterations or function evaluations. In this section the number of function evaluations is kept at 50 000 (not including the function evaluations during initialization) for all the five algorithms.

In the following experiments, we performed 30 independent runs on each test problem. Figure 5, Figure 6, Figure 7 and Figure 8 show the box plots (McGill, Tukey, & Larsen, 1978) of NNIA against PESA-II, NSGA-II, SPEA2 and MISA based on the Coverage of two sets. In the following, **I** denotes the solution set obtained by NNIA, **P** denotes the solution set obtained by PESA-II, **S** denotes the solution set obtained by SPEA2, **N** denotes the solution set obtained by NSGA-II, and **M** denotes the solution set obtained by MISA.

The comparison between NNIA and PESA-II in the coverage of two sets shows that most of the values of $I_C(I,P)$ and $I_C(P,I)$ for the five DTLZ problems are greater than 0.5, therefore, the majority solutions obtained by PESA-II are weakly dominated by the solutions obtained by NNIA (Especially for DTLZ2, all the PESA-II's solutions are weakly dominated by NNIA's ones over 30 independent runs), while the majority solutions obtained by NNIA are also weakly dominated by the solutions obtained by PESA-II.

The box plots of the other eight problems show that only minority solutions are weakly dominated by each other. As the analysis in Zitzler, Thiele, Laumanns, Fonseca, and da Fonseca (2003), $0 < I_C(A,B) < 1$ and $0 < I_C(B,A) < 1$ shows neither A weakly dominates B nor B weakly dominates A, that is, A and B are incomparable. But if only the values of coverage be considered, the box plots of $I_C(I,P)$ are higher than the corresponding box plots of $I_C(P,I)$ in SCH, DEB, the five ZDT problems and the five DTLZ problems, while the box plot of $I_C(P,I)$ is higher than the corresponding box plot of $I_C(I,P)$ only in KUR. $I_C(I,P)$ denotes the ratio of the number of solutions obtained by PESA-II which are weakly dominated by the solutions obtained by NNIA to the total number of the solu-

Figure 6. Statistical Values of the Coverage of the two sets obtained by NNIA and NSGA-II in solving the 13 problems. The 13 plots denote the results of the 13 problems respectively. In each plot, the left box represents the distribution of $I_C(I,N)$ and the right box represents the distribution of $I_C(N,I)$.

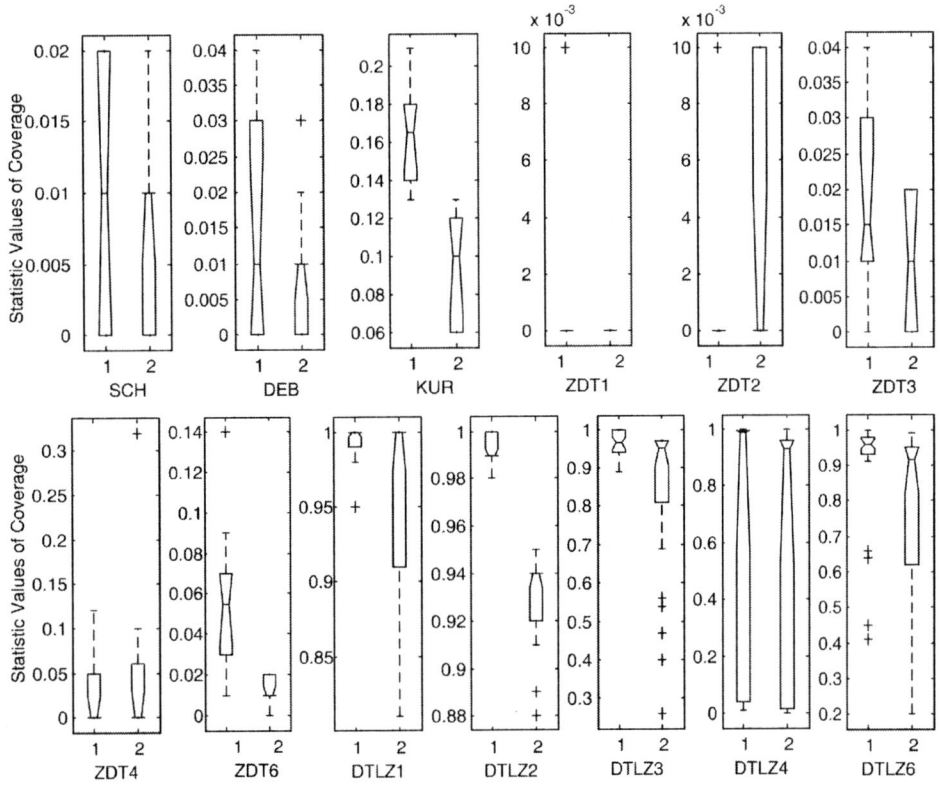

tions obtained by PESA-II in a single run. So in a sense (but neither ▷ –compatible nor ▷ –complete), NNIA did better than PESA-II in SCH, DEB, the five ZDT problems and the five DTLZ problems while PESA-II did better than NNIA in KUR as far as the Coverage is concerned.

The 13 plots denote the results of the 13 problems respectively. In each plot, the left box represents the distribution of $I_C(I,S)$ and the right box represents the distribution of $I_C(S,I)$.

The comparison between NNIA and NSGA-II and the comparison between NNIA and SPEA2 in terms of the Coverage are similar to the comparison between NNIA and PESA-II. But NNIA did better than NSGA-II in SCH, DEB, KUR, ZDT1, ZDT3, ZDT6 and the five DTLZ problems while NSGA-II did better than NNIA in ZDT2, ZDT4. Meanwhile, NNIA did better than SPEA2 in SCH, DEB, ZDT4, ZDT6 and the five DTLZ problems while SPEA2 did better than NNIA in KUR, ZDT2, and ZDT3 as far as the Coverage is concerned.

The 13 plots denote the results of the 13 problems respectively. In each plot, the left box represents the distribution of $I_C(I,M)$ and the right box represents the distribution of $I_C(M,I)$.

The comparison between NNIA and MISA shows that for the five ZDT problems and the five DTLZ problems, the majority solutions obtained by MISA are weakly dominated by the solutions obtained by NNIA. But the majority solutions obtained by NNIA are weakly dominated by the solutions obtained by MISA only in DTLZ1, DTLZ2, and DTLZ3. We estimate that NNIA did

Figure 7. Statistical values of the coverage of the two sets obtained by NNIA and SPEA2 in solving the 13 problems

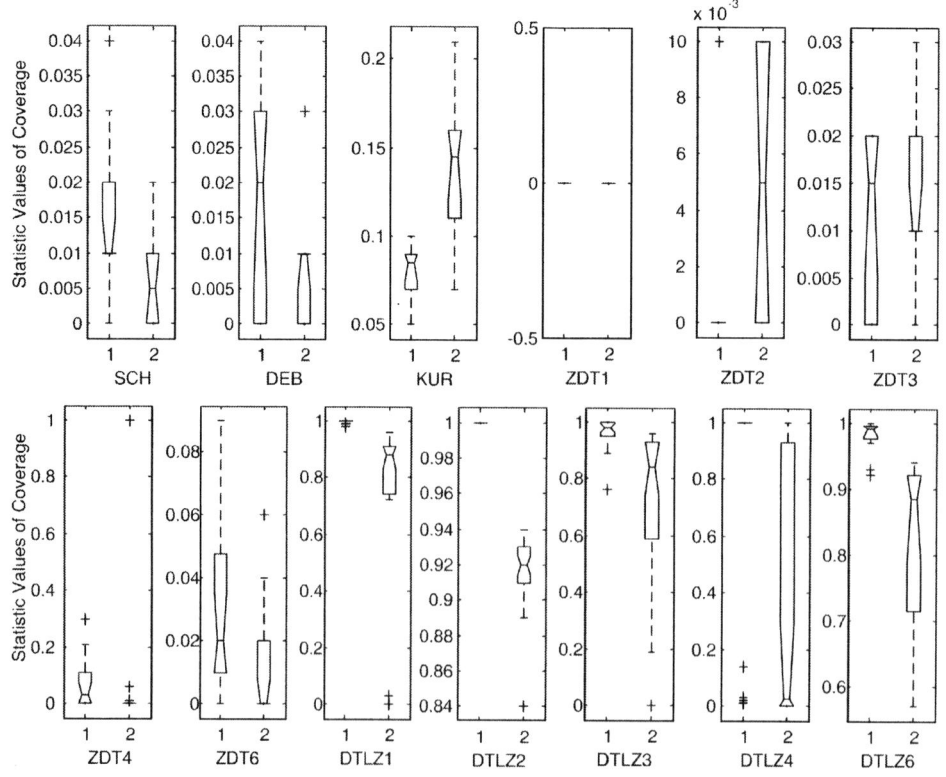

better than MISA in all the problems as far as the Coverage is concerned because the box plots of $I_C(I,M)$ are higher than the corresponding box plots of $I_C(M,I)$ for all the test problems. The main limitation of MISA may be its binary representation. Since the test problems that we are dealing with have continuous spaces, real encoding should be preferred to avoid problems related to Hamming cliffs and to achieve arbitrary precision in the optimal solution (Khare, Yao & Deb, 2003). We think it is not appropriate to compare the performance of a binary-coded algorithm with respect to a real-coded algorithm, but MISA's special operators (two types of mutation in Step 8 and Step 9 of MISA) were designed for antibodies represented by binary strings. However, in a sense, MISA has the ability to approximate these real-coded algorithms by using the binary representation with enough coding length.

Figure 9 shows the box plots based on the Convergence metric over 30 independent runs for the 13 problems.

Box plots are used to illustrate the distribution of these samples. In a notched box plot the notches represent a robust estimate of the uncertainty about the medians for box-to-box comparison. Symbol '+' denote for outliers. The 13 rows (a) to (m) denote the results of the 13 problems, respectively. The left figure of each row representing the distribution of the values of the Convergence metric obtained by NNIA, PESA-II, NSGA-II, SPEA2 and MISA. For most of the problems, the box plots of MISA are obviously higher than the other four algorithms. In order to show the comparison among NNIA,

Figure 8. Statistical Values of the Coverage of the two sets obtained by NNIA and MISA in solving the 13 problems

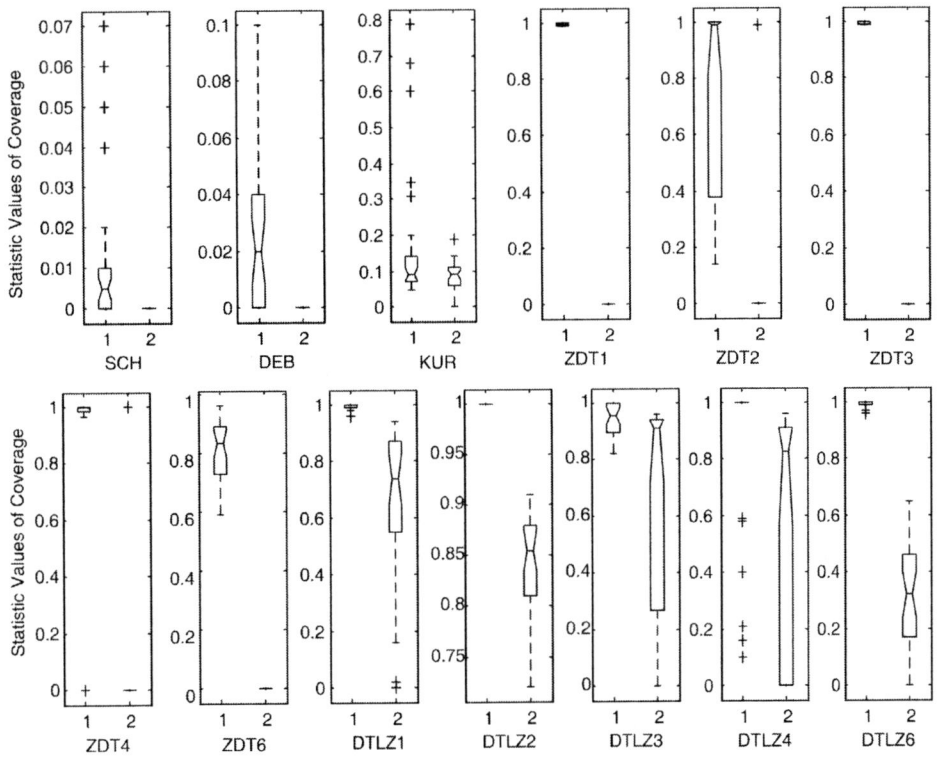

PESA-II, NSGA-II and SPEA2 clearly, we show the distribution of the measure values obtained by the four algorithms in the right figures.

Figure 9 shows that, for the three first low-dimensional problems, all the five algorithm can obtain the values less than 10^{-2} in almost all the 30 independent runs. For the five ZDT problems, DTLZ2, DTLZ4 and DTLZ6, the differences between the corresponding values obtained by NNIA, PESA-II, NSGA-II and SPEA2 are small. Hereinto, NNIA did a little better than others in ZDT1, ZDT4, ZDT6, and DTLZ2. PESA-II did a little better than others in ZDT3 and DTLZ6. NNIA and PESA-II obtained similar values in ZDT2. NNIA, NSGA-II and SPEA2 obtained similar values in DTLZ4. For DTLZ1 and DTLZ3, NNIA did much better than the other four algorithms even though DTLZ1 and DTLZ3 have ($11^{|x_M|}$ − 1) and ($3^{|x_M|}$ − 1) local Pareto-optimal fronts, respectively. (Deb, Thiele, Laumanns & Zitzler, 2001) and (Khare, Yao & Deb, 2003) claimed that for DTLZ3, both NSGA-II and SPEA2 could

Figure 9. Statistical values of the convergence metric obtained by NNIA, PESA-II, NSGA-II, SPEA2, and MISA in solving the 13 problems

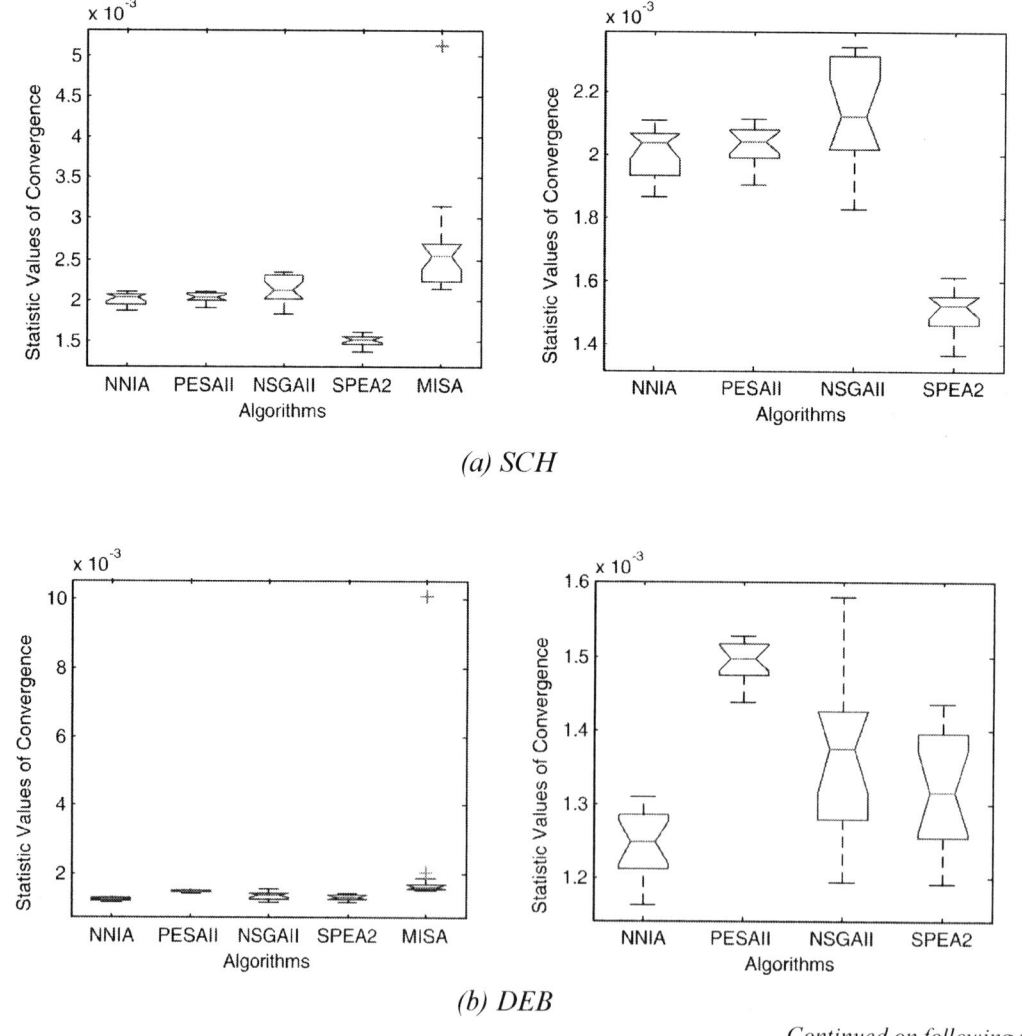

(a) SCH

(b) DEB

Continued on following page

Figure 9. continued

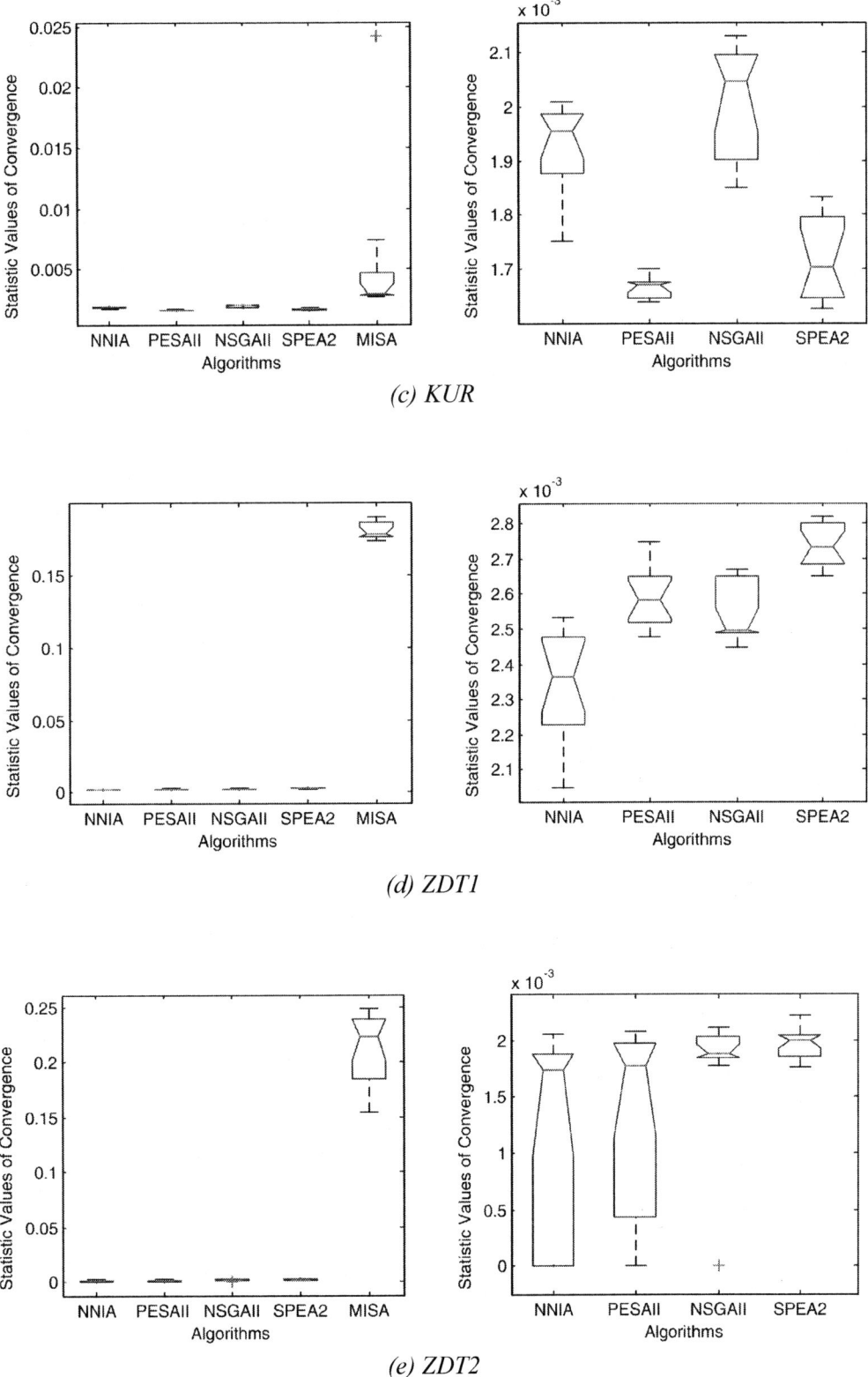

(c) KUR

(d) ZDT1

(e) ZDT2

Continued on following page

Figure 9. continued

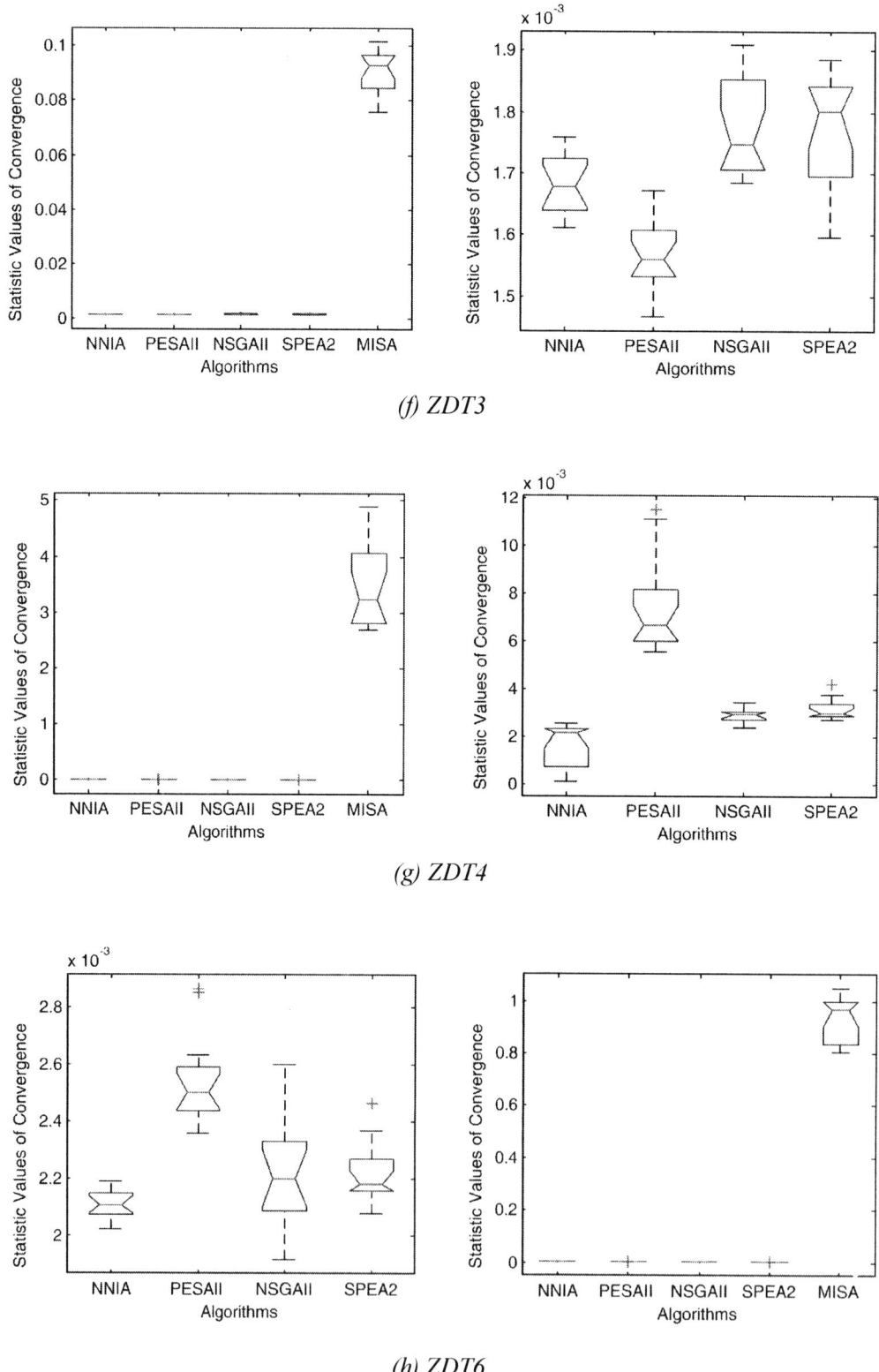

(f) ZDT3

(g) ZDT4

(h) ZDT6

Continued on following page

Figure 9. continued

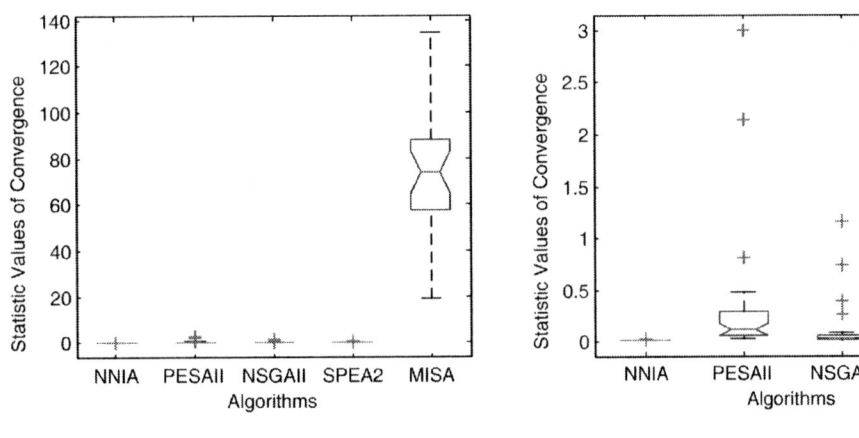

(i) DTLZ1

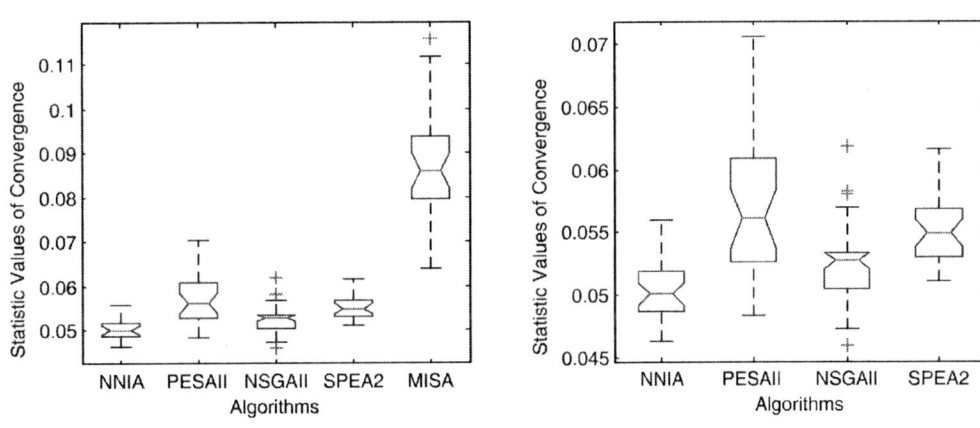

(j) DTLZ2

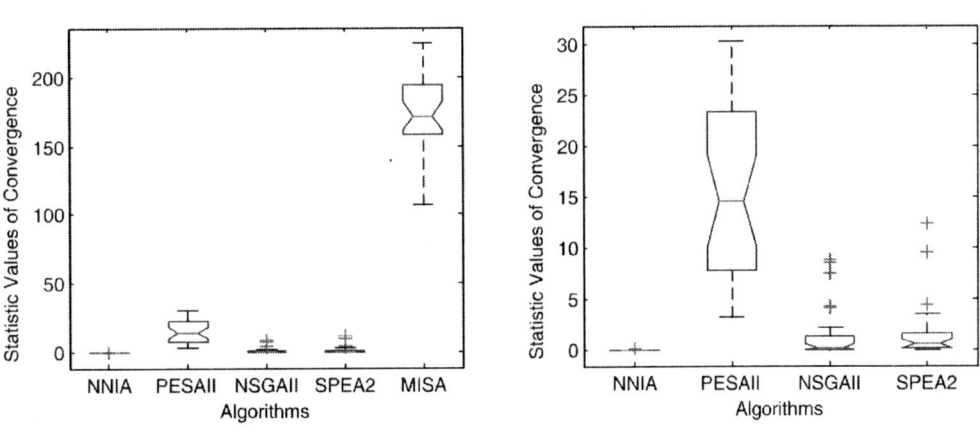

(k) DTLZ3

Continued on following page

Figure 9. continued

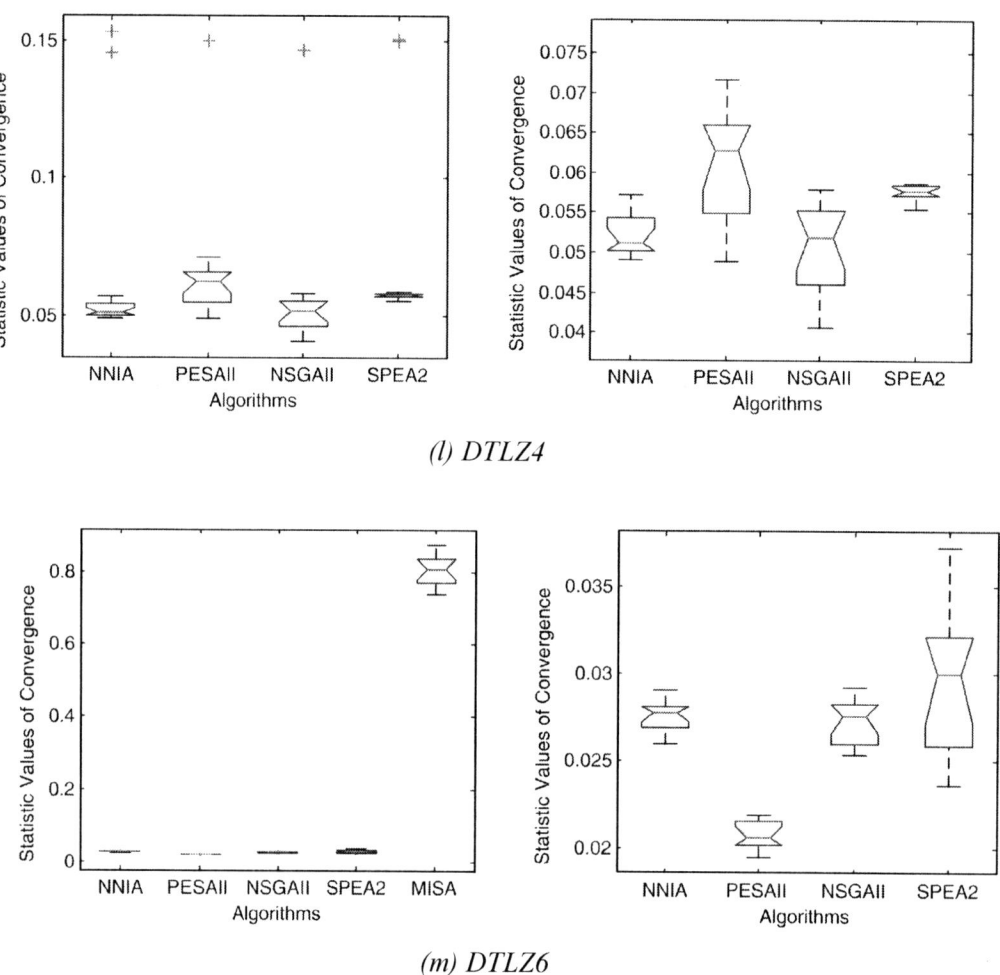

(l) DTLZ4

(m) DTLZ6

not quite converge on to the true Pareto-optimal fronts in 500 generations (50 000 function evaluations). We have found that PESA-II also did badly in solving DTLZ3, but NNIA did very well. Overall, as far as the Convergence metric is concerned, NNIA did best in DEB, ZDT1, ZDT4, ZDT6, DTLZ1, DTLZ2 and DTLZ3 (7 out of the 13 problems).

Figure 10 shows the box plots based on the Spacing metric over 30 independent runs for the 13 problems.

Box plots are used to illustrate the distribution of these samples. In a notched box plot the notches represent a robust estimate of the uncertainty about the medians for box-to-box comparison. Symbol '+' denote for outliers. The 13 plots (a) to (m) denote the results of the 13 problems, respectively.

Figure 10 shows that SPEA2 did best in nine problems in terms of the diversity metric Spacing. SPEA2 used an expensive archive truncation procedure whose worst run-time complexity is $O(N^3)$, where N is the number of nondominated individuals. PESA-II and MISA reduced their nondominated individuals using a hyper-grid based scheme, whose grid size was a crucial factor (Khare, Yao & Deb, 2003). NNIA reduced

Multi-Objective Optimization Using Artificial Immune Systems

Figure 10. Statistical values of the spacing metric obtained by NNIA, PESA-II, NSGA-II, SPEA2, and MISA in solving the 13 problems

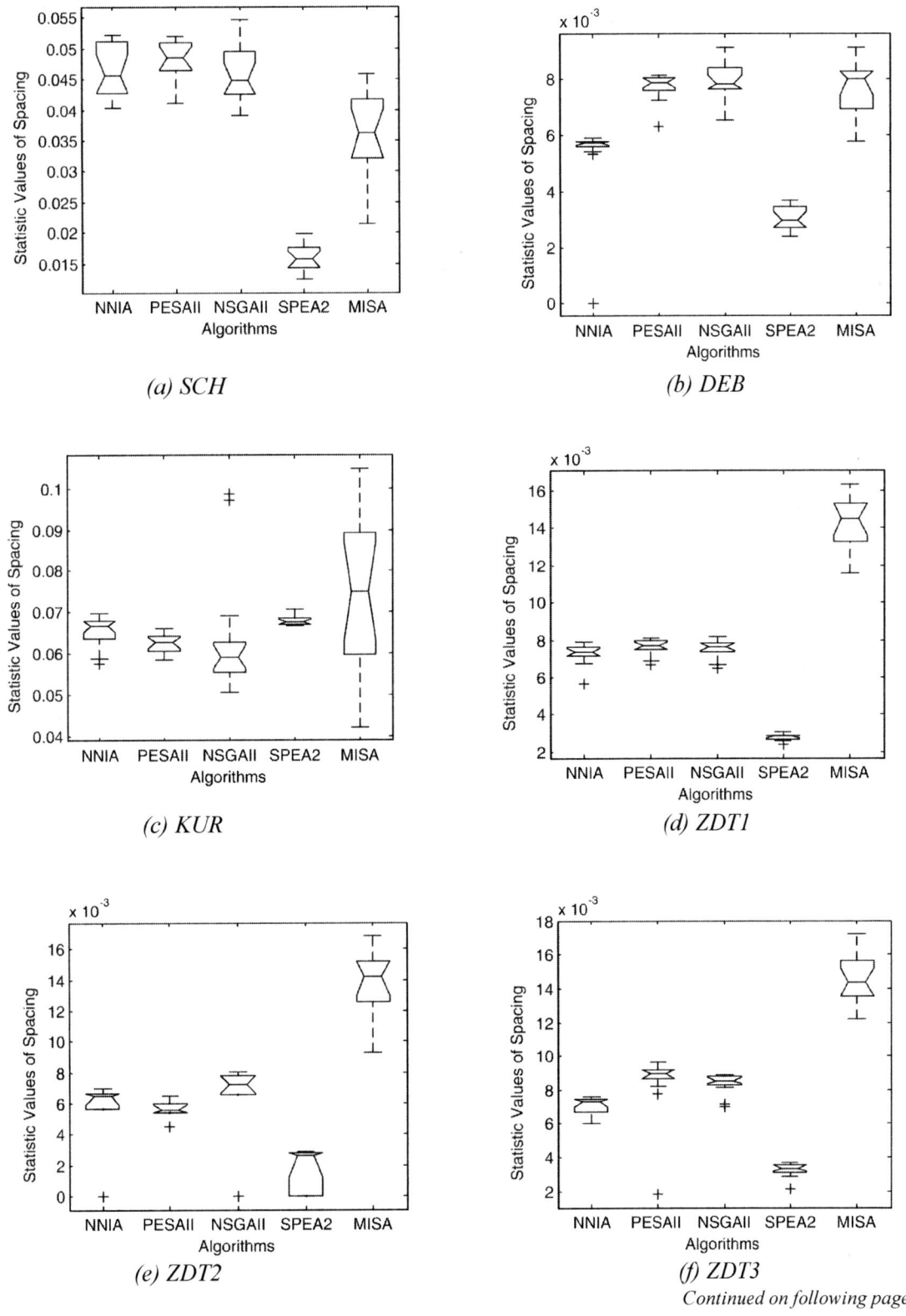

(a) SCH

(b) DEB

(c) KUR

(d) ZDT1

(e) ZDT2

(f) ZDT3

Continued on following page

Figure 10. continued

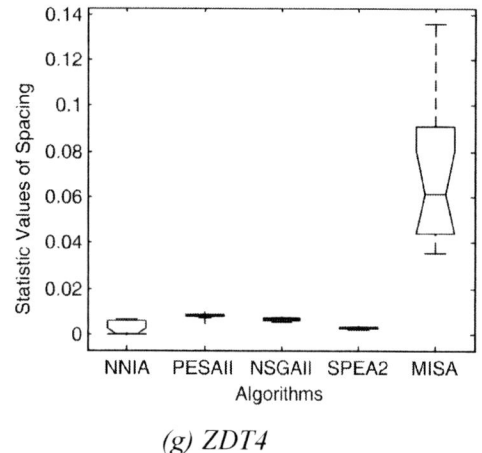

(g) ZDT4

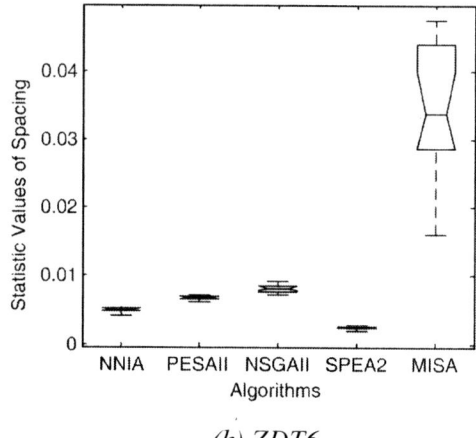

(h) ZDT6

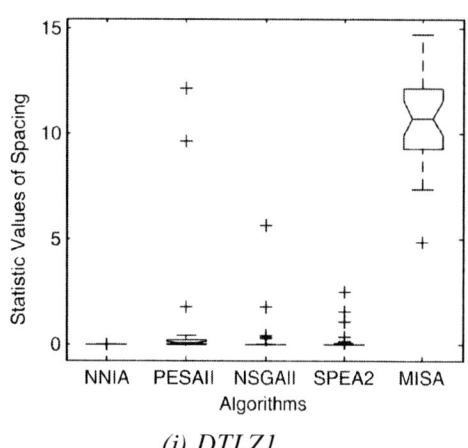

(i) DTLZ1

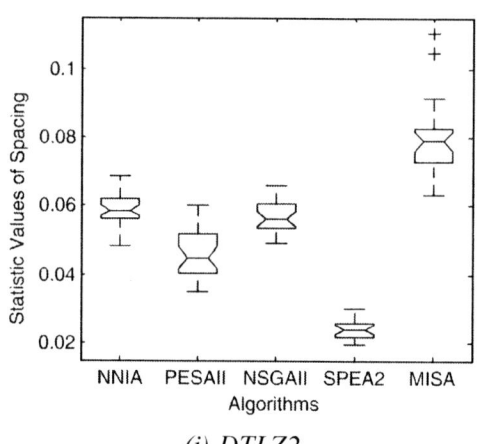

(j) DTLZ2

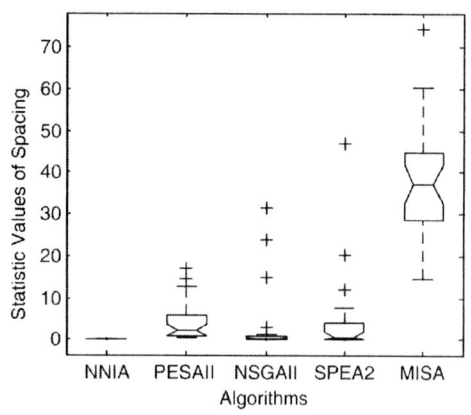

(k) DTLZ3

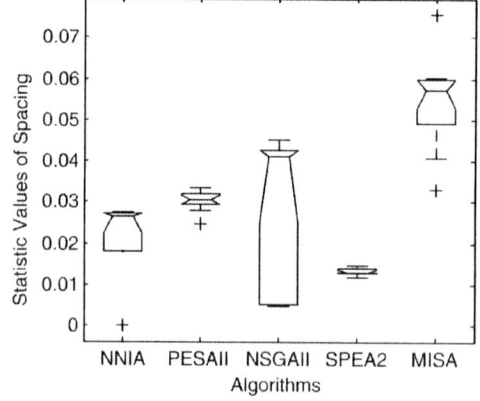

(l) DTLZ4

Continued on following page

Figure 10. continued

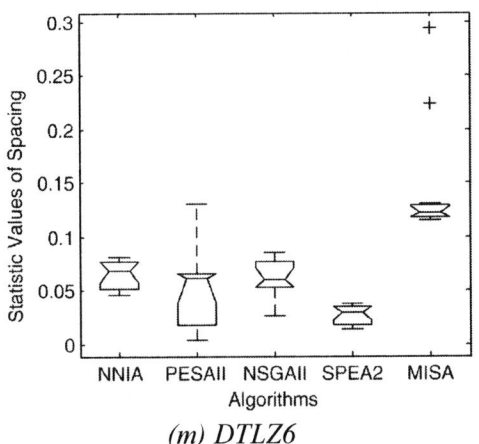

(m) DTLZ6

nondominated solutions using the crowded comparison procedure (Deb, Pratap, Agarwal & Meyarivan, 2002), whose worst run-time complexity is only $O(N\log(N))$. Except SPEA2, the box plots of Spacing obtained by NNIA are lower than those obtained by NSGA-II, PESA-II and MISA in DEB, ZDT1, ZDT3, ZDT4, ZDT6, DTLZ1, DTLZ3 and DTLZ4 (eight out of the 13 problems), while PESA-II did best (except SPEA2) in ZDT2, DTLZ2 and DTLZ6, NSGA-II did best (except SPEA2) in KUR, and MISA did best (except SPEA2) in SCH. For DTLZ1 and DTLZ3, NNIA did best in all five algorithms because the other four algorithms could not quite converge on to the true Pareto-optimal fronts. Overall, SPEA2 is the best algorithm in diversity maintenance, but the differences between the values of Spacing obtained by NNIA, PESA-II and NSGA-II are unconspicuous.

Overall considering the experimental results, we can conclude that

1. For the three low-dimensional problems, all the five algorithms were capable to approximate the true Pareto-optimal fronts.
2. For DTLZ2, DTLZ4, DTLZ6 and the five ZDT problems, NNIA did best in four out of the eight problems in terms of the Convergence metric. SPEA2 did best in seven out of the eight problems in terms of diversity of solutions. Except SPEA2, NNIA did best in six out of the eight problems in terms of diversity of solutions.
3. For DTLZ1 and DTLZ3 problems, NSGA-II, SPEA2, PESA-II and MISA could not quite converge on to the true Pareto-optimal fronts in 50 000 function evaluations, but NNIA were capable to approximate the true Pareto-optimal fronts.

The difference between NNIA and NSGA-II lies in their individual selection methods before heuristic search (recombination and mutation). In the experiments, both NNIA and NSGA-II adopt the same heuristic search operators (simulated binary crossover and polynomial mutation). Therefore, the better performance of NNIA in contrast to NSGA-II is resulted from the unique nondominated neighbor-based selection method cooperating with the proportional cloning, which makes the less-crowded individuals have more chances to do heuristic search. NNIA, PESA-II, SPEA2 and MISA are different in their different ways to do selection and archive maintenance. NNIA also outperformed PESA-II, SPEA2 and MISA in convergence for majority of the test problems. Depending on these empirical comparisons, we conclude that the nondominated neighbor-based selection method is effective, and NNIA is an effective algorithm for solving MOPs.

Comparison of NNIA with and without Recombination

Most of the existing immune inspired optimization algorithms, especially some pure clonal selection algorithms, did not use recombination. However, we think that recombination should not be forbidden in AIS community. Some immunologists have claimed that recombination is a mode of receptor editing used by the B cell antibodies to improve

Figure 11. Statistical values of the coverage of the two sets obtained by NNIA with and without SBX, in solving the 13 problems

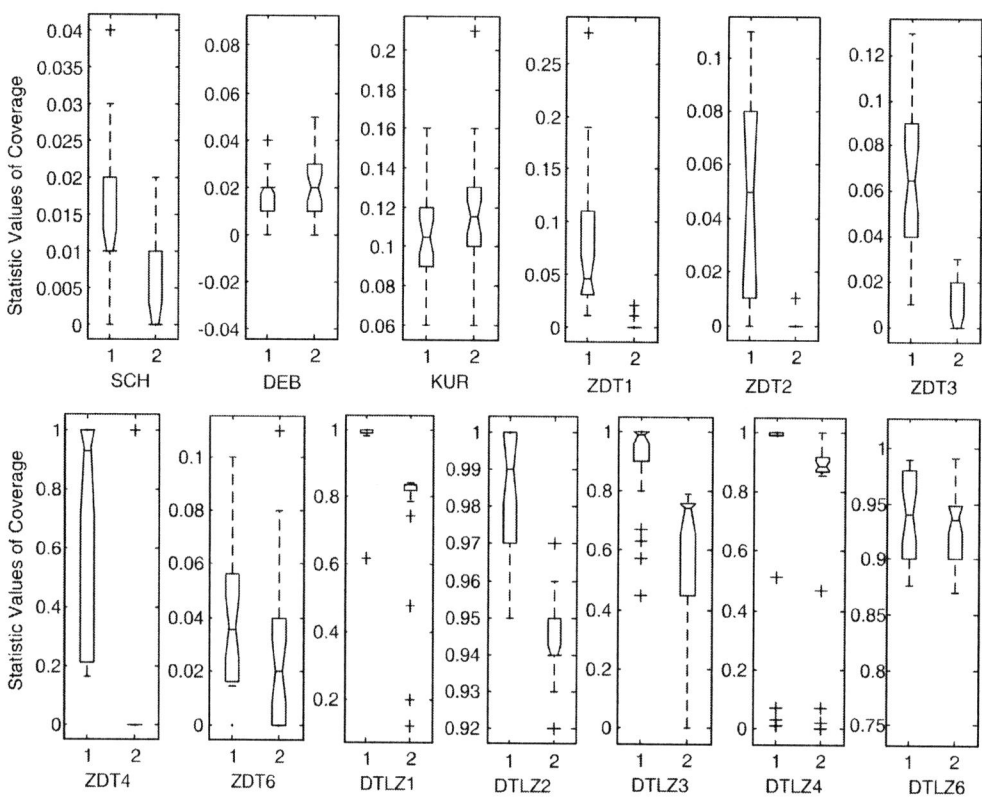

their affinity (George & Gray, 1999). de Castro and Von Zuben (2002) also claimed that genetic recombination and mutation are the two central processes involved in the production of antibodies, even though they did not use recombination in their pure clonal selection algorithm CLONALG according to the clonal selection theory (Burnet, 1959).

In the experiments, the simulated binary crossover (SBX) was introduced as the recombination operator. SBX has been adopted in many MOEA literatures (Deb and Jain, 2002; Deb, Pratap, Agarwal, & Meyarivan, 2002; Khare, Yao, & Deb, 2003; Zitzler, Laumanns, & Thiele, 2002). In order to identify the improvement produced by SBX, we performed the proposed algorithm with SBX (denoted by NNIA) and without SBX (denoted by NNIA-X) 30 independent runs on each test problem, respectively. The parameter settings are the same as the previous section. Figure 11 illustrates the box plots based on the Coverage of the two sets obtained by NNIA and NNIA-X. Here, I denotes the solution set obtained by NNIA; I^{-X} denotes the solution set obtained by NNIA-X.

Here, box plots are used to illustrate the distribution of these samples. In a notched box plot the notches represent a robust estimate of the uncertainty about the medians for box-to-box comparison. Symbol '+' denote for outliers. The 13 plots denote the results of the 13 problems respectively. In each plot, the left box represents the distribution of $I_C(I, I^{-X})$ and the right box represents the distribution of $I_C(I^{-X}, I)$.

The comparison between NNIA and NNIA-X in Coverage shows that

- For ZDT1, ZDT2, ZDT3, ZDT4, DTLZ1, DTLZ2, DTLZ3 and DTLZ4, the box plots of $I_C(I,I^{-X})$ are obviously higher than the corresponding box plots of $I_C(I^{-X},I)$. Therefore, NNIA did much better than NNIA-X in solving these eight problems as far as the coverage is concerned.
- For SCH, ZDT6 and DTLZ6, the box plots of $I_C(I,I^{-X})$ are slightly higher than the corresponding box plots of $I_C(I^{-X},I)$. Therefore, NNIA did a little better than NNIA-X in solving these three problems.
- For DEB and KUR, the box plots of $I_C(I^{-X},I)$ are slightly higher than the corresponding box plots of $I_C(I,I^{-X})$. Therefore, NNIA-X did a little better than NNIA in solving these two problems.

Overall, NNIA did better than NNIA-X in solving 11 out of the 13 problems. NNIA-X only did a little better than NNIA in solving the two low-dimensional problems DEB and KUR.

Based on the empirical results, we did not abandon the recombination in our algorithm because our aim was to construct a useful algorithm for multi-objective optimization rather than a pure clonal selection algorithm. Furthermore, the recombination of genes involved in the production of antibodies differs somewhat from the recombination of parental genes in sexual reproduction used in genetic algorithms. In the former, the recombination on a clone is performed as a crossover between the clone and a random selected active antibody. It realized replacing at random some gene segments of the clone by the corresponding ones of the selected active antibody. The latter involves the crossover of two parents to generate offspring. However, the similarity between them is also obviously, because the similarity between biological evolution and the production of antibodies is even more striking as claimed in de Castro and Von Zuben (2002).

CONCLUDING REMARKS

NSGA-II, SPEA, PAES and some other MOEAs can be considered as different MOEAs because they adopt different ways to do selection (or fitness assignment) and population maintenance in solving multi-objective optimization problems. The essential difference between IDCMA and them is the different selection technique. In IDCMA, the fitness value of each individual is determined by the distance between the individual and one nondominated individual found so far. Only partial individuals around the Nondominated individual (in decision space) are selected to do local search. So in a single generation, IDCMA only performs a local search in the niche around the nondominated individual which has been selected for fitness assignment. The essential difference between IDCMA and MISA is also in their different selection methods and population maintenance strategies. MISA clones all the nondominated individuals without selection, and reduces their nondominated individuals using a hyper-grid based scheme, whose grid size was a crucial factor. But IDCMA selects only partial individuals based on the values of Ab-Ab affinity to do clone and mutation, and prunes the nondominated individuals while maintaining its characteristics via cluster analysis.

IDCMA provided a novel fitness assignment method based on the Ab-Ab affinity which is a custom distance measure. IDCMA is characterized by its unique fitness assignment strategy based on the Ab-Ab affinity and by its enhanced local research around nondominated individuals found so far using the Cloning operation. The performance comparison between IDCMA and some well-known MOEAs based on nine combinatorial test problems showed that IDCMA had a good performance in converging to approximate Pareto-optimal fronts with a good distribution for most of the test problems.

But the IDCMA which adopts binary string representation and a small population size had difficulties in converging to the true Pareto-optimal front and obtaining the well-distributed solutions simultaneously for some continuous problems with high variable dimensions (e.g. ZDT6). So we described another multi-objective immune algorithm NNIA for solving continuous multi-objective optimization problems.

In NNIA, the fitness value of nondominated individuals is assigned as the crowding-distance. The selection technique only performs on nondominated individuals and selects minority isolated individuals to clone proportionally to crowding-distance values, recombine and mutation. Some immunologists claimed that repertoire diversity of antibody underlies the immune response however the majority of antibodies do not play any active role during the immune response (Baranzini, Jeong, Butunoi, et al., 1999; Cziko, 1995; Parkin Cohen, 2001; Pannetier, Even, & Kourilsky, 1995). NNIA simulated this mechanism by selecting only the minority of nondominated individuals with greater crowding-distance values as active antibodies, and performing the proportional cloning, recombination, and hypermutation only on these active antibodies. It realized the enhanced local search around the active antibodies which are the less-crowded individuals in objective space.

In contrast to NSGA-II, the nondominated neighbor-based selection and proportional cloning make the less-crowded individuals have more chances to do recombination and mutation. So in a single generation, NNIA pays more attention to the less-crowded regions of the current trade-off front. The essential difference between NNIA and MISA is in their different selection methods and population maintenance strategies as well as individual representation methods. MISA adopts binary representation, clones all the nondominated individuals (and feasible individuals for constraint problems), and applies two types of mutation to the clones and other "not so good" individuals, respectively. MISA updates its external population by using the grid based techniques used in PAES which need a crucial parameter, the number of grid cells. The difference between NNIA and VAIS may be also lies in their selection and population maintenance strategies. VAIS adopts the flowchart of opt-aiNet and the fitness assignment method in SPEA2 with some simplification. VAIS maintains its external population (memory population) using the suppression mechanism like opt-aiNet based on the Euclidean distance in objective space and a threshold for suppression. We can also find some similar points between NNIA and PESA-II, PAES, SPEA2, e.g. storing the nondominated individuals previously found externally and reducing the number of nondominated individuals stored without destroying the characteristics of the trade-off front, because our algorithm is constructed inspired from them.

The main contribution of this study to MO field may be its unique selection technique. The selection technique only selects minority isolated nondominated individuals based on their crowding-distance values. The selected individuals are then cloned proportionally to their crowding-distance values before heuristic search. By using the nondominated neighbor-based selection and proportional cloning, the new algorithm realizes the enhanced local search in the less-crowded regions of the current trade-off front. Depending on the enhanced local search, NNIA can solve MOPs with a simple procedure. The experimental study on NNIA, SPEA2, NSGA-II, PESA-II and MISA in solving three low-dimensional problems, five ZDT problems and five DTLZ problems has shown that NNIA was able to quite converge to the true Pareto-optimal fronts in solving most of the test problems. More important, for the complicated problems DTLZ1 and DTLZ3, NNIA did much better than the other four algorithms. Depending on these empirical comparisons, we concluded that the nondominated neighbor-based selection method is effective, and NNIA is an effective algorithm for solving multi-objective optimization problems.

FUTURE RESEARCH DIRECTIONS

Some literatures have implied that the MOEAs based on Pareto-dominance will be useless along the increasing of the number of objectives as there is no way to discriminate among the different individuals (Benedetti, Farina, & Gobbi, 2006; Deb, 2001). In order to clarify the scalability of NNIA, it is interesting to perform a set of explanatory experiments intending to dissect this issue from a practical point of view.

Another issue should be addressed in the future research is the population size self-adaptive strategy. These algorithms with a small population size have difficulties in converging to the true Pareto-optimal front and obtaining the well-distributed solutions simultaneously for some complicated problems. The dependence between the problem complexity and the population size required to be solved correctly. However, to estimate the correct population size for a given problem cannot be done a priori as the complexity of the problem generally can not be inferred advanced.

Most of the existing artificial immune system algorithms for multi-objective optimization are inspired from clonal selction principle. Some immunological theories are not well explored in the field of multi-objective optimization, such as Negative Selection and Danger Theory. These immune models have been employed successfully in other fields of engineering, and an investigation of their potential for multi-objective optimization may be an interesting direction of the future research.

ACKNOWLEDGMENT

This work was supported by the National Natural Science Foundation of China (Grant No. 60703107), the National High Technology Research and Development Program (863 Program) of China (No. 2006AA01Z107), the National Basic Research Program (973 Program) of China (Nos. 2001CB309403 and 2006CB705700) and the Graduate Innovation Fund of Xidian University (Grant No. 05004).

REFERENCES

Abbas, A. K., Lichtman, A. H., & Pober, J. S. (2000). *Cellular and molecular immunology* (4th ed.). New York: W B Saunders Co.

Benedetti, A., Farina, M., & Gobbi, M. (2006) Evolutionary multi-objective industrial design: The case of a racing car tire-suspension systems. *IEEE Transactions on Evolutionary Computation, 10*(3), 230-244.

Beyer, H. G. & Schwefel, H. P. (2002). Evolution strategies: A comprehensive introduction. *Journal Natural Computing, 1*(1), 3-52.

Burnet, F. M. (1959). *The clonal selection theory of acquired immunity.* Cambridge University Press.

Campelo, F., Guimaraes, F. G., & Igarashi, H (2007). Overview of artificial immune systems for multi-objective optimization. In *Proceedings of the 4th International Conference on Evolutionary Multi-Criterion Optimization, EMO 2007. Lecture notes in computer science* (Vol. 4403, pp. 937–951). Springer

Campelo, F., Guimaraes, F. G., Saldanha, R. R., Igarashi, H., Noguchi, S., Lowther, D. A., & Ramirez, J. A. (2004). A novel multi-objective immune algorithm using nondominated sorting. In *Proceedings of the 11th International IGTE Symposium on Numerical Field Calculation in Electrical Engineering*, Seggauberg, Austria.

Carter, J. H. (2000). The immune system as a model for pattern recognition and classification. *Journal of the American Medical Informatics Association, 7*(3), 28–41.

Coello Coello, C. A. (2003). Evolutionary multi-objective optimization: Current and future challenges. *Advances in soft computing-engineering, design and manufacturing* (pp. 243-256). Springer-Verlag.

Coello Coello, C. A., & Cortes, N. C. (2002, September 9-11). An approach to solve multi-objective optimization problems based on an artificial immune system. In *Proceedings of the First International Conference on Artificial Immune Systems, ICARIS2002* (pp. 212-221), University of Kent at Canterbury, UK.

Coello Coello, C. A. & Cortes, N. C. (2005). Solving multi-objective optimization problems using an artificial immune system. *Genetic Programming and Evolvable Machines, 6*, 163-190.

Coello Coello, C. A., Rivera, D. C., & Cortes, N. C. (2003). Use of an artificial immune system for job shop scheduling. In *Proceedings of the Second International Conference on Artificial Immune Systems (ICARIS)*, Napier University, Edinburgh, UK.

Coello Coello, C. A. & Pulido, G. T. (2001). Multi-objective optimization using a micro-genetic algorithm. In *Proceedings of the Genetic and Evolutionary Computation Conference (GECCO-2001)* (pp. 274-282). San Francisco: Morgan Kaufmann Publishers.

Coello Coello, C. A., Van Veldhuizen, D. A., & Lamont, G. B. (2002). Evolutionary algorithms for solving multi-objective problems. New York: Kluwer Academic Publishers.

Corne, D. W., Jerram, N. R., Knowles, J. D., & Oates, M. J. (2001). PESA-II: Region-based selection in evolutionary multi-objective optimization. In *Proceedings of the Genetic and Evolutionary Computation Conference (GECCO-2001)* (pp. 283-290). San Francisco: Morgan Kaufmann Publishers.

Corne, D. W., Knowles, J. D., & Oates, M. J. (2000). The Pareto-envelope based selection algorithm for multi-objective optimization. Parallel problem solving from nature-PPSN VI, Lecture notes in computer science (pp. 869-878). Springer

Cutello, V., Narzisi, G., & Nicosia, G. (2005). A class of Pareto archived evolution strategy algorithms using immune inspired operators for ab-initio protein structure prediction. In *Proceedings of the Third European Workshop on Evolutionary Computation and Bioinformatics, EvoWorkshops 2005-EvoBio 2005*, Lausanne, Switzerland. *Lecture notes in computer science* (Vol. 3449, pp. 54-63).

Cutello, V., Narzisi, G., Nicosia, G., & Pavone, M. (2005). Clonal selection algorithms: A comparative case study using effective mutation potentials. In *Proceedings of 4th International Conference on Artificial Immune Systems, ICARIS 2005*, Banff, Canada. *Lecture notes in computer science* (Vol. 3627, pp. 13-28).

Cutello, V., Nicosia, G., & Pavone, M. (2004). Exploring the capability of immune algorithms: A characterization of hypemutation operators. In *Proceedings of Third International Conference on Artificial Immune Systems, ICARIS2004*, Catania, Italy. *Lecture notes in computer science* (Vol. 3239, pp. 263-276).

Deb, K. (1999). Multi-objective genetic algorithms: Problem difficulties and construction of test problems. *Evolutionary Computation, 7*(3), 205-230.

Deb, K. (2001). *Multi-objective optimization using evolutionary algorithms*. Chichester, UK: John Wiley & Sons.

Deb, K. & Beyer, H. G. (2001). Self-adaptive genetic algorithms with simulated binary crossover. *Evolutionary Computation, 9*(2), 197-221.

Deb, K. & Jain, S. (2002). *Running performance metrics for evolutionary multi-objective optimization* (Tech. Rep. No. 2002004). KanGAL, Indian Institute of Technology, Kanpur 208016, India.

Deb, K., Pratap, A., Agarwal, S., & Meyarivan, T. (2002). A fast and elitist multi-objective genetic algorithm: NSGA-II. *IEEE Transactions on Evolutionary Computation, 6*(2), 182-197.

Deb, K., Thiele, L., Laumanns, M., & Zitzler, E. (2001). *Scalable multi-objective optimization test problems* (Tech. Rep. No. 112). Computer Engineering and Networks Laboratory (TIK), Swiss Federal Institute of Technology (ETH), Zurich, Switzerland.

Deb, K., Thiele, L., Laumanns, M., & Zitzler, E. (2002). Scalable multi-objective optimization test problems. In *Proceedings of Congress on Evolutionary Computation, CEC 2002* (Vol.1, pp. 825-830). IEEE Service Center

de Castro, L. N., & Timmis, J. (2002a). *Artificial immune systems: A new computational intelligence approach*. Heidelberg, Germany: Springer-Verlag.

de Castro, L. N. & Timmis, J. (2002b). An artificial immune network for multimodal function optimization. In *Proceedings of the 2002 Congress on Evolutionary Computation, CEC' 02* (Vol. 1, pp. 699-704).

de Castro, L. N. & Von Zuben, F. J. (2002). Learning and optimization using the clonal selection principle. *IEEE Transactions on Evolutionary Computation, 6*(3), 239-251.

Du, H. F., Gong, M. G., Jiao, L. C., & Liu, R. C. (2005). A novel artificial immune system algorithm for high-dimensional function numerical optimization. *Progress in Natural Science, 15*(5), 463–471.

Fieldsend, J., Everson, R. M., & Singh, S. (2003). Using unconstrained elite archives for multi-objective optimization. *IEEE Transactions on Evolutionary Computation, 7*(3), 305-323.

Fonseca, C. M. & Fleming, P. J. (1995). An overview of evolutionary algorithms in multi-objective optimization. *Evolutionary Computation, 3*(1), 1-16.

Forrest, S., Perelson, A. S., Allen, L., & Cherukuri, R. (1994). Self-nonself discrimination in a computer. In *Proceedings of the IEEE Symposium on Research in Security and Privacy* (pp. 202-212). Los Alamitos, CA: IEEE Computer Society Press.

Freschi, F. & Repetto, M. (2005). Multi-objective optimization by a modified artificial immune system algorithm. In *Proceedings of the 4th International Conference on Artificial Immune Systems, ICARIS 2005. Lecture notes in computer science* (Vol. 3627, pp. 248-261). Springer.

Fukuda, T., Mori, K., & Tsukiyama, M. (1993). Immune networks using genetic algorithm for adaptive production scheduling. In *Proceedings of the 15th IFAC World Congress* (Vol. 3, pp. 57-60).

Garrett, S. M. (2004). Parameter-free, Adaptive clonal selection. In *Proceedings of IEEE Congress on Evolutionary Computing, CEC 2004* (pp. 1052-1058), Portland, Oregon.

Garrett, S. M. (2005). How do we evaluate artificial immune systems. *Evolutionary Computation, 13*(2), 145-178.

Goldberg, D. E. (1989). *Genetic algorithms in search, optimization, and machine learning*. Reading, Massachusetts: Addison-Wesley.

Gong, M. G., Jiao, L. C., Du, H. F., & Wang, L. (2005). An artificial immune system algorithm for CDMA multiuser detection over multi-path channels. In *Proceedings of the Genetic and Evolutionary Computation Conference (GECCO-2005)* (pp. 2105-2111),Washington, D.C.

Gonzalez, F., Dasgupta, D., & Kozma, R. (2002). Combining negative selection and classification techniques for anomaly detection. In *Proceedings of the Special Sessions on Artificial Immune Systems in Congress on Evolutionary Computation, IEEE World Congress on Computational Intelligence*, Honolulu, Hawaii.

Hajela, P. & Lin, C.Y. (1992). Genetic search strategies in multicriterion optimal design. *Structural Optimization, 4*, 99–107.

Hajela, P., Yoo, J., & Lee, J. (1997). GA based simulation of immune networks-applications in structural optimization. *Journal of Engineering Optimization.*

Hart, E., & Ross, P. (1999). The evolution and analysis of a potential antibody library for use in job-shop scheduling. *New ideas in optimization* (pp. 185–202). McGraw-Hill.

Hart, E. & Timmis, J. (2005). Application areas of AIS: The past, the present and the future. In *Proceedings of the 4th International Conference on Artificial Immune Systems, ICARIS 2005. Lecture notes in computer science* (Vol. 3627, pp. 483-497). Springer

Horn, J. & Nafpliotis, N. (1993). *Multi-objective optimization using the niched Pareto genetic algorithm* (Tech. Rep.) IlliGAL Report 93005, Illinois Genetic Algorithms Laboratory, University of Illinois, Urbana, Champaign.

Igel, C., Hansen, N., & Roth, S. (2007). Covariance matrix adaptation for multi-objective optimization. *Evolutionary Computation, 15*(1), 1-28.

Ishida, Y. (1990). Fully distributed diagnosis by PDP learning algorithm: Towards immune network PDP model. In *Proceedings of the International Joint Conference on Neural Networks: 777–782*

Jacob, C., Pilat, M. L., Bentley, P. J., & Timmis, J. (Eds.) (2005). *Artificial immune systems: Proceedings of the fourth international conference on artificial immune systems, ICARIS 2005.* Lecture notes in computer science (Vol. 3627). Banff, Alberta, Canada: Springer-Verlag.

Jiao, L. C., Gong, M. G., Shang, R. H., Du, H. F., & Lu, B. (2005). Clonal selection with immune dominance and anergy based multi-objective optimization. In *Proceedings of the Third International Conference on Evolutionary Multi-Criterion Optimization, EMO 2005.* Guanajuato, Mexico: Springer-Verlag, *Lecture notes in computer science* (Vol. 3410, pp. 474-489).

Jiao, L. C., Liu, J., & Zhong, W. C. (2006). An organizational coevolutionary algorithm for classification. *IEEE Transactions on Evolutionary Computation, 10*(1), 67-80.

Jiao, L. C. & Wang, L. (2000). A novel genetic algorithm based on immunity. *IEEE Transactions on Systems, Man and Cybernetics, Part A, 30*(5), 552-561.

Khare, V., Yao, X., & Deb, K. (2003). Performance scaling of multi-objective evolutionary algorithms. In *Proceedings of the Second International Conference on Evolutionary Multi-Criterion Optimization, EMO 2003. Lecture notes in computer science* (Vol. 2632, pp. 376-390). Springer-Verlag

Knowles, J. D. & Corne, D. W. (2000). Approximating the nondominated front using the Pareto archived evolution strategy. *Evolutionary Computation, 8*(2), 149-172.

Knowles, J., Thiele, L., & Zitzler, E. (2006). *A tutorial on the performance assessment of stochastic multi-objective optimizers* (Rev. ed.) (Tech. Rep. No. 214), Computer Engineering and Networks Laboratory (TIK), Swiss Federal Institute of Technology (ETH), Zurich, Switzerland.

Kursawe, F. (1991). A variant of evolution strategies for vector optimization. *Parallel problem solving from nature-PPSN* I. *Lecture notes in computer science* (Vol. 496, pp. 193-197). Springer-Verlag

Luh, G. C., Chueh, C. H., & Liu, W. W. (2003). MOIA: Multi-objective immune algorithm. *Engineering Optimization, 35*(2), 143-164.

Luh, G. C., Chueh, C. H., & Liu, W. W. (2004). Multi-objective optimal design of truss structure with immune algorithm. *Computers and Structures, 82*, 829–844.

McGill, R., Tukey, J. W., & Larsen, W. A. (1978). Variations of boxplots. *The American Statistician, 32*, 12-16.

Nicosia, G., Cutello, V., Bentley, P. J., & Timmis, J. (Eds.) (2004). Artificial immune systems. In *Proceedings of The Third International Conference on Artificial Immune Systems, ICARIS 2004*, Catania, Italy. *Lecture notes in computer science* (Vol. 3239). Springer-Verlag

Rudolph, G. (1998). On a multi-objective evolutionary algorithm and its convergence to the Pareto set. In *Proceedings of the 5th IEEE Congress on Evolutionary Computation, CEC 1998* (pp. 511-516). Piscataway, New Jersey: IEEE Service Center.

Schaffer, J. D. (1984). *Multiple objective optimization with vector evaluated genetic algorithms.* Unpublished doctoral thesis, Vanderbilt University.

Schott, J. R. (1995). *Fault tolerant design using single and multictiteria gentetic algorithm optimization.* Unpublished master's thesis, Massachusetts Institute of Technology, Cambridge.

Srinivas, N. & Deb, K. (1994). Multi-objective optimization using nondominated sorting in genetic algorithms. *Evolutionary Computation, 2*(3), 221-248.

Tarakanov, A. & Dasgupta, D. (2000). A formal model of an artificial immune system. *BioSystems, 55*(1/3), 151-158.

Timmis, J., Neal, M., & Hunt, J. (2000). An artificial immune system for data analysis. *Biosystems, 55*(1/3), 143–150.

Van Veldhuizen, D. A. (1999). *Multi-objective evolutionary algorithms: Classification, analyses, and new innovations.* Unpublished doctoral thesis. Presented to the Faculty of the Graduate School of Engineering of he Air Force Institute of Technology. Air University.

Van Veldhuizen, D. A. & Lamont, G. B. (2000a). Multi-objective optimization with messy genetic algorithms. In *Proceedings of the 2000 ACM Symposium on Applied Computing* (pp. 470-476), Villa Olmo, Como, Italy.

Van Veldhuizen, D. A. & Lamont, G. B. (2000b). On measuring multi-objective evolutionary algorithm performance. In *Proceedings of the 2000 IEEE Congress on Evolutionary Computation, CEC 2000* (Vol. 1, pp. 204-211). Piscataway, New Jersey: IEEE Service Center.

White, J. A. & Garrett, S. M. (2003). Improved pattern recognition with artificial clonal selection. In *Proceedings of the Second International Conference on Artificial Immune Systems (ICARIS)*, Napier University, Edinburgh, UK.

Zitzler, E. (1999). *Evolutionary algorithms for multi-objective optimization: Methods and applications,* Swiss Federal Institute of Technology Zurich. Submitted for publication.

Zitzler, E., Deb, K., & Thiele, L. (2000). Comparison of multi-objective evolutionary algorithms: Empirical results. *Evolutionary Computation, 8*(2), 173-195.

Zitzler, E., Laumanns, M., & Thiele, L. (2002). SPEA2: Improving the strength Pareto evolutionary algorithm. Evolutionary Methods for Design, Optimization and Control with Applications to Industrial Problems, Athens, Greece, pages 95-100.

Zitzler, E. & Thiele, L. (1998). Multi-objective optimization using evolutionary algorithms—A comparative case study. Parallel problem solving from nature-PPSN V. *Lecture notes in computer science* (pp. 292-301). Springer

Zitzler, E. & Thiele, L. (1999). Multi-objective evolutionary algorithms: A comparative case study and the strength Pareto approach. *IEEE Transactions on Evolutionary Computation, 3*(4), 257-271.

Zitzler, E., Thiele, L., Laumanns, M., Fonseca, C. M., & da Fonseca, V. G. (2003). Performance assessment of multi-objective optimizers an analysis and review. *IEEE Transactions on Evolutionary Computation, 7*(2), 117-132.

ADDITIONAL READING

Abbas, A. K., Lichtman, A. H., & Pober, J. S. (2000). Cellular and molecular immunology (4th ed.). New York: W B Saunders Co.

Aickelin, U. & Cayzer, S. (2002). The danger theory and its application to artificial immune systems. In *Proceedings of the 1st International Conference on Artificial Immune Systems*, University of Kent at Canterbury, England.

Aickelin, U., Bentley, P., Cayzer, S., Kim, J. & McLeod, J. (2003). Danger theory: The Link between AIS and IDS. In *Proceedings of the 2nd International Conference on Artificial Immune Systems*, Edinburgh, UK.

Campelo, F., Guimaraes, F. G., & Igarashi, H (2007). Overview of artificial immune systems for multi-objective optimization. In *Proceedings of the 4th International Conference on Evolutionary Multi-Criterion Optimization, EMO 2007. Lecture notes in computer science* (Vol. 4403, pp. 937-951). Springer

Campelo, F., Guimaraes, F. G., Saldanha, R. R., Igarashi, H., Noguchi, S., Lowther, D. A., & Ramirez, J. A. (2004). A novel multi-objective immune algorithm using nondominated sorting. In *Proceedings of the 11th International IGTE Symposium on Numerical Field Calculation in Electrical Engineering*, Seggauberg, Austria.

Coello Coello, C. A. & Cortes, N. C. (2002). An approach to solve multi-objective optimization problems based on an artificial immune system. In *Proceedings of the First International Conference on Artificial Immune Systems, ICARIS2002* (pp. 212-221), University of Kent at Canterbury, UK.

Coello Coello, C. A. & Cortes, N. C. (2005). Solving multi-objective optimization problems using an artificial immune system. *Genetic Programming and Evolvable Machines, 6*, 163-190.

Coello Coello, C. A., Rivera, D. C., & Cortes, N. C. (2003). Use of an artificial immune system for job shop scheduling. In *Proceeding of the Second International Conference on Artificial Immune Systems (ICARIS)*, Napier University, Edinburgh, UK.

Cutello, V., Narzisi, G., & Nicosia, G. (2005). A class of Pareto archived evolution strategy algorithms using immune inspired operators for ab-initio protein structure prediction. In *Proceedings of the Third European Workshop on Evolutionary Computation and Bioinformatics, EvoWorkshops 2005-EvoBio 2005*, Lausanne, Switzerland. Lecture notes in computer science (Vol. 3449, pp. 54-63).

Dasgupta, D. & Forrest, S. (1999). Artificial immune systems in industrial applications. In *Proceedings of the Second International Conference on Intelligent Processing and Manufacturing of Materials*, Hawaii.

Dasgupta, D., Ji, Z., & Gonzalez, F. (2003). Artificial immune system (AIS) research in the last five years. In *Proceedings of CEC 2003: IEEE Congress on Evolutionary Computation* (pp.123–130)

Dasgupta, D., KrishnaKumar, K., & Barry, M. (2004). Negative selection algorithm for aircraft fault detection. In *Proceedings of the 3rd International Conference on Artificial Immune Systems*, Catania, Italy. Lecture notes in computer science (Vol. 3239, pp. 1–13)

de Castro, L. N. & Timmis, J. (2002a). *Artificial immune systems: A new computational intelligence approach*. Heidelberg, Germany: Springer-Verlag.

de Castro, L. N. & Timmis, J. (2002b). An artificial immune network for multimodal function optimization. In *Proceedings of the 2002 Congress on Evolutionary Computation, CEC' 02* (Vol. 1, pp. 699-704).

de Castro, L. N. & Von Zuben, F. J. (2002). Learning and optimization using the clonal selection principle. *IEEE Transactions on Evolutionary Computation, 6*(3), 239-251.

Farmer, J. D., Packard, N. H., & Perelson, A. S. (1986). The immune system, adaptation, and machine learning. *Physica D, 2*(1–3), 187–204.

Forrest, S. & Hofmeyr, S. A. (2001). Immunology as information processing. In L. A. Segel & I. Cohen (Eds.), *Design principles for the immune system and other distributed autonomous systems*. New York: Oxford University Press.

Freschi, F. & Repetto, M. (2005). Multi-objective optimization by a modified artificial immune system algorithm. In *Proceedings of the 4th International Conference on Artificial Immune Systems, ICARIS 2005. Lecture notes in computer science* (Vol. 3627, pp. 248-261). Springer.

Garrett, S. M. (2005). How do we evaluate artificial immune systems. *Evolutionary Computation, 13*(2), 145-178.

Gasper, A. & Collard, P. (1999). From GAs to artificial immune systems: Improving adaptation in time dependent optimization. In *Proceedings of the Congress on Evolutionary Computation (CEC 99)*. IEEE press.

Hart, E. & Timmis, J. (2005). Application areas of AIS: The past, the present and the future. In *Proceedings of the 4th International Conference on Artificial Immune Aystems, ICARIS 2005. Lecture notes in computer science* (Vol. 3627, pp. 483-497). Springer.

Hofmeyr, S. & Forrest, S. (1999). Immunity by design: An artificial immune system. In *Proceedings of the Genetic and Evolutionary Computation Conference (GECCO)* (pp. 1289-1296). San Francisco: Morgan-Kaufmann.

Jiao, L. C., Gong, M. G., Shang, R. H., Du, H. F., & Lu, B. (2005). Clonal selection with immune dominance and anergy based multi-objective optimization. In *Proceedings of the Third International Conference on Evolutionary Multi-Criterion Optimization, EMO 2005*, Guanajuato, Mexico. *Lecture notes in computer science* (Vol. 3410, pp. 474-489). Springer-Verlag

Jiao, L. C. & Wang, L. (2000). A novel genetic algorithm based on immunity. *IEEE Transactions on Systems, Man and Cybernetics, Part A, 30*(5), 552-561.

Kim, J. & Bentley, P. J. (2001). Towards an artificial immune system for network intrusion detection: An investigation of clonal selection with a negative selection operator. In *Proceedings of the 2001 Congress on Evolutionary Computation* (Vol. 2, pp. 1244-1252), Seoul Korea.

Luh, G. C., Chueh, C. H., & Liu, W. W. (2003). MOIA: Multi-objective immune algorithm. *Engineering Optimization, 35*(2), 143-164.

Luh, G. C., Chueh, C. H., & Liu, W. W. (2004). Multi-objective optimal design of truss structure with immune algorithm. *Computers and Structures, 82*, 829–844.

Matzinger, P. (1994). Tolerance danger and the extended family. *Annual Reviews of Immunology, 12*, 991-1045.

Tarakanov, A. O., Skormin, V. A., & Sokolova, S. P. (2003). Immunocomputing: Principles and Applications. New York: Springer-Verlag.

Warrender, C., Forrest, S., & Legal, L. (2001). Effective feedback in the immune system. In *Proceedings of the Genetic and Evolutionary Computation Conference Workshop Program* (pp. 329–332). Morgan Kaufman.

Chapter VI
Lexicographic Goal Programming and Assessment Tools for a Combinatorial Production Problem

Seamus M. McGovern
U.S. DOT National Transportation Systems Center, USA

Surendra M. Gupta
Northeastern University, USA

ABSTRACT

NP-complete combinatorial problems often necessitate the use of near-optimal solution techniques including heuristics and metaheuristics. The addition of multiple optimization criteria can further complicate comparison of these solution techniques due to the decision-maker's weighting schema potentially masking search limitations. In addition, many contemporary problems lack quantitative assessment tools, including benchmark data sets. This chapter proposes the use of lexicographic goal programming for use in comparing combinatorial search techniques. These techniques are implemented here using a recently formulated problem from the area of production analysis. The development of a benchmark data set and other assessment tools is demonstrated, and these are then used to compare the performance of a genetic algorithm and an H-K general-purpose heuristic as applied to the production-related application.

INTRODUCTION

More and more manufacturers are acting to recycle and remanufacture their post-consumed products due to new and more rigid environmental legislation, increased public awareness, and extended manufacturer responsibility. A crucial first step is disassembly. Disassembly is defined as the methodical extraction of valuable parts, subassemblies, and materials from discarded products through a series of operations. Recently, disassembly has gained a great deal of attention in the literature due to its role in environmentally conscious manufacturing. A disassembly line system faces many unique challenges; for example, it has significant inventory problems because of the disparity between the demands for certain parts or subassemblies and their yield from disassembly. These many challenges are reflected in its formulation as a multicriteria decision making problem.

Line balancing (ordering assembly/disassembly tasks on a line to achieve some objective) is critical in minimizing the use of valuable resources (e.g., time and money) invested and in maximizing the level of automation and the quality of parts or materials recovered (Figure 1). The Disassembly Line Balancing Problem (DLBP) seeks a sequence of parts for removal from an end of life product that minimizes the resources for disassembly and maximizes the automation of the process and the quality of the parts or materials recovered. This chapter first mathematically models the multicriteria DLBP, which belongs to the class NP-complete, necessitating use of specialized solution techniques. Combinatorial optimization is an emerging field that combines techniques from applied mathematics, operations research, and computer science to solve optimization problems over discrete structures. Due to the suboptimal nature of these searches, a method is needed to access different combinatorial optimization techniques. Lexicographic goal programming is proposed to provide a hierarchical search structure, while quantitative tools including a benchmark data set are introduced. The DLBP is then solved using two combinatorial optimization methods: a genetic algorithm (GA) and the hunter-killer (H-K) general-purpose heuristic.

LITERATURE REVIEW

Key to addressing any engineering problem is to understand how complex or easy it is, what it shares with similar problems, and appropriate methods to obtain reasonable solutions. For these reasons, a background in optimization and algorithms is valuable. Tovey (2002) provides a well-structured review of complexity, NP-hardness, NP-hardness proofs (including the concise style of Garey & Johnson, 1979), typical NP-hard problems, the techniques of specialization, forcing, padding, and gadgets, mathematical programming versus heuristics, and other complexity classifications. Rosen (1999) provides a useful text in the general area of discrete mathematics including set theory, logic, algorithms, graph theory, counting, set theory and proofs. Papadimitriou and Steiglitz (1998) is the de-facto text on combinatorial optimization as is Garey and Johnson (1979) in the area of NP-completeness. Holland (1975) is credited with developing the genetic algorithm. Osman and Laporte (1996) provide a well-researched paper on all forms of metaheuristics, the basic concepts of each, and references to applications. A follow-on paper by Osman (2004) is more compact and also more current.

A major part of manufacturing and assembly operations, the *assembly line* is a production line where material moves continuously at a uniform rate through a sequence of workstations where assembly work is performed. With research papers going back to the 1950's, the Assembly Line Balancing problem is well defined and fairly well understood. While having significant differences from assembly line balancing, the recent development of DLBP requires that related problems be fully investigated and understood in order to better define DLBP and to obtain guidance in the search for appropriate methodologies to solve it. Gutjahr and Nemhauser (1964) first described a solution to the Assembly Line Balancing problem, while Erel and Gokcen (1964) developed a modified version by allowing for *mixed-model* lines (assembly lines used to assemble different models of the same product). Suresh, Vinod, and Sahu (1996) first presented a genetic algorithm to provide a near-optimal solution to the Assembly Line Balancing problem. *Tabu search* is used in balancing assembly lines in Lapierre, Ruiz, and Soriano (2006) using SALB-I with instances from the literature (*Arcus 1* and *2*) and a case study from industry. Hackman, Magazine, and Wee (1989) proposed a *branch-and-bound* heuristic for the SALB-I problem. Ponnambalam, Aravindan, and Naidu (1999) compared line-balancing heuristics with a quantitative evaluation of six assembly line balancing techniques.

Many papers have discussed the different aspects of product recovery. Brennan, Gupta, and Taleb (1994) and Gupta and Taleb (1994) investigated the problems associated with disassembly planning and scheduling. Torres, Gil, Puente, Pomares, and Aracil (2004) reported a study for nondestructive automatic disassembly of personal computers. Gungor and Gupta (1999b, 1999c, 2002, 2001) presented the first introduction to disassembly line balancing and developed an algorithm for solving the DLBP in the presence of failures with the goal of assigning tasks to workstations in a way that probabilistically minimizes the cost of defective parts. For a review of environmentally conscious manufacturing and product recovery see Gungor and Gupta (1999a). For a comprehensive review of disassembly sequencing see Lambert (2003) and Lambert and Gupta (2005). McGovern, Gupta, and Kamarthi (2003) first proposed combinatorial optimization techniques for the DLBP.

MODELING THE MULTI-CRITERIA PRODUCTION PROBLEM

The desired solution to a DLBP instance consists of an ordered sequence (i.e., *n*-tuple) of work elements (also referred to as tasks, components, or parts). For example, if a solution consisted of the eight-tuple ⟨5, 2, 8, 1, 4, 7, 6, 3⟩, then component 5 would be removed first, followed by component 2, then component 8, and so on.

While different authors use a variety of definitions for the term "balanced" in reference to assembly (Elsayed & Boucher, 1994) and disassembly lines, we propose the following definition (McGovern et al., 2003; McGovern & Gupta, 2003) that considers the total number of workstations *NWS* and the station times (i.e., the total processing time requirement in workstation *j*) ST_j; this definition will be used consistently throughout this chapter:

Definition: *A disassembly line is optimally balanced when the fewest possible number of workstations is needed and the variation in idle times between all workstations is minimized. This is mathematically described by*

Minimize *NWS*

Figure 1. Multicriteria selection procedure

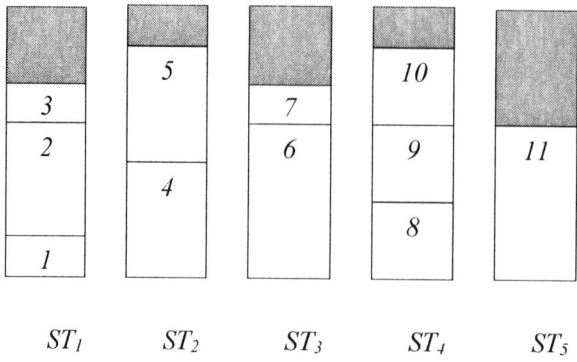

then

Minimize [max (ST_x) − min (ST_y)] ∀ $x, y \in \{1, 2, ..., NWS\}$

This is done while meeting any constraints, including precedence constraints. Line balancing can be visualized in Figure 1 with the boxes representing workstations (five here), the total height of the boxes indicating cycle time *CT* (the maximum time available at each workstation), the numbered boxes representing each part (1 through 11 here) and proportionate in height to each part removal time, and the gray area indicative of the idle time.

Minimizing the sum of the workstation idle times *I*, which will also minimize the total number of workstations, is described by,

$$I = \sum_{j=1}^{NWS} (CT - ST_j) \quad (1)$$

Line balancing seeks to achieve perfect balance (i.e., all idle times equal to zero). When this is not achievable, either Line Efficiency (LE) or the Smoothness Index (SI) is often used as a performance evaluation tool (Elsayed & Boucher, 1994). SI rewards similar idle times at each workstation, but at the expense of allowing for a large (suboptimal) number of workstations. This is because SI compares workstation elapsed times to the largest ST_j instead of to *CT*. (SI is very similar in format to the sample standard deviation from the field of statistics, but using max$(ST_j) | j \in \{1, 2, ..., NWS\}$ rather than the mean of the station times.) LE rewards the minimum number of workstations but allows unlimited variance in idle times between workstations because no comparison is made between ST_j's. The balancing method developed by McGovern et al. (2003; McGovern & Gupta, 2003) seeks to simultaneously minimize the number of workstations while ensuring that idle times at each workstation are similar, though at the expense of the generation of a nonlinear objective function. A resulting minimum numerical value is the more desirable solution, indicating both a minimum number of workstations and similar idle times across all workstations. The measure of balance *F* is represented as,

$$F = \sum_{j=1}^{NWS} (CT - ST_j)^2 \quad (2)$$

Note that mathematically, Formula (2) effectively makes Formula (1) redundant due to the fact that it concurrently minimizes the number of workstations. This new method should be effective with traditional assembly line balancing problems as well.

Theorem: *Let PRT_k be the part removal time for the kth of n parts where CT is the maximum amount of time available to complete all tasks assigned to each workstation. Then for the most efficient distribution of tasks, the minimum (optimal) number of workstations, NWS^* satisfies,*

$$NWS^* \geq \left\lceil \frac{\sum_{k=1}^{n} PRT_k}{CT} \right\rceil \quad (3)$$

Proof: *If the inequality is not satisfied, then there must be at least one workstation completing tasks requiring more than CT of time, which is a contradiction.* □

Subsequent bounds are shown to be true in a similar fashion and are presented throughout the chapter without proof.

The upper bound (worst case) for the number of workstations is given by,

$$NWS_{nom} = n \quad (4)$$

Therefore

$$\left\lceil \frac{\sum_{k=1}^{n} PRT_k}{CT} \right\rceil \leq NWS \leq n \qquad (5)$$

The lower bound on F is given by,

$$F^* \geq \left(\frac{I}{NWS^*}\right)^2 \cdot NWS^* \qquad (6)$$

while the upper bound is described by,

$$F_{nom} = \sum_{k=1}^{n} (CT - PRT_k)^2 \qquad (7)$$

therefore,

$$\left(\frac{I}{NWS^*}\right)^2 \cdot NWS^* \leq F \leq \sum_{k=1}^{n} (CT - PRT_k)^2 \qquad (8)$$

A hazard measure was developed to quantify each solution sequence's performance, with a lower calculated value being more desirable. This measure is based on binary variables that indicate whether a part is considered to contain hazardous material (the binary variable is equal to one if the part is hazardous, else zero) and its position in the sequence. A given solution sequence hazard measure is defined as the sum of hazard binary flags multiplied by their position in the solution sequence, thereby rewarding the removal of hazardous parts early in the part removal sequence. This measure H is represented as,

$$H = \sum_{k=1}^{n} (k \cdot h_{PS_k})$$

$$h_{PS_k} = \begin{cases} 1, hazardous \\ 0, otherwise \end{cases} \qquad (9)$$

where PS_k identifies the kth part in the solution sequence; that is, for solution ⟨3, 1, 2⟩, PS_2 = 1. The lower bound on the hazardous part measure is given by,

$$H^* = \sum_{p=1}^{|HP|} p \qquad (10)$$

where the set of hazardous parts is defined as,

$$HP = \{k : h_k \neq 0 \ \forall \ k \in P\} \qquad (11)$$

where P set of n part removal tasks, and its cardinality can be calculated with,

$$|HP| = \sum_{k=1}^{n} h_k \qquad (12)$$

For example, a product with three hazardous parts would give an H^* value of 1 + 2 + 3 = 6. The upper bound on the hazardous part measure is given by,

$$H_{nom} = \sum_{p=n-|HP|+1}^{n} p \qquad (13)$$

or alternatively,

$$H_{nom} = (n \cdot |HP|) - |HP| \qquad (14)$$

For example, three hazardous parts in a product having a total of twenty would give an H_{nom} value of 18 + 19 + 20 = 57 or equivalently, H_{nom} = (20 · 3) – 3 = 60 – 3 = 57. Formulae (10), (13), and (14) are combined to give,

$$\sum_{p=1}^{|HP|} p \leq H \leq \sum_{p=n-|HP|+1}^{n} p = (n \cdot |HP|) - |HP| \qquad (15)$$

Also, a demand measure was developed to quantify each solution sequence's performance, with a lower calculated value being more desirable. This measure is based on positive integer values that indicate the quantity required of this part after it is removed—or zero if it is not desired—and its position in the sequence. Any given solution sequence demand measure is defined as the sum of the demand value multiplied by their position in the sequence, rewarding the removal of high demand parts early in the part removal sequence. This measure D is represented as,

$$D = \sum_{k=1}^{n}(k \cdot d_{PS_k})$$
$$d_{PS_k} \in N, \forall PS_k \quad (16)$$

The lower bound on the demand measure (D^*) is given by Formula (16) where,

$$d_{PS_1} \geq d_{PS_2} \geq ... \geq d_{PS_n} \quad (17)$$

For example, three parts with demands of 4, 5, and 6 respectively would give a best-case value of $(1 \cdot 6) + (2 \cdot 5) + (3 \cdot 4) = 28$. The upper bound on the demand measure (D_{nom}) is given by Formula (16) where,

$$d_{PS_1} \leq d_{PS_2} \leq ... \leq d_{PS_n} \quad (18)$$

For example, three parts with demands of 4, 5 and 6 respectively would give a worst-case value of $(1 \cdot 4) + (2 \cdot 5) + (3 \cdot 6) = 32$.

Finally, a direction measure was developed to quantify each solution sequence's performance, with a lower calculated value indicating minimal direction changes and a more desirable solution. This measure is based on a count of the direction changes. Integer values represent each possible direction (typically $r = \{+x, -x, +y, -y, +z, -z\}$; in this case $|r| = 6$). These directions are expressed as,

$$r_{PS_k} = \begin{cases} +1, direction + x \\ -1, direction - x \\ +2, direction + y \\ -2, direction - y \\ +3, direction + z \\ -3, direction - z \end{cases} \quad (19)$$

and are easily expanded to other or different directions in a similar manner. The direction measure R is represented as,

$$R = \sum_{k=1}^{n-1} R_k$$
$$R_k = \begin{cases} 1, r_{PS_k} \neq r_{PS_{k+1}} \\ 0, otherwise \end{cases} \quad (20)$$

The lower bound on the direction measure is given by,

$$R^* = |r| - 1 \quad (21)$$

For example, for a given product containing six parts that are installed/removed in directions $r_k = (-y, +x, -y, -y, +x, +x)$ the resulting best-case value would be $2 - 1 = 1$ (e.g., one possible R^* solution containing the optimal, single-change of product direction would be: $\langle -y, -y, -y, +x, +x, +x \rangle$). In the specific case where the number of unique direction changes is one less than the total number of parts n, the upper bound on the direction measure would be given by,

$$R_{nom} = |r| \text{ where } |r| = n - 1 \quad (22)$$

Otherwise, the measure varies depending on the number of parts having a given removal direction and the total number of removal directions. It is bounded by,

$$|r| \leq R_{nom} \leq n - 1 \text{ where } |r| < n - 1 \quad (23)$$

For example, six parts installed/removed in directions $r_k = (+x, +x, +x, -y, +x, +x)$ would give an R_{nom} value of 2 as given by the lower bound of Formula (23) with a solution sequence of $\langle +x, +x, -y, +x, +x, +x \rangle$. Six parts installed/removed in directions $r_k = (-y, +x, -y, -y, +x, +x)$ would give an R_{nom} value of $6 - 1 = 5$ as given by the upper bound of Formula (23) with a solution sequence of $\langle -y, +x, -y, +x, -y, +x \rangle$ for example.

In the special case where each part has a unique removal direction, the measures for R^* and R_{nom} are equal and are given by,

$$R^* = R_{nom} = n - 1 \text{ where } |r| = n \quad (24)$$

Note that the optimal and nominal hazard, demand, and direction formulae are dependent upon favorable precedence constraints that will allow for generation of these optimal or nominal measures. Finally, note that McGovern and Gupta (2006a) have proven that the DLBP is NP-complete.

The combinatorial optimization techniques described here make use of these many criteria in a lexicographic form (detailed in the next section) to address the multicriteria aspects of DLBP. Since measure of balance is the primary consideration in this chapter, additional objectives are only considered subsequently; that is, the methodologies first seek to select the best performing measure of balance solution; equal balance solutions are then evaluated for hazardous part removal positions; equal balance and hazard measure solutions are evaluated for high-demand part removal positions; and equal balance, hazard measure and high-demand part removal position solutions are evaluated for the number of direction changes. This priority ranking approach was selected over a weighting scheme for its simplicity, ease in reranking the priorities, ease in expanding or reducing the number of priorities, due to the fact that other weighting methods can be readily addressed at a later time, and primarily to enable unencumbered *efficacy* (a method's effectiveness in finding good solutions) *analysis* of the combinatorial optimization methodologies and problem data instances under consideration.

LEXICOGRAPHIC GOAL PROGRAMMING FOR USE IN SOLUTION METHODOLOGY EVALUATION

One of the ways in which the complexity of DLBP manifests itself is with the multiple, often conflicting objectives (as defined in the previous section). The field of *multiple-criteria decision making* (MCDM) provides a variety of means for addressing the selection of a solution where several objectives exist. The bulk of MCDM methods involve multicriteria versions of linear programming (LP) problems. Since DLBP requires integers exclusively as its solution, it cannot be formulated as an LP. Additionally, since the objective described by Formula (2) is nonlinear, DLBP is not linear either (a requirement of LP, though this can be remedied using a version of the descriptions in the previous formal Definition). Also, many MCDM methods rely on *weighting*. These weights are in proportion to the importance of each objective. Weights were not desirable for this study since any results would be expected to be influenced by the weights selected. While this is appropriate for an application of the methodologies in this study to an applied problem and using experts to select the appropriate weights, here weighting would only serve to add an additional level of complexity to the comprehension of the problem and the proposed solutions. In addition, since the research in this study is not applied to a particular, unique disassembly situation but rather to the DLBP in general, the assignment of weighting values would be completely arbitrary and hence add little if any value to the final analysis of any results. Finally, the use of weights may not adequately reflect the generalized performance of the combinatorial optimization methods being studied; nuances in the methods, the data, and the weights themselves may generate atypical, unforeseen, or non-repeatable results. For these reasons, a simplified process was developed to select the best solution. Based on the priorities listed, the balance is the primary objective used to search for an optimal solution (note the use of "less than" and "less than or equal to" signs in Figure 2 indicating the desire for the better solution to be on the left side of the inequality since we are seeking to minimize all measures). Given multiple optimum extreme points in F, early removal of hazardous parts is then considered. Given multiple optimum extreme points in *F* and *H*, early removal of high-demand parts is considered next. Finally, given multiple optimum extreme points in *F*, *H*, and *D*, adjacent removal of parts with equivalent part removal directions is considered. This process is shown in pseudo-code format in Figure 2 where the most recent solution generated is given by *new_solution* while the best solution visited thus far in the search is given by *best_solution* with *.F*, *.H*, *.D*, and *.R* indicating the respective solution's numerical measures from formulae (2), (9), (16), and (20).

This process has its basis in two MCDM techniques:

The *feasible region* in an LP problem (and in DLBP) is usually a multidimensional subset of $\mathbf{R}^z$ containing an infinite (finite in DLBP due to its integer nature) number of points. Because it is formed by the intersection of a finite number of *closed half-spaces* (defined by $\leq$ and $\geq$, that is, the inequality constraints) and *hyperplanes* (equality constraints) it is *polyhedral*. Thus, the feasible region is *closed* and *convex* with a finite number of extreme points. The Simplex method (Hillier & Lieberman, 2005) for solving LPs exploits the polyhedral properties in the sense that the optimal solutions can be found without having to examine all of the points in the feasible region. Taking the steepest *gradient* following each point examined accomplishes this. Conventional LP algorithms and software terminate their search once the first optimal extreme point is found (in our example, once the first F^* is found). They fail to identify alternative optima if they exist. In general, an LP instance may have one or more optimal extreme points and one or more *unbounded edge(s)* (though the latter would not be expected of DLBP since it should be contained within the *convex hull* of a *polytope*, that is, a finite region of *n*-dimensional space enclosed by a finite number of hyperplanes). The optimal set is the *convex combination* (i.e., the set of all the points) of all optimal extreme points and points on unbounded edges. It is therefore desired to test all optimal extreme points. This can be done by *pivoting* and is performed using what is known

Figure 2. Multicriteria selection procedure

```
Procedure BETTER_SOLUTION (new_solution, best_solution) {
IF      (new_solution.F < best_solution.F
        ∨
        (new_solution.F ≤ best_solution.F ∧
        new_solution.H < best_solution.H)
        ∨
        (new_solution.F ≤ best_solution.F ∧
        new_solution.H ≤ best_solution.H ∧
        new_solution.D < best_solution.D)
        ∨
        (new_solution.F ≤ best_solution.F ∧
        new_solution.H ≤ best_solution.H ∧
        new_solution.D ≤ best_solution.D ∧
        new_solution.R < best_solution.R)){
                RETURN (TRUE)
        }
        RETURN (FALSE)
}
```

as a *Phase III bookkeeping system*. Determining all alternative optima is enabled in a similar way using the routine shown in Figure 2 (as long as the combinatorial optimization technique in question is able to visit those extreme points).

A second MCDM technique that the process in Figure 2 borrows from is *preemptive (lexicographic) goal programming* (GP). GP was initially conceived by Charnes, Cooper, and Ferguson (1955) and Charnes and Cooper (1961) and conceptualizes objectives as *goals* then assigns priorities to the achievement of these goals. In preemptive GP, goals are grouped according to priorities. The goals at the highest priority level are considered to be infinitely more important than goals at the second priority level, and the goals at the second priority level are considered to be infinitely more important than goals at the third priority level, and so forth (note that a search can effectively terminate using GP if a high priority goal has a unique solution; as a result, lower order goals would not have the opportunity to influence the GP-generated solution). This process can be readily seen in Figure 2 where "infinitely more important" is enforced using the "less than or equal to" ($\leq$) symbol.

This chapter makes use of the term "optimal" to describe the best solution. It should be noted that in the field of MCDM this term is changed to "efficient" (also, *noninferior, nondominated,* or *Pareto-optimum*) where there is no unique solution that maximizes all objectives simultaneously. With this understanding, "optimal" will continue to be used to refer to the best answer possible for a given instance and meeting the criteria set in Figure 2.

ASSESSMENT TOOLS

While the disassembly line is the best choice for automated disassembly of returned products, finding the optimal balance for a disassembly line is computationally intensive with exhaustive search quickly becoming prohibitively large. Combinatorial optimization techniques provide a general algorithmic framework that can be applied to this optimization problem. Although combinatorial optimization holds promise in solving DLBP, one of the concerns when using heuristics is the idea that very little has been rigorously established in reference to their performance; developing ways of explaining and predicting their performance is considered to be one of the most important challenges currently facing the fields of optimization and algorithms (Papadimitriou & Steiglitz, 1998). These challenges exist in the variety of evaluation criteria available, a lack of data sets for testing (disassembly-specific instances are addressed in Section 5.5), and a lack of performance analysis tools. In this section, mathematical and graphical tools for quantitative and qualitative performance analysis are developed and reviewed, focusing on analytical methodologies used in evaluating both of the combinatorial optimization searches used here.

Graphical Analysis Tools

Charts and tables provide an intuitive view into the workings and performance of solution-generating techniques. Both are used here to enhance the qualitative understanding of a methodology's execution and status of its terminal state as well as to allow for a comparison of relative performance with instance size and when compared to other methodologies.

The tables are used to observe the solution of any single instance. The tables used here present a solution in the following format: the sequence n-tuple is listed in the first row, followed by the corresponding part removal times, then the workstation assignments, then the hazard values, followed by the demand values, and finally the direction values (note that the direction representation $\{+x, -x, +y, -y, +z, -z\}$ is changed from $\{+1, -1, +2, -2, +3, -3\}$ as portrayed in the McGovern and Gupta (2006b) formulae to $\{0, 1, 2, 3, 4, 5\}$

for purposes of software engineering). To improve readability, the columns are shaded corresponding to the workstation assignment using alternating shades of gray. Use of this format (i.e., table) allows for study of the final solution state as well as potentially enabling improvements in algorithm performance due to insights gained by this type of observation.

The second graphical format used to allow for qualitative study of techniques and their solutions consists of a graphical comparison of known best- and worst-case results with the results/averaged results (deterministic techniques/stochastic techniques; since methodologies with a probabilistic component—such as would be found with evolutionary algorithms—can be expected to generate different answers over multiple runs) of a solution technique under consideration. The charts are used to observe multiple, varying-size solutions of the DLBP *A Priori* instances. Multiple charts are used to display the various performance measures, which are demonstrated here with the DLBP *A Priori* benchmark data sets of sizes $8 \leq n \leq 80$. The near-optimal solutions coupled with the known optimal and nominal solutions for all instance sizes under study provides a method, not only for comparing the methodologies to the best and worst cases, but to other methodologies as well. Computational complexity is portrayed using time complexity (analysis of the time required to solve a particular size instance of a given problem) while *space complexity* (analysis of the computer memory required to solve a particular size instance of a given problem; Rosen, 1999) is not considered. All time complexities are provided in *asymptotic notation* (*big-Oh*, *big-Omega*, and *big-Theta*) when commonly known or when calculated where able. "Time complexity" typically refers to worst-case runtimes, while in the numerical results portion of this chapter, the runtimes provide a qualitative description of the studied methodologies, so the experimentally determined time complexities are presented with the understanding that the information is the average-case time complexity of the particular software written for the problem used with a specific instance. In this chapter the charts used include: number of workstations with optimal, balance measure with optimal, normalized balance measure with optimal and nominal, hazard measure with optimal and nominal, demand measure with optimal and nominal, direction measure with optimal and nominal, average-case time complexity with third-order and exhaustive growth curves, and average-case time complexity curves in detail. Note that "number of workstations" and "idle time" measures are analogous (e.g., one can be calculated from the other) so only "number of workstations" is calculated and displayed here. Also, while "number of workstations" and "balance" are both calculated in various ways and displayed in separate graphs, they are strongly related as well. Both are presented to allow insight into the search processes and further quantify the efficacy of their solutions; however, it should be noted that, for example, a solution optimal in balance must also obviously be optimal in the number of workstations.

Note that with the graphs depicting third-order (i.e., $O(n^3)$) and exhaustive (i.e., $O(n!)$) growth curve graphics (as seen in Figure 14), the actual average-case time complexity curve under consideration is often not even readily visible. Even so, average-case time complexity with the third-order and exhaustive growth curves helps to show how relatively fast all of these techniques are, while the average-case time complexity graphics (Figure 15) defines the methodologies' speed and rate of growth in even more detail.

Though not demonstrated in this chapter, it is often of value to make use of overlaid linear or polynomial fitted regression lines to better provide graphical information for analysis of some of these very fast heuristics. When a heuristic's software is configured to time down to 1/100th of a second or slower, it should be recognized that many applications of heuristics are able to run on that order (or in some cases even faster); therefore, average-case time complexity curves may give the appearance of making dramatic steps up or down when this is actually more of an aberration of the order of the timing data that is collected. For that reason, showing the average-case time complexity with its regression line displays both the actual data and more importantly, the shape of the time growth in n.

In order to make the balance results comparable in magnitude to all other measures and to allow for more legible graphical comparisons with worst-case calculations in the charts, the effects of squaring portions of Formula (2) can be compensated for by taking the square root of the resulting F, F^*, or F_{nom}. This will subsequently be referred to in this study as *normalizing* (to reflect the concept of a reduction in the values to a common magnitude). While using Formula (2) is desirable to emphasize the importance of a solution's balance as well as to drive stochastic search processes towards the optimal solution, normalization allows for a more intuitive observation of the relative merits of any two solutions. For example, two solutions having an equal number of workstations (e.g., $NWS = 3$) but differing balance such as $I_j = \langle 1, 1, 4 \rangle$ and $I_j = \langle 2, 2, 2 \rangle$ (optimal balance) would have balance values of 18 and 12 respectively, while the normalized values would stand at 4.24 and 3.46, still indicating better balance with the latter solution, but also giving a sense of the relative improvement that solution provides, which the measure generated by Formula (2) lacks.

Efficacy Index Equations

The primary mathematical tool developed for quantitative analysis is shown in Formula (25). This will subsequently be referred to as the *efficacy index* (McGovern & Gupta, 2006b). The efficacy index EI_x (where x is some metric under consideration, e.g., F) is the ratio of the difference between a calculated measure and its worst-case measure to the measure's *sample range* (i.e., the difference between the best-case measure and the worst-case measure as given by: $\max(X_y) - \min(X_z) \mid y, z \in \{1, 2, \ldots, |X|\}$ from the area of statistical quality control) expressed as a percentage and described by

$$EI_x = \frac{100 \cdot (x_{nom} - x)}{x_{nom} - x^*} \qquad (25)$$

This generates a value between 0% and 100%, indicating the percentage of optimum for any given measure and any given combinatorial optimization methodology being evaluated. For example, the efficacy index formula for balance would read

$$EI_F = \frac{100 \cdot (F_{nom} - F)}{F_{nom} - F^*}$$

where the subscript *nom* represents the worst-case bound (nominal) for a given data set and the superscript * represents the best-case bound (optimal) for a given data set.

For the study of multiple data sets, probability theory presents us with the concept of a *sample mean*. The sample mean of a method's efficacy index can be calculated using

$$\overline{EI}_x = \left(\sum_{i=1}^{y} \frac{100 \cdot (x_{nom} - x_i)}{x_{nom} - x^*} \right) \Big/ y \qquad (26)$$

where y is the sample size (the number of data sets). While Formula (25) provides individual data set size efficacy indices—especially useful in demonstrating worst and best case as well as trends with instance size—Formula (26) allows a single numerical value that provides a quantitative measure of the location of the data center in a sample.

Statistical Regression

Performed but not demonstrated in here, an additional quantitative tool may be borrowed from the field of statistics. *Simple linear regression* and *correlation* (using the *sample coefficient of determination*), and *polynomial regression* and its associated *coefficient of multiple determination* can be used to quantify the accuracy of the curves and to provide the regression equation. The chart containing the combinatorial optimization methodologies with the third-order and exhaustive growth curves was used not only to provide a qualitative, graphical comparison, but also (along with the detailed time complexity curves) to determine the *degree* (*order*) of the fitted polynomial regression curve. Once the order was observed by comparison, either a linear or a polynomial regression model was selected and the regression equation was then automatically calculated by mathematical software (using, for example, an EXCEL 2000 spreadsheet software function), as was the coefficient of determination. The heuristic methodologies used here were either first (linear) or second order. As part of the quantitative portion of this research, this corresponds to average-case time complexities of $O(n)$ or $O(n^2)$.

Statistical Coefficient of Determination

The coefficient of determination was the final portion of the quantitative component of the study. This value represents the portion of the *variation* in the collected data explained by the fitted curve. The coefficient of determination is then multiplied by 100 to illustrate the adequacy of the fitted regression model, indicating the percentage of variation time that can be attributed to the size of the data set. The closer the value comes to 100%, the more likely it is an accurate model. While the coefficients of the polynomial regression model are of interest in presenting as accurate a growth curve model as possible, of greater value in this study is the order of the model since the largest exponent is the only variable of interest in complexity theory.

Performance Assessment Experimental Benchmark Data Set

Any solution methodology needs to be applied to a collection of test cases to demonstrate its performance as well as its limitations. Benchmark data sets are common for many NP-complete problems, such as *Oliver30* and *RY48P* for application to the Traveling Salesman Problem and *Nugent15/20/30*, *Elshafei19*, and *Krarup30* for the Quadratic Assignment Problem. Unfortunately, because of their size and their design, most of these existing data sets have no known optimal answer and new solutions are not compared to the optimal solution, but rather the best solution to date. In addition, since DLBP is a recently defined problem, no appropriate benchmark data sets exist.

This size-independent *a priori* benchmark data set was generated (McGovern & Gupta, 2004) based on the following. Since, in general, solutions to larger and larger instances cannot be verified as optimal (due to the time complexity of exhaustive search), it is proposed that instances be generated in such a way as to always provide a known solution. This was done by using part removal times consisting exclusively of prime numbers further selected to ensure that no permutations of these part removal times allowed for any equal summations (in order to reduce the number of possible optimal solutions). For example, part removal times (PRT_k, where k typically identifies a part or sequence position) 1, 3, 5, and 7, and CT = 16 would have minimum idle time solutions of not only one 1, one 3, one 5, and one 7 at each workstation, but various additional combinations of these as well since $1 + 7 = 3 + 5 = ½ CT$. Subsequently, the chosen instances were made up of parts with removal times of 3, 5, 7, and 11, and CT = 26. As a result, the optimal balance for all subsequent instances would consist of a perfect balance of precedence-preserving permutations of 3, 5, 7, and 11 at each workstation with idle times of zero. (Note that the cardinality of the set of part removal times $|PRT| \leq n$ since PRT_k is *onto* mapped to *PRT*, though not necessarily *one-to-one*, since multiple parts may have equal part removal times; that is, PRT_k is a *surjection* and may or may not be a *bijection* to *PRT*.)

As demonstrated in Table 1, to further complicate the data (i.e., provide a large, feasible search space), only one part was listed as hazardous and this was one of the parts with the largest part removal time (the last one listed in the original data). In addition, one part (the last listed, second largest part removal time component) was listed as being demanded. This was done so that only the hazardous and the demand sequencing would be demonstrated while providing a slight solution sequence disadvantage to any purely greedy methodology (since two parts with part removal times of 3 and 5 are needed along with the parts with the larger part removal times to reach the optimal balance F^*, assigning hazard and high-demand attributes to those parts with smaller part removal times may prevent some methodologies from artificially obtaining an F^* sequence). From each part removal time size, the first listed part was selected to have a removal direction differing from the other parts with the same part removal time. This was done to demonstrate direction selection while requiring any solution-generating methodology to move these first parts of each part removal time size encountered to the end of the sequence (i.e., into the last workstation) in order to obtain the optimal part direction value of $R^* = 1$ (assuming the solution technique being evaluated is able to successfully place the hazardous and demanded parts towards the front of the sequence).

Also, there were no precedence constraints placed on the sequence, a deletion that further challenges any method's ability to attain an optimal solution (by maximizing the feasible search space). This has the added benefit of more precisely modeling the restricted version of the decision version (i.e., non-optimization) of DLBP seen in McGovern and Gupta (2006a).

Hazard values are given by,

$$h_k = \begin{cases} 1, & k = n \\ 0, & otherwise \end{cases} \quad (27)$$

with demand values given by,

$$d_k = \begin{cases} 1, & k = \dfrac{n \cdot (|PRT|-1)}{|PRT|} \\ 0, & otherwise \end{cases} \quad (28)$$

and part removal direction values given by,

$$r_k = \begin{cases} 1, \\ 0, \end{cases}$$

$$k = 1, \dfrac{n}{|PRT|}+1, \dfrac{2n}{|PRT|}+1,\ldots,\dfrac{(|PRT|-1)\cdot n}{|PRT|}+1$$
$$otherwise$$

$$(29)$$

Since $|PRT| = 4$ in this chapter, each part removal time is generated by,

$$PRT_k = \begin{cases} 3, & 0 < k \leq \dfrac{n}{4} \\ 5, & \dfrac{n}{4} < k \leq \dfrac{n}{2} \\ 7, & \dfrac{n}{2} < k \leq \dfrac{3n}{4} \\ 11, & \dfrac{3n}{4} < k \leq n \end{cases} \quad (30)$$

Known optimal results include balance measure $F^* = 0$, hazardous part measure $H^* = 1$,

Table 1. DLBP A Priori data for n = 12

Part ID	1	2	3	4	5	6	7	8	9	10	11	12
PRT	3	3	3	5	5	5	7	7	7	11	11	11
Hazardous	0	0	0	0	0	0	0	0	0	0	0	1
Demand	0	0	0	0	0	0	0	0	1	0	0	0
Direction	1	0	0	1	0	0	1	0	0	1	0	0

demanded part measure $D^* = 2$, and part removal direction measure $R^* = 1$.

A data set containing parts with equal part removal times and no precedence constraints will result in multiple optimum extreme points. Using probability theory (counting sample points using the generalized multiplication rule covering n operations), it can be seen in Table 2 (and detailed in McGovern & Gupta, 2004) that the number of solutions optimal in all objectives goes from less than 8.3% of n at $n = 4$, to 0.12% at $n = 8$, dropping to effectively 0% at $n = 16$; as n grows, the percentage of optimal solutions gets closer and closer to zero.

The final configuration of the benchmark as used here was 19 instances with instance size distributed from $n = 8$ to $n = 80$ in steps of $|PRT| = 4$. The size and range of the instances is considered appropriate, with small ns tested—which decreases the *NWS* value and tends to exaggerate less than optimal performance—as well as large, which demonstrates time complexity growth and efficacy changes with n.

H-K HEURISTIC

Heuristic Search Background

Exhaustive search techniques (e.g., pure depth-first or pure breadth-first) will fail to find a solution to any but the smallest instances within any practical length of time. *Blind search, weak search, naïve search,* and *uninformed search* are all terms used to refer to algorithms that use the simplest, most intuitive method of searching through a search space, whereas *informed search* algorithms use heuristics to apply knowledge about the structure of the search space. An uninformed search algorithm is one that does not take into account the specific nature of the problem. This allows uninformed searches to be implemented in general, with the same implementation able to be used in a wide range of problems. Uninformed searches include exhaustive search and H-K. H-K seeks to take advantage of the benefits of uninformed search while addressing the exhaustive search drawbacks of runtime growth with instance size.

Heuristic Motivation and Introduction

Exhaustive search is optimal because it looks at every possible answer. While an optimal solution can be found, this technique is impractical for all but the simplest combinatorial problems due to the explosive growth in search time. In many physical search applications (e.g., antisubmarine warfare, search and rescue) exhaustive search is not possible due to time or sensor limitations. In these cases, it becomes practical to sample the search space and operate under the assumption that, for example, the highest point of land found during the conduct of a limited search is either is the highest point in a given search area or is reasonably near the highest point. The proposed search technique (McGovern & Gupta, 2004) in this chapter works by sampling the exhaustive solution set; that is, search the solution space in a method similar to an exhaustive search but in a pattern that skips solutions (conceptually similar to the STEP functionality in a FOR loop as found in computer programming) to significantly minimize the search space (Figure 3; the shading indicates solutions visited, the border represents the search space).

Table 2. Comparison of possible solutions to optimal solutions for a given n using the DLBP A Priori data

n	n!	Number optimal in balance	Number optimal in all	Percentage optimal in balance	Percentage optimal in all
4	24	24	2	100.00%	8.33%
8	40,320	9,216	48	22.86%	0.12%
12	479,001,600	17,915,904	10,368	3.74%	0.00%
16	2.09228E+13	1.10075E+11	7,077,888	0.53%	0.00%

Figure 3. Exhaustive search space and the H-K search space and methodology

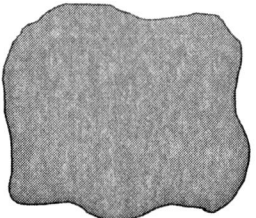
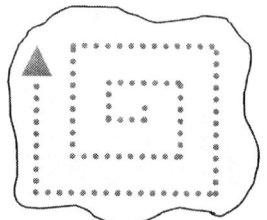

This pattern is analogous to the radar acquisition search pattern known as "spiral scan," the search and rescue pattern of the "expanding square," or the antisubmarine warfare aircraft "magnetic anomaly detector (MAD) hunting circle." Once the solution is generated, the space can be further searched with additional applications of the H-K heuristic (with modifications from the previous H-K) or the best-to-date solution can be further refined by performing subsequent local searches (such as 2-opt or smaller, localized H-K searches). Depending on the application, H-K can be run once, multiple times on subsequent solutions, multiple times from the same starting point using different skip measure (potentially as a multiprocessor application using parallel algorithms or as a grid computing application), multiple times from a different starting point using the same skip measure (again, potentially as a multiprocessor or grid computing application), or followed up with an H-K or another, differing local search on the best or several of the best suboptimal solutions generated. While termination normally takes place after all sequences are generated for a given skip size, termination can also be effected based on time elapsed or once finding a solution that is within a predetermined bound. H-K can also be used as the first phase of a hybrid algorithm or to hot start another methodology (e.g., to provide the initial population in a GA). One interesting use for H-K is application to the unusual problem where quantifying a small improvement (i.e., a greedy decision, such as would be found in ant colony optimization where the ant agents build a solution incrementally and, therefore, need to know which of the available solution elements reflects an improvement) is not possible or is not understood, or where the incremental greedy improvements may not lead to a global optima. Finally, H-K would also be useful in quickly gathering a sampling of the solution space to allow for a statistical or other study of the data (e.g., H-K could enable the determination of the approximate worst-case and best-case solutions

Figure 4. DLBP H-K results at n = 5 and ψ = 2

$PS_k = \langle 1, 2, 3, 4, 5 \rangle$
$PS_k = \langle 1, 2, 5, 3, 4 \rangle$
$PS_k = \langle 1, 4, 2, 3, 5 \rangle$
$PS_k = \langle 1, 4, 5, 2, 3 \rangle$
$PS_k = \langle 1, 4, 5, 3, 2 \rangle$
$PS_k = \langle 3, 1, 2, 4, 5 \rangle$
$PS_k = \langle 3, 1, 4, 2, 5 \rangle$
$PS_k = \langle 3, 1, 4, 5, 2 \rangle$
$PS_k = \langle 3, 4, 1, 2, 5 \rangle$
$PS_k = \langle 3, 4, 1, 5, 2 \rangle$
$PS_k = \langle 3, 4, 5, 1, 2 \rangle$
$PS_k = \langle 5, 1, 2, 3, 4 \rangle$
$PS_k = \langle 5, 1, 4, 2, 3 \rangle$
$PS_k = \langle 5, 3, 1, 2, 4 \rangle$
$PS_k = \langle 5, 3, 1, 4, 2 \rangle$
$PS_k = \langle 5, 3, 4, 1, 2 \rangle$

as well as solution efficacy indices *mean*, *median*, and *mode*).

The *skip size* ψ, or more generally ψ_k (the kth element's skip measure; i.e., for the solution's third element, visit every 2nd possible task for $\psi_3 = 2$) can be as small as ψ = 1 or as large as ψ = n. Since ψ = 1 is equivalent to exhaustive search and ψ = n generates a trivial solution (it returns only one solution, that being the data in the same sequence as it is given to H-K, that is, $PS_k = \langle 1, 2, 3, \ldots, n \rangle$; also, in the single-phase H-K this solution is already considered by any value of ψ), in general all skip values can be further constrained as

$$2 \leq \psi_k \leq n - 1 \qquad (31)$$

Depending on structural decisions, H-K can take on a variety of forms, from a classical optimization algorithm in its most basic form, to a general evolutionary algorithm with the use of multiple H-K processes, to a *biological* or *natural process algorithm* by electing random functionality. In order to demonstrate the method and show some of its limitations, in this chapter the most basic form of the H-K heuristic is used: one process (though visiting the data twice, in forward and in reverse order), constant starting point of $PS_k = \langle 1, 1, 1, \ldots, 1 \rangle$ (since the solution set is a permutation, there are no repeated items; therefore, the starting point is effectively $PS_k = \langle 1, 2, 3, \ldots, n \rangle$), constant skip type (i.e., each element in the solution sequence is skipped in the same way), constant maximum skip size (although different skip sizes are used throughout each H-K run, and no follow-on solution refinement.

The H-K Process and DLBP Application

As far as the H-K process itself, since it is a modified exhaustive search allowing for solution sampling, it searches for solutions similar to depth-first search iteratively seeking the next permutation iteration—allowing for skips in the sequence—in lexicographic order. In the basic H-K and with ψ = 2, the first element in the first solution would be 1, the next element considered would be 1, but since it is already in the solution, that element would be incremented and 2 would be considered and be acceptable. This is repeated for all of the elements until the first solution is generated. In the next iteration, the initial part under consideration would be incremented by 2 and, therefore, 3 would be considered and inserted as the first element. Since 1 is not yet in the sequence, it would be placed in the second position, 2 in the third, and so forth. For DLBP H-K this is further modified to test the proposed sequence part addition for precedence constraints. If all possible parts for a given solution position fail these checks, the remainder of the positions are not further inspected, the procedure falls back to the previously successful solution addition, increments it by 1, and continues. These processes are repeated until all allowed items have been visited in the first solution position (and by default, due to the nested nature of the search, all subsequent solution positions). For example, with $n = 4$, $P = \{1, 2, 3, 4\}$, and no precedence constraints, instead of considering the $4! = 24$ possible permutations, only five are considered by the single-phase H-K with $\psi = 2$ and using forward-only data: $PS_k = \langle 1, 2, 3, 4 \rangle$, $PS_k = \langle 1, 4, 2, 3 \rangle$, $PS_k = \langle 3, 1, 2, 4 \rangle$, $PS_k = \langle 3, 1, 4, 2 \rangle$, and $PS_k = \langle 3, 4, 1, 2 \rangle$. With $n = 5$, $P = \{1, 2, 3, 4, 5\}$, and no precedence constraints, instead of considering the $5! = 120$ possible permutations, only 16 are considered by the single-phase H-K with $\psi = 2$ and using forward-only data as demonstrated in Figure 4.

All of the parts are maintained in a tabu-type list. Each iteration of the DLBP H-K generated solution is considered for feasibility. If it is ultimately feasible in its entirety, DLBP H-K then looks at each element in the solution and places that element using the Next-Fit (NF) rule (from the Bin-Packing problem application; once a bin has no space for a given item attempted to be packed into it, that bin is never used again even though a later, smaller item may appear in the list and could fit in the bin (see Hu & Shing, 2002). DLBP H-K puts the element under consideration into the current workstation if it fits. If it does not fit, a new workstation is assigned and previous workstations are never again considered. Although NF does not perform as well as First-Fit, Best-Fit, First-Fit-Decreasing, or Best-Fit-Decreasing when used in the general Bin-Packing problem, it is the only one of these rules that will work with a DLBP solution sequence due to the existence of precedence constraints (see McGovern & Gupta, 2005 for a DLBP implementation of First-Fit-Decreasing). When all of the work elements have been assigned to a workstation, the process is complete and the balance, hazard, demand and direction measures are calculated. The best of all of the inspected solution sequences is then saved as the problem solution. Although the actual software implementation for this study consisted of a very compact recursive algorithm, in the interest of clarity, the general DLBP H-K procedure is presented here as a series of nested loops (Figure 5, where ISS_k is the binary flag representing the tabu-type list; set to 1 if part k is in the solution sequence, and FS is the feasible sequence binary flag; set to 1 if the sequence is feasible).

Skip size affects various measures including the efficacy indices and time complexity. The general form of the skip-size to problem-size relationship is formulated as

$$\psi_k = n - \Delta\psi_k \tag{32}$$

where $\Delta\psi$ represents the kth element's delta skip measure; difference between problem size n and skip size ψ_k (i.e., for $\Delta\psi = 10$ and $n = 80$, $\psi = 70$).

Early tests of time complexity growth with skip size suggest another technique to be used as part of H-K search. Since any values of ψ that are larger than the chosen skip value for a given H-K instance were seen to take significantly less processing time, considering all larger skip values should also be considered in order to increase the search space at the expense of a minimal increase in search time. In other words, H-K can be run repeatedly on a given instance using all skip values from a smallest ψ (selected based upon time complexity considerations) to the largest (i.e., $n - 1$ per Formula (31)) without a significant time penalty. In this case, any ψ_k would be constrained as

$$n - \Delta\psi_k \leq \psi_k \leq n - 1$$

where $1 \leq \Delta\psi_k \leq n - 2$ \qquad (33)

If this technique is used (as it is here), it should also be noted that multiples of ψ visit the same solutions; for example, for $n = 12$ and $2 \leq \psi \leq 10$, the four solutions considered by $\psi = 10$ are also visited by $\psi = 2$ and $\psi = 5$.

In terms of time complexity, the rate of growth has been observed to be exponential in the in-

Figure 5. The DLBP H-K procedure

```
Procedure DLBP_H-K {
        SET ISS_k := 0 ∀ k∈P
        SET FS := 1

        PS_1 := 1 to n, skip by ψ_1
                SET ISS_PS1 := 1

                PS_2 := 1 to n, skip by ψ_2
                        WHILE      (ISS_PS2 == 1 ∨
                                    PRECEDENCE_FAIL ∧
                                    not at n)
                                Increment PS_2 by 1

                        IF      ISS_PS2 == 1
                        THEN SET FS := 0
                        ELSE SET ISS_PS2 := 1
                           :
                        IF      FS == 1
                                PS_n := 1 to n skip by ψ_n
                                        WHILE      (ISS_PSn == 1 ∨
                                                    PRECEDENCE_FAIL ∧
                                                    not at n)
                                                Increment PS_n by 1

                                        IF      ISS_PSn == 0
                                        THEN evaluate solution PS
                           :
                        IF      FS == 1
                        THEN SET ISS_PS2 := 0
                        ELSE SET FS := 1

                SET ISS_PS1 := 0
                SET FS := 1
}
```

verse of ψ. The average-case time complexity of H-K is then listed as $O(b^b)$ in skip size, where $b = 1/\psi$. Due to the nature of H-K, the number of commands executed in the software do not vary based on precedence constraints, data sequence, greedy or probabilistic decision making, improved solutions nearby, and so forth, so the worst case is also $O(b^b)$, as is the best case (big-Omega of $\Omega(b^b)$), and, therefore, a tight bound exists, which is $\Theta(b^b)$. As used in the Numerical Comparison section below (forward and reverse data, $1 \leq \Delta\psi \leq 10$, and resulting skip sizes of $n - 10 \leq \psi \leq n - 1$), the average-case time complexity of DLBP H-K curve is listed as $O(n^2)$ or polynomial complexity. The deterministic, single iteration nature of H-K also indicates that the process would be no faster than this, so it is expected that the time complexity lower bound is $\Omega(n^2)$ and, therefore, the H-K appears to have an asymptotically tight bound of $\Theta(n^2)$ as configured here.

GENETIC ALGORITHM

GA Model Description

A genetic algorithm (a parallel neighborhood, stochastic-directed search technique) provides an environment where solutions continuously crossbreed, mutate, and compete with each other until they evolve into an optimal or near-optimal solution (Holland, 1975). Due to its structure and search method, a GA is often able to find a global solution, unlike many other heuristics that use hill climbing to find a best solution nearby resulting only in a local optima. In addition, a GA does not need specific details about a problem nor is the problem's structure relevant; a function can be linear, nonlinear, stochastic, combinatorial, noisy and so forth.

GA has a solution structure defined as a *chromosome*, which is made up of *genes* and generated by two *parent* chromosomes from the *pool* of solutions, each having its own measure of *fitness*. New solutions are generated from old using the techniques of *crossover* (sever parents genes and swap severed sections) R_x and *mutation* (randomly vary genes within a chromosome) R_m. Typically, the main challenge with any genetic algorithm implementation is determining a chromosome representation that remains valid after each generation.

For DLBP the chromosome (solution) consisted of a sequence of genes (parts). A pool, or *population*, of size N was used. Only feasible disassembly sequences were allowed as members of the population or as offspring. The fitness was computed for each chromosome using the method for solution performance determination (i.e., in lexicographic order using F, H, D, then R).

The time complexity is a function of the number of generations, the population size N, and the chromosome size n. As such, the runtime is seen to be on the order of $n \cdot N \cdot$ (number of generations). Since both the population and the number of generations are considered to stay constant with instance size, the best-case time complexity of GA is seen to have an asymptotic lower bound of $\Omega(n)$. Because the worst-case runtime also requires no more processing time than $T(n) \propto n \cdot N \cdot$ (number of generations), the worst-case time complexity of GA has the asymptotic upper bound $O(n)$, so GA therefore exhibits a tight time complexity bound of $\Theta(n)$.

DLBP-Specific Genetic Algorithm Architecture

The GA for DLBP was constructed as follows (McGovern & Gupta, 2007). An initial, feasible population was randomly generated and the fitness of each chromosome in this generation was calculated. An even integer of $R_x \cdot N$ parents was randomly selected for crossover to produce $R_x \cdot N$ offspring (offspring make up ($R_x \cdot N \cdot 100$)% of each generation's population). (Note that often GA's use fitness values rather than random selection for crossover; the authors found that random selection made creation of children that were duplicates of each other or of parents less likely and allowed for a more diverse population.) An elegant crossover, the precedence preservative crossover (PPX) developed by Bierwirth, Mattfeld, and Kopfer (1996) was used to create the offspring. As shown in Figure 6, PPX first creates a mask (one for each child, every generation). The mask consists of random 1s and 2s indicating which parent part information should be taken from. If, for example, the mask for child 1 reads 22121112, the first two parts (i.e., from left to right) in parent 2 would make up the first two genes of child 1 (and these parts would be stricken from the parts available to take from both parent 1 and 2); the first available (i.e., not stricken) part in parent 1 would make up gene three of child 1; the next available part in parent 2 would make up gene four of child 1; the next three available parts in parent 1 would make up genes five, six, and seven of child 1; the last part in parent 2 would make up gene eight of

Figure 6. PPX example

Parent 1:	1 3 2 6 5 8 7 4		Parent 1:	1 3 2 6 5 8 7 4	
Parent 2:	1 2 3 5 6 8 7 4	⇒	Parent 2:	1 2 3 5 6 8 7 4	⇒
Mask:	2 2 1 2 1 1 1 2		Mask:	2 2 1 2 1 1 1 2	
Child:			Child:	1 2	
Parent 1:	x 3 x 6 5 8 7 4		Parent 1:	x x x 6 5 8 7	
Parent 2:	x x 3 5 6 8 7 4	⇒	Parent 2:	x x x 5 6 8 7 4	⇒
Mask:	1 2 1 1 1 2		Mask:	2 1 1 1 2	
Child:	1 2 3		Child:	1 2 3 5	
Parent 1:	x x x 6 x 8 7 4		Parent 1:	x x x x x x x 4	
Parent 2:	x x x x 6 8 7 4	⇒	Parent 2:	x x x x x x x 4	
Mask:	1 1 1 2		Mask:	2	
Child:	1 2 3 5 6 8 7		Child:	1 2 3 5 6 8 7 4	

child 1. This technique is repeated using a new mask for child 2.

After crossover, mutation is randomly conducted. Mutation was occasionally (based on the R_m value) performed by randomly selecting a single child then exchanging two of its disassembly tasks while ensuring precedence is preserved. The $R_x \cdot N$ least-fit parents are removed by sorting the entire parent population from worst-to-best based on fitness.

Since the GA saves the best parents from generation to generation and it is possible for duplicates of a solution to be formed using PPX, the solution set could contain multiple copies of the same answer resulting in the algorithm potentially becoming trapped in a local optima. This becomes more likely in a GA with solution constraints (such as precedence requirements) and small populations, both of which are seen in the study in this chapter. To avoid this, DLBP GA was modified to treat duplicate solutions as if they had the worst fitness performance (highest numerical value), relegating them to replacement in the next generation. With this new ordering, the best unique $(1 - R_x) \cdot N$ parents were kept along with all of the $R_x \cdot N$ offspring to make up the next generation then the process was repeated.

DLBP-Specific GA Qualitative Modifications

DLBP GA was modified from a general GA in several ways (Figure 7). Instead of the worst portion of the population being selected for crossover as is often the case in GA, in DLBP GA all of the population was (randomly) considered for crossover. This better enables the selection of nearby solutions (i.e., solutions similar to the best solutions to-date) common in many scheduling problems. Also, mutation was performed only on the children in DLBP GA, not the worst parents as is typical in a general GA. This was done to address the small population used in DLBP GA and to counter PPX's tendency to duplicate parents. Finally, duplicate children are sorted in DLBP GA to make their deletion from the population likely since there is a tendency for the creation of duplicate solutions (due to PPX) and due to the small population saved from generation to generation.

DLBP-Specific GA Quantitative Modifications

While the matter of population sizing is a controversial research area in evolutionary computing,

Figure 7. The DLBP GA procedure

```
Procedure DLBP_GA {
        INITIALIZE_DATA              {Load data: part removal times, etc.}

    SET count := 1                   {count is the generation counter}

    FOR N DO:                        {Randomly create an initial population}
        DO:
            RANDOMLY_CREATE_CHROMOSOME
        WHILE (PRECEDENCE_FAIL)
        CALC_FITNESS                 {Establish the initial solution's fitness}

    SET num_parents := N * R_x       {Determine number of parents for reproduction}
                                     {Ensure an even number of parents}
    SET num_parents := 2 * (num_parents / 2)
                                     {Note: num_parents is typed as an integer}
    DO:                              {Run GA for MAX_GENERATIONS}
        RANDOMIZE_PARENTS            {Randomly order the parents for breeding}

        FOR num_parents DO:          {Perform crossover using PPX}
            CROSSOVER

        IF FLIP(R_m) DO:             {FLIP equals 1 R_m % of the time, else 0}
            MUTATE_CHILD             {Randomly select and mutate a child}

        REMOVE_LEAST_FIT             {Sort: best parents to the last positions}
        REMOVE_REPEATS               {Duplicate answers to the front and resort}
        CHILDREN_TO_POOL             {Add children to the population}

        FOR N DO:
            CALC_FITNESS             {Calculate each solution's fitness}

        count := count + 1           {Next generation}
    WHILE (count < MAX_GENERATIONS)

    SAVE the last chromosome as the best_solution
}
```

here a small population was used (20) to minimize data storage requirements and simplify analysis while a large number of generations were used (10,000) to compensate for this small population while not being so large as to take an excessive amount of processing time. This was also done to avoid solving all cases to optimality since it was desirable to determine the point at which the DLBP GA performance begins to break down and how that breakdown manifests itself.

A 60% crossover was selected based on test and analysis. Developmental testing indicated that a 60% crossover provided better solutions and did so with one-third less processing time than, for example 90%. Previous assembly line balancing literature that indicated best results have typically been found with crossover rates of from 0.5 to 0.7 also substantiated the selection of this lower crossover rate. A mutation was performed about one percent of the time. Although some texts recommend 0.01% mutation while applications in journal papers have used as much as 100% mutation, it was found that 1.0% gave excellent algorithm performance for the Disassembly Line Balancing Problem.

NUMERICAL COMPARISON AND QUALITATIVE ANALYSIS

The evolutionary algorithm and the uninformed heuristic were run on the DLBP *A Priori* experimental instances (with size varying between $8 \leq n \leq 80$) with the results comparatively analyzed in this section. For H-K, all cases were calculated using a varying delta skip of $1 \leq \Delta\psi \leq 10$ with the resulting skip sizes of $n - 10 \leq \psi \leq n - 1$; the software was set up so that it would not attempt any skip size smaller than $\psi = 3$ (to avoid exhaustive or near-exhaustive searches with small instances). In addition, the DLBP *A Priori* data sets were run with the data in forward and reverse for H-K. For GA, all tests were performed using a population size of 20, mutation rates of 1.0%, 10,000 generations, and crossover rates of 60%. Note that, due to the averaging of the results given by the process with stochastic characteristics (DLBP GA), many of the reported results are not purely discrete.

Table-Based Qualitative Assessment

From Section 5.1, the table-based qualitative analysis tool is demonstrated. The DLBP H-K technique can be seen below (Table 3) on the DLBP *A Priori* data presented forward and reverse at $n = 12$ and $3 \leq \psi \leq 11$ (note that without the minimum allowed value of $\psi = 3$, skip values would include $2 \leq \psi \leq 11$). DLBP H-K was able to find a solution optimal in the number of workstations, balance, and hazard (though not demand or direction). The solution found came from the reverse set and consisted of $NWS^* = 3$, $F^* = 0$, $H^* = 1$, $D = 10$ (optimal value is $D^* = 2$), and $R = 2$ (optimal value is $R^* = 1$).

An example of a GA metaheuristic solution can be seen below with $n = 12$ (Table 4). While there is more than one optimal solution for the *A Priori* instances, GA was able to regularly find one of the multiple optimum extreme points (three workstations and $F^* = 0$, $H^* = 1$, $D^* = 2$, and $R^* = 1$).

Graph-Based Qualitative Assessment and Quantitative Analysis Using Efficacy Indices and Regression

Next, a qualitative comparison was performed using the graph-based format. Quantitative analysis

Table 3. H-K solution using the A Priori instance at $n = 12$ and $3 \leq \psi \leq 11$ (data presented in forward and reverse order)

Part ID	12	2	5	8	11	1	4	7	10	9	6	3
PRT	11	3	5	7	11	3	5	7	11	7	5	3
Workstation	1	1	1	1	2	2	2	2	3	3	3	3
Hazardous	1	0	0	0	0	0	0	0	0	0	0	0
Demand	0	0	0	0	0	0	0	0	0	1	0	0
Direction	0	0	0	0	0	1	1	1	1	0	0	0

Table 4. Typical GA solution using the A Priori instance at n = 12

Part ID	12	9	5	3	8	11	6	2	4	10	7	1
PRT	11	7	5	3	7	11	5	3	5	11	7	3
Workstation	1	1	1	1	2	2	2	2	3	3	3	3
Hazardous	1	0	0	0	0	0	0	0	0	0	0	0
Demand	0	1	0	0	0	0	0	0	0	0	0	0
Direction	0	0	0	0	0	0	0	0	1	1	1	1

was enabled first by calculating the efficacy indices and then through the experimental determination of average-case time complexity using linear or polynomial regression. Note that the curves also appear to rather sharp increases and decreases. This is due to a combination of discrete values being connected by straight lines (i.e., with no smoothing) and due to the scale of those parameters' charts, rather than being indicative of any data anomalies.

The first study performed was a measure of each of the technique's calculated number of workstations as compared to the optimal. As shown in Figure 8, both of the methods performed very well in workstation calculation, staying within 2 workstations of optimum for all data set sizes tested. On the full range of data ($8 \leq n \leq 80$), DLBP H-K found solutions with NWS^* workstations up to $n = 12$, then solutions with $NWS^* + 1$ workstations through data set 11 ($n = 48$), after which it stabilized at $NWS^* + 2$. From Formula (25) H-K's efficacy index in number of workstations started at an optimal $EI_{NWS} = 100\%$, dropped to a low of $EI_{NWS} = 92\%$, then continuously climbed through to $EI_{NWS} = 97\%$ with an efficacy index sample mean in number of workstations of $\overline{E}_{NWS} = 96\%$. DLBP GA's efficacy index in number of workstations went from a high of 100%, down to 94% then stabilized between 97% and 98%. Overall, as given by Formula (26), DLBP GA shows an efficacy index sample mean in number of workstations of 97%.

In terms of the calculated measure of balance, again, both of the methods are seen to perform very well and significantly better than the worst case (as given by formula (7)). Best case is found uniformly at $F = 0$, as illustrated by Figure 9. However, examining the balance in greater detail provides some insight into the different techniques.

DLBP H-K and GA tend to decrease similarly and in a step function fashion (note, however, that even their normalized balance performance actually improves overall with instance size as a percentage of worst case as indicated by their improved efficacy indices with instance size; see Figure 10). This is to be expected; for H-K this has to do with the fact that as the instance size grows, a lower and lower percentage of the search space is investigated (assuming the skip size range is not allowed to increase with instance size, which is the case in this chapter). For GA, efficacy falls off with instance size because (unlike, for example, many hill-climbing and *r*-optimal processes that continue to search until no better nearby solution can be found) GA is set up to terminate after a fixed number of generations (in addition, GA's population does not increase with increases in instance size).

While increases in H-K's balance measure are seen with increases in data set size, as a percentage

Figure 8. Workstation calculations for each DLBP combinatorial optimization method

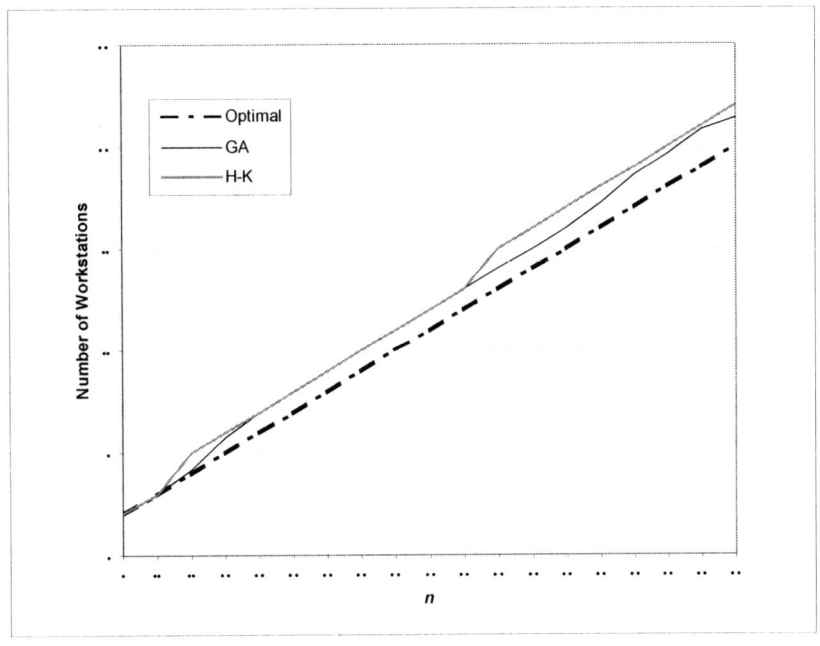

Figure 9. Detailed DLBP combinatorial optimization methods' balance performance

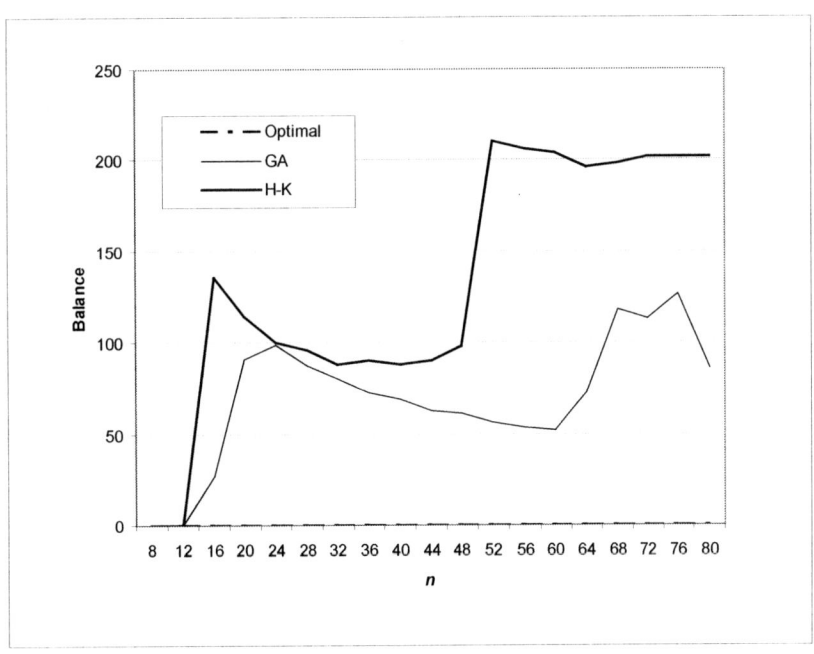

Figure 10. Normalized DLBP combinatorial optimization methods' balance performance

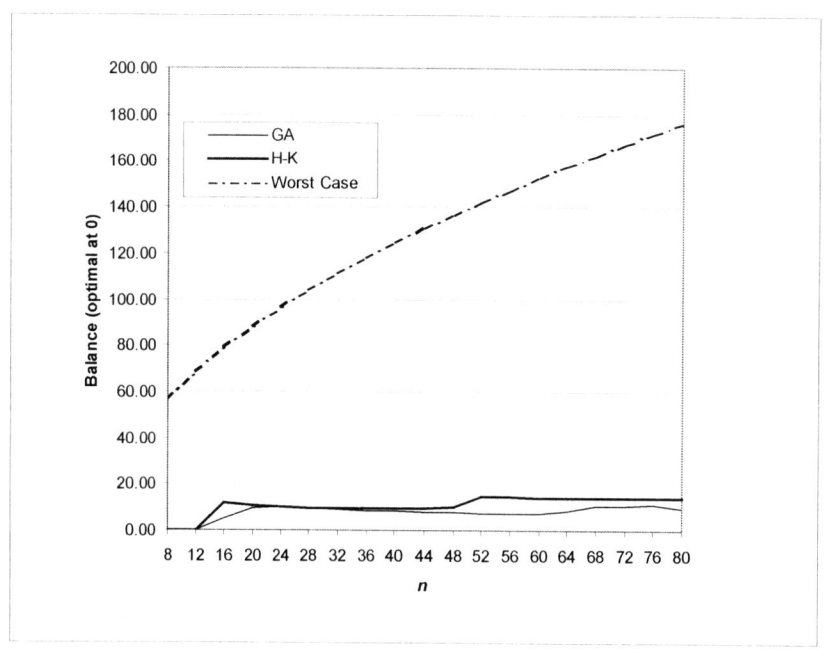

of the overall range from best case to worst case, the normalized balance measure tends to decrease (i.e., improve) with increases in the data set size. The normalized balance efficacy index dropped from a high of $EI_F = 100\%$ to a low of $EI_F = 85\%$ at data set 3 ($n = 16$) then slowly climbed to $EI_F = 92\%$ giving a sample mean of $\overline{E}_F = 92\%$. With DLBP GA, the normalized balance efficacy index started as high as 100% then dropped to 93% to 95%; it was never lower than 89% and had a sample mean of 94%. An instance size of $n = 16$ was seen to be the point at which the optimally balanced solution was not consistently found for the selected N and number of generations. Although DLBP GA's performance decreased with instance size, it can be seen in Figure 10 that the solution found, while not optimal, was very near optimal and when normalized, roughly paralleled the optimal balance curve.

The hazard measure results are as expected since hazard performance is designed to be deferential to balance and affected only when a better hazard measure can be attained without adversely affecting balance. The hazard measure tends to get worse with problem size using DLBP GA, with its efficacy index dropping relatively constantly from 100% to 60% and having a sample mean of $\overline{E}_H = 84\%$. The hazardous part was regularly suboptimally placed by DLBP H-K as well. Hazardous-part placement stayed relatively consistent with problem size (though effectively improving as compared to the worst case, as illustrated by Figure 11). The hazard measure's efficacy index fluctuates, similarly to a sawtooth wave function, between $EI_H = 57\%$ and $EI_H = 100\%$, giving a sample mean of $\overline{E}_H = 90\%$.

With DLBP GA, the demand measure gets worse at a slightly more rapid rate than the hazardous-part measure—as is expected due to the multicriteria priorities—with its efficacy index dropping from 100% to 45% (with a low of 42%) and having a sample mean of $\overline{E}_D = 78\%$ (Figure 12). DLBP H-K also suboptimally placed the high-demand part, and also at a higher rate than

Figure 11. DLBP combinatorial optimization methods' hazard performance

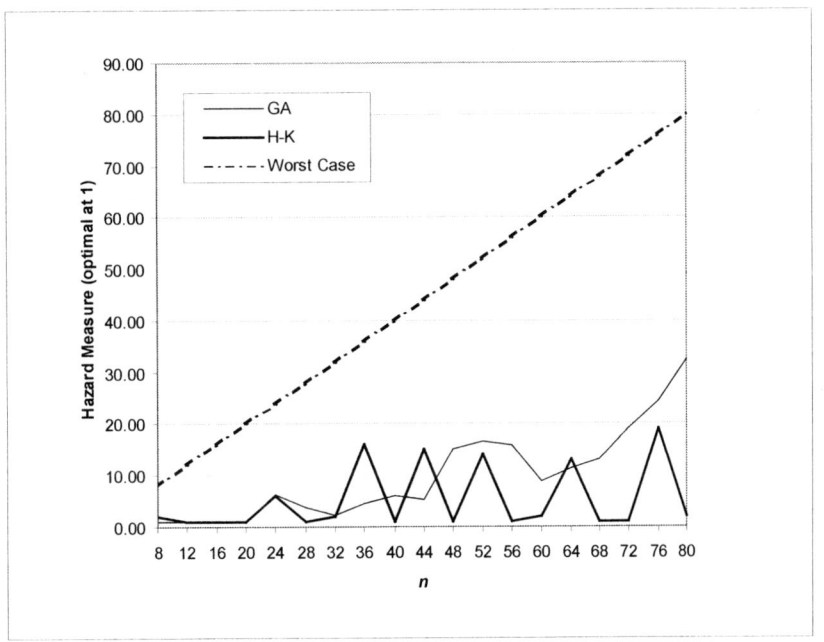

the hazardous part. Its efficacy index fluctuates between $EI_D = 7\%$ and $EI_D = 103\%$ (due to better than optimal placement in position $k = 1$ at the expense of hazard placement). Its resulting demand measure sample mean is $\overline{E}_D = 49\%$.

With part removal direction structured as to be deferential to balance, hazard, and demand, the two methodologies were seen to decrease in performance in a haphazard fashion. This decrease in performance is seen both when compared to the best case and when compared to the worst case (Figure 13). Again, these results are as expected due the prioritization of the multiple objectives. Though the part removal direction efficacy gets as high as $EI_R = 86\%$ with the H-K implementation, by data set 5 ($n = 24$) it has dropped to $EI_R = 0\%$ and never rises higher again than $EI_R = 43\%$, resulting in a sample mean of $\overline{E}_R = 20\%$. Using the GA, the part removal direction measure gets worse at a more rapid rate than the demand measure, again attributed to the multicriteria priorities, with its efficacy index dropping as low as 17% (at data set 15 where $n = 64$) and having a sample mean of $\overline{E}_R = 49\%$.

Finally, time complexity was examined using the *A Priori* data. Both of the techniques were seen to be very fast (Figure 14) and each is seen to be faster than third order.

Using DLBP GA, runtime increased very slowly with instance size. A linear model was used to fit the curve with the linear regression equation calculated to be $T(n) = 0.0327n + 1.5448$ with a coefficient of determination of 0.9917 indicating 99.17% of the total variation is explained by the calculated linear regression curve. The growth of $0.0327n + 1.5448$ provides an experimentally derived result for the average-case time complexity of DLBP GA on the DLBP *A Priori* data sets as $O(n)$ or *linear complexity* (Rosen, 1999). This is in agreement with the theoretical calculations.

With DLBP H-K, the regression equation was calculated to be $T(n) = 0.0033n^2 - 0.0002n + 0.2893$. The small coefficients are indicative of the slow runtime growth in instance size. The coefficient of

Figure 12. DLBP combinatorial optimization methods' demand performance

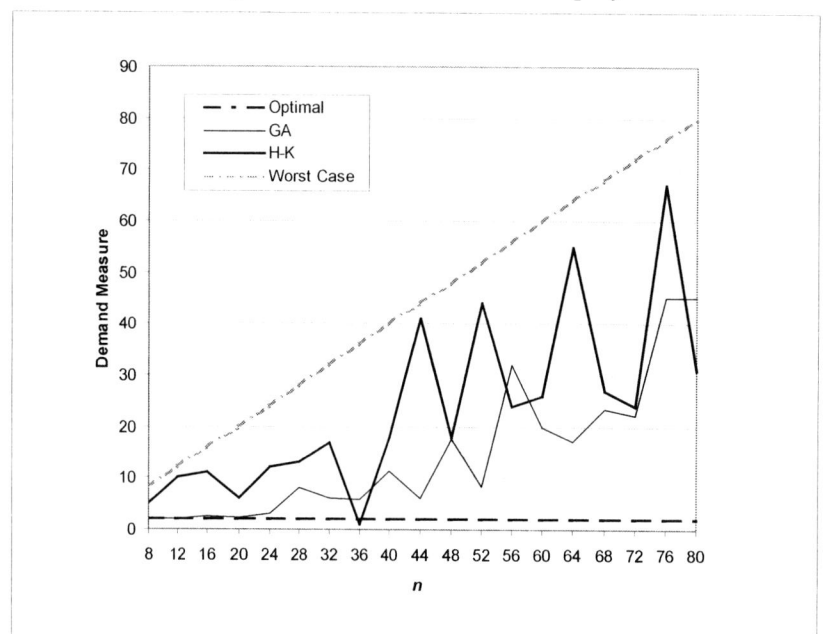

Figure 13. DLBP combinatorial optimization methods' part removal direction performance

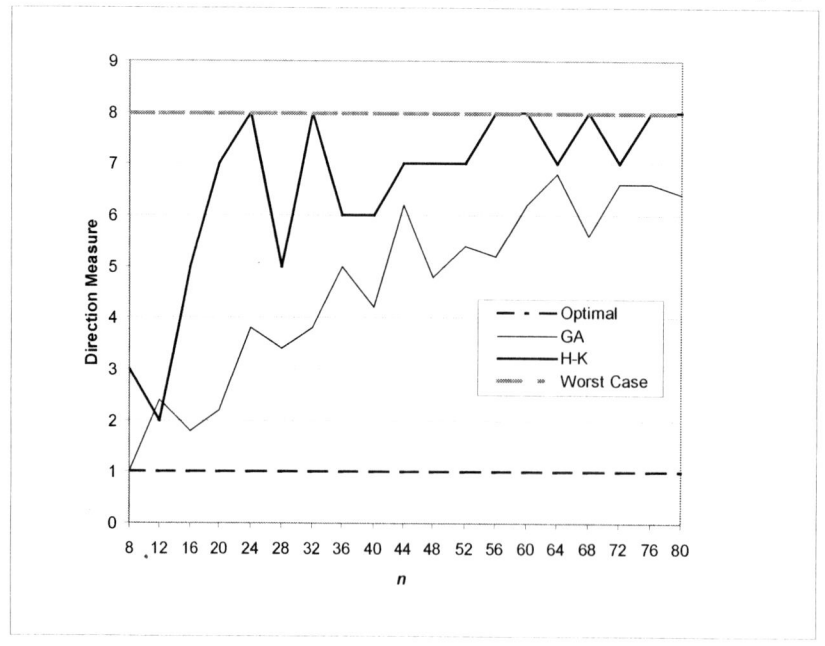

determination is calculated to be 0.9974, indicating 99.74% of the total variation is explained by the calculated regression curve. With a 2nd-order polynomial regression model used to fit the H-K curve, the average-case time complexity of DLBP H-K curve (with forward and reverse data, $1 \leq \Delta\psi \leq 10$, and resulting skip sizes of $n - 10 \leq \psi \leq n - 1$) is listed as $O(n^2)$ or polynomial complexity. The deterministic, single iteration nature of H-K also indicates that the process would be no faster than this, so it is expected that the time complexity lower bound is $\Omega(n^2)$ and, therefore, the H-K appears to have an asymptotically tight bound of $\Theta(n^2)$ as configured here. This empirical result is also in agreement with the theoretical complexity determination.

The runtimes can be examined in greater detail in Figure 15. While DLBP GA was seen to be very fast due to its linear growth, at some point it may be necessary to increase GA's population or number of generations to allow for the generation of adequate solutions and this will of course increase its runtime. DLBP H-K was also very fast, even with $\Delta\psi$ varying from 1 to 10 and with forward and reverse data runs (the anomaly seen in the H-K curve in Figure 15 is due to a software rule that dictated that all ψ could be as small as $n - 10$, but no less than $\psi = 3$, to prevent exhaustive or near-exhaustive searches at small n). The H-K process grows approximately exponentially in $1/\psi$, taking, for example from 0.02 seconds at $\psi = 5$ (actually $5 \leq \psi \leq 11$) up to just under 20 seconds at $\psi = 2$ (i.e., $2 \leq \psi \leq 11$ and 19.34 seconds) with $n = 12$ and forward and reverse data (exhaustive search was seen to take almost 25 minutes (24.61 minutes) on the same size data).

Although less than optimal, these results are not unusual for heuristics run against this data set. These suboptimal results are not indicative of poor heuristic performance but are, more likely, indicative of a successful DLBP *A Priori* benchmark data set design. The DLBP *A Priori* benchmark data is especially designed to challenge the solution-finding ability of a variety of combinatoric solution-generating techniques to enable a thorough quantitative evaluation of

Figure 14. Time complexity of DLBP combinatorial optimization methods

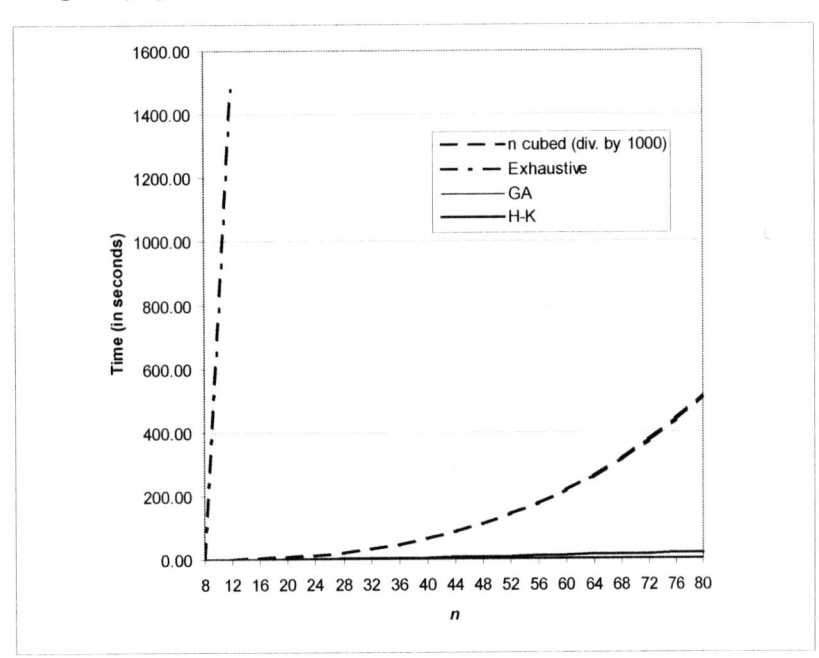

Figure 15. Detailed time complexity of DLBP combinatorial optimization methods

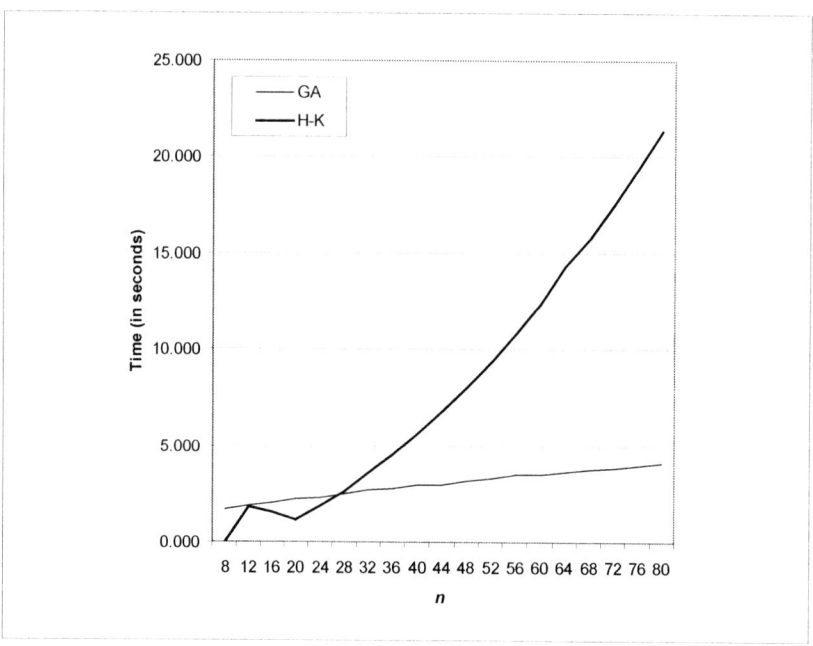

various method's performances in different areas (McGovern & Gupta, 2004). Suboptimal solutions typically result when this specially designed set of instances is processed, even at seemingly small n values. For each of these methodologies, their DLBP-specific engineering element of searching exclusively for precedence-preserving solution n-tuples means that the inclusion or addition of precedence constraints will reduce the search space and increasingly move any of these methods towards the optimal solution.

A smaller ψ or (as with GA and other search techniques) the inclusion of precedence constraints will increasingly move the DLBP H-K method towards the optimal solution. The time complexity performance of DLBP H-K provides the tradeoff benefit with the technique's near-optimal performance, demonstrating the moderate increase in time required with problem size, which grows markedly slower than the exponential growth of exhaustive search. Runtime performance can be improved by increasing skip size and by running the data in one direction only while the opposite (i.e., decreasing skip size and running different versions of the data, including running the data in forward and reverse order) would be expected to increase solution efficacy. Note that, as a newly developed methodology, other modifications may decrease runtime and/or increase solution efficacy as well. With DLBP GA runtime performance can be improved by reducing the number of generations or reducing the population, while the opposite is true for improving other measures of performance; that is, increase the number of generations or increase the population to improve efficacy indices.

Each of the collected quantitative values was then compiled into one table for reference and comparison (Table 5). This table contains each of the combinatorial optimization methodologies researched here and lists their number of workstations, balance, hazard, demand and part removal

Table 5. Summary of quantitative measures for both methodologies

	$\overline{EI}_{NWS}$	$\overline{EI}_{F(norm)}$	$\overline{EI}_H$	$\overline{EI}_D$	$\overline{EI}_R$	$T(n)$	big-Oh
Exhaustive	100%	100%	100%	100%	100%	$1.199n!$	$O(n!)$
GA	97%	94%	84%	78%	49%	$0.033n$	$O(n)$
H-K	96%	92%	90%	49%	20%	$0.003n^2$	$O(n^2)$

direction sample mean efficacy indices; regression model average-case experimentally determined time complexity; and associated asymptotic upper bound (experimentally determined average case using the DLBP *A Priori* data).

The shading provides a quick reference to performance, with darker shades indicating worsening performance. While Exhaustive Search is included in the table, none of its row elements are considered for shading since its purpose in the table is as the benchmark for comparison. Note that the balance measure sample mean efficacy index is based on the normalized balance. This is done in the interest of providing a more appropriate and consistent scale across the table.

FUTURE DIRECTIONS

Directions for future research can be described as follows:

- It may be of interest to vary the multicriteria ordering of the objectives; two possibilities include a re-ordering of the objectives based on expert domain knowledge, and a comparison of all permutations of the objectives in search of patterns or unexpected performance improvements or decreases
- While the multiple-criteria decision making approach used here made use of preemptive goal programming, many other methodologies are available and should be considered to decrease processing time, for an overall or selective efficacy improvement, or to examine other promising methods including weighting schemes
- It may be of interest to make use of the promise of H-K in generating uninformed solutions from throughout the search space through the use of H-K to hot start GA
- Throughout the research, complete disassembly was assumed; while this is of great theoretical interest (since it allows for a worst-case study in terms of problem complexity and it provides consistency across the problem instances and methodologies), in practical applications it is not necessarily desired, required, practical, or efficient—recommend that future studies consider the more applied problem that allows for incomplete or partial disassembly
- Per the prior recommendation and an earlier one, different multicriteria ordering of the objectives could simplify the determination of the optimal level of incomplete disassembly; for example, if the main objective is to remove several demanded parts of a product containing hundreds of parts, by making the demand measure a higher priority objective than the balance, it may be found that these parts can be removed relatively early on in the disassembly process thereby allowing the process to terminate significantly earlier in the case of partial disassembly

This concludes some suggestions for future research. In addition to the items listed above, any further developments and applications of recent methodologies to multicriteria decision making, the H-K algorithm or GA or the Disassembly Line Balancing Problem that will help to extend the research in these areas may be appropriate.

CONCLUSION

In this chapter, a new multi-objective optimization problem was reviewed and used to demonstrate the development of several performance assessment techniques and the use of lexicographic goal programming for comparison and analysis of combinatoric search methodologies. From the field of combinatorial optimization, an evolutionary algorithm and an uninformed general-purpose search heuristic were selected to demonstrate these tools. Quantitative and qualitative comparison was performed using tables, graphs and efficacy measures with varying instance sizes and using exhaustive search as a time and performance benchmark. Each of the methodologies performed very well—though consistently suboptimally—with the different performance assessment techniques demonstrating a variety of performance subtleties that show no one technique to be ideal in all applications. While these results are solely dependent on the *A Priori* data set instances used, this data set appears to have successfully posed—even with multiple optimum extreme points—a nontrivial challenge to the methodologies and in all instance sizes, providing at least an initial indication that the data set does meet its design expectations and does not contain any unforeseen nuances that would render it a weak benchmark for this type of NP-complete combinatorial problem.

REFERENCES

Bierwirth, C., Mattfeld, D. C., & Kopfer, H. (1996). On permutation representations for scheduling problems. In H. M. Voigt, W. Ebeling, I. Rechenberg, & H.-P. Schwefel (Eds.), *Parallel problem solving from nature -- PPSN IV, Lecture notes in computer science* (pp. 310-318). Berlin, Germany: Springer-Verlag.

Brennan, L., Gupta, S. M., & Taleb, K. N. (1994). Operations planning issues in an assembly/disassembly environment. *International Journal of Operations and Production management, 14*(9), 57-67.

Charnes, A. & Cooper, W. W. (1961). *Management models and industrial applications of linear programming.* New York: John Wiley and Sons.

Charnes, A., Cooper, W. W., & Ferguson, R. O. (1955). Optimal estimation of executive compensation by linear programming. *Management Science, 1*(2), 138-151.

Elsayed, E. A. & Boucher, T. O. (1994). *Analysis and control of production systems.* Upper Saddle River, New Jersey: Prentice Hall.

Erel, E. & Gokcen, H. (1964). Shortest-route formulation of mixed-model assembly line balancing problem. *Management Science, 11*(2), 308-315.

Garey, M. & Johnson, D. (1979). *Computers and intractability: A guide to the theory of NP completeness.* San Francisco, CA: W. H. Freeman and Company.

Güngör, A. & Gupta, S. M. (1999a). A systematic solution approach to the disassembly line balancing problem. In *Proceedings of the 25th International Conference on Computers and Industrial Engineering* (pp. 70-73), New Orleans, Louisiana.

Güngör, A. & Gupta, S. M. (1999b). Disassembly line balancing. In *Proceedings of the 1999 Annual Meeting of the Northeast Decision Sciences Institute* (pp. 193-195), Newport, Rhode Island.

Güngör, A. & Gupta, S. M. (1999c). Issues in environmentally conscious manufacturing and product recovery: A survey. *Computers and Industrial Engineering, 36*(4), 811-853.

Güngör, A. & Gupta, S. M. (2001). A solution approach to the disassembly line problem in the presence of task failures. *International Journal of Production Research, 39*(7), 1427-1467.

Güngör, A. & Gupta, S. M. (2002). Disassembly line in product recovery. *International Journal of Production Research, 40*(11), 2569-2589.

Gupta, S. M. & Taleb, K. (1994). Scheduling disassembly. *International Journal of Production Research, 32*(8), 1857-1866.

Gutjahr, A. L. & Nemhauser, G. L. (1964). An algorithm for the line balancing problem. *Management Science, 11*(2), 308-315.

Hackman, S. T., Magazine, M. J., & Wee, T. S. (1989). Fast, effective algorithms for simple assembly line balancing problems. *Operations Research, 37*(6), 916-924.

Hillier, F. S. & Lieberman, G. J. (2005). *Introduction to operations research.* New York: McGraw-Hill.

Holland, J. H. (1975). *Adaptation in natural and artificial systems.* Ann Arbor, MI: University of Michigan Press.

Hu, T. C. & Shing, M. T. (2002). *Combinatorial algorithms.* Mineola, NY: Dover Publications.

Lambert, A. D. J. (2003). Disassembly sequencing: A survey. *International Journal of Production Research, 41*(16), 3721-3759.

Lambert, A. J. D. & Gupta, S. M. (2005). *Disassembly modeling for assembly, maintenance, reuse, and recycling.* Boca Raton, FL: CRC Press (Taylor & Francis).

Lapierre, S. D., Ruiz, A., & Soriano, P. (2006). Balancing assembly lines with tabu search. *European Journal of Operational Research, 168*(3), 826-837.

McGovern, S. M. & Gupta, S. M. (2003). Greedy algorithm for disassembly line scheduling. In *Proceedings of the 2003 IEEE International Conference on Systems, Man, and Cybernetics* (pp. 1737-1744), Washington, D.C.

McGovern, S. M. & Gupta, S. M. (2004). Combinatorial optimization methods for disassembly line balancing. In *Proceedings of the 2004 SPIE International Conference on Environmentally Conscious Manufacturing IV* (pp. 53-66), Philadelphia, Pennsylvania.

McGovern, S. M. & Gupta, S. M. (2005). Local search heuristics and greedy algorithm for balancing the disassembly line. *The International Journal of Operations and Quantitative Management, 11*(2), 91-114.

McGovern, S. M. & Gupta, S. M. (2006a). Computational complexity of a reverse manufacturing line. In *Proceedings of the 2006 SPIE International Conference on Environmentally Conscious Manufacturing VI* (CD-ROM), Boston, Massachusetts.

McGovern, S. M. & Gupta, S. M. (2006b). Performance metrics for end-of-life product processing. In *Proceedings of the 17th Annual Production & Operations Management Conference* (CD-ROM) Boston, Massachusetts.

McGovern, S. M., & Gupta, S. M. (2007). A balancing method and genetic algorithm for disassembly line balancing. *European Journal of Operational Research, 179*(3), 692-708.

McGovern, S. M., Gupta, S. M., & Kamarthi, S. V. (2003). Solving disassembly sequence planning problems using combinatorial optimization. In *Proceedings of the 2003 Northeast Decision Sciences Institute Conference* (pp. 178-180), Providence, Rhode Island.

Osman, I. H. (2004). Metaheuristics: Models, design and analysis. In *Proceedings of the Fifth Asia Pacific Industrial Engineering and Management Systems Conference* (pp. 1.2.1-1.2.16), Gold Coast, Australia.

Osman, I. H. & Laporte, G. (1996). Metaheuristics: A bibliography. *Annals of Operations Research, 63,* 513-623.

Papadimitriou, C. H. & Steiglitz, K. (1998). *Combinatorial optimization: Algorithms and complexity.* Mineola, NY: Dover Publications.

Ponnambalam, S. G., Aravindan, P., & Naidu, G. M. (1999). A comparative evaluation of assembly line balancing heuristics. *The International Journal of Advanced Manufacturing Technology, 15,* 577-586.

Rosen, K. H. (1999). *Discrete mathematics and its applications.* Boston, MA: McGraw-Hill.

Suresh, G., Vinod, V. V., & Sahu, S. (1996). A genetic algorithm for assembly line balancing. *Production Planning and Control, 7*(1), 38-46.

Torres, F., Gil, P., Puente, S. T., Pomares, J., & Aracil, R. (2004). Automatic PC disassembly for component recovery. *International Journal of Advanced Manufacturing Technology, 23*(1-2), 39-46.

Tovey, C. A. (2002). Tutorial on computational complexity. *Interfaces, 32*(3), 30-61.

ADDITIONAL READING

Agrawal, S. & Tiwari, M. K. (2008). A collaborative ant colony algorithm to stochastic mixed-model u-shaped disassembly line balancing and sequencing problem. *International Journal of Production Research, 46*(6), 1405-1429.

Aho, A. V., Hopcroft, J. E., & Ullman, J. D. (1974). *The design and analysis of computer programs.* Reading, MA: Addison-Wesley.

Altekin, F. T. (2005). *Profit oriented disassembly line balancing.* Unpublished doctoral dissertation, Middle East Technical University, Ankara, Turkey.

Altekin, F. T., Kandiller, L., & Ozdemirel, N. E. (2008). Profit-oriented disassembly-line balancing. *International Journal of Production Research, 46*(10), 2675-2693.

Bautista, J. & Pereira, J. (2002). Ant algorithms for assembly line balancing. In M. Dorigo (Ed.), *ANTS 2002, LNCS 2463* (pp. 65-75). Berlin, Germany: Springer-Verlag.

Das, S. K. & Naik, S. (2002). Process planning for product disassembly. *International Journal of Production Research, 40*(6), 1335-1355.

Dorigo, M., Maniezzo, V., & Colorni, A. (1996). The ant system: Optimization by a colony of cooperating agents. *IEEE Transactions on Systems, Man, and Cybernetics–Part B, 26*(1), 1-13.

Duta, L., Filip, F. G., & Henrioud, J. M. (2002). Automated disassembly: Main stage in manufactured products recycling. In *Proceedings of the 4th International Workshop on Computer Science and Information Technologies* (CD-ROM), Patras, Greece.

Duta, L., Filip, F. G., & Henrioud, J. M. (2005). Applying equal piles approach to disassembly line balancing problem. In *Proceedings of the 16th IFAC World Congress* (CD-ROM), Prague, Czech Republic.

Franke, C., Basdere, B., Ciupek, M., & Seliger, S. (2006). Remanufacturing of mobile phones - Capacity, program and facility adaptation planning. *Omega, 34*(6), 562-570.

Glover, F. (1989). Tabu search, Part I. *ORSA Journal of Computing, 1*(3), 190-206.

Glover, F. (1990). Tabu search, Part II. *ORSA Journal of Computing, 2*(1), 4-32.

Güngör, A. & Gupta, S. M. (1997). An evaluation methodology for disassembly processes. *Computers and Industrial Engineering, 33*(1), 329-332.

Güngör, A. & Gupta, S. M. (1998). Disassembly sequence planning for products with defective parts in product recovery. *Computers and Industrial Engineering, 35*(1-2), 161-164.

Güngör, A. & Gupta, S. M. (2001). Disassembly sequence plan generation using a branch-and-bound algorithm. *International Journal of Production Research, 39*(3), 481-509.

Gupta, S. M., Evren, E., & McGovern, S. M. (2004). Disassembly sequencing problem: A case study of a cell phone. In *Proceedings of the 2004 SPIE International Conference on Environmentally Conscious Manufacturing IV* (pp. 43-52), Philadelphia, Pennsylvania.

Gupta, S. M. & Güngör, A. (2001). Product recovery using a disassembly line: Challenges and solution. In *Proceedings of the 2001 IEEE International Symposium on Electronics and the Environment* (pp. 36-40), Denver, Colorado.

Gupta, S. M. & McGovern, S. M. (2004). Multi-objective optimization in disassembly sequencing problems. In *Proceedings of the 2nd World Conference on Production & Operations Management and the 15th Annual Production & Operations Management Conference* (CD-ROM), Cancun, Mexico.

Hong, D. S. & Cho, H. S. (1997). Generation of robotic assembly sequences with consideration of line balancing using simulated annealing. *Robotica, 15,* 663-673.

Hopper, E. & Turton, B. C. H. (2000). An empirical investigation of meta-heuristic and heuristic algorithms for a 2D packing problem. *European Journal of Operational Research, 128*(1), 34-57.

Huang, Y. M. & Liao, Y.-C. (2006). Optimum disassembly process with genetic algorithms for a compressor. In *Proceedings of the ASME 2006 Design Engineering Technical Conferences and Computers and Information in Engineering Conference* (CD-ROM), Philadelphia, Pennsylvania.

Iori, M. (2003). *Metaheuristic algorithms for combinatorial optimization problems.* Unpublished doctoral dissertation, University of Bologna, Bologna, Italy.

Kekre, S., Rao, U. S., Swaminathan, J. M., & Zhang, J. (2003). Reconfiguring a remanufacturing line at Visteon, Mexico. *Interfaces, 33*(6), 30-43.

Kongar, E. & Gupta, S. M. (2002a). A genetic algorithm for disassembly process planning. In *Proceedings of the 2002 SPIE International Conference on Environmentally Conscious Manufacturing II* (pp. 54-62), Newton, Massachusetts.

Kongar, E. & Gupta, S. M. (2002b). A multi-criteria decision making approach for disassembly-to-order systems. *Journal of Electronics Manufacturing, 11*(2), 171-183.

Kongar, E., Gupta, S. M., & McGovern, S. M. (2003). Use of data envelopment analysis for product recovery. In *Proceedings of the 2003 SPIE International Conference on Environmentally Conscious Manufacturing III* (pp. 219-231), Providence, Rhode Island.

Kotera, Y. & Sato, S. (1997). An integrated recycling process for electric home appliances. *Mitsubishi Electric ADVANCE, September,* 23-26.

Lambert, A. J. D. (1999). Linear programming in disassembly/clustering sequence generation. *Computers and Industrial Engineering, 36*(4), 723-738.

Lambert, A. J. D. (2002). Determining optimum disassembly sequences in electronic equipment. *Computers and Industrial Engineering, 43*(3), 553-575.

Lambert, A. J. D. & Gupta, S. M. (2002). Demand-driven disassembly optimization for electronic products. *Journal of Electronics Manufacturing, 11*(2), 121-135.

Lapierre, S. D. & Ruiz, A. B. (2004). Balancing assembly lines: An industrial case study. *Journal of the Operational Research Society, 55*(6), 589–597.

Lee, D.-H., Kang, J.-G., & Xirouchakis, P. (2001). Disassembly planning and scheduling: Review and further research. *Journal of Engineering Manufacture, 215*(B5), 695-709.

McGovern, S. M., & Gupta, S. M. (2003). 2-opt heuristic for the disassembly line balancing problem. In *Proceedings of the SPIE International Conference on Environmentally Conscious Manufacturing III* (pp. 71-84), Providence, Rhode Island.

McGovern, S. M. & Gupta, S. M. (2004a). Demanufacturing strategy based upon metaheuristics. In *Proceedings of the 2004 Industrial Engineering Research Conference* (CD-ROM), Houston, Texas.

McGovern, S. M. & Gupta, S. M. (2004b). Metaheuristic technique for the disassembly line balancing problem. In *Proceedings of the 2004 Northeast Decision Sciences Institute Conference* (pp. 223-225), Atlantic City, New Jersey.

McGovern, S. M., & Gupta, S. M. (2004c). Multi-criteria ant system and genetic algorithm for end-of-life decision making. In *Proceedings of the 35th Annual Meeting of the Decision Sciences Institute* (pp. 6371-6376). Boston, Massachusetts.

McGovern, S. M. & Gupta, S. M. (2005a). Stochastic and deterministic combinatorial optimization solutions to an electronic product disassembly flow shop. In *Proceedings of the Northeast Decision Sciences Institute – 34th Annual Meeting* (CD-ROM), Philadelphia, Pennsylvania.

McGovern, S. M. & Gupta, S. M. (2005b). Uninformed and probabilistic distributed agent combinatorial searches for the unary NP-complete disassembly line balancing problem. In *Proceedings of the 2005 SPIE International Conference on Environmentally Conscious Manufacturing V* (pp. 81-92), Boston, Massachusetts.

McGovern, S. M. & Gupta, S. M. (2006a). Ant colony optimization for disassembly sequencing with multiple objectives. *The International Journal of Advanced Manufacturing Technology, 30*(5-6), 481-496.

McGovern, S. M. & Gupta, S. M. (2006b). Deterministic hybrid and stochastic combinatorial optimization treatments of an electronic product disassembly line. In K. D. Lawrence, G. R. Reeves, & R. Klimberg (Eds.), *Applications of management science, Vol. 12*, (pp. 175-197). North-Holland, Amsterdam: Elsevier Science.

McGovern, S. M., Gupta, S. M., & Nakashima, K. (2004). Multi-criteria optimization for non-linear end of lifecycle models. In *Proceedings of the Sixth Conference on EcoBalance* (pp. 201-204). Tsukuba, Japan.

McMullen, P. R. & Frazier, G. V. (1998). Using simulated annealing to solve a multi-objective assembly line balancing problem with parallel workstations. *International Journal of Production Research, 36*(10), 2717-2741.

McMullen, P. R. & Tarasewich, P. (2003). Using ant techniques to solve the assembly line balancing problem. *IIE Transactions, 35*, 605-617.

Merkle, D. & Middendorf, M. (2000). An ant algorithm with a new pheromone evaluation rule for total tardiness problems. In *Proceedings of Real-World Applications of Evolutionary Computing, EvoWorkshops 2000: EvoSTIM* (pp. 287-296), Edinburgh, Scotland.

Moore, K. E., Güngör, A., & Gupta, S. M. (1996). Petri net models of flexible and automated manufacturing systems: A survey. *International Journal of Production Research, 34*(11), 3001-3035.

Moore, K. E., Güngör, A., & Gupta, S. M. (2001). Petri net approach to disassembly process planning for products with complex AND/OR precedence relationships. *European Journal of Operational Research, 135*(2), 428-449.

O'Shea, B., Kaebernick, H., Grewal, S. S., Perlewitz, H., Müller, K., & Seliger, G. (1999). Method for automatic tool selection for disassembly planning. *Assembly Automation, 19*(1), 47-54.

Pinedo, M. (2002). *Scheduling theory, algorithms and systems.* Upper Saddle River, New Jersey: Prentice-Hall.

Prakash & Tiwari, M. K. (2005). Solving a disassembly line balancing problem with task failure using a psychoclonal algorithm. In *Proceedings of the ASME 2005 International Design Engineering Technical Conferences & Computers and Information in Engineering Conference* (CD-ROM), Long Beach, California.

Reingold, E. M., Nievergeld, J., & Deo, N. (1977). *Combinatorial algorithms: Theory and practice.* Englewood Cliffs, NJ: Prentice-Hall.

Scholl, A. (1995). *Balancing and sequencing of assembly lines.* Heidelberg, Germany: Physica-Verlag.

Schultmann, F. & Rentz, O. (2001). Environment-oriented project scheduling for the dismantling of buildings. *OR Spektrum, 23,* 51-78.

Sodhi, M. S. & Reimer, B. (2001). Models for recycling electronics end-of-life products. *OR Spektrum, 23,* 97-115.

Taleb, K. N., Gupta, S. M., & Brennan, L. (1997). Disassembly of complex products with parts and materials commonality. *Production Planning and Control, 8*(3), 255-269.

Tang, Y., Zhou, M.-C., & Caudill, R. (2001a). A systematic approach to disassembly line design. In *Proceedings of the 2001 IEEE International Symposium on Electronics and the Environment* (pp. 173-178), Denver, Colorado.

Tang, Y., Zhou, M.-C., & Caudill, R. (2001b). An integrated approach to disassembly planning and demanufacturing operation. *IEEE Transactions on Robotics and Automation, 17*(6), 773-784.

Thilakawardana, D., Driscoll, J., & Deacon, G. (2003a). A forward-loading heuristic procedure for single model assembly line balancing. In *Proceedings of the 17th International Conference on Production Research* (CD-ROM), Blacksburg, Virginia.

Thilakawardana, D., Driscoll, J., & Deacon, G. (2003b). Assembly line work assignment using a front loading genetic algorithm. In *Proceedings of the 17th International Conference on Production Research* (CD-ROM), Blacksburg, Virginia.

Tiacci, L., Saetta, S., & Martini, A. (2003). A methodology to reduce data collection in lean simulation modeling for the assembly line balancing problem. In *Proceedings of Summer Computer Simulation Conference 2003* (pp. 841-846), Montreal, Canada.

Tiwari, M. K., Sinha, N., Kumar, S., Rai, R., & Mukhopadhyay, S. K. (2001). A petri net based approach to determine the disassembly strategy of a product. *International Journal of Production Research, 40*(5), 1113-1129.

Toffel, M. W. (2002). End-of-life product recovery: Drivers, prior research, and future directions. In *Proceedings of the INSEAD Conference on European Electronics Take-Back Legislation: Impacts on Business Strategy and Global Trade,* Fontainebleau, France.

Veerakamolmal, P. & Gupta, S. M. (1998). Optimal analysis of lot-size balancing for multiproducts selective disassembly. *International Journal of Flexible Automation and Integrated Manufacturing, 6*(3&4), 245-269.

Veerakamolmal, P. & Gupta, S. M. (1999). Analysis of design efficiency for the disassembly of modular electronic products. *Journal of Electronics Manufacturing, 9*(1), 79-95.

Wang, H., Niu, Q., Xiang, D., & Duan, G. (2006). Ant colony optimization for disassembly sequence planning. In *Proceedings of the ASME 2006 Design Engineering Technical Conferences and Computers and Information in Engineering Conference* (CD-ROM), Philadelphia, Pennsylvania.

Wang, H., Xiang, D., Duan, G., & Song, J. (2006). A hybrid heuristic approach for disassembly/recycle applications. In *Proceedings of the Sixth International Conference on Intelligent Systems Design and Applications* (pp. 985-995), Jinan, Shandong, China,.

Zeid, I., Gupta, S. M., & Bardasz, T. (1997). A case-based reasoning approach to planning for disassembly. *Journal of Intelligent Manufacturing, 8*(2), 97-106.

Chapter VII
Evolutionary Population Dynamics and Multi-Objective Optimisation Problems

Andrew Lewis
Griffith University, Australia

Sanaz Mostaghim
University of Karlsruhe, Germany

Marcus Randall
Bond University, Australia

ABSTRACT

Problems for which many objective functions are to be simultaneously optimised are widely encountered in science and industry. These multi-objective problems have also been the subject of intensive investigation and development recently for metaheuristic search algorithms such as ant colony optimisation, particle swarm optimisation and extremal optimisation. In this chapter, a unifying framework called evolutionary programming dynamics (EPD) is examined. Using underlying concepts of self organised criticality and evolutionary programming, it can be applied to many optimisation algorithms as a controlling metaheuristic, to improve performance and results. We show this to be effective for both continuous and combinatorial problems.

INTRODUCTION

Due to the large number of applications in science and industry, multi-objective optimisation using evolutionary algorithms (MOEAs) have been increasingly studied during the last decade (Coello Coello, Van Veldhuizen, & Lamont, 2002; Deb, 2001; Zitzler, 1999). There are many issues to be resolved for effective use of MOEAs, such as developing new algorithms to obtain solutions with good diversity and convergence, designing metrics for measuring the quality of the achieved solutions, producing test functions in static and dynamic environments. Any new development in these areas is valuable for scientific and industrial applications. However, solving large-scale problems with a large number of objectives is still a major challenge (Deb, 2001; Purshouse & Flemming, 2003).

In this chapter, we outline the development and use of evolutionary population dynamics (EPD) as a metaheuristic for population based optimisation algorithms. These include, but are not limited to, ant colony optimisation (ACO) (Dorigo, 1999), Extremal Optimisation (EO) (Boettcher & Percus, 2000) and Particle Swarm Optimisation (PSO) (Eberhart & Kennedy, 1995). This approach can be applied to both continuous and combinatorial problems for single-valued and multi-objective problems.

MULTI-OBJECTIVE ORIENTED METAHEURISTICS

As preliminary background, we describe three well-known metaheuristics: particle swarm optimisation, ant colony optimisation and extremal optimisation. The general mechanics of each method is briefly outlined along with how they have been applied to multi-objective optimisation.

Particle Swarm Optimisation

PSO is motivated from the simulation of social behaviour of animals (Eberhart & Kennedy, 1995; Englebrecht, 2005; Kennedy & Eberhart, 1995). PSO is a population-based technique, similar in some respects to evolutionary algorithms, except that potential solutions (called particles) move, rather than evolve, through the search space. The rules or particle dynamics, which govern this movement, are inspired by models of swarming and flocking. Each particle has a position and a velocity, and experiences linear spring-like attractions towards two guides:

1. The best position attained by that particle so far (local guide), and
2. The best position found by the swarm as a whole (global guide),

where "best" is in relation to evaluation of an objective function at that position. The global guide therefore enables information sharing between particles, whilst the local guides serve as individual particle memories.

The optimisation process is iterative. At each iteration the acceleration vectors of all the particles are calculated based on the positions of the corresponding guides. Then this acceleration is added to the velocity vector. The updated velocity is constricted so that the particles progressively slow down, and this new velocity is used to move the individual from the current to the new position.

Due to the success of particle swarm optimisation in single objective optimisation, in recent years more attempts have been made to extend PSO to the domain of multi-objective problems (Alvarez-Benitez, Everson & Fieldsend, 2005; Mostaghim, 2005; Mostaghim & Teich, 2003; Parsopoulos & Vrahatis, 2002). The main challenge in multi-objective particle swarm optimisation (MOPSO) is to select the global and local guides such that the swarm is guided towards the Pareto optimal front and maintains sufficient diversity. In MOPSO, the set of nondominated solutions must be used to determine the global guide for each particle. Selecting, or constructing, the guide from this set for each particle of the population is a very difficult yet important problem for attaining convergence and diversity of solutions. Several methodologies in MOPSO for selecting the global guide and their influences on the convergence and diversity of solutions are being explored (Alvarez-Benitez et al., 2005; Fieldsend & Singh, 2002; Ireland, Lewis, Mostaghim & Lu,

2006; Mostaghim, 2005; Reyes-Sierra & Coello Coello, 2006).

In the early stage of developing MOPSO algorithms, Parsopulos and Vrahatis (2002) modified the idea of vector evaluated genetic algorithm (VEGA) to MOPSO. Their algorithm was based on an aggregated objective function, changing the multi-objective problem to that of a single objective. Hu and Eberhart (2002) proposed a method in which only one objective was optimized at a time. Their method is efficient for problems with a low number of objectives and problems which are not sensitive to the order of objectives. Recently, most research in the area of MOPSO has concentrated on the selection of the global guide for each individual. Mostaghim and Teich (2003) introduced the Sigma method for guiding particles towards the Pareto front, Ireland et al. (2006) have suggested an artificial, constructed guide, and Fieldsend and Singh (2002) use an elite archive. Coello Coello and Lechuga (2002) suggest using a random selection and a repository for saving the nondominated solutions. Alvarez-Benitez et al. (2005) have introduced a selection schema for solutions that dominate many particles for use as global guides. In recent work, the task of selecting the local guide has been demonstrated by Branke and Mostaghim (2006) to be as important as selecting the global guide.

Practical application of MOPSO is in its early stages. There are a number of hybrid MOPSO algorithms for solving real-world problems, for example Mostaghim and Halter (2006), and Parallel MOPSO has been proposed recently by Mostaghim, Branke, and Schmeck (2006). For a more extensive treatment of MOPSO and PSO techniques in general, the reader is referred to Reyes-Sierra and Coello Coello (2006).

Ant Colony Optimisation

Ant colony optimisation (ACO) (Dorigo, 1999) is a population optimisation paradigm encompassing a range of metaheuristics based on the evolutionary mechanics of natural ant colonies. These techniques have been applied extensively to benchmark problems such as the travelling salesman problem (TSP), the job sequencing problem and the quadratic assignment problem. Work on more complex problems that have difficult constraints, in such areas as transportation and telecommunications, has also been undertaken (Dorigo, 1999). Like other evolutionary algorithms, populations of solutions evolve over time. The major difference is that ACO represents a set of constructive techniques, that is, each ant at each step of the generalised algorithm adds a component (such as the next city for the TSP) to its solution. Using simulated chemical or pheromone markers as a collective form of self-adaptation, populations produce increasingly better solutions.

In terms of multi-objective optimisation, an illustrative sample of work will be surveyed here. A good overview of this topic is found in Garcia-Martinez, Cordon, and Herrera (2007). In the main, ACO has been used to solve specific instances of multi-objective problems. These problems are from diverse areas, ranging from multidimensional TSPs and vehicle routing problems to sharemarket portfolio selection and planning water irrigation channels. While they have been tailored to these problems, the main theme has been the use of different colonies to optimise each objective function.

Garcia-Martinez, Cordon, and Herrera (2004, 2007) compare a number of published multi-objective ant colony optimisation (MOACO) methods on a single set of bi-criteria TSPs. These methods are from Mariano and Morales (1999), Iredi, Merkle, and Middendorf (2001), Gambardella, Taillard, and Agazzi (1999) and Doerner, Gutjahr, Hartl, and Strauss (2004). For the first of these (named Multiple Objective Ant-Q (MOAQ)), families of ants are used to optimise each objective. Each ant of the family learns from its same number in the preceding family. Additionally, infeasible solutions are penalised. Iredi et al. (2001) propose two methods they call BicriterionAnt and BicriterionMC. Both use different pheromone repositories for the two objective functions. The main difference is that the former allows its ants to update both repositories while the latter will update one or the other (at each step of an iteration). Doerner et al. (2004) use a variation on the idea of separate colonies in a scheme called COMPETants. After each iteration of the algorithm, the better performing colony gets a greater number of ants for the next generation. In contrast, the multiple ant colony system of Gambardella et al. (1999) uses a single pheromone matrix for each colony, but uses multiple visibility heuristics.

The results of Garcia-Martinez et al. (2004) indicate the MOACOs could return better sets of solutions (in terms of the Pareto front) than other more specialised algorithms (specifically NSGA-II and SPEA2). Apart from COMPETants and MOAQ, the MOACOs performed equally well.

Population ACO (PACO)[a] has also been used to solve multiple objective optimisation problems (Guntsch & Middendorf, 2003). Rather than keeping separate colonies of ants for each objective function, PACO creates different subpopulations to update each of the pheromone matrices (one for each objective). A variation of this is crowding PACO (CPACO) (Angus, 2006) in which a population, without subpopulations, is maintained. Each solution of the current population of ants is compared (in terms of solution quality) to a subset of the population. Given that two solutions are approximately similar, the old population member will be replaced if the other dominates it. Using a set of bicriteria TSPs, it was shown that that CPACO was able to outperform PACO.

Extremal Optimisation

EO is a relatively new metaphor for solving functional and combinatorial optimisation problems. It is based on the Bak-Sneppen model for self-organised criticality (Bak, Tang, & Wiesenfeld, 1987; Bak & Sneppen, 1993). To date only a limited number of combinatorial problems have been solved with this method. As it is relatively new in the field, compared to other techniques such as ACO, genetic algorithms (Goldberg, 1989) and PSO, there exists wide scope to apply and extend this heuristic.

Boettcher and Percus (1999, 2000, 2003) describe the general tenets of EO. Nature can be seen as an optimising system in which the aim is to allow competitive species to populate environments. In the course of the evolutionary process, successful species will have the ability to adapt to changing conditions while the less successful will suffer and may become extinct. This notion extends to the genetic level as well. Poorly performing genes are replaced using random mutation. Over time, if the species does not become extinct, its overall fitness will increase.

As EO is an emerging metaheuristic, relatively little has been done on it in connection with multi-objective optimisation. Galski, de Sousa, Ramos and Muraoka (2007) present an EO algorithm to find the optimal design of a simplified configuration of a thermal control system for a spacecraft platform. The objectives are to minimise the difference between target and actual temperatures on radiation panels as well as to minimise battery heater power dissipation. Using EO, two possible solutions to their test problem were found. As the authors combined both objectives into a single function, the designs were really only able to satisfy the first objective. Future designs will optimise both objectives using a Pareto front approach.

EVOLUTIONARY POPULATION DYNAMICS

The optimisation process is, at its core, a process of gradual improvement. In general, some trial solution to a problem is proposed, measured against some objective scale, and algorithmic means are applied to transform the solution to some ideal solution. It is a simple, but insightful, observation that the trial solution evolves. Early optimisation methods drew on a foundation of mathematical and geometric methods to search for particular solutions to systems of equations: the classical methods of gradient descent and direct search. In recent years practitioners have sought inspiration from nature, giving rise to such methods as genetic algorithms, evolutionary programming methods, swarm intelligence, ant colony algorithms and immune system simulation. Some of the most powerful heuristics are modelled on direct observation of the processes of evolution of species. Populations of solutions are manipulated to mimic evolutionary adaptation, in which species gradually become more suited to their environment or, to put it in optimisation terms, alter their characteristics (parameters) to become better adapted to the environmental pressures (objectives) imposed upon them.

The evolutionary programming methods of Fogel (1962) are a simple, robust and highly parallel approach to implementing these concepts. This class of methods in evolutionary computation apply a random mutation to each member of a population, generating a single offspring. However, unlike several other approaches, no recombination operators are applied. Some form of selection takes place, and half the combined population of parents and offspring enter the next generation. It is important to note that this is a phylogenetically-oriented approach: population members are considered as representative of species, not individual members within those species; hence the lack of recombination operators which mimic sexual reproduction.

The theory of self-organised criticality can give additional insight into emergent complexity in nature. Bak (1996) contends that the critical state is "the most efficient state that can actually be reached dynamically". Understanding "efficient" to mean "well-adapted", this holds promise of another means to improve population fitness. In this state, a population in an apparent equilibrium evolves episodically in spurts, a phenomenon known as punctuated equilibrium. Local change may affect any other element in the system, and this delicate balance arises without any external, organizing force.

Key to understanding the mechanics of the method is the observation that evolution progresses by selecting against the few most poorly adapted species rather than by expressly breeding those species best adapted to their environment. So the algorithms derived by reference to Bak's work do not have as their main aim the direct improvement of individual solutions, but the improvement of the population, as a whole, by removing poor solutions from it.

Using these concepts, an algorithm has been developed: evolutionary programming using self organizing criticality (EPSOC). This proved to be quite successful when applied to a range of real-world optimisation problems (Lewis, Abramson, & Peachey, 2003). Since EPSOC's operation is basically to apply EPD to some population of solutions, and several contemporary multi-objective optimisation methods are based on manipulation of populations, potentially EPD could be applied as a controlling metaheuristic to improve their performance. In this work its application to ACO, EO and PSO is described, but it should be evident that it is equally applicable to a wide range of population-based algorithms.

We first describe the mechanics of EPSOC, and then how the integration with other optimisation algorithms is achieved.

EPSOC

EPSOC (Lewis et al., 2003) is a relatively new metaheuristic that follows the method of Fogel (1962) but with an additional selection operator from the Bak-Sneppen model. The steps of the algorithm are given in Algorithm 1.

Each set of values defining a trial solution is independent of all others. Therefore, the evaluation of trial solutions can be performed concurrently. Since the evaluation of the objective function

Algorithm 1. The EPSOC algorithm

1: Initialise a random, uniformly-distributed population, and evaluate each trial solution
2: **for** a preset number of iterations **do**
3:    Sort the population by objective function value
4:    Select a set, B, of the worst members of the population. For each member of B, add to the set its two nearest neighbours in solution space that are not already members of the set, or from the best half of the sorted population
5:    Reinitialise the solutions of the selected set, B. For all other members of the population, apply some (generally small) random, uniformly distributed mutation.
6:    Evaluate each new trial solution.
7:    **for** each of the trial solutions **do**
8.   **if** it has a better objective function value than its original **then** retain it.
9.   **end for**
10: **end for**
11: **end**

Figure 1. Functional structure of EPD applied to population based methods

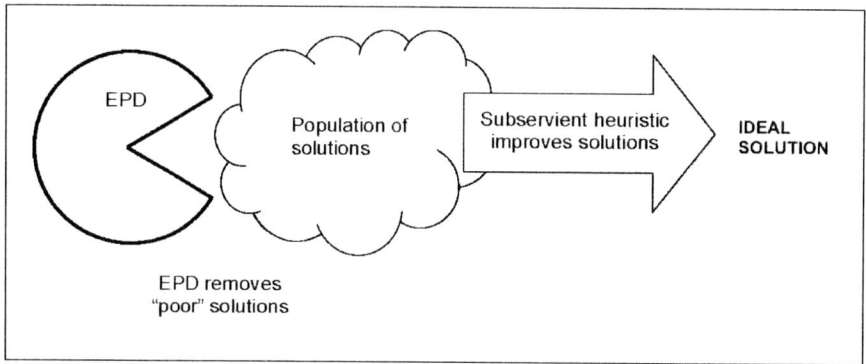

generally dominates the execution time, extremely high parallel efficiency can be achieved.

EPSOC is a straightforward implementation of the nearest-neighbour, punctuated equilibrium model as an optimisation algorithm. It is novel in that, by considering the trial solution vectors as defining a location in an n-dimensional space, the spatial behavior of the model is realised naturally. The algorithm has a high degree of greediness as it maintains a large elite (half the total population). This can be viewed as a constructive operator. It encourages gradual improvement in the better half of the population. Over time, the mutated population members move into the protected half of the population. Thus the median of the population moves toward better objective function values.

Applying EPD

The development of EPSOC allows us to investigate the use of standard metaheuristics (such as ACO, EO and PSO) as subservient heuristics to it. We aim to demonstrate that this hybrid approach may be used on a range of real-world problems.

A large component of this work is the determination of the allocation of sufficient parallel computing resources to the hybrid components.

Figure 2. Functional structure of EPSOC and EO hybrid (© 2006 IEEE Used with permission)

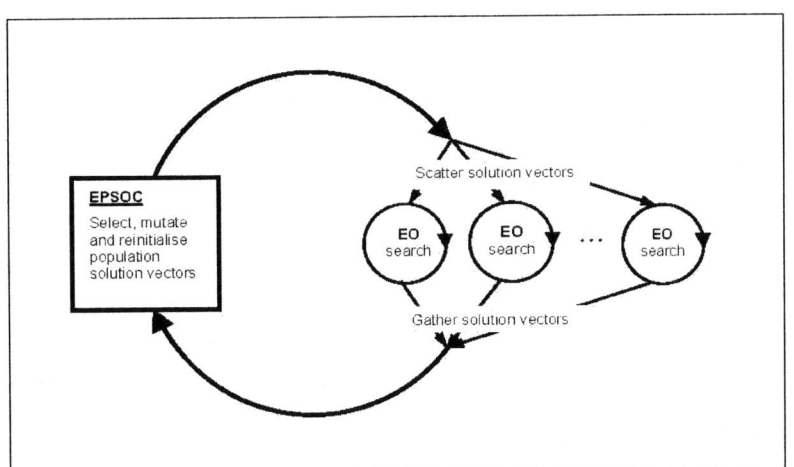

To apply EPD it is, of course, necessary to have a subject population. For optimisation algorithms that are inherently population based, such as ACO[b] and PSO, EPD can be directly applied to their internal population. This is conceptually illustrated in Figure 1. The algorithmic power of the subservient heuristic acts on the population and gradually improves it. It can be expected that the median of the population will tend to move towards generally "better" solutions. Simultaneously, EPD acts to remove the least fit solutions. By this means the motion of the population median, as a measure of the overall population fitness, will be accelerated, leading to faster convergence rates.

However, if the method is *not* population based, as with EO, a population on which EPD can act must be constructed. This is achieved by initiating a collection of several, independent searches using the subheuristic. The resulting "population" is subject to EPSOC's evolutionary population dynamics and, at each iteration, each member of the population carries out a metaheuristic algorithm search for some number of internal iterations to deliver an improved solution. This hybrid approach is effectively a *nested loop* of the two individual methods. For the example considered here, using EO, both components of the hybrid have a user-specified, maximum iteration count for their termination criterion. The hybrid algorithm is thus simple, robust and easy to control. The conceptual operation of the hybrid (using EO as the example subservient heuristic) is illustrated in Figure 2.

EPD has been used to good effect in combination with EO (Randall & Lewis, 2006), applied to a single objective problem. To extend this approach for application to multi-objective problems presents a further complication. EPD assumes the population is ranked by fitness—the least fit solutions being replaced. However, in multi-objective optimisation, as previously stated, there are no single best and worst solutions. Correctly selecting poor solutions for elimination has a great impact on the convergence of algorithms and quality of solutions obtained. Here we examine several techniques for applying EPD to multi-objective problems and therefore develop a new methodology to solve large-scale multi-objective optimisation problems.

MOPSO and EPD

One possible combination of MOPSO and EPD is shown in Algorithm 2. In order to find the poor

Algorithm 2. MOPSO+EPD Algorithm

---
1. **Initialisation**: Initialise population P_t, $t = 0$:
2. **Evaluation**: Evaluate(P_t)
3. **Renew Poor Solutions**:
$TotalHV$ = ComputeHyperVolume(P_t)
for i = 1 to N do
   HV_i = ComputeHyperVolume $(\vec{x}_i^t)$
   if $HV_i < TH$ then
     Renew $(\vec{x}_i^t)$
   end if
end for
4. **Update**: A_{t+1} = Update(P_t, A_t)
5. **Move**: P_{t+1} = Move(P_t, A_t)
6. **Termination**: Unless a termination criterion is met $t = t + 1$ and goto Step 2
---

particles in the population, a hypervolume metric can be used. This metric can, in fact, be any quantitative measurement for convergence and diversity of solutions. Hypervolume is the volume between a particle and a reference point in the objective space (Figure 3). For finding the poor solutions, the total hypervolume of the population is calculated by $TotalHV$ = ComputeHyperVolume(P_t). Then the hypervolume of every single particle is computed as HV_i and being compared to a threshold value called TH. This value can be set by using the $TotalHV$ to be one third of the total hypervolume. If a solution is categorised as poor that solution must be renewed (Step 3 in the Algorithm 2). The way a particle is renewed has a large impact on the solutions obtained. The two simple ways are:

1. Find a random new position for the particle. This is like adding a turbulence factor to the poor solutions.
2. Find a new position close to the particles in the Archive.

An alternative approach might be to use the Euclidian distance of the solution point from the Pareto front. In Figure 4 point "A" can be considered to be a distance from the Pareto front defined by the vector shown. If, for example, a weighted centroid guide particle method had been used in a MOPSO algorithm (Ireland et al., 2006), these distances would also be readily available for determining ranking, those points furthest from the Pareto front being considered the "worst".

Finally, it may be possible to rank solutions by comparing them using some aggregated objective function (AOF) that provides a single measure of fitness. The use of simple, weighted-sum AOFs has been shown to have significant difficulties finding all Pareto-dominant solutions, particularly for nonconvex Pareto fronts (Koski, 1985) and their use has been widely deprecated. However, since the solutions of particular interest are not the "best", approximating the Pareto front, but the "worst" these considerations should not have significant effect. Care should be taken to use an AOF of the form of equation (1).

$$P_s(\alpha_1,\ldots,\alpha_n;\omega_1,\ldots,\omega_n) = \left(\frac{\omega_1 \alpha_1^s + \ldots + \omega_n \alpha_n^s}{\omega_1 + \ldots + \omega_n} \right)^{\frac{1}{s}} \quad (1)$$

where α_i are the solution variables, ω_i are the preference weights, and s is a compensation fac-

Figure 3. Total Hypervolume (totalHV) of the population and the Hypervolume of the particle i (HV). "ref" indicates the reference point

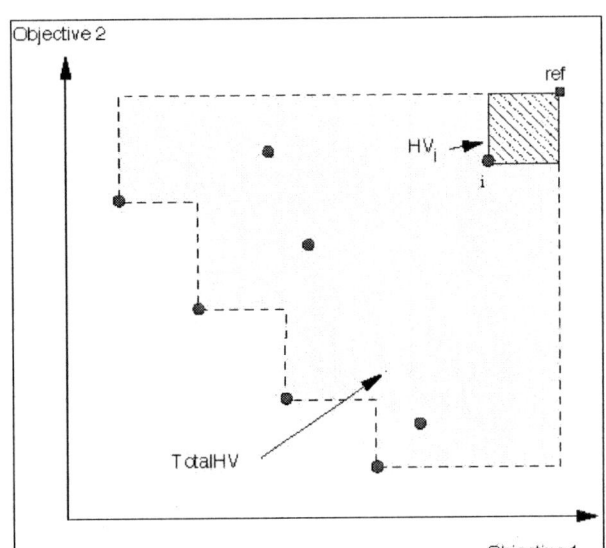

tor allowing specification of the degree to which compromise solutions are preferred over those in which one objective excels to the exclusion of others (Scott & Antonsson, 2005), protecting such solutions from premature removal.

Which of these various methods to use for specific problems remains an open question.

There also remains the issue of what constitutes a "nearest neighbour" to the points selected for removal in step 4 of the EPSOC algorithm. Current practice has dictated that these neighbouring points be selected on the basis of Euclidian distance in parameter space, with the caveat that members of a large "archive" of preserved solutions—not the archive storing the approximation to the Pareto front but a large set, often half the population, chosen by rank to make the algorithm greedy—not be removed. For application to multi-objective problems, this latter condition can be altered to protect the archive members only. Use of distance in objective space may also be worthy of consideration.

COMPUTATIONAL EXAMPLE

EPD has been successfully applied to EO solving combinatorial problems in single objectives (Randall & Lewis, 2006). In this experiment the multidimensional knapsack problem (MKP), an extension of the classical knapsack problem, was used as a test case. For this problem, a mix of items must be chosen that satisfy a series of weighting constraints whilst maximizing the collective utility of the items. Equations (2)-(4) show the 0-1 ILP model.

$$\text{Maximise} \sum_{i=1}^{N} P_i x_i \qquad (2)$$

s.t.

$$\sum_{j=1}^{N} w_{ij} x_j \leq b_i \qquad \forall i \quad 1 \leq i \leq M \qquad (3)$$

$$x_i \in \{0,1\} \qquad \forall i \quad 1 \leq i \leq N \qquad (4)$$

Figure 4. Distance from Pareto front to determine ranking

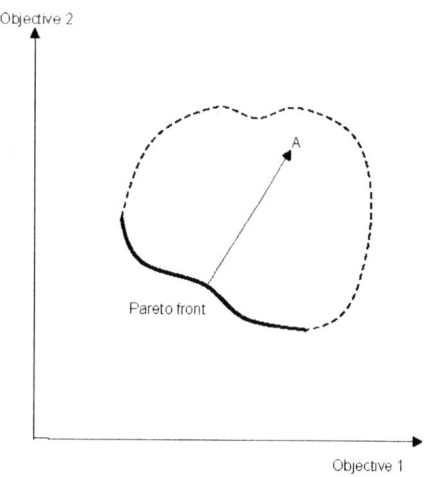

where: x_i is 1 if item i is included in the knapsack, 0 otherwise, P_i is the profit of including item i in the knapsack, N is the total number of items, w_{ij} is the weight of item j in constraint i, M is the number of constraints, and b_i is the total allowable weight according to constraint i.

A number of standard MKP problem instances from the World OR-Library (Beasley, 2007) were used as test cases. The problem instance descriptions are given in Table 1.

These problem instances have been used in previous tests of ACO algorithms (Randall, 2005). In those tests, ACO was able to find the global optimum in 4 of the 6 cases, only achieving results of 12380 on mknap3 (0.2%) and 10137 on mknap4 (-4.5%). EO was used by itself, and allowed to run for 500,000 iterations, to ensure achieving the best solution of which the algorithm was capable. Best and median results obtained over a number of trials, and the average actual number of iterations required to obtain the results, are shown in Table 2.

Using EO with EPD, loop counts for the nested loop were determined empirically, from preliminary experiments, and then set the same for all tests. There is, perhaps, potential for tuning these parameters using self-adaptation (Meyer-Nieberg & Beyer, 2007). However, observation of the convergence history of the hybrid algorithm tends to suggest that the gains from this may not be great. A typical convergence profile (for mknap6) for 100 iterations of EPSOC using 1000, 5000 and 50,000 iterations of EO are shown in Figure 5. The overall shape of each trace is determined by the EPSOC component and shows generally rapid initial convergence, followed by stagnation. Tests using 1000 iterations of the EPSOC component showed no benefit from allowing it a larger numbers of iterations. The effect of changing the number of iterations for the inner EO component is primarily apparent in the lower starting values for the traces. By allowing EO to search further even the first iteration of the hybrid algorithm is improved.

Table 1. MKP problem instance descriptions (© 2006 IEEE Used with permission)

Problem Name	N	M	Optimal Value
mknap1	6	10	3800
mknap2	20	10	6120
mknap3	28	10	12400
mknap4	39	5	10618
mknap5	50	5	6339
mknap6	60	5	6954

From Figure 5 it may be observed that the final result is obtained in less than 100 outer loop iterations for any number of inner loop iterations tested, that is, using at most 100 iterations for the outer and at least 1000 for the inner loop would be adequate to achieve good results in minimal time. For this reason these limits were chosen for use for each of the test cases. The EPSOC component was given a population of 10 to manipulate, that is, 10 simultaneous EO searches were executed on parallel computing resources at each iteration of the outer loop of the algorithm. The results achieved by the EO algorithm with EPD are given in Table 3.

Comparison of results showed that EO with EPD achieved equal or better results than EO alone on almost all tests cases (in one case it was slightly worse, with a difference of only 1%). On all test cases EO with EPD also achieved its results in less time. On average, EO required 80% more time to obtain generally poorer results. The results using EO with EPD were also compared with tests using unmodified ACO. EO with EPD was been found to deliver near-optimal results faster than the existing ACO algorithm, and the relative speed of the algorithm could be expected to improve for larger problem sizes. Further results of these experiments are given elsewhere (Randall & Lewis, 2006).

The experiment described, using EPD with EO on the multidimensional knapsack problem, is analogous to applying EPD to a single objective optimisation algorithm to solve a multi-objective problem using an aggregated objective function. As such, it may prove instructive for this approach to the solution of multi-objective optimisation problems.

To illustrate the use of EPD with Pareto dominance algorithms for the solution of multidimensional problems, a standard test problem (Zitzler, Deb, & Thiele, 1999) was chosen. The objective functions were:

Figure 5. Convergence histories of EO with EPD for mknap6 (© 2006 IEEE Used with permission)

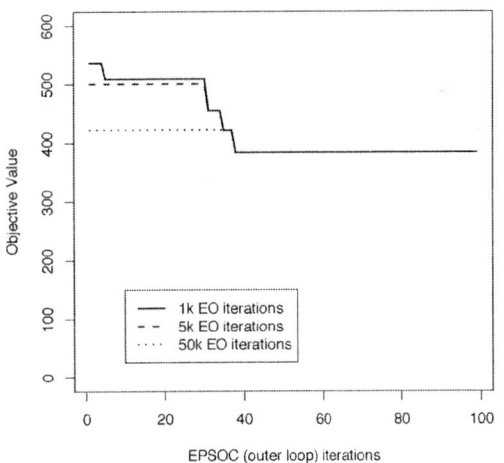

Table 2. Test results for EO only (© 2006 IEEE Used with permission)

Problem Name	Best result	Iterations taken	Median result	Iterations taken
mknap1	3800	9140	3800	9140
mknap2	6040	166304	5980	7080
mknap3	12180	161089	12180	161089
mknap4	9083	287120	9022	197651
mknap5	6097	172585	6003	31215
mknap6	6650	119523	6583	169988

$$f_1(x) = x_1$$
$$f_2(x) = g(x) \cdot h(f_1, g)$$

where the choice of the *h* and *g* functions dictate the shape of the Pareto front. For the experiment shown here, equations (5) and (6) are used. These yield a convex Pareto front.

$$g(x) = 1 + \frac{9}{N-1} \sum_{n=2}^{N} x_n \quad (5)$$

$$h(f_1, g) = 1 - \sqrt{\frac{f_1}{g}} \quad (6)$$

The dimension of parameter space, N, was 30. A swarm size of 100 was used and the Sigma selection method determined the guide points. At each iteration of the MOPSO algorithm, points removed from the population by EPD were reinitialised by selecting a member from the archive and initialising a point randomly distributed in a region surrounding the location of the chosen archive member in parameter space.

As the population evolves, nondominated solutions accumulate in the archive. In a sense, the number of unique solutions in the archive, the "best" solutions found to date, is a measure of the quality of the algorithm's output. This was found, in this case, to be the chief difference between a standard MOPSO algorithm run with identical conditions, and the MOPSO algorithm with EPD.

Table 3. Test results of EO with EPD (© 2006 IEEE Used with permission)

Problem Name	Value obtained
mknap1	3800
mknap2	6040
mknap3	12210
mknap4	10052
mknap5	6107
mknap6	6570

Traces of the archive size for standard MOPSO and MOPSO with EPD are shown in Figure 6.

When individual solutions in the archives of each algorithm were compared, their locations and objective function values were quite similar. As can be seen in Figure 5, in the early stages there is little to distinguish the performance of the two algorithms. However, MOPSO with EPD gradually starts to accumulate more archive members—more "good" solutions. As more and more points are transferred from "poor" areas closer to the evolving approximation to the Pareto front, an increasing number find better solutions, enter the nondominated set—the approximation to the Pareto front—and are captured in the archive. Towards the end of the program's execution, this trend rapidly accelerates, as MOPSO with EPD fills in more of the Pareto front, yielding a more detailed description of its shape.

The previous examples show the use of EPD with the EO and MOPSO algorithms. Despite references to the "EPSOC algorithm" it should be noted that EPD is not a new algorithm, competing with other, state-of-the-art algorithms. It is, instead a novel, complementary technique that can be applied to these algorithms. To emphasise this point, the following example demonstrates application of EPD to the widely-used nondominated sorting genetic algorithm, NSGA-II (Deb, Agrawal, Pratab, & Meyarivan, 2000).

NSGA-II sorts a population of solutions according to their degree of nondomination. That is, all nondominated solutions in the population are given rank 1. Removing the rank 1 individuals from consideration, those individuals that are nondominated in the remainder of the population are given rank 2, and so on. Elitism is introduced by comparing the current population at each iteration with the previously found best nondominated solutions. Conventional processes of tournament selection, recombination and mutation are used to evolve the population.

Since NSGA-II is a population-based algorithm, EPD can be applied directly to the subject

Figure 6. History of archive size for standard MOPSO and MOPSO + EPD

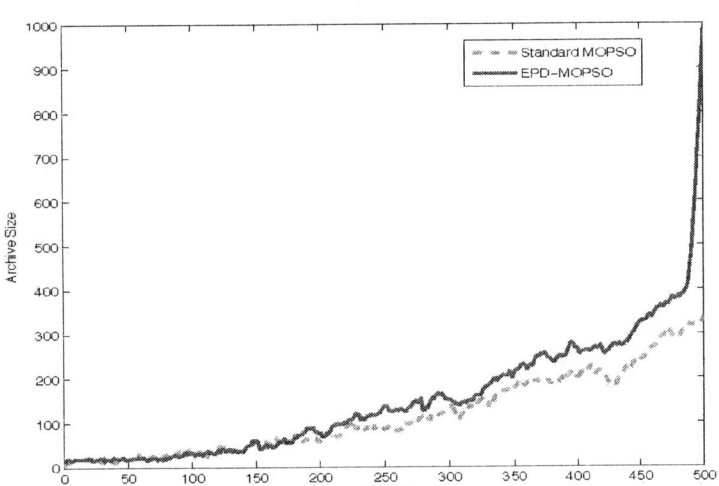

population, as in the previous MOPSO example. At each iteration, *nbad* of the lowest ranked population members are removed, along with their nearest neighbour in solution space. Nearest neighbours are avoided if they fall in the upper half of the ranked population, preserving the elitism of the parent algorithm. The removed individuals are replaced by new individuals initialised close to randomly chosen rank 1 individuals.

This modified algorithm was compared with the unmodified code using five standard, multi-objective test problems (Deb et al., 2000). Details of the problem formulations are given in Table 4. All test case parameters were real-valued. Each problem was run for 10 different, random seeds for both modified and original code. The number of iterations was limited to 50.

Often plots showing several runs are confusing and misleading. Sometimes it is impossible to pick out points from a specific run in those plots. In order to illustrate the results of 10 runs, the best (first) and the median (fifth) attainment surfaces (Knowles, 2005) have been plotted. The results of multiple runs build up a set of points that can approximately represent the union of all goals achieved (independently) in the multiple runs. The best attainment surface is a collection of points which build a nondominated set. The second attainment surface is a set of points which are weakly dominated by the first one. The median surface illustrates an average summary of the obtained results in 10 runs. These attainment surfaces have been produced by diagonal sampling as in Knowles (2005). The attainment surfaces for the best results and median results obtained are plotted in Figures 7a-e and 8a-e respectively.

From the figures, it may be seen that the algorithm using EPD uniformly delivers better results than the unmodified algorithm. This is, however, for a limited number of iterations. If the two algorithms were allowed to run further, they were found to converge to essentially the same set of Pareto optimal solutions. EPD appears to confer an advantage in that the set of solutions approximating the Pareto front more rapidly converge toward "reasonably good" solutions. Thereafter, the unmodified algorithm catches

Table 4. The test problems used. All objective functions are to be minimised

Name	n	Variable Bounds	Objective Functions	Type
ZDT1	30	$[0,1]$	$f_1(\mathbf{x}) = x_1$ $f_2(\mathbf{x}) = g(\mathbf{x})[1 - \sqrt{x_1/g(\mathbf{x})}]$ $g(\mathbf{x}) = 1 + 9(\sum_{i=2}^{n} x_i)/(n-1)$	Convex
ZDT2	30	$[0,1]$	$f_1(\mathbf{x}) = x_1$ $f_2(\mathbf{x}) = g(\mathbf{x})[1 - (x_1/g(\mathbf{x}))^2]$ $g(\mathbf{x}) = 1 + 9(\sum_{i=2}^{n} x_i)/(n-1)$	non-convex
ZDT3	30	$[0,1]$	$f_1(\mathbf{x}) = x_1$ $f_2(\mathbf{x}) = g(\mathbf{x})[1 - \sqrt{x_1/g(\mathbf{x})} - \frac{x_1}{g(\mathbf{x})} \sin(10\pi x_1)]$ $g(\mathbf{x}) = 1 + 9(\sum_{i=2}^{n} x_i)/(n-1)$	
ZDT4	10	$x_1 \in [0,1]$ $x_i \in [-5,5]$ $i = 2,...,n$	$f_1(\mathbf{x}) = x_1$ $f_2(\mathbf{x}) = g(\mathbf{x})[1 - \sqrt{x_1/g(\mathbf{x})}]$ $g(\mathbf{x}) = 1 + 10(n-1) + \sum_{i=2}^{n}[x_i^2 - 10\cos(4\pi x_i)]$	non-convex
ZDT6	10	$[0,1]$	$f_1(\mathbf{x}) = 1 - \exp(-4x_1)\sin^6(4\pi x_1)$ $f_2(\mathbf{x}) = g(\mathbf{x})[1 - (f_1(\mathbf{x})/g(\mathbf{x}))^2]$ $g(\mathbf{x}) = 1 + 9[(\sum_{i=2}^{n} x_i)/(n-1)]^{0.25}$	non-convex non-uniform

up, as the algorithm with EPD does not refine the obtained solutions any more effectively.

These results are similar to those found in previous applications of the EPSOC algorithm, for example, to a bin-packing problem (Mathieu, 2005). They suggest that hybridisation of algorithms using EPD with local search techniques may be quite profitable, though this remains a topic for future investigation.

CONCLUDING REMARKS AND FUTURE RESEARCH DIRECTIONS

The use of evolutionary population dynamics (EPD) as a controlling metaheuristic for population based optimisation algorithms is a recent development. As briefly outlined in this chapter, there are a number of open questions regarding the most effective means for its application. This work

Evolutionary Population Dynamics and Multi-Objective Optimisation Problems

Figures 7a and 7b. Best results for ZDT1 and ZDT2 respectively

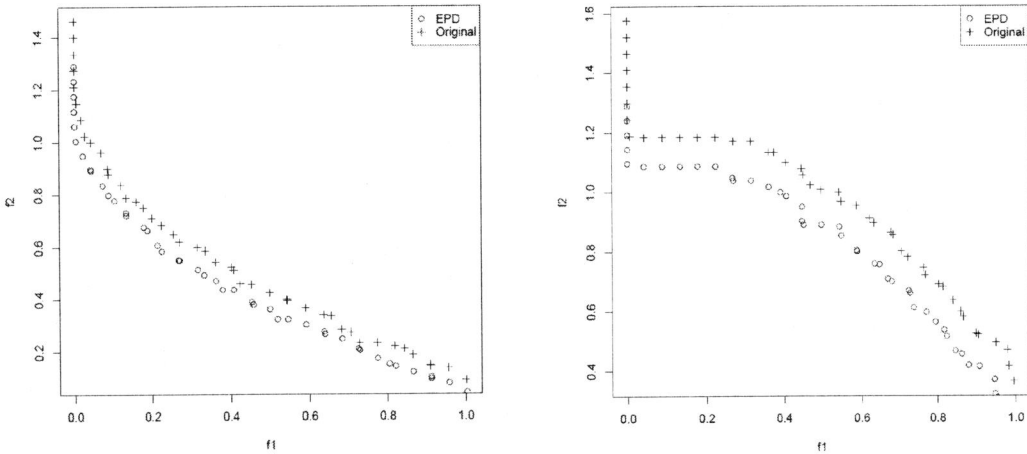

Figures 7c and 7d. Best results for ZDT3 and ZDT4 respectively

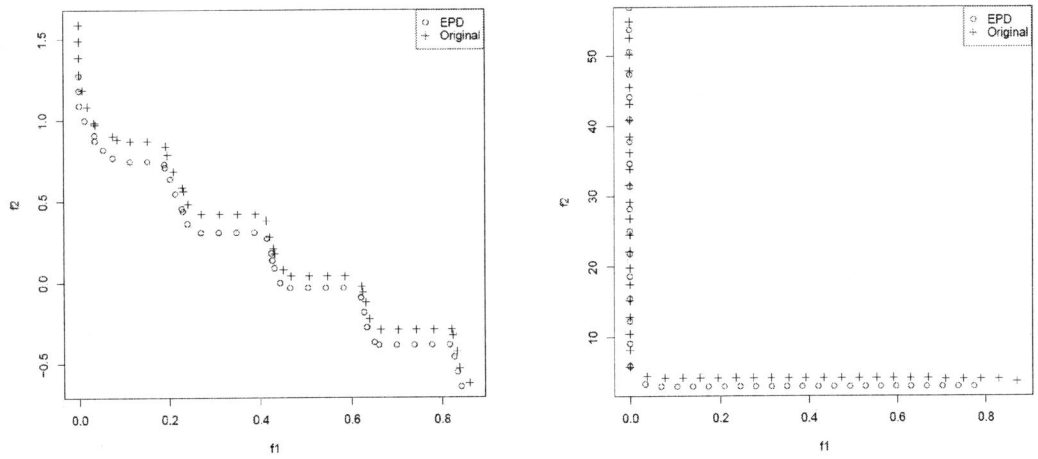

Figures 7e. Best results for ZDT6

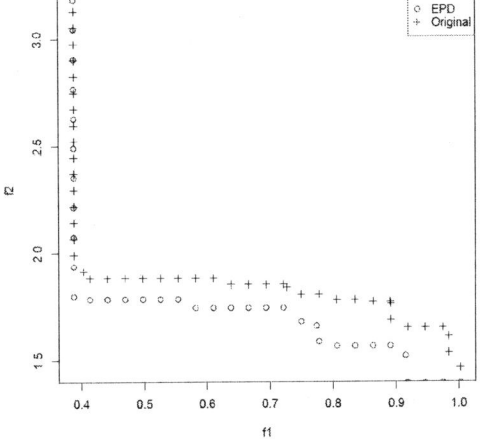

Figures 8a and 8b. Median results for ZDT1 and ZDT2 respectively

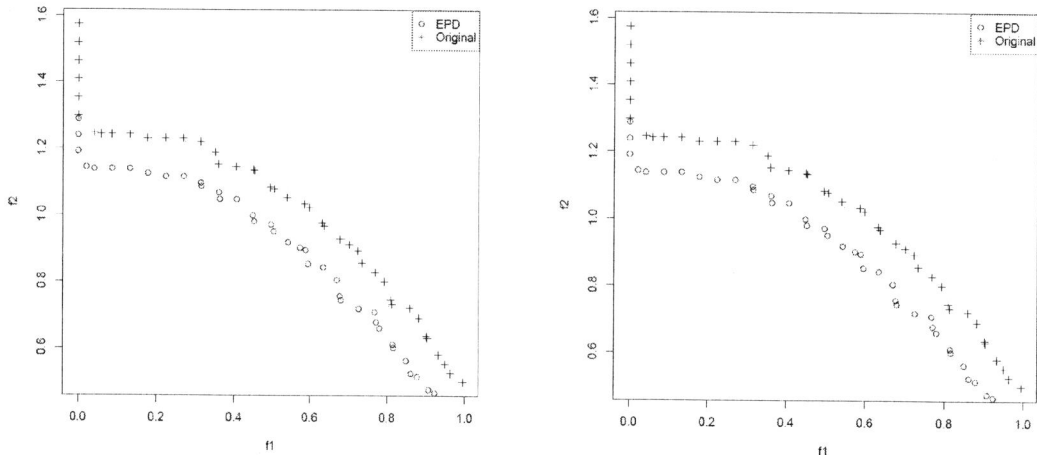

Figures 8c and 8d. Median results for ZDT3 and ZDT4 respectively

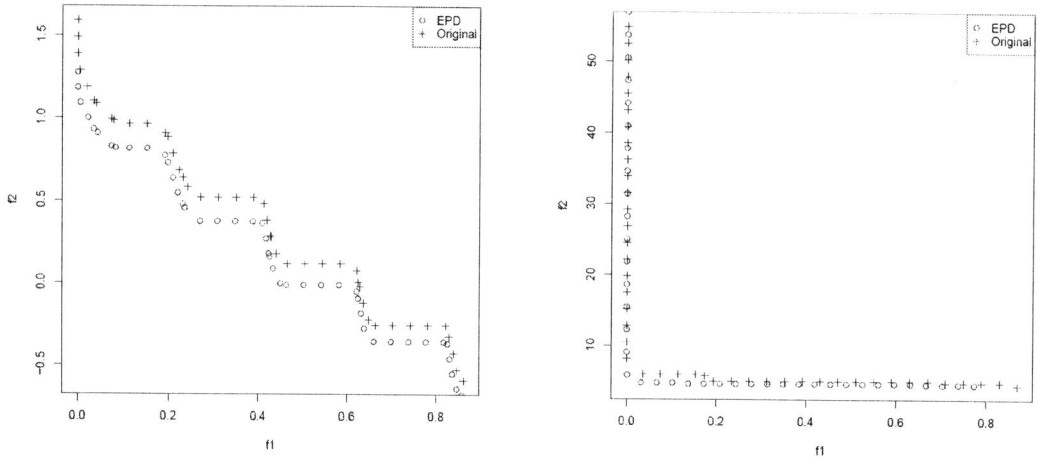

Figures 8e. Median results for ZDT6

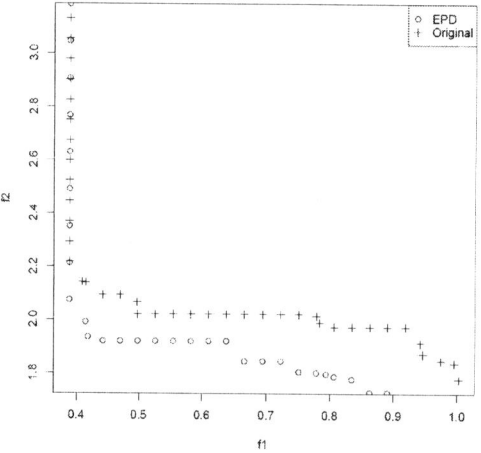

has sought to describe some of the fundamental concepts underpinning this novel paradigm, the rationale behind its use, and some practical suggestions for its implementation. Some of the potential benefits of its use—better solutions derived more rapidly—have been demonstrated from preliminary experimental results. As has been shown, this concept can be applied to both continuous and combinatorial problems for single valued and multi-objective problems. While designed for use with population based algorithms, a suggested methodology for applying the concept to other types of algorithms has also been described, and its efficacy demonstrated.

This is a newly emerging approach and, while early results have been very encouraging, considerable work remains to examine and understand the performance, emergent behaviour and expected outcomes of its use in an expanding range of applications. EPD therefore has a great scope for further improvement and refinement. We believe that the following lines of investigation could prove profitable:

- **Methods of selection of "poor" solutions for removal:** As outlined in the body of the chapter, three alternatives can be envisaged:
  1. Comparison using hypervolume metrics
  2. Measurement of Euclidean distance to the Pareto front (or some "Utopia Point", as used in several performance metrics)
  3. Ranking of solutions by use of an Aggregated Objective Function (AOF)

  In addition to these three, the ranking methods of the algorithms themselves can be used. For example, NSGA-II sorts individuals in its population by means of degree of domination. This ranking was implicitly used in the computational experiments applying EPD to NSGA-II described.

- **Methods for determination of "nearest neighbours" – during selection of solutions for removal:** At present a large (half the entire population) subset of solutions is protected from removal as part of the greedy elitism. The effect of reducing this to members of the archive approximating the Pareto optimal set, across a range of algorithms and test problems, has yet to be determined.

- **Methods of re-initialisation of points removed from the population at each iteration by the application of EPD:** The experiments described here use simple methods of random re-initialisation of trial solutions in regions "close" to known, good solutions. These approaches were chosen on the basis of limited, empirical comparison with uniformly random re-initialisation. More sophisticated approaches, and a more systematic comparison of emergent behaviour, may prove beneficial.

- **The possible benefits of the use of self-adaptation:** Self-adaptation is when an algorithm optimises its own control parameters while it is solving a problem. In the case of EPD, the possible parameters include the number of iterations of inner and outer loops; number of *nbad* trial solutions to be removed (where appropriate); and the number of neighbouring points.

- **The hybridisation of EPD-manipulated algorithms with techniques of local search:** This promises significant advantages in a number of areas, particularly in achieving computational efficiency.

ACKNOWLEDGMENT

The authors wish to thank David Ireland for his assistance in generating the experimental results described in this work.

REFERENCES

Alvarez-Benitez, J., Everson, R., & Fieldsend, J. (2005). A MOPSO algorithm based exclusively on Pareto dominance concepts. In C. Coello Coello, A. Aguirre & E. Zitzler (Eds.), *Evolutionary multi-criterion optimisation: Vol. 3410. Lecture notes in computer science* (pp. 459–473). Berlin: Springer-Verlag.

Angus, D. (2006). Crowding population-based ant colony optimisation for the multi-objective travelling salesman problem. In P. Sloot, G. van Albada, M. Bubak, & A. Referthen (Eds.), *2nd IEEE international e-science and grid computing conference (Workshop on biologically-inspired optimisation methods for parallel and distributed architectures: Algorithms, systems and applications)*. Piscataway: IEEE-Press.

Bak, P. (1996). *How nature works*. New York: Springer-Verlag.

Bak, P. & Sneppen, K. (1993). Punctuated equilibrium and criticality in a simple model of evolution. *Physical Review Letters, 71*, 4083–4086.

Bak, P., Tang, C., & Wiesenfeld, K. (1987). Self-organized criticality: An explanation of 1/f noise. *Physical Review Letters, 59*, 381–384.

Beasley, J. (2007). *OR-library*. Retrieved February 10, 2008, from http://people.brunel.ac.uk/mastjjb/jeb/info.html.

Boettcher, S. & Percus, A. (1999). Extremal optimisation: Methods derived from co-evolution. In W. Banzhaf, J. Daida, A. Eiben, M. Garzon, V. Honavar, M. Jakiela, & R. Smith (Eds.), *Genetic and evolutionary computation conference* (pp. 825–832). San Francisco: Morgan Kaufmann.

Boettcher, S. & Percus, A. (2000). Nature's way of optimizing, *Artificial Intelligence, 119*, 275–286.

Boettcher, S. & Percus, A. (2003). Extremal optimisation: An evolutionary local search algorithm. In H. Bhargava & N. Ye (Eds.), *8th INFORMS computer society conference: Vol. 21. Interfaces in computer science and operations research* (pp. 61–78). Norwell, MA: Kluwer Academic Publishers.

Branke, J. & Mostaghim, S. (2006). About selecting the personal best in multi-objective particle swarm optimisation. In T. Runarsson, H. Beyer, E. Burke, J. Merelo Guervos, L. Darrell Whitley, & X. Yao (Eds.), *Parallel problem solving from nature: Vol. 4193. Lecture notes in computer science* (pp. 523–532). Berlin: Springer-Verlag.

Coello Coello, C. & Lechuga, M. (2002). MOPSO: A proposal for multiple objective particle swarm optimisation. In D. Fogel, M. El-Sharkawi, X. Yao, G. Greenwood, H. Iba. P. Marrow, & M. Shackleton (Eds.), *Congress on evolutionary computation* (pp. 1051–1056). Piscataway: IEEE-Press.

Coello Coello, C., Van Veldhuizen, D., & Lamont, G. (2002). *Evolutionary algorithms for solving multi-objective problems*. Norwell, MA: Kluwer Academic Publishers.

Deb, K. (2001). *Multi-objective optimisation using evolutionary algorithms*. New York: John Wiley and Sons.

Deb, K., Agrawal, S., Pratab, A., & Meyarivan, T. (2000). *A fast elitist non-dominated sorting genetic algorithm for multi-objective optimisation: NSGA-II*. (KanGAL Rep. No. 200001), Kanpur, India: Indian Institute of Technology.

Doerner, K., Gutjahr, W., Hartl, R., & Strauss, C. (2004). Pareto ant colony optimisation: A metaheuristic approach to multi-objective portfolio selection. *Annals of Operations Research, 131*, 79–99.

Dorigo, M. & Di Caro, G. (1999). The ant colony optimisation meta-heuristic. In D. Corne, M. Dorigo, & F. Glover (Eds.), *New ideas in optimisation* (pp. 11–32). London: McGraw-Hill.

Eberhart, R. & Kennedy, J. (1995). A new optimizer using particle swarm theory. *6th international symposium on micro machine and human science* (pp. 39–43). Piscataway: IEEE-Press.

Engelbrecht, A. (2005). *Fundamentals of computational swarm intelligence*. New York: John Wiley and Sons.

Fieldsend, J. & Singh, S. (2002). A multi-objective algorithm based upon particle swarm optimisation, An efficient data structure and turbulence. In X. Tao (Ed.), *The U.K. workshop on computational intelligence* (pp. 34–44).

Fogel, L. (1962). Autonomous automata. *Industrial Research, 4*, 14–19.

Galski, R., de Sousa, F., Ramos, F., & Muraoka, I. (2007). Spacecraft thermal design with the generalized extremal optimisation algorithm. *Inverse Problems in Science and Engineering, 15*, 61–75.

Gambardella, L., Taillard, E., & Agazzi, G. (1999). MACS-VRPTW - A multiple ant colony system for vehicle routing problems with time windows. In D. Corne, M. Dorigo, & F. Glover (Eds.), *New ideas in optimisation* (pp. 63–76). London: McGraw-Hill.

Garcia-Martinez, C., Cordón, O., & Herrera, F. (2004). An empirical analysis of multiple objective ant colony optimisation algorithms for the bi-criteria TSP. In M. Dorigo, M. Birattari, C. Blum, L. Gambardella, F. Mondada, & T. Stützle (Eds.), *4th international workshop on ant colony optimisation and swarm intelligence: Vol. 3172. Lecture notes in computer science* (pp. 61–72). Berlin: Springer-Verlag.

Garcia-Martinez, C., Cordón, O., & Herrera, F. (2007). A taxonomy and an empirical analysis of multiple objective ant colony optimisation algorithms for bi-criteria TSP. *European Journal of Operational Research, 180*, 116–148.

Goldberg, D. (1989). *Genetic algorithms in search, optimisation and machine learning*. Reading, MA: Addison Wesley.

Guntsch, M. & Middendorf, M. (2003). Solving multi-criteria optimisation problems with population-based ACO. In G. Goos, J. Hartmanis, & J. van Leeuwen (Eds.), *Second international conference on evolutionary multi-criterion optimisation: Vol. 2632. Lecture notes in computer science* (pp. 464–478). Berlin: Springer-Verlag.

Hu, X. & Eberhart, R. (2002). Multi-objective optimisation using dynamic neighborhood particle swarm optimisation. In D. Fogel, M. El-Sharkawi, X. Yao, G. Greenwood, H. Iba. P. Marrow, & M. Shackleton (Eds.), *Congress on evolutionary computation* (pp. 1677–1681). Piscataway: IEEE-Press.

Iredi, S., Merkle, D., & Middendorf, M. (2001). Bi-criterion optimisation with multi colony ant algorithms. In E. Zitzler, K. Deb, L. Thiele, C. Coello Coello, & D. Corne (Eds.), *First international conference on evolutionary multi-criterion optimisation: Vol. 1993. Lecture notes in computer science* (pp. 359–372). Berlin: Springer-Verlag.

Ireland, D., Lewis, A., Mostaghim, S., & Lu, J. (2006). Hybrid particle guide selection methods in multi-objective particle swarm optimisation. In P. Sloot, G. van Albada, M. Bubak, & A. Referthen (Eds.), *2nd international e-science and grid computing conference (Workshop on biologically-inspired optimisation methods for parallel and distributed architectures: Algorithms, systems and applications)*. Piscataway: IEEE-Press.

Kennedy, J. & Eberhart, R. (1995). Particle swarm optimisation. *International conference on neural networks* (pp. 1942–1948). Piscataway: IEEE-Press.

Knowles, J. (2005). A summary-attainment-surface plotting method for visualizing the performance of stochastic multi-objective optimizers. In *Proceedings of the 5th International Conference* on *Intelligent Systems Design and Applications* (pp. 552–557).

Koski, J. (1985). Defectiveness of weighting method in multicriterion optimisation of structures. *Communications in Applied Numerical Methods, 1*, 333–337.

Lewis, A., Abramson, D., & Peachey, T. (2003). An evolutionary programming algorithm for automatic engineering design. In R. Wyrzykowski, J. Dongarra, M. Paprzycki, & J. Wasniewski (Eds.), *5th international conference on parallel processing and applied mathematics: Vol. 3019. Lecture notes in computer science* (pp. 586–594). Berlin: Springer-Verlag.

Mariano, C. & Morales, E. (1999). *A multiple objective ant-Q algorithm for the design of water distribution irrigation networks* (Tech. Rep. HC-9904), Mexico City: Instituto Mexicano de Tecnologia del Agua.

Mathieu, O. (2005). *Utilisation d'algorithmes évolutionnaires dans le cadre des problèmes d'empaquetage d'objets*. Unpublished master's thesis, Facultes Universitaires Notre-Dame de la Paix Namur, Brussels.

Meyer-Nieberg, S. & Beyer, H. (2007). Self-adaptation in evolutionary algorithms. In F. Lobo, C. Lima, & Z. Michalewicz (Eds.), *Parameter settings in evolutionary algorithms: Vol. 54. Studies in computational intelligence* (pp. 47–76). Berlin: Springer-Verlag.

Mostaghim, S. (2005). *Multi-objective evolutionary algorithms: Data structures, Convergence and, diversity*. Unpublished doctoral thesis, University of Paderborn, Paderborn.

Mostaghim, S. & Teich, J. (2003). Strategies for finding good local guides in multi-objective particle swarm optimisation. *Swarm intelligence symposium* (pp. 26–33). Piscataway: IEEE-Press.

Mostaghim, S. & Halter, W. (2006). Bilevel optimisation of multi-component silicate melts using particle swarm optimisation. In D. Fogel (Ed.), *Congress on evolutionary computation* (pp. 4383–4390). Piscataway: IEEE-Press.

Mostaghim, S., Branke, J., & Schmeck, H. (2006). *Multi-objective particle swarm optimisation on computer grids* (Tech. Rep. No. 502). Karlsruhe, Germany: University of Karlsruhem, AIFB Institute.

Parsopoulos, K. & Vrahatis, M. (2002). Particle swarm optimisation method in multi-objective problems. In B. Panda (Ed.), *Symposium on applied computing* (pp. 603–607). New York: ACM Press.

Purshouse, R. & Fleming, P. (2003). Evolutionary multi-objective optimisation: An exploratory analysis. In R. Sarker, R. Reynolds, H. Abbass, K. Tan, B. McKay, D. Essam, & T, Gedeon (Eds.), *Congress on evolutionary computation* (pp. 2066–2073). Piscataway: IEEE-Press.

Randall, M. (2005). A dynamic optimisation approach for ant colony optimisation using the multidimensional knapsack problem. In H. Abbass, T. Bossamaier, & J. Wiles (Eds.), *Recent advances in artificial life* (pp. 215–226). Singapore: World Scientific.

Randall, M. & Lewis, A. (2006). An extended extremal optimisation model for parallel architectures. In P. Sloot, G. van Albada, M. Bubak, & A. Referthen (Eds.), *2nd international e-science and grid computing conference (Workshop on biologically-inspired optimisation methods for parallel and distributed architectures: Algorithms, systems and applications)*. Piscataway: IEEE-Press.

Reyes-Sierra, M. & Coello Coello, C. (2006). Multi-objective particle swarm optimizers: A survey of the state-of-the-art. *International Journal of Computational Intelligence Research, 2*, 287–308.

Scott, M. & Antonsson, E. (2005). Compensation and weights for trade-offs in engineering design:

Beyond the weighted sum. *Journal of Mechanical Design, 127,* 1045–1055.

Zitzler, E. (1999). *Evolutionary algorithms for multi-objective optimisation: Methods and applications.* Unpublished doctoral thesis, Swiss Federal Institute of Technology (ETH).

Zitzler, E., Deb, K., & Thiele, L. (1999). Comparison of multi-objective evolutionary algorithms on test functions of different difficulty. In A. Wu (Ed.), *Genetic and evolutionary computation conference (Workshop Program)* (pp. 121–122).

ADDITIONAL READING

This chapter draws on a number of different fields. In order to gain a greater understanding of these, the following references are provided over and beyond those in the References list; metaheuristic search algorithms overview (Back, Fogel, & Michalewicz, 1999; Bonabeau, Dorigo, & Theraulaz, 1999; Ebehart, Simpson, & Dobbins, 1996; Eberhart, Shi, & Kennedy, 2001; Michalewicz & Fogel, 2004), ACO (Dorigo, Maniezzo, & Colorni, 1996; Dorigo & Stützle, 2004; Dorigo & Stützle, 2003; Guntsch & Middendorf, 2002; López-Ibáñez, Paquete, & Stützle, 2004), EO (Boettcher, 2000; Boettcher & Percus, 2001), PSO (Clerc, 2006; Kennedy & Eberhart, 1999), multi-objective optimisation (Coello Coello, 2006a; Coello Coello, 1999; Coello Coello, 2000; Coello Coello, 2006b; Collette & Siarry, 2004; Deb, 2000; Deb & Jain, 2004; Deb, Thiele, Laumanns, & Zitzler, 2005; Zitzler & Thiele, 1999).

Back, T., Fogel, D., & Michalewicz, Z. (Eds.). (1997). *Handbook of evolutionary computation.* Oxford: Oxford University Press.

Bonabeau, E., Dorigo, M., & Theraulaz, G. (1999). *Swarm intelligence.* Oxford: Oxford University Press.

Boettcher, S. (2000). Extremal optimisation—Heuristics via co-evolutionary avalanches. *Computing in Science & Engineering, 2,* 75–82.

Boettcher, S. & Percus, A. (2001). Optimisation with extremal dynamics. *Physics Review Letters, 86,* 5211–5214.

Clerc, M. (2006). *Particle swarm optimisation.* UK: ISTE Publishing Company.

Coello Coello, C. (1999). A comprehensive survey of evolutionary-based multi-objective optimisation techniques. *Knowledge and Information Systems, 1,* 269–308.

Coello Coello, C. (2000). Handling preferences in evolutionary multi-objective optimisation: A survey. *Congress on evolutionary computation* (pp. 30–37). Piscataway: IEEE Computer Society Press.

Coello Coello, C. (2006a). 20 years of evolutionary multi-objective optimisation: What has been done and what remains to be done. In G. Yen & D. Fogel (Eds.), *Computational intelligence: Principles and practice* (pp. 73–88). Piscataway: IEEE-Press.

Coello Coello, C. (2006b). The EMOO repository: A resource for doing research in evolutionary multi-objective optimisation. *IEEE Computational Intelligence Magazine, 1,* 37–45.

Coello Coello, C., Toscano Pulido, G. & Salazar Lechuga, S. (2002). An extension of particle swarm optimisation that can handle multiple objectives. *The workshop on multiple objective metaheuristics.*

Collette, Y. & Siarry, P. (2004). *Multi-objective optimisation: Principles and case studies (Decision Engineering).* Berlin: Springer-Verlag.

Deb, K. (2000). Multi-objective evolutionary optimisation: Past, present and future. In I. Parmee (Ed.), *Evolutionary design and manufacture* (pp. 225–236). Berlin: Springer-Verlag.

Deb, K. & Jain, S. (2004). Evaluating evolutionary multi-objective optimisation algorithms using running performance metrics. In K. Tan, M. Lim, X. Yao, & L. Wang (Eds.), *Recent advances in simulated evolution and learning* (pp. 307–326). Singapore: World Scientific Publishers.

Deb, K., Thiele, L., Laumanns, M., & Zitzler, E. (2005). Scalable test problems for evolutionary multi-objective optimisation. In A. Abraham, L. Jain, & R. Goldberg (Eds.), *Evolutionary multi-objective optimisation: Theoretical advances and applications* (pp. 105–145). Berlin: Springer-Verlag.

Dorigo, M. & Stützle, T. (2003). The ant colony optimisation metaheuristic: Algorithms, applications, and advances. In F. Glover & G. Kochenberger (Eds.), *Handbook of metaheuristics* (pp. 251–285). Norwell, MA: Kluwer Academic Publishers.

Dorigo, M. & Stützle, T. (2004). *Ant colony optimisation*. Cambridge, MA: MIT Press.

Dorigo, M., Maniezzo, V., & Colorni, A. (1996). The ant system: Optimisation by a colony of cooperating agents. *IEEE Transactions on Systems, Man and Cybernetics – Part B, 26*, 29–41.

Englebrecht, A. (2006). *Fundamentals of computational swarm intelligence*. New Jersey: Wiley.

Eberhart, R., Simpson, P., & Dobbins, R. (1996). *Computational intelligence PC Tools* (1st ed.). Boston, MA: Academic Press Professional.

Eberhart, R., Shi, Y., & Kennedy, J. (2001). *Swarm intelligence*. San Fransisco: Morgan Kauffman.

Guntsch, M. & Middendorf, M. (2002). A population based approach for ACO. In S. Cagnoni, J. Gottlieb, E. Hart, M. Middendorf, & G. Raidl (Eds.), *Applications of evolutionary computing: Vol. 2279. Lecture notes in computer science* (pp. 72–81). Berlin: Springer-Verlag.

Kennedy, J. & Eberhart, R. (1999). The particle swarm: Social adaptation in information-processing systems. In D. Corne, M. Dorigo, & F. Glover (Eds.), *New ideas in optimisation* (pp. 379–387). London: McGraw-Hill.

López-Ibáñez, M., Paquete, L., & Stützle, T. (2004). On the design of ACO for the biobjective quadratic assignment problem. In M. Dorigo, M. Birattari, C. Blum, L. Gambardella, F. Mondada, & T. Stützle (Eds.), *4th international workshop on ant colony optimisation and swarm intelligence: Vol. 3172. Lecture notes in computer science* (pp. 61–72). Berlin: Springer-Verlag.

Michalewicz, Z. & Fogel, D. (2004). *How to solve it: Modern heuristics*. Berlin: Springer-Verlag.

Zitzler, E. & Thiele, L. (1999). Multi-objective evolutionary algorithms: A comparative case study and the strength Pareto approach. *IEEE Transactions on Evolutionary Computation, 3*, 257–271.

ENDNOTES

[a] PACO uses a population of solutions to derive its pheromone matrix, rather than directly from the solution components.

[b] In terms of ACO, PACO and its variants are the most suitable for EPD. This is because we can apply its mechanisms can be applied to the population of pheromone deriving solutions.

Section II
Applications

Chapter VIII
Multi-Objective Evolutionary Algorithms for Sensor Network Design

Ramesh Rajagopalan
Syracuse University, USA

Chilukuri K. Mohan
Syracuse University, USA

Kishan G. Mehrotra
Syracuse University, USA

Pramod K. Varshney
Syracuse University, USA

ABSTRACT

Many sensor network design problems are characterized by the need to optimize multiple conflicting objectives. However, existing approaches generally focus on a single objective (ignoring the others), or combine multiple objectives into a single function to be optimized, to facilitate the application of classical optimization algorithms. This restricts their ability and constrains their usefulness to the network designer. A much more appropriate and natural approach is to address multiple objectives simultaneously, applying recently developed multi-objective evolutionary algorithms (MOEAs) in solving sensor network design problems. This chapter describes and illustrates this approach by modeling two sensor network design problems (mobile agent routing and sensor placement), as multi-objective optimization problems, developing the appropriate objective functions and discussing the tradeoffs between them. Simulation results using two recently developed MOEAs, viz., EMOCA (Rajagopalan, Mohan, Mehrotra, & Varshney, 2006) and NSGA-II (Deb, Pratap, Agarwal, & Meyarivan, 2000), show that these MOEAs successfully discover multiple solutions characterizing the tradeoffs between the objectives.

INTRODUCTION

A sensor network is typically composed of a large number of sensor nodes, each of which may carry out simple computations as well as communicate with each other and a *fusion center* (that carries out global inferences) via wired or wireless channels (Shen, Srisathapornphat, & Jaikaeo, 2001; Tilak, Abu-Ghazaleh, & Heinzelman, 2002). Sensor networks can solve difficult monitoring and control problems by exploiting the cooperative effort of multiple sensor nodes, and have been used for myriad applications including military surveillance, homeland security, chemical/biological detection, facility monitoring, reconnaissance and environmental monitoring.

Many sensor network design problems involve the simultaneous consideration of multiple objectives, such as maximizing the lifetime and the information extracted from the network, while minimizing energy consumption, latency and deployment costs. These problems and the associated objective functions are described in Section 2.

The application of *multi-objective optimization* (MOO) techniques in sensor network design problems remains largely unexplored. Existing sensor network design approaches (e.g., Tilak et al. 2002; Yu, Krishnamachari, & Prasanna, 2004) (1) optimize only one objective while treating the others as constraints or (2) convert the multi-objective optimization problem into a single objective optimization problem, that is, they attempt to minimize a weighted sum of the various objective functions, using weights that represent relative "preference strengths." In the absence of a reliable and accurate preference vector, the optimal solution obtained by a weighted approach is highly subjective. The implications of choosing a certain set of preference weights may not be clear to the user until the solution is generated, and a user's intuition cannot be relied on to give weights that accurately correspond to the true preferences of the user. By contrast, an MOO approach, which optimizes all objectives simultaneously and obtains multiple solutions, is more useful for effective decision making. The user can evaluate these solutions based on qualitative higher-level information and make an informed choice, rather than being restricted to a choice implied by prior selection of preference weight values.

Multi-objective evolutionary algorithms simultaneously pursue the search for multiple solutions with varying emphases on different objective functions, and have recently been successfully applied to various MOO problems (Deb 2001; Deb, Pratap, Agarwal, & Meyarivan, 2000; Knowles & Corne, 1999; Zitzler, Laumanns, & Thiele, 2001), outperforming other algorithms such as the weighted sum approach, motivating their application to sensor network design problems, as discussed in the rest of this chapter. In particular, two sensor network design problems (mobile agent routing, and sensor placement) are formulated as MOO problems, and it is shown that they can be solved effectively employing multi-objective evolutionary algorithms.

Section 2 presents a detailed description of sensor network design problems, the main challenges involved, and prior work. Section 3 describes multi-objective evolutionary algorithms used for solving sensor network design problems. Section 4 discusses the mobile agent routing problem, with simulation results. Section 5 describes the sensor placement problem for target detection, along with simulation results. Section 6 discusses postprocessing of solutions obtained by MOEAs. Future research directions and conclusions are presented in Sections 7 and 8 respectively.

BACKGROUND ON SENSOR NETWORK DESIGN

Wireless sensor networks (WSNs) have been used for numerous applications including military surveillance, health monitoring and environmental monitoring. In military applications, sensor networks can be used for target detection, localization, and tracking. In health monitoring, sensor nodes can monitor the health of a patient and can also assist disabled patients. In environment monitoring, sensors monitor quantities such as temperature and pressure, and can also detect and localize abnormal events such as release of a toxic air pollutant.

In a WSN, the sensors could be scattered randomly in harsh environments (such as a battlefield) or deterministically placed at specified locations in hospitable situations. The sensors coordinate among themselves to form a communication network such as a single multihop network or a hierarchical organization with several clusters and "cluster heads". The cluster heads are powerful sensor nodes with higher battery power and computation capability compared to normal sensor nodes. Each cluster head fuses the data from sensors within its cluster and transmits the fused data to the base station or sink.

The sensors periodically sense the data, process it and transmit it to the base station or cluster head. The frequency of data reporting and the number of sensors which report data usually depends on the specific application. A comprehensive survey on wireless sensor networks is presented in Akyldiz, Su, Sankarasubramanian, and Cayirci, (2002) and Tubaishat and Madria (2003). Some features of sensor networks that render sensor network design challenging are:

1. Sensor nodes are prone to hardware failure and energy depletion and hence fault tolerance is a very important issue in sensor network design.
2. Sensor nodes are severely constrained in their energy, computation, and storage capabilities.
3. Sensor networks may contain hundreds or thousands of nodes and hence the network design should be scalable.
4. Sensor nodes could be mobile and the topology of the network may change rapidly.
5. Data transmission in sensor networks should incorporate the effect of the channel noise and radio propagation effects.
6. Sensor networks are data centric and the death of a few nodes may render the network dysfunctional.

Sensor network design is highly application specific and the design should address constraints imposed by the battery power, sensor failures, and topology changes. Recently, several researchers have developed techniques required to address the above challenges (Akyildiz et al., 2002; Heinzelman, Chandrakasan, & Balakrishnan, 2002; Shen, Srisathapornphat, & Jaikaeo, 2001).

MULTI-OBJECTIVE OPTIMIZATION PROBLEMS IN SENSOR NETWORKS

Many sensor network design problems involve the simultaneous optimization of multiple objectives, as shown in Table 1. These problems are described in the rest of this section.

Sensor Placement Problem

The goal of the sensor placement problem is to determine optimal locations of sensors for maximizing the information collected from the sensor network. For instance, in a target detection problem, the sensors should be placed such that the target detection probability is maximized. But equally important are factors such as the cost of the network and energy consumption of the network. Intuitively, deploying more sensors would improve the detection probability of the system while increasing the energy consumption and deployment cost. The resulting tradeoffs between the objectives are outlined below.

Table 1. Example multi-objective optimization problems in sensor networks

Problem	Objectives
Sensor placement for target detection	Detection probability, deployment cost, and energy consumption
Mobile agent routing	Detection accuracy, path loss, and energy consumption
Data aggregation	Data accuracy, latency, and lifetime
Area coverage	Lifetime, coverage, and deployment cost

Detection Probability

The detection probability is an indicator of the efficiency of the sensor network in determining the presence of the target. Ideally, the network should achieve a detection probability close to 1.

Deployment Cost

In a homogeneous sensor network, the deployment cost is proportional to the number of sensors deployed in the network. In a heterogeneous sensor network, the deployment cost is given by $C = \sum_{i=1}^{N} C_i T_i$ where N is the total number of nodes, C_i is the cost of a node of type i, and T_i is the number of nodes of type i.

Energy Consumption

In a target detection problem, sensors transmit their data to the sink where it is processed. The transmission of data involves energy consumption at the sensors which is a function of the distance between the sensor and the sink. The energy consumption of the network is computed as the sum of the energy expended at each sensor in the network.

Related Work

Several researchers have investigated the sensor placement problem focusing on detection and coverage. A recent survey on algorithms for sensor networks with focus on sensor deployment and coverage, routing, and sensor fusion is presented in Sahni and Xu (2004). Two noteworthy contributions on this problem are by Dhillon, Chakrabarty, and Iyengar (2002) and Clouqueur, Phipatanasuphorn, Ramanathan, and Saluja (2003). Dhillon et al. (2002) have considered the sensor placement problem for grid coverage. They have developed an iterative sensor placement algorithm for coverage optimization under the constraints of terrain properties. The sensor model for target detection used in Dhillon et al. (2002) does not consider the physics of the phenomenon or the measurement noise. Clouqueur et al. (2003) have solved the sensor placement problem for distributed target detection. They have developed a sequential deployment algorithm which terminates when a satisfactory detection performance is achieved. They have focused on deployment cost and detection performance while ignoring energy efficiency. Kar and Banerjee (2003) solve the problem of deploying a minimal number of homogenous sensors to cover a plane with a connected sensor network. The main goal of their approach is to minimize the number of sensors while guaranteeing coverage and connectivity. All of these works have considered the sensor deployment problem for single objective optimization in which the focus was on maximizing the detection performance or minimizing the deployment cost. In addition, energy efficiency has not been considered by several existing placement strategies.

Jourdan and de Weck (2004) have investigated the optimization of sensor network layout for maximizing the coverage and lifetime of the network. They model the sensor layout problem as a multi-objective optimization problem characterizing the tradeoffs between coverage and lifetime of the network. They propose a multi-objective genetic algorithm for obtaining Pareto-optimal solutions. Ferentinos and Tsiligiridis (2007) solve a multi-objective sensor network design problem in which sensors are selectively activated and a specific set of nodes are selected as cluster heads to monitor an agricultural area. The objectives are to optimize energy consumption and application requirements such as uniformity of the sensor measurements while incorporating constraints on the connectivity of the network. They combine the multiple objectives using weights that represent the relative priorities of various objectives, and use a genetic algorithm for solving the resulting single-objective optimization problem. Though their approach is interesting, it does not provide Pareto-optimal solutions characterizing the tradeoffs between the objectives. In addition, the system designer has to determine the weights *a priori* which might be infeasible if the relative priorities of different objectives are unknown. Raich and Liszkai (2003) have solved the sensor placement problem for structural damage detection. They formulated a multi-objective optimization problem involving maximization of the diagnostic information collected by the sensors and minimization of the number of sensors. They solved the multi-objective optimization problem using a nondominated sorting genetic algorithm (NSGA). It would be interesting to investigate the performance of recently developed MOEAs such as NSGA-II, SPEA-II, and EMOCA on this problem.

Mobile Agent Routing

In distributed detection problems, transmission of non-critical data consumes battery power and network bandwidth. To circumvent this problem, Qi, Iyengar, and Chakrabarty (2001) have proposed the concept of *Mobile Agent based Distributed Sensor Networks* (MADSNs) where a mobile agent selectively visits the sensors and incrementally fuses the data. It has been found that mobile agent implementation saves almost 90% of data transmission time since it avoids raw data transmissions. The objective of the mobile agent routing problem is to compute mobile agent routes for maximizing the detection accuracy while minimizing the path loss and energy consumption.

Detection Accuracy

In target detection problems, the detection accuracy of a route is computed as the sum of the detected signal energies of all nodes along the route. A higher detection accuracy would enable the sink to draw appropriate inferences about the location and type of the target.

Path Loss

Each link of the mobile agent route is associated with a path loss, which represents the signal attenuation due to free space propagation, and should be minimized to guarantee reliable communication. The path loss of a route is computed as the sum of path loss along each link of the route.

Energy Consumption

The energy consumption of a route is equal to the total energy expended at each sensor along the route in data processing and transmission.

Related Work

One of the key challenges in the design of MADSNs is the security of the data as the mobile agent visits different nodes. The data collected by the mobile agent from the sensors are susceptible to physical attacks by hostile agents. Security issues in MADSNs are investigated in Berkovits, Guttman, and Swarup (1998) and Sander and Tschudin (1998).

The main advantages of using mobile agents are presented in Lange and Oshima (1999). These include: reducing latency in data transmission, autonomous and asynchronous operation, energy efficient distributed information retrieval, and parallel processing. The applications of mobile agents include e-commerce, target detection, localization and classification, and battlefield surveillance. The conditions under which a MADSN performs better than a distributed sensor network are analyzed in Qi et al. (2001).

The sequence and the number of sensors on the route traversed by a mobile agent determine the detection accuracy, energy consumption and path loss of the route and also characterizes the overall performance of the MADSN. Algorithms based on local closest first (LCF) and global closest first (GCF) heuristics (Qi et al., 2001) have been used to compute mobile agent routes for distributed data fusion. These approaches provide satisfactory results for small network sizes with systemically deployed sensors. The performance of these algorithms deteriorates as the network size grows and the sensor distributions become more complicated. These approaches consider only spatial distances between sensor nodes for route computation, whereas other important factors in target detection applications include the detected energy level and link power consumption. Satisfactory routes cannot be obtained when some of these factors are ignored.

Wu, Rao, Barhen, Iyengar, Vaishnavi, Qi, and Chakrabarty (2004) combine three objectives: the communication cost, the path loss and the detected signal energy level into a single function optimized using a genetic algorithm that outperforms the LCF and GCF strategies. Though this approach provides good results, it does not assist the system designer in obtaining the Pareto-optimal solutions. A more appropriate approach is to model the mobile agent routing problem as a multi-objective optimization problem where evolutionary MOO algorithms can be used for obtaining the Pareto-optimal solutions.

Data Aggregation

Data aggregation is defined as the process of aggregating the data from multiple sensors to eliminate redundant transmission and provide fused information to the sink (Rajagopalan & Varshney, 2006). Data aggregation usually involves the fusion of data from multiple sensors at intermediate nodes and transmission of the aggregated data to the sink. Data aggregation attempts to collect the most critical data from the sensors and make it available to the sink in an energy efficient manner with minimum data latency. It is critical to develop energy efficient data aggregation algorithms so that network lifetime is enhanced while maximizing the data accuracy and minimizing the latency involved in data transmission. These terms are defined below.

Data Accuracy

The definition of data accuracy depends on the specific application for which the sensor network is designed. For instance, in a target localization problem, the estimate of target location at the sink determines the data accuracy.

Network Lifetime

Network lifetime is defined as the number of data aggregation rounds until a specified percentage of sensors are depleted of their battery power. For instance, in applications where the time that all nodes operate together is vital, lifetime is defined as the number of rounds until the first sensor is drained of its energy.

Latency

Latency is defined as the delay involved in data transmission, routing and data aggregation. It can be measured as the time delay between the data packets received at the sink and the data generated at the sensor nodes.

Related Work

A recent survey of data aggregation techniques in sensor networks is presented in Rajagopalan and Varshney (2006). The architecture of the sensor network plays a vital role in the performance of different data aggregation protocols. In flat networks, each sensor node plays the same role and is equipped with approximately the same battery power. The "sensor protocol for information via negotiation" (SPIN) (Kulik, Heinzelman, & Balakrishnan, 2001) can be classified as a push based diffusion protocol in flat networks. The sources flood the data when they detect an event while the sink subscribes to the sources through enforcements. Compared to flooding, SPIN incurs much less energy consumption (a factor of 3.5) and is able to distribute 60% more data per unit energy. One of the main advantages of SPIN is that topological changes are localized, since each node only requires the knowledge of its single-hop neighbors. The main disadvantage of SPIN is its inability to guarantee data delivery.

In flat networks, the failure of a sink node may result in the breakdown of the entire network. In addition, flat networks do not utilize node heterogeneity for improving energy efficiency. Hence, in view of scalability and energy efficiency, several hierarchical data aggregation approaches have been proposed. Hierarchical data aggregation involves data fusion at special nodes called cluster heads or leader nodes, which reduces the number of messages transmitted to the sink. This improves the energy efficiency of the network. Heinzelman et al. (2002) were the first to propose an energy conserving cluster formation protocol called "low energy adaptive clustering hierarchy" (LEACH). The LEACH protocol is distributed and sensor nodes organize themselves into clusters for data fusion. LEACH improves the system lifetime and data accuracy of the network but it assumes that all sensors have enough power to reach the sink if needed. In other words, each sensor has the capability to act as a cluster head and perform data fusion. This assumption might not be valid with energy-constrained sensors.

Lindsey, Raghavendra, and Sivalingam (2002) presented a chain-based data aggregation protocol called "power efficient data gathering protocol for sensor information systems (PEGASIS)". In PEGASIS, nodes are organized into a linear chain for data aggregation. The nodes can form a chain by employing a greedy algorithm or the sink can determine the chain in a centralized manner. The PEGASIS protocol has considerable energy savings compared to LEACH.

Ding, Cheng, and Xue (2003) have proposed an energy aware distributed heuristic to construct and maintain a data aggregation tree in sensor networks. The main advantage of their approach is that sensors with higher residual power have a higher chance to become a nonleaf tree node.

In sensor networks, the data gathered by spatially close sensors are usually correlated. Cristescu, Beferull-Lozano, and Vetterli (2004) have studied the problem of network correlated data gathering. When sensors use source-coding strategies, this leads to a joint optimization problem which involves optimizing rate allocation at the nodes and the transmission structure. Slepian-Wolf coding and joint entropy coding with explicit communication have been investigated in the context of data gathering. An optimal Slepian-Wolf rate allocation scheme has been proposed in (Cristescu et al., 2004). In this scheme, the node closest to the sink codes data at a rate equal to its unconditioned entropy. All other nodes code at a rate equal to their respective entropies conditioned on all nodes which are closer to the sink than themselves. The main disadvantage of this scheme is that each sensor requires global knowledge of the network in terms of distances between all nodes.

Area Coverage

In area coverage problems, the main goal of the sensor network is to collectively monitor or cover a region of interest. Coverage is a measure of quality of service of the sensor network. In most studies, it is assumed that the sensing range of a sensor can be specified as a disk and the sensor covers the area of the disk. Area coverage can be defined as the fraction of the whole monitoring area covered by all sensors in the network. In area coverage problems, there are multiple objectives of interest including coverage, network lifetime, and the deployment cost. Deploying more sensors would increase the coverage of the network but would also result in an increase in deployment cost.

To guarantee that the sensor network covers the whole area, each location of interest in the monitoring region should be within the sensing range of at least one sensor. This can be accomplished by activating a subset of sensors which covers every location of interest while the other sensors can be scheduled in sleep mode to conserve power (Cardei, MacCallum, Cheng, Min, Jia, Li, & Du, 2002). This approach prolongs the lifetime of the network while ensuring a prespecified area coverage.

Related Work

A recent survey on energy efficient coverage problems in sensor networks is presented in Cardei and Wu (2006). In Cardei et al. (2002) and Slijepcevic and Potkonjak (2001), a large number of sensors is deployed for area monitoring. The proposed approach divides the sensor nodes into disjoint sets such that each set can monitor the area independently. These sets are activated successively such that at any given time only one of the sets is active while all other sets are in the sleep mode. Zhang and Hou (2003) have considered the joint problem of guaranteeing coverage and network connectivity. A set of active nodes is defined as connected if each pair of nodes is within the transmission range of each other. They have shown that if the communication range of a sensor is at least twice the sensing range, a complete coverage of a convex region guarantees connectivity of the active nodes.

A sensor network has a coverage degree k if every point of interest in the region is within the sensing range of at least k sensors. A k-connected network guarantees network connectivity when atmost k-1 sensors are removed from the network. Wang, Xing, Zhang, Lu, Pless, and Gill (2003) investigated the k-coverage problem and showed that when the communication range is at least twice the sensing range, a k-covered network will result in a k-connected network. They proposed a coverage configuration protocol which can dynamically configure the sensor network to provide the required coverage degree.

The objective of the point coverage problem is to deploy sensors to cover a set of points in the region of interest. Cardie and Du (2005) have solved the point coverage problem in which a certain number of points or targets need to be monitored. The objective of the problem is that every target should be monitored by at least one sensor at each instant. The sensors in the network are divided into disjoint sets such that every set completely covers all targets. In Cardie and Du (2005), the disjoint set cover problem is shown to be NP complete and the problem is reduced to a maximum flow problem which is solved using an integer programming approach.

PRIOR WORK: MULTIPLE OBJECTIVES IN SENSOR NETWORK DESIGN

Current sensor network design approaches optimize only one objective while treating the others as constraints, and hence the results of various possible tradeoffs between multiple objectives are not considered. The following are examples of prior work in sensor network design and applications that address tradeoffs between multiple objectives.

1. **Data aggregation:** Boulis, Ganeriwal, and Srivastava (2003) have studied the energy-accuracy tradeoffs for periodic data aggregation problems in sensor networks. They have considered a problem in which the sensors provide periodic estimates of the environment. A distributed estimation algorithm has been developed which uses the "max" aggregation function. The key idea of their approach is a threshold-based scheme where the sensors compare their fused estimates to a threshold to make a decision regarding transmission. However, in the absence of prior information about the physical environment, setting the threshold is a nontrivial task. The threshold can be used as a tuning parameter to characterize the tradeoff between accuracy and energy consumption. Although, they discuss the tradeoff between accuracy and energy consumption, they do not consider minimization of energy consumption as an explicit objective, that is, they do not address the problem of finding multiple solutions (representing different tradeoff choices between different objectives). The main advantage of the approach proposed in Boulis et al. (2003) is that it does not depend on a hierarchical structure for performing data aggregation. Instead, every node has the global information about the aggregated data. The main disadvantage of the approach is that the functionality of the fusion algorithm depends on the aggregation function. Hence the fusion algorithm is not applicable for a wide range of aggregation functions such as "average", "count" or "min".
2. **Infrastructure design:** Tilak et al. (2002) have studied infrastructure tradeoffs in sensor networks. The infrastructure refers to the number of sensors, the deployment method, and the capabilities of the sensors. Tilak et al. (2002) have demonstrated that a denser infrastructure usually leads to a large number of collisions and congestion in the network which results in an increase in the data latency. Hence, increasing the number of sensors to a large extent may deteriorate the performance of the network. They conclude that a congestion control mechanism is required to ensure that the data transmission does not exceed the capacity of the network. They have analyzed the effect of sensor density and deployment strategy on the performance of the network in terms of accuracy, latency, throughput and energy efficiency. They considered three deployment strategies: random deployment, regular deployment such as grid and planned deployment. An example of planned deployment is biasing the sensor deployment to provide higher density in areas where the event is more likely to occur. Their experiments showed that planned deployment performs better than regular and random deployment in terms of data accuracy. However, this increase in data accuracy comes at the cost of an increase in energy consumption. They have evaluated data accuracy and energy consumption measures independently, and their approach does not provide multiple solutions that assist the decision maker in analyzing the tradeoffs.
3. **Data gathering:** Yu, Krishnamachari, and Prasanna (2004) have studied the energy-latency tradeoffs in real time applications where the goal is minimization of energy consumption subject to a specified latency constraint. They have proposed a packet-scheduling scheme based on an iterative numerical optimization algorithm that optimizes the overall energy dissipation of the sensors in the aggregation tree. There is no guarantee on the convergence speed

of the iterative algorithm. In addition, the packet-scheduling scheme assumes that the structure of the aggregation tree is known *a priori*. A pseudo-polynomial time approximation algorithm has been developed based on dynamic programming. The main drawback of the algorithm is that each node has to wait for information from all of its child nodes before performing data aggregation. This might increase the associated latency. An interesting extension of this problem would be to model the data-gathering problem as a multi-objective optimization problem optimizing energy consumption and latency simultaneously.

4. **Target tracking:** Pattem, Poduri, and Krishnamachari (2003) have proposed four sensor activation schemes for characterizing the tradeoffs between tracking quality and energy efficiency for target tracking in sensor networks: naive activation, random activation, selective activation with prediction, and duty-cycled activation. In the naive activation scheme, all sensors in the network are in the active mode continuously sensing the target. This approach results in the worst energy efficiency while providing the best tracking quality. In the randomized activation strategy, each sensor is active with probability p. The selective activation strategy activates a small subset of nodes at a given time. This set of nodes predicts the position of the target at the next time instant, and hands over the responsibility of tracking to another set of nodes which can track the target at the next time instant. In duty-cycled activation, all sensors in the network periodically switch states (active vs. inactive) with a regular duty cycle. Simulation results showed that selective activation is highly energy efficient with near-optimal tracking quality when compared to the other activation schemes. However, though the activation schemes characterize various energy-quality tradeoff choices, each produces only a single solution.

MULTI-OBJECTIVE OPTIMIZATION ALGORITHMS

MOO algorithms attempt to obtain a set of solutions that *approximates* the Pareto front for the problem. Some well-known nonevolutionary MOO algorithms include: normal-boundary intersection method (NBI), normal constraint method (NC), Timmel's population based method (TPM), and Schaffler's stochastic method (SSM). These approaches are described in detail in (Shukla & Deb, 2005). The SSM method requires the objective functions to be twice continuously differentiable. It is a gradient descent approach where the direction of descent is obtained by solving a quadratic subproblem. The TPM method is a population based stochastic approach for obtaining the Pareto-optimal solutions of a differentiable multi-objective optimization problem. The NBI and NC methods are mathematical programming approaches in which multiple searches are performed from a uniformly distributed set of points in the objective space.

The nonevolutionary approaches described earlier were compared with NSGA-II on various test problems in Shukla and Deb (2005). Their simulations showed that nonevolutionary approaches were unsuccessful in solving complex problems involving multi-modality, disconnectedness, and nonuniform density of solutions in the Pareto-front. In such problems, NSGA-II obtained solutions with better convergence and diversity when compared to the nonevolutionary approaches. The solutions obtained by non-evolutionary approaches are not necessarily Pareto-optimal. The SSM method is computationally slow in obtaining a well-distributed solution set and in many problems it obtains only a part of the entire Pareto-front. The TPM approach requires fine tuning of parameters for every problem and is also computationally inefficient. Hence, in our work we do not consider nonevolutionary approaches.

We have applied three evolutionary algorithms for solving the sensor network design problems: weight based genetic algorithm (WGA), NSGA-II, and EMOCA. WGA is a classical MOO algorithm while NSGA-II and EMOCA are multi-objective evolutionary algorithms. In the rest of this section, we briefly describe these algorithms.

Weight Based Genetic Algorithm

The weight based genetic algorithm is a classical MOO approach in which the user specifies the weights or priorities associated with different objectives. Each objective function is associated with a weight value w_i. The weights are chosen such that, $0 \leq w_i \leq 1$ and $\sum_{i=1}^{k} w_i = 1$ where k is the number of objectives. A genetic algorithm is employed to optimize a weighted combination of the normalized values of the objectives. Each solution is assigned a fitness value based on the weighted combination of the objectives. In order to obtain multiple Pareto-optimal solutions, the GA is run each time with a different weight vector. The WGA employs binary tournament selection and an elitist steady-state replacement strategy. Some of the disadvantages of WGA are:

1. Choosing a uniformly distributed set of weight vectors is not assured to sample different regions of the Pareto front for the problem.
2. Distinct weight vectors may lead to the same Pareto-optimal solution.
3. Some Pareto-optimal solutions will never be found if the Pareto front is non-convex.

Multi-Objective Evolutionary Algorithms (MOEAs)

MOEAs simultaneously evolve multiple solutions, explicitly considering the task of obtaining diverse solutions in parallel (Deb 2001; Zitzler, 1999). This section briefly describes two recently developed MOEAs: EMOCA and NSGA-II.

EMOCA is similar to NSGA-II in that both algorithms use a nondomination ranking approach to classify the solutions in the population into different fronts. The main difference between EMOCA and NSGA-II is that EMOCA uses a probabilistic approach based on diversity-rank in determining whether or not an offspring individual is accepted into the new population in the replacement selection phase. In EMOCA, convergence is emphasized by Pareto-ranking, whereas diversity is maintained among the solutions of the population by invoking the use of a *diversity rank* in the selection and replacement phase. We first define the following terms which are used in various stages of NSGA-II and EMOCA.

Non-domination rank: As in Deb et al. (2000), $rank(x) = j$ in a population X iff $x \in F_j$, where fronts $F_1, F_2 ... F_{i+1}$ are inductively defined as follows:

$$F_1 = \{x \in X | \forall y \in X : \neg(y \gg x)\};$$

$$F_{i+1} = \{x \in X | \forall y \in X - (F_1 \cup F_2 \cup ... \cup F_i) : \neg(y \gg x)\} \quad (1)$$

In other words, elements of front 1 are not dominated by any other elements in X; and elements in front $(i+1)$ are dominated only by elements in fronts 1 to i.

Crowding distance: To obtain an estimate of the density of the solutions surrounding a particular solution x_i of a front, we compute the average distance of two solutions on either side of solution x_i along each objective. This gives the crowding distance of solution x_i (Deb et al., 2000), defined as

$$\psi(x_i) = \sum_{m=1}^{M} \xi_m(x_i) \quad (2)$$

where (see equation (3)).
$g = \min (f_m(x_j) - f_m(x_k))$ where $x_i \neq x_j \neq x_k \in F$ and $f_m(x_j) > f_m(x_i) > f_m(x_k) j, k$

Equation (2).

$$\xi_m(x_i) = \begin{cases} \infty & \text{if} \quad \forall x_j, f_m(x_i) < f_m(x_j) \quad \text{or} \quad \forall x_k, f_m(x_k) < f_m(x_i) \\ \dfrac{g}{h} & \text{otherwise} \end{cases}$$

and

$h = \max(f_m(x_j) - f_m(x_k))$ where $x_j \neq x_k \in X$ and $f_m(x_j) > f_m(x_k)$ j, k

Description of NSGA-II

NSGA-II is based on a nondomination ranking approach where solutions in a population are ranked based on the fronts they belong to as defined in (1). The different stages of the algorithm are described next.

Mating population generation: NSGA-II uses binary tournament selection to fill the mating population. Each solution is assigned a fitness value equal to its *nondomination rank*. If two solutions participating in the binary tournament have the same nondomination rank, the solution with the higher crowding distance (better diversity) is chosen as the winner.

New pool generation: A new pool is generated consisting of all parents and all offspring.

Trimming new pool: A nondominated sorting is performed on all solutions of the new pool. The new population is filled with solutions of different nondominated fronts $F_1, F_2, ..., F_n$ as defined in (1) starting from F_1 and proceeding until the last allowable front. If there exists more solutions in the last front than the remaining slots (v) available in the population, the solutions in the last front are sorted based on the crowding distance. The first v elements of the sorted list are inserted into the new population.

Description of EMOCA

EMOCA addresses the convergence and diversity issues by using nondomination rank and diversity rank in multiple stages of the algorithm. The individual steps of EMOCA are described next.

Mating population generation: EMOCA employs binary tournament selection to fill the mating population. Each solution is assigned a fitness value equal to the sum of its *non-domination rank* and *diversity rank*. The diversity rank is defined below:

Diversity rank: The solutions are sorted and ranked based on the crowding distance. The solution with the highest crowding distance is assigned the best (lowest) diversity rank.

New pool generation: A "New Pool" is generated consisting of all the parents and some of the offspring. To generate the new pool, an offspring O is compared with one of its parents P which is randomly chosen among its two parents. The result of the comparison governs the probability with which O is inserted into the new pool as summarized in Table 2.

Trimming new pool: The new pool is sorted based on the primary criterion of nondomination rank and the secondary criterion of diversity rank. In other words, solutions with the same non-domination rank are compared based on diversity rank. The new population will consist of the first μ elements of the sorted list containing solutions grouped into different fronts: $F_1, F_2, ..., F_n$ as defined in (1).

Table 2. Acceptance probabilities of offspring for different scenarios. P>>O indicates P dominates O. P≈O indicates that P and O are mutually nondominating.

Non-domination comparison	Crowding distance comparison	Prob(O is accepted)
$P>>O$	$\psi(O) > \psi(P)$	$1 - e^{\psi(P) - \psi(O)}$
$P>>O$	$\psi(P) \geq \psi(O)$	0
$O>>P$		1
$P\approx O$	$\psi(O) \geq \psi(P)$	1
$P\approx O$	$\psi(P) > \psi(O)$	0

Archiving strategy: EMOCA maintains an archive (with fixed size) of nondominated solutions at every generation. When the archive is full, a new nondominated solution can replace an existing archive element with lower crowding distance.

Most of the metrics proposed for evaluating the convergence of an MOEA require prior knowledge of the Pareto-optimal front. When the Pareto-optimal front is unavailable, three metrics we invoke in this chapter are the *C-metric*, the *domination metric* and *the spacing (S) metric*. The *C-metric* and *domination metric* are pairwise comparison metrics while the *S metric* determines the diversity of the Pareto front. These metrics are described in Rajagopalan et al. (2006).

MOBILE AGENT ROUTING IN SENSOR NETWORKS

In this section, we employ the mobile agent routing problem as a vehicle to illustrate the application of MOO framework for distributed sensor network design.

Mobile Agent Distributed Sensor Network (MADSN) Architecture

In distributed detection problems, transmission of noncritical data consumes battery power and network bandwidth. To circumvent this problem, Qi et al. (2001) have proposed the concept of *Mobile Agent based Distributed Sensor Networks* (MADSNs) where a *mobile agent* selectively visits the sensors and incrementally fuses the data. It has been found that mobile agent implementation saves almost 90% of data transmission time since it avoids raw data transmissions.

The measurements from sensors which are close to the target and receive strong signals from the target are highly useful for the fusion process. Hence in MADSNs, the sensors which are close to the target with high-detected signal energies are first identified before the fusion step. The identification of such sensor nodes reduces the complexity and amount of data for fusion. Hence, the objective of MADSNs is to compute a route for the mobile agent through such sensor nodes by using the detected signal energies of different sensors. The mobile agent visits the sensors in the route and performs data fusion at these nodes.

In a hierarchical MADSN (Rajagopalan, Mohan, Varshney, & Mehrotra, 2005b), shown in Figure 1, sensor nodes within the communication range of each other form a cluster, using algorithms such as those in Chan and Perrig (2004). The sensors within each cluster form a completely connected graph. Each sensor in a cluster communicates with its *cluster head*. The cluster heads form a completely connected graph: they can communicate with each other and with the fusion

Figure 1. Hierarchical MADSN architecture: The arrows indicate the wireless communication links

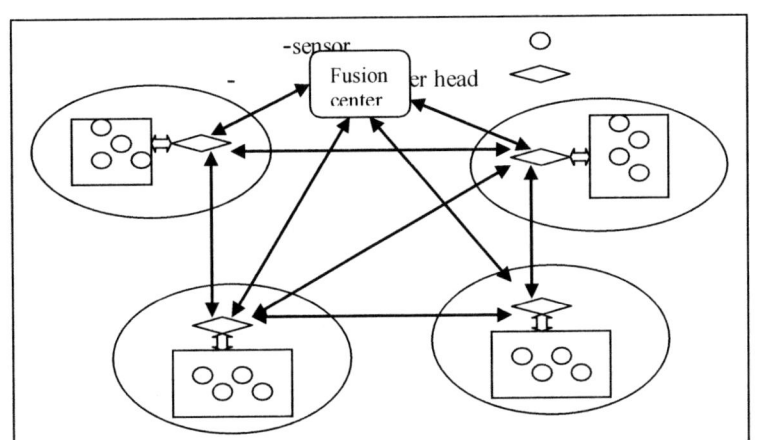

center. Elements of the network are connected through wireless communication links.

We consider the task of routing a mobile agent in a hierarchical MADSN. The mobile agent (dispatched from the fusion center) visits a sequence of cluster heads and a sequence of sensors within the corresponding clusters, collects data and then returns to the fusion center. The goal of mobile agent routing is to find paths for the mobile agent for making accurate decisions in target detection and classification, maximizing the information obtained from multiple sensors. Targets are assumed to be stationary, and the routes are computed only once at the cluster heads and the fusion center.

Each sensor node in the MADSN is associated with two parameters: detected signal energy and energy consumption. These quantities determine the energy consumption and detection accuracy of the path. The path loss is a function of the distance between the sensors and is associated with each edge of the graph representing the MADSN. Hence, the order of sensors on the path traversed by the mobile agent determines the path loss. These quantities have a significant influence on the performance of the MADSN (Wu et al., 2004).

The cluster heads and the fusion center have predetermined knowledge necessary for computing the route, such as the geographical locations (through GPS interfaces) and transmitting/receiving parameters of the sensor nodes. The fusion center computes an intercluster path consisting of a noncyclic sequence of a subset of cluster heads. Each cluster head in the intercluster path also computes a path consisting of a noncyclic sequence of a subset of sensor nodes within its cluster.

Problem Formulation

Our goals are to: (a) minimize energy consumption, (b) minimize path loss, and (c) maximize total detected signal energy. These objectives are briefly discussed in the next section.

Energy Consumption

Sensors are equipped with limited battery power and the total energy consumption of the sensor network is a critical consideration. The energy consumption of a path P is the sum of the energy expended at each sensor node along the path. If $(n_0, n_1, n_2, ..., n_l)$ denotes the sequence of nodes along a path P, then the total energy consumption $E(P)$ is given by:

$$E(P) = \sum_{k=0}^{l} \{((t_{ak} + t_{pk}) \times H_k^2) + (P_{tk} \times t_m)\}$$

where t_{ak} and t_{pk} indicate the data acquisition time and data processing time for node k, H_k denotes the operational power level which is square of the operational frequency and P_{tk} denotes the transmission power of node k (Wu et al., 2004). The partially integrated data at each sensor is stored in a packet of size K bits. The messages transmitted between adjacent sensors along a path P include the mobile agent code of size M bits and the data of size K bits. The message transmission time t_m over a wireless link of P is given by

$t_m = (M+K)/B$

where B is the bandwidth of the link.

Path Loss

Wireless communication links need to be established between neighboring sensor nodes as the mobile agent traverses the path. The received signal level may not be acceptable if it is below a certain threshold due to path loss. The path loss represents the signal attenuation due to free space propagation, and should be minimized to guarantee reliable communication.

The well-known Friss free space propagation model (Friss, 1947), expresses the relation between the power P_{rj} received by sensor j and the power P_{ti} transmitted by sensor i as:

$$P_{rj} = \frac{P_{ti} \times G_{ti} \times G_{rj} \times \lambda^2}{4\pi^2 \times d_{ij}^2 \times \beta}$$

where G_{ti} is the gain of transmitting sensor i, G_{rj} is the gain of the receiving sensor j, λ is the wavelength, d_{ij} is the Euclidean distance between the coordinates of sensors i and j, and β is the system loss factor. The path loss associated with the corresponding wireless link is (in dB):

$PL_{i,j} = 10 \times \log(P_{ti}/P_{rj})$

The total path loss along a path is the sum of the path losses associated with each link along the path. The total path loss for a path P is calculated as

$$PL(P) = \sum PL_{i,j} = \sum_{i=0}^{l-1} PL_{n_i, n_{i+1}}$$

where l is the total number of nodes along the path.

Detection Accuracy

High detection accuracy is also an important goal for accurate inference about the target. Each sensor detects a certain amount of energy $e_k(u)$, emitted by a target. If K_o is the energy emitted by a target at location $u = (x_t, y_t)$, the signal energy $e_k(u)$ measured by a sensor i is

$e_k(u) = K_o/(1 + \alpha\, d_i^p)$,

where d_i is the Euclidean distance between the target location and sensor location, p is the signal decay exponent that takes values between 2 and 3, and α is an adjustable constant. For our simulations, we chose $\alpha = 1$. A path P is a non-cyclic sequence of sensor nodes within a set of selected clusters of the hierarchical MADSN. The fusion center decides the sequence of clusters the mobile agent should visit based on the representative energy of the cluster head. The sum of the detected signal energy along a path P is defined as

$$DE(P) = \sum_{i=1}^{l} E_i$$

where E_i is the representative energy of the ith sensor. The representative energy accounts for faulty sensors and is computed using two different approaches: randomized median filtering (RMF) and randomized censored averaging (RCA). In the RMF approach, the representative energy of a sensor i is computed as the median of the detected signal energies of a randomly chosen set of neighboring sensors of the ith sensor. In the RCA approach, the cluster head chooses m neighboring sensors of sensor i, drops the r highest and r lowest values among the set of m $e_k(u)$'s and averages the remaining $m-2r$ values to compute the representative energy. A detailed description of these approaches is presented in (Rajagopalan et al., 2005b).

Problem Representation and Genetic Operators

We have applied EMOCA, NSGA-II and WGA with identical problem representation and genetic operators for solving the mobile agent routing problem discussed in the previous section.

Representation

Each individual in the population is a sequence of sensor nodes to be visited by the mobile agent, represented as a sequence of cluster-head and labels of sensors within clusters, for example, (*ch1, s7, s6, ch2, s8, s1, s9, ch3, s5, s11*) denotes that *s7* and *s6* are sensors traversed in the cluster with cluster-head *ch1*. For each individual, path computation proceeds as follows:

a. The fusion center computes an intercluster path between the cluster heads. The initial path consists of a random noncyclic sequence of a subset of cluster heads.
b. Each cluster head in the intercluster path computes an intracluster path consisting of a random noncyclic sequence of a subset of sensor nodes within its cluster.

Crossover

Two-point crossover is applied for intracluster and intercluster paths, removing duplicate occurrences of sensors. If a sensor or cluster head occurs multiple times in the child path, only the first occurrence is retained and all further occurrences of that sensor are removed. Figure 2 shows an example of the application of two-point crossover for the intercluster case.

We performed simulations on heterogeneous sensor networks with different number of sensors and various sensor distribution patterns. The data processing time and power level of each sensor are chosen randomly from the specified ranges. The sensors were randomly deployed (uniform distribution) in the network. Targets were placed at random locations in the sensor field.

Simulations were conducted with a population size of 100, a crossover probability of 0.9 and a mutation probability of 0.1. We executed EMOCA, NSGA-II, and WGA for 1000 generations over 30 trials each corresponding to a different random initialization. Execution of the algorithms beyond

Figure 2. Example of intercluster crossover

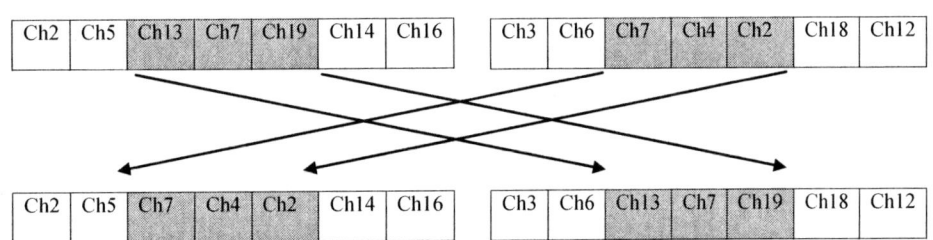

Figure 3. Projections showing the nondominated solutions obtained by EMOCA, NSGA-II, and WGA along two of the three objectives (energy consumption and detected signal energy) for a 200 node MADSN in one trial

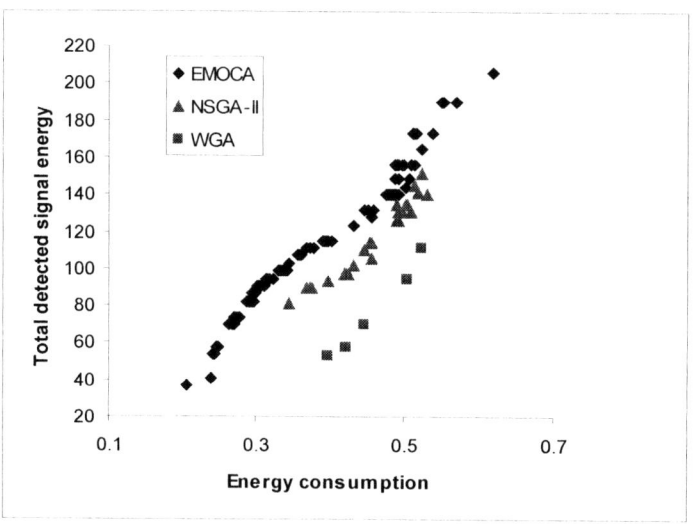

Figure 4. Mutually nondomination solutions obtained by EMOCA for a 200 node MADSN in one trial

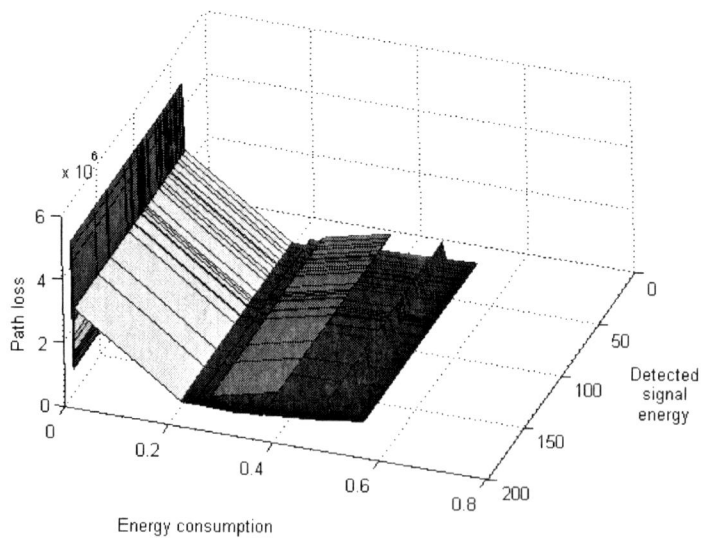

1000 generations resulted in no significant improvement. In our simulations, small variations (in population size, crossover probability, and mutation probability) did not have a significant impact on the performance of the algorithms.

Figure 3 shows the nondominated solutions obtained by EMOCA, NSGA-II, and WGA with the randomized censored averaging approach (Rajagopalan et al., 2005b). From Figure 3, we observe that EMOCA and NSGA-II discover sev-

Table 4. EMOCA (E) vs. WGA (W) using C, Dom and S metrics: The mean and standard deviation (SD) correspond to results averaged over 30 trials

Problem parameters: (no. of targets, clusters, sensors per cluster)	Randomized median filtering								Randomized censored averaging							
	C(W,E) C(E,W) Mean SD		Dom(E,W) Mean SD		S(E) Mean SD		S(W) Mean SD		C(W,E) C(E,W) Mean SD		Dom(E,W) Mean SD		S(E) Mean SD		S(W) Mean SD	
1,5,20	0 0.79	0 0.02	1	0	0.002 0.001	0.17 0.03			0 0.87	0 0.01	1	0	0.005 0.001	0.46 0.01		
2,10,20	0 0.84	0 0.05	1	0	0.02 0.01	0.13 0.06			0 0.93	0 0.07	1	0	0.012 0.002	0.36 0.05		
2,10,30	0 0.89	0 0.03	1	0	0.006 0.003	0.21 0.05			0 0.89	0 0.05	1	0	0.011 0.006	0.34 0.06		
3,10,40	0 0.96	0 0.08	1	0	0.01 0.002	0.26 0.01			0 0.96	0 0.02	1	0	0.008 0.001	0.25 0.04		
3,20,25	0 0.96	0 0.031	1	0	0.02 0.004	0.18 0.03			0 0.96	0 0.02	1	0	0.035 0.008	0.48 0.03		
4,30,20	0 0.97	0 0.05	1	0	0.06 0.003	0.15 0.07			0 0.97	0 0.01	1	0	0.05 0.003	0.53 0.01		
5,20,35	0 0.99	0 0.01	1	0	0.03 0.005	0.36 0.01			0 0.99	0 0.01	1	0	0.03 0.009	0.61 0.05		
5,20,40	0 0.98	0 0.01	1	0	0.02 0.006	0.37 0.05			0 0.98	0 0.01	1	0	0.05 0.007	0.48 0.03		
5,30,30	0 0.95	0 0.03	1	0	0.05 0.01	0.34 0.06			0 0.95	0 0.03	1	0	0.06 0.001	0.37 0.09		

eral nondominated solutions with higher quality compared to WGA. The nondominated solutions obtained by EMOCA and NSGA-II have detected signal energies ranging between 40 and 200 units with energy consumption ranging between 0.2 and 0.6 units. On the other hand, the solutions obtained by WGA have a detected signal energy ranging between 50 and 70 units with energy consumption in the range of 0.4 to 0.5 units. The figure also shows that EMOCA obtains solutions with better quality compared to NSGA-II. Figure 4 shows the collection of mutually nondominating solutions obtained by EMOCA.

Tables 4 and 5 compare EMOCA with WGA and NSGA-II respectively in terms of different metrics. The results show that EMOCA obtains solutions with better quality and diversity compared to WGA and NSGA-II.

Figures 5 and 6 show the mobile agent routes obtained by EMOCA and WGA respectively. For clarity, we show the path obtained in a cluster. Figure 5 shows that the route obtained by EMOCA consists of sensors in the target neighborhood, which maximizes the detection accuracy. The optimization strategy of EMOCA makes the mobile agent capable of visiting nodes in the target neighborhood while finding an energy saving route. Figure 6 shows that the route discovered by WGA consists of many sensors which are far away from the target signifying a low detection

Table 5. EMOCA (E) vs. NSGA-II (N) using C, Dom and S metrics: The mean and standard deviation (SD) correspond to results averaged over 30 trials

Problem parameters: (no. of targets, clusters, sensors per cluster)	Randomized median filtering								Randomized censored averaging							
	C(N,E) C(E,N)		Dom(E,N)		S(E)		S(N)		C(N,E) C(E,N)		Dom(E,N)		S(E)		S(N)	
	Mean	SD	Mean	SD	Mean	SD	Mean	SD	Mean	SD	Mean	SD	Mean	SD	Mean	SD
1,5,20	0.005 0.95	0.001 0.05	0.67	0.04	0.002 0.001	0.07 0.03			0.004 0.81	0 0.04	0.70	0.01	0.005 0.001	0.26 0.08		
2,10,20	0.16 0.84	0.03 0.01	0.85	0.01	0.02 0.01	0.09 0.05			0.10 0.78	0.07 0.03	0.73	0.09	0.012 0.002	0.16 0.03		
2,10,30	0.11 0.86	0.09 0.05	0.93	0.02	0.006 0.003	0.02 0.01			0.05 0.76	0.03 0.04	0.86	0.08	0.011 0.006	0.14 0.06		
3,10,40	0.16 0.87	0.07 0.01	0.75	0.06	0.01 0.002	0.13 0.03			0.18 0.75	0.01 0.06	0.75	0.03	0.008 0.001	0.09 0.05		
3,20,25	0.08 0.83	0.03 0.04	0.72	0.07	0.02 0.004	0.38 0.04			0.13 0.82	0.07 0.03	0.77	0.06	0.035 0.008	0.18 0.07		
4,30,20	0.11 0.77	0.06 0.07	0.77	0.02	0.06 0.003	0.10 0.06			0.21 0.86	0.07 0.05	0.81	0.08	0.05 0.003	0.13 0.09		
5,20,35	0.09 0.83	0.04 0.06	0.84	0.08	0.03 0.005	0.26 0.08			0.19 0.84	0.03 0.01	0.74	0.02	0.03 0.009	0.55 0.06		
5,20,40	0.15 0.86	0.05 0.03	0.79	0.05	0.02 0.006	0.27 0.07			0.06 0.81	0.04 0.05	0.79	0.05	0.05 0.007	0.28 0.02		
5,30,30	0.28 0.74	0.06 0.05	0.68	0.03	0.05 0.01	0.14 0.03			0.23 0.82	0.02 0.01	0.72	0.03	0.06 0.001	0.25 0.04		

Figure 5. Visualization of the mobile agent route computed by EMOCA for a 30 node cluster. CH indicates the cluster head and the arrows indicate the mobile agent route. The circles denote the sensors.

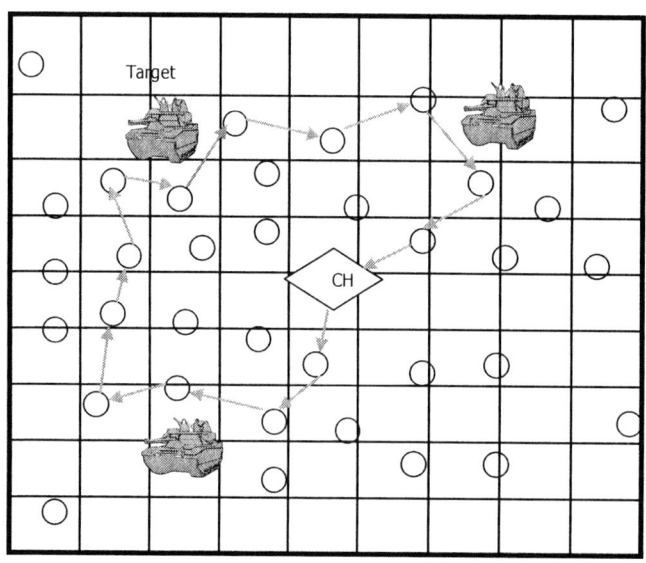

Figure 6. Visualization of the mobile agent route computed by WGA for a 30 node cluster. CH indicates the cluster head and the arrows indicate the mobile agent route. The circles denote the sensors.

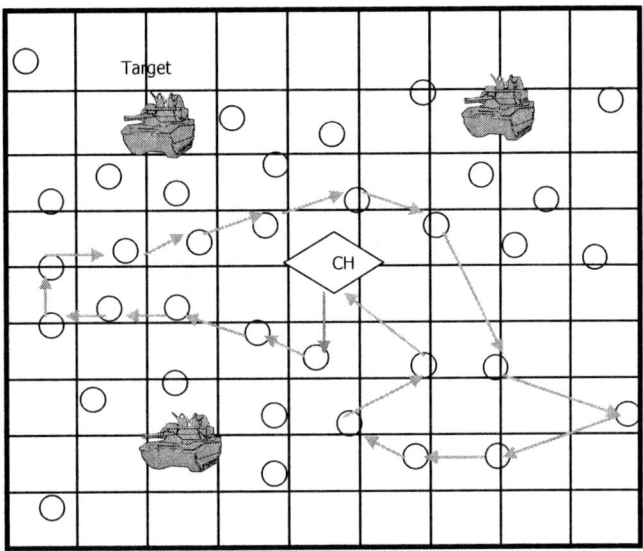

accuracy of the route. In addition, the route consists of more hops when compared to the route obtained by EMOCA. This results in an increase in energy consumption and path loss. This shows that the route obtained by EMOCA has a better quality than WGA.

From our simulation results, we conclude that multi-objective evolutionary algorithms such as EMOCA and NSGA-II were useful in obtaining mobile agent routes characterizing the tradeoffs between different objectives such as detection accuracy, path loss, and energy consumption.

SENSOR PLACEMENT FOR ENERGY EFFICIENT TARGET DETECTION

This section describes the sensor placement problem for energy efficient target detection.

Problem Formulation

Consider a grid of area $a \times b$ where sensor locations correspond to the center of a cell $C(i, j)$ of unit area in the grid whose coordinates are (x_i, y_j). Collaboratively, the sensors need to solve a binary hypothesis testing problem: H_1 - that corresponds to target present or H_0 - that corresponds to target absent. The main problem is to maximize the probability of global target detection; f_1. However, as discussed earlier, the following two objectives are also important.

- Minimize the total energy dissipated in the sensor network; f_2
- Minimize the total number of sensors to be deployed; f_3

Detailed description of objective functions f_1 and f_2 are presented below. The third criterion is obvious. Target detection depends on the fusion methodology used in the network. The two approaches are: data level fusion and decision fusion and the functions f_1 and f_2 depend on these two methodologies.

Probability of Target Detection

Our development of this objective function is based on (Niu, Varshney, & Cheng, 2006). The signal power emitted by the target decays as the distance from the target increases. If K_o is the energy emitted by a target at location $u = (x_t, y_t)$, the signal energy e_i measured by a sensor is given by $e_i(u) = \dfrac{k_0}{1 + \alpha d_i^p}$ where d_i is the Euclidean distance between the target and the sensor location, p is the signal decay exponent that takes values between 2 and 3, and α is an adjustable constant. Our goal is to maximize the average probability of collaborative target detection where the average is over all possible target locations in the grid. We assume that the probability of target T appearing in cell $C(i, j)$ is given by the uniform distribution, that is, $P(T \in C(i, j)) = \dfrac{1}{a \times b}$. Let Л$(S,T,i,j)$ be the probability of detecting the target, located at $C(i, j)$ by the set S of s sensors. Then, the average probability of target detection is:

$$P_{avg}(\text{detecting } T|S) = \sum_{i=0}^{a-1} \sum_{j=0}^{b-1} Л(S,T,i,j) \times P(T \in C(i,j)),$$
$$= \dfrac{1}{a \times b} \times \sum_{i=0}^{a-1} \sum_{j=0}^{b-1} Л(S,T,i,j)$$

The following section describes the calculation of Л(S,T,i,j) and its dependence on the fusion models.

Data Level Fusion Model: Calculation of Л(S,T,i,j)

In data-level fusion, the fusion center gathers the energy measurements from other sensors, fuses the energy measurements and compares the sum to a threshold λ to detect the presence of a target. The energy measurement at the fusion center, from a sensor i, consists of two components: $e_i(u)$ if target is present (0 if no target in the region) and $N_i = n_i^2$ where n_i denotes the noise. We assume that for all sensors, n_i is Gaussian with mean 0 and variance 1. The global probability of target detection Л(S,T,i,j) and false alarm P_f are given by,

$$Л(S,T,i,j) = \text{Prob}\left[\sum_{i=1}^{s}(e_i(u) + N_i) \geq \lambda\right] = \text{Prob}\left[\sum_{i=1}^{s} N_i \geq (\lambda - \sum_{i=1}^{s} e_i u))\right], \text{ and } P_f = \text{Prob}\left[\sum_{i=1}^{s} N_i \geq \lambda\right]$$

Decision Fusion Model: Calculation of Л(S,T,i,j)

In decision fusion, each sensor compares its energy measurement to a threshold to arrive at a local decision about the presence of a target. The ith sensor transmits the local binary decision I_i to the fusion center; $i=1,2,\ldots,s$. Since the local sensors transmit only binary data, the fusion center does not have the knowledge of detection probabilities at local sensors. In the absence of this information, the fusion center treats the decisions from the sensors equally and evaluates $\Lambda = \sum_{i=1}^{s} I_i$ and compares it against a threshold γ. If the target is absent, Λ follows a binomial distribution and the probability of false alarm at the fusion center is given by

$$P_f = \sum_{i=\gamma}^{s} \binom{s}{i} p_f^i (1-p_f)^{n-i}$$

where p_f is the probability of false alarm at a local sensor which is identical across all local sensors if we use identical local thresholds. If a target is present, the detection probabilities at the local sensors are not identical since p_{di} at sensor i is a function of the distance d_i. The probability of detection at sensor i, that is, Prob$(I_i=1)$ is given by $p_{di} = \text{Prob}[N_i + e_i(u) \geq \eta]$. If the number of sensors is sufficiently large, we can employ the asymptotic approximation derived by Niu et al. (2006) to calculate P_d. The local decisions I_i follow a Bernoulli distribution with p_{di} as the probability of success. Since the local decisions are mutually independent, when s is large, we can use the central limit theorem (Papoulis, 1984) to obtain P_d. The distribution function of Λ approaches a Gaussian distribution with mean μ and variance σ^2, where

$$\mu = E[\Lambda] = \sum_{i=1}^{s} E[I_i] = \sum_{i=1}^{s} p_{di}$$

$$\sigma^2 = \text{var}[\Lambda] = \sum_{i=1}^{s} \text{var}[I_i] = \sum_{i=1}^{s} p_{di}(1 - p_{di})$$

The detection probability at the fusion center is given by

$$Л(S,T,i,j) \cong Q((\eta-\mu)/\sigma),$$

where $Q(.)$ is the complementary distribution function of the standard Gaussian.

Energy Cost Analysis

The second objective is to minimize the total energy dissipated in the network. We use the first order radio model discussed in (Heinzelman, Chandrakasan, & Balakrishnan, 2002). In this model, a radio dissipates E_{elec} = 50 nJ/bit for the transmitter or receiver circuitry and $\in_{amp}$ = 100 pJ/bit/m² for the transmitter amplifier. The equations used to calculate transmission energy and receiving energy at a sensor i for a k-bit message are:

- Transmission: $E_t(k, d_i) = E_{elec} \times k + \in_{amp} \times k \times d_i^2$
- Reception: $E_r(k) = E_{elec} \times k$

where d_i is the distance between the ith sensor location and the fusion center. We employ different strategies to calculate the total energy dissipation for the data-level fusion and decision fusion models. These methodologies are described below

Data Level Fusion Model: Calculation of Total Energy

For the data-level fusion model, we employ "power efficient gathering in sensor information systems" (PEGASIS) methodology that is near optimal for data gathering applications in sensor networks (Lindsey et al., 2002). The main idea of PEGASIS is to form a chain among sensor nodes so that each node will receive data from and transmit data to one of its neighbors. Gathered data is transmitted from node to node, fused at each node and eventually a designated node transmits the fused data to the base station or the fusion center. Let E_{ci} denote the energy consumed by a sensor node i in the chain.

$$E_{ci} = E_t(k, d_{ij}) + E_r(k)$$

where d_{ij} is the distance between sensor i and sensor j. The total energy consumption of the sensor network is given by

$$E = \sum_{i=1}^{n} E_{ci}$$

where n is the total number of sensors in the network.

Decision Fusion Model: Calculation of Total Energy

In decision fusion, the presence or absence of a target is just encoded in one bit and transmitted to the fusion center. Let $E_c(k,d_i)$ denote the energy consumed by the sensor node i for communication with the fusion center.

$$E_c(k,d_i) = E_t(k,d_i) + E_r(k)$$

The total energy consumption of the sensor network is given by $E = \sum_{i=1}^{n} E_c(k,d_i)$.

Problem Representation and Genetic Operators

Each individual specifies the arrangement of a group of sensors as a vector of genes. Each gene represents the (x, y) coordinates of the sensor locations in the grid. Since the number of sensors to be deployed is one of the objectives, we allow the algorithms to evolve variable length individuals. The base station is placed at a fixed location far away from the sensors. We have employed a two-point crossover operator where the crossover points are chosen independently in the parents. The mutation step consists of a random perturbation of the co-ordinates of each sensor in a chromosome with a probability of *1/number of sensors*.

Simulations were conducted with a population size of 100, a crossover probability of 0.9 and a mutation probability of 0.1. Small variations in these parameters did not result in significant difference in the performance of the algorithms. For the sensor placement problem, we fix the maximum number of sensors N_{max}=100 for both data-level fusion and decision fusion methods. For decision fusion, we impose an additional constraint on the minimum number of sensors, N_{min}=10. This is a reasonable assumption, since we might need at least 10 sensors to achieve significant coverage in a surveillance region with large number of sensor locations. We executed EMOCA, NSGA II, and WGA for 1000 generations over 30 trials each corresponding to a different random initialization. Execution beyond 1000 generations resulted in no significant improvements. We randomly chose 100 weight vectors in the interval [0, 1] for the WGA. Random choice of weight vectors is appropriate in the absence of any specific relationship between the spacing of Pareto optimal solutions and the spacing of weight vectors.

Simulation Results

We performed simulations on a 10 × 10 grid for different values of global false alarm probability viz., P_f = 0.1, 0.01, and 0.001, for both data-level fusion and decision fusion models. The results presented in Table 6 and Table 7 show that the nondominated solutions obtained by EMOCA have better quality and diversity compared to those obtained by NSGA-II and WGA.

Table 6 shows that a large fraction of solutions obtained by WGA are dominated by EMOCA. For instance, a particular nondominated solution obtained by EMOCA has a detection probability of 0.99 and an energy consumption of 0.29 Joules with 41 sensors. On the other hand, a solution obtained by WGA has a detection probability of 0.43, and an energy consumption of 0.68 Joules with 54 sensors. Our results showed that for the solutions obtained by EMOCA, the average detection probability increases with the number of sensors and reaches 1.0 (100%) with as few as 40 sensors whereas WGA requires almost 75 sensors. Figure 7 shows the Pareto-optimal surface obtained by EMOCA on the data-level fusion model.

POSTPROCESSING OF SOLUTIONS OBTAINED BY A MOO ALGORITHM

In some applications, the decision maker might have a rough idea of the relative priorities associ-

Table 6. EMOCA (E) vs. WGA using C, Dom and S metrics: The mean and standard deviation (SD) correspond to results averaged over 30 trials

Fusion model	C(N,E)		C(E,N)		Dom(E,N)		S(N)		S(E)	
	Mean	SD	Mean	SD	Mean	SD	Mean	SD	Mean	SD
Data level fusion	0.15	0.05	0.77	0.08	0.60	0.03	0.09	0.01	0.05	0.02
Decision fusion	0	0	0.744	0.04	1	0	0.13	0.07	0.09	0.05

Table 7. EMOCA (E) vs. NSGA-II (N) using C, Dom and S metrics: The mean and standard deviation (SD) correspond to results averaged over 30 trials

Fusion model	C(WGA,E)		C(E,WGA)		Dom(E,WGA)		S(WGA)		S(E)	
	Mean	SD	Mean	SD	Mean	SD	Mean	SD	Mean	SD
Data level fusion	0.08	0.01	0.84	0.03	0.75	0.06	0.29	0.04	0.05	0.02
Decision fusion	0	0	0.81	0.05	1	0	0.43	0.05	0.09	0.05

Figure 7. Pareto optimal surface obtained by EMOCA for the data-level fusion model

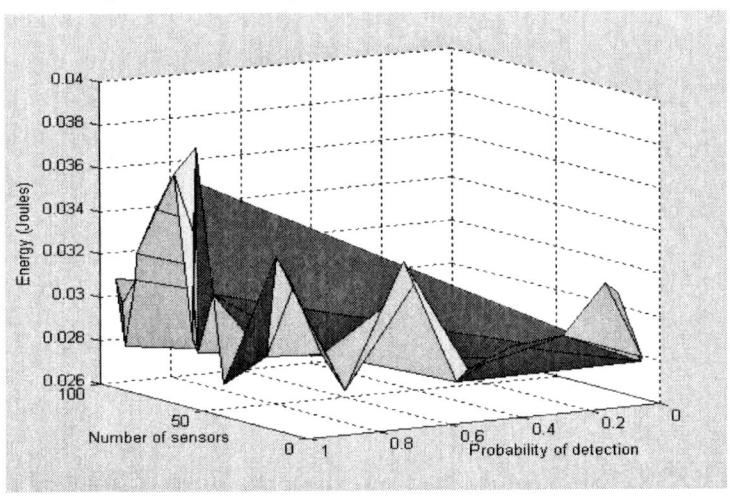

ated with different objectives. In such scenarios, it would be necessary to guide the decision maker towards a single or a small set of solutions from the numerous nondominated solutions obtained by MOO algorithms.

Voronoi diagrams have been used for solving numerous difficult problems in computational geometry. A survey of Voronoi diagrams is presented in (Aurenhammer, 1991). We propose a new approach using the Voronoi diagram for the post processing of solutions obtained by MOEAs. In this method, we employ a weighted objective approach for the selection of a solution among several nondominated solutions obtained by the algorithm. For each nondominated solution, the objective function f_i is multiplied by a weight w_i. For a three objective problem, the weight vector $\{w_1, w_2, w_3\}$ is chosen such that $0 \leq w_1, w_2, w_3 \leq 1$, $w_1+w_2+w_3 =1$. The weighted objective function values are then added together to evaluate the fitness of the nondominated solutions. The solution with the best fitness is identified. The procedure is repeated for different weight vectors. We chose several uniformly spaced weight vectors in the interval [0, 1]. We then employ a Voronoi tessellation approach for the identified solutions in the weight vector space. Several researchers have investigated the computational complexity of Voronoi diagrams as a function of the number of points (n) and dimensionality of the space (d).

Figure 8. Voronoi cells associated with the nondominated solutions for the sensor placement problem

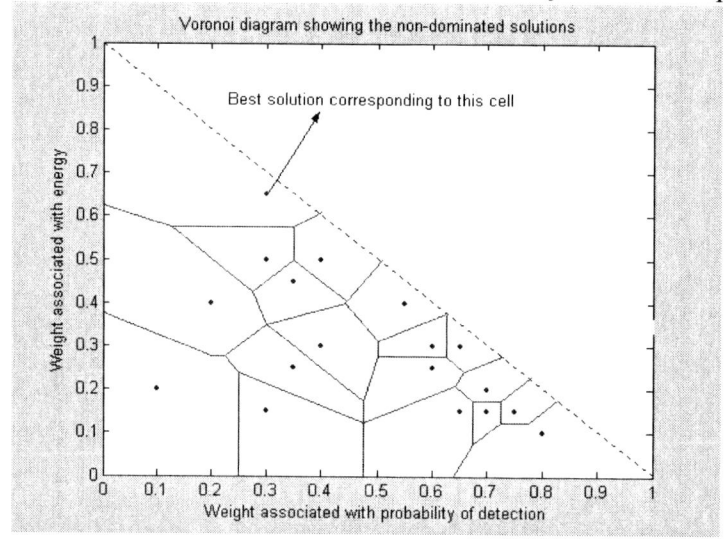

In a two dimensional space, the computational complexity for constructing the Voronoi diagram is $O(n)$. However, for $d \geq 3$, the construction of Voronoi diagrams becomes complex. For MOO problems with a large number of objectives, the algorithm proposed in (Boissonnat et al., 1995) can be used for the post processing of Pareto-optimal solutions. This is a randomized incremental algorithm that adds points sequentially to construct the Voronoi diagram in d dimensional space with time complexity,

$$O\left(n^{\left\lceil \frac{d}{2} \right\rceil} + n \log n\right)$$

Figure 8 shows the Voronoi tessellation of the nondominated solutions obtained by EMOCA for the sensor placement problem. If the decision maker can express a relative preferences among various objectives in terms of the weight vector, then a corresponding solution can be chosen from the associated Voronoi cell. The main advantages of the Voronoi approach are:

1. A precise weight vector is not necessary for the decision maker to choose a particular solution among the several nondominated solutions obtained. Approximate knowledge of weights would be sufficient to select a solution.
2. If additional higher level information about the relative priorities of different objectives becomes available, it is not necessary to rerun the algorithm. The decision maker can simply choose an alternative solution best suited for the new weights.

The Voronoi approach clearly shows the advantages of using MOEAs as opposed to single objective optimization algorithms. For instance, a single objective optimization approach whose main goal is to optimize probability of detection would obtain only one solution. Such a solution can also be obtained by assigning a weight vector of $\{1,0\}$ and choosing a solution from Figure 8 corresponding to the weight vector. However, MOEAs obtain multiple solutions which correspond to several choices of the weight vector. In general, a user may have no basis for deciding what choice of preference weights is most appropriate for the problem at hand; with the Voronoi approach, greater clarity is available to evaluate the tradeoff regions where each Pareto-optimal solution is most preferable to the user.

FUTURE RESEARCH DIRECTIONS

Many sensor network design problems (such as target detection, localization and tracking) are multi-objective in nature and the framework developed in this chapter can be used to solve such problems. For instance, the sensor selection problem for efficient target localization involves two conflicting objectives: maximization of estimation accuracy and minimization of energy consumption by selecting the minimal number of sensors to report data. Hence, this problem can be modeled as a multi-objective optimization problem and solved using multi-objective evolutionary algorithms to characterize the tradeoffs between estimation accuracy and energy consumption.

Post processing of the solutions obtained by MOEAs remains an open research problem and very little work has been pursued along this direction. In problems where the Pareto-front consists of a very large number of solutions, the development of post processing approach will enable the system designer to choose a small subset of solutions which closely matches the user preferences.

Another interesting issue is the integration of user preferences into MOEAs. The main theme is to bias the search based on user preferences. This technique helps in obtaining a preferred set of solutions in the Pareto-optimal front. Some recent research in this direction has been described in (Deb et al., 2000) and significant scope exists for future work.

For the mobile agent routing problem, future work could incorporate the stochastic nature of the wireless channels and the obstacles in the environment in order to model the communication cost along a route. This would involve development of new objective functions to capture such stochastic effects. Another interesting aspect would be to consider the mobility of the sensors for solving the mobile agent routing problem. This would present new challenges in terms of updating the routes based on the locations of the sensors.

In this chapter, we solved unconstrained MOO problems. However, sensor networks problems have constraints on energy consumption, data accuracy, and data latency. Hence, it would be useful to model the sensor network design problems as constrained multi-objective optimization problems. For instance, in the sensor placement problem, we could minimize the deployment cost while maximizing the detection probability, subject to constraints on the energy consumption and connectivity of the network. This would require developing mathematical models for the constraints and designing new constrained MOEAs for solving the problem.

CONCLUSION

In this chapter, we have described the multi-objective nature of different sensor network design problems. The two main issues involved in solving MOO problems in sensor networks are: (1) Development of appropriate mathematical models for the objectives involved (2) Design of efficient MOEAs for solving the optimization problem. We illustrated this approach via two sensor network design problems: mobile agent routing and sensor placement. We presented and used suitable mathematical models for the objective functions such as detection probability, energy consumption and communication cost. We used two recently proposed MOEAs: EMOCA and NSGA-II and compared their performance with a weighted genetic algorithm. We proposed a new approach employing Voronoi diagrams for post processing of solutions obtained by an MOEA. This approach is very useful for selecting a solution even in the absence of precise knowledge of the relative priorities between different objectives.

REFERENCES

Akyldiz, I., Su, W., Sankarasubramanian Y., & Cayirci E. (2002). A survey on sensor networks. *IEEE Communications Magazine, 40*(8), 102-14.

Berkovits, S., Guttman, J. D., & Swarup, V. (1998) Authentication for mobile agents mobile agents and security. In G. Vigna (ed.), (pp. 114- 136), Springer-Verlag.

Boulis, A., Ganeriwal, S., & Srivastava, M. B. (2003). Aggregation in sensor networks: An energy-accuracy tradeoff. *Ad Hoc Networks, 1,* 317-331.

Cardei, M. & Du, D.Z. (2005). Improving wireless sensor network lifetime through power aware organization. *ACM Wireless Networks, 11* (3), 333-40.

Cardei, M. & Wu, J. (2006). Energy efficient coverage problems in wireless ad hoc sensor networks. *Computer Communications, 29*(4), 413-420.

Cardei, M., MacCallum, D., Cheng, X., Min, M., Jia, X., Li, D., & Du, D. Z. (2002). Wireless sensor networks with energy efficient organization. *Journal of Interconnection Networks, 3*(3-4), 213-229.

Chan, H. & Perrig, A. (2004). ACE: An emergent algorithm for highly uniform cluster formation. In *Proceedings of 2004 European Workshop on Sensor Networks* (pp.154-171).

Clouqueur, T., Phipatanasuphorn, V., Ramanathan, P., & Saluja, K.K. (2003). Sensor deployment strategy for detection of targets traversing a region. *Mobile Networks and Applications, 8*(4), 453-61.

Cristescu, R., Beferull-Lozano, B., & Vetterli, M. (2004). On network correlated data gathering. *IEEE INFOCOM, 4*(4), 2571-82.

Das, I. & Dennis, J. E. (1998). Normal-boundary intersection: A new method for generating the Pareto surface in nonlinear multicriteria optimization problems. *SIAM J. Optimization, 8,* 631-657.

Deb, K. (2001). *Multi-objective optimization using evolutionary algorithms.* England: Wiley and Sons.

Deb, K., Pratap, A., Agarwal, S., & Meyarivan, T. (2000). A fast and elitist multi-objective genetic algorithm: NSGA-II. In *Proceedings Parallel Problem Solving from Nature VI.* (pp. 849-858).

Ding, M., Cheng, X., & Xue, G. (2003). Aggregation tree construction in sensor networks. *IEEE 58th Vehicular Technology Conference, 4*(4), 2168-2172.

Ferentinos, K. P. & Tsiligiridis, T. A. (2007). Adaptive design optimization of wireless sensor networks using genetic algorithms. *Computer Networks: The International Journal of Computer and Telecommunications Networking, 51*(4), 1031-51.

Friss, H. T. (1946). A note on a simple transmission formula. In *Proceedings of the Institute of Radio Engineers, Vol. 34* (pp. 254-56).

Heinzelman, W., Chandrakasan, A., & Balakrishnan, H. (2000). Energy-efficient communication protocol for wireless micro sensor networks. In *Proceedings of Hawaii Conference on System Sciences.*

Heinzelman, W. R., Chandrakasan, A. P., & Balakrishnan, H. (2002). An application-specific protocol architecture for wireless microsensor networks. *IEEE Trans Wireless Communications, 1*(4), 660-670.

Jourdan, D. B. & de Weck, O. L. (2004). Layout optimization for a wireless sensor network using a multi-objective genetic algorithm. In *Proceedings of the IEEE 59th Vehicular Technology Conference, Vol. 5* (pp. 2466-70).

Kar, K. & Banerjee, S. (2003). Node placement for connected coverage in sensor networks. In *Proceedings WiOpt: Modeling and Optimization in Mobile, Ad Hoc and Wireless Networks.*

Knowles, J. D. & Corne, D. W. (1999). The Pareto archived evolution strategy: A new baseline algorithm for multi-objective optimization. *In Proceedings of the 1999 congress on Evolutionary Computation* (pp. 98-105).

Kulik, J., Heinzelman, W. R., & Balakrishnan, H. (2002). Negotiation-based protocols for disseminating information in wireless sensor networks. *Wireless Networks, 8*, 169-185.

Lange, D. B. & Oshima, M. (1999). Seven good reasons for mobile agents. *Comm. ACM, 42*(3), 88-89.

Lindsey, S., Raghavendra, C., & Sivalingam, K. M. (2002). Data gathering algorithms in sensor networks using energy metrics. *IEEE Transactions on Parallel and Distributed Systems, 13*(9), 924-35.

Miettinen, K. (1999). *Nonlinear multi-objective optimization.* Boston: Kluwer.

Niu, R., Varshney, P., & Cheng, Q. (2006). Distributed detection in a large wireless sensor network. *International Journal on Information Fusion, 7*(4), 380-394.

Papoulis, A. (1984). *Probability, random variables, and stochastic processes.* McGraw-Hill.

Pattem, S., Poduri, S., & Krishnamachari, B. (2003). Energy-quality tradeoffs for target tracking in wireless sensor networks. In *Proceedings Information Processing in Sensor Networks* (pp. 32-46).

Qi, H., Iyengar, S. S., & Chakrabarty, K. (2001). Multi-resolution data integration using mobile agents in distributed sensor networks. *IEEE Transactions on Systems, Man and Cybernetics Part C: Applications and Rev., 31*(3), 383-391.

Raich, A. M. & Liszkai, T. R. (2003). Multi-objective genetic algorithms for sensor layout optimization in structural damage detection. In *Proceedings of the Artificial Neural Networks in Engineering Conference* (pp. 889-894).

Rajagopalan, R., Mohan, C. K., Mehrotra, K. G., & Varshney, P. K. (2005a). An evolutionary multi-objective crowding algorithm: Benchmark test function results. In *Proceedings 2nd Indian International Conference on Artificial Intelligence* (pp.1488-1506), Pune, India.

Rajagopalan, R., Mohan, C. K., Varshney, P. K., & Mehrotra, K. G. (2005b). Multi-objective mobile agent routing in wireless sensor networks. In *Proceedings IEEE Congress on Evolutionary Computation* (Vol. 2, pp.1730-1737).

Rajagopalan, R., Mohan, C. K., Varshney, P. K., & Mehrotra, K. G. (2005c). Sensor placement for energy efficient target detection in wireless sensor networks: A multi-objective optimization approach. In *Proceedings of the 39th Annual Conference on Information Sciences and Systems,* Baltimore, Maryland.

Rajagopalan, R., Mohan, C. K., Mehrotra, K. G., & Varshney, P. K. (2006). EMOCA: An evolutionary multi-objective crowding algorithm. *Journal of Intelligent Systems.*

Rajagopalan, R. & Varshney, P. K. (2006). Data aggregation techniques in sensor networks: A survey. *IEEE Communications Surveys and Tutorials, 8*(4), 48-63.

Rakowska, J., Haftka, R. T., & Watson, L. T. (1991). Tracing the efficient curve for multi-objective control-structure optimization. *Computing Systems in Engineering, 2*(6), 461-471.

Sahni, S. & Xu, X. (2005). Algorithms for wireless sensor networks. *International Journal on Distributed Sensor Networks, 1*, 35-56.

Sander, T. & Tschudin, C. (1998) Protecting mobile agents against malicious hosts mobile agent and security. In G. Vigna (Ed.), (pp. 44-60), Springer-Verlag.

Schott, J. R. (1995). *Fault tolerant design using single and multi-criteria genetic algorithm optimization.* Unpublished master's thesis, Department of Aeronautics and Astronautics, Massachusetts Institute of Technology.

Shen C., Srisathapornphat C., & Jaikaeo C., (2001). Sensor information networking architecture and applications. *IEEE Personal Communications,* 52–59.

Slijepcevic, S. & Potkonjak, M. (2001). Power efficient organization of wireless sensor networks. In *Proceedings of the IEEE International Conference on Communications* (pp. 472-476).

Tilak, S., Abu-Ghazaleh, N., & Heinzelman, W. (2002). Infrastructure tradeoffs for sensor networks. In *Proceedings ACM 1st International Workshop on Sensor Networks and Applications* (pp. 49-58).

Tubaishat, M. & Madria, S. (2003). Sensor networks: An overview. *IEEE Potentials,* 22(2), 20- 23.

Wang, X., Xing, G., Zhang, Y., Lu, C., Pless, R., & Gill, C. D. (2003). Integrated coverage and connectivity configuration in wireless sensor networks. In *Proceedings of the First ACM Conference on Embedded Networked Sensor Systems* (pp. 28-39).

Wu, Q., Rao, N. S. V., Barhen, J., Iyengar, S. S., Vaishnavi, V. K., Qi, H., & Chakrabarty, K. (2004). On computing mobile agent routes for data fusion in distributed sensor networks. *IEEE Transactions on Knowledge and Data Engineering,* 16(6), 740-753.

Yu, Y., Krishnamachari, B., & Prasanna, V.K. (2004). Energy-latency tradeoffs for data gathering in wireless sensor networks. In *Proceedings IEEE INFOCOM* (pp. 244-55).

Zhang, H. & Hou, J. C. (2003). Maintaining sensing coverage and connectivity in large sensor networks (Tech. Rep. UIUC, UIUCDCS-R-2003-2351).

Zitzler, E., (1999). *Evolutionary algorithms for multi-objective optimization: Methods and applications.* Unpublished doctoral dissertation, Zurich, Switzerland: Swiss Federal Institute of Technology.

Zitzler, E., Laumanns, M., & Thiele, L. (2001). *SPEA2: Improving the strength Pareto evolutionary algorithm* (Tech. Rep. No. 103) Swiss Federal Institute of Technology.

ADDITIONAL READING

Multi-Objective Evolutionary Algorithms

Coello Coello, C. A. (2000). An updated survey of GA-based multi-objective optimization techniques. *ACM computing Surveys,* 32(2), 109-143.

Coello Coello, C. A., Van Veldhuizen, D. A., & Lamont, G. B. (2002). *Evolutionary algorithms for solving multi-objective optimization problems.* New York: Kluwer Academic Publishers.

Deb, K. (1999). Multi-objective genetic algorithms: Problem difficulties and construction of test functions. *Evolutionary Computation,* 7, 205-230.

Dhillon, S. S. Chakrabarty, K. & Iyengar, S. S. (2002). Sensor placement for grid coverage under imprecise detections. In *Proceedings Fifth International Conference on Information Fusion* (pp. 1581-87).

Fonseca, C. M. & Fleming, P. J. (1993). Genetic algorithms for multi-objective optimization: Formulation, discussion and generalization. In *Proceedings of the fifth international conference on Genetic Algorithms* (pp. 416-423).

Hajela, P. & Lin, C. Y. (1992). Genetic strategies in multicriterion optimal design. *Structural Optimization, 4*, 99-207.

Horn, J., Nafpliotis, N., & Goldberg, D. E. (1994). A niched pareto genetic algorithm for multi-objective optimization. In *Proceedings of the first IEEE conference on Evolutionary Computation* (Vol.1, pp. 82-87).

Knowles, J. D. & Corne, D. W. (2000). Approximating the nondominated front using the Pareto Archived Evolution Strategy. *Evol. Computation, 8*(2), 149-172.

Rajagopalan, R., Mohan, C. K., Mehrotra, K. G., & Varshney, P. K. (2004). Evolutionary multi-objective crowding algorithm for path computations. In *Proceedings of the Fifth International Conference on Knowledge Based Computer Systems* (pp. 46-65).

Schaffer, J. D. (1985). Multi-objective optimization with vector evaluated genetic algorithms. In *Proceedings of an International Conference on Genetic Algorithms and their Applications* (pp. 93-100).

Veldhuizen, D.V. (1999). Multi-objective evolutionary algorithms: Classifications, analyses and new innovations, PhD thesis, Air Force Institute of Technology, Ohio, Technical Report AFIT/DS/ENG/99-01.

Zitzler, E., Thiele, L., Laumanns, M., Fonseca, C. M., & da Fonseca, V. G. (2003). Performance assessment of multi-objective optimizers: An Analysis and Review. *IEEE Trans. Evolutionary Computation, 7*(2), 117-132.

Sensor Networks

Carle, J. & Simplot, D. (2004). Energy efficient area monitoring by sensor networks, *IEEE Computer, 37*(2), 40–46.

Chakrabarty, K., Iyengar, S. S., Qi, H., & Cho, E. (2002). Grid coverage for surveillance and target location in distributed sensor networks. *IEEE Transactions on Computers, 51*, 1448-1453.

Chakrabarty, K., Iyengar, S. S., Qi, H., & Cho, E. (2001). Coding theory framework for target location in distributed sensor networks. In *Proceedings of the International Symposium on Information Technology: Coding and Computing* (pp. 130-134).

Chen, B., Jamieson, K., Balakrishnan, H., & Morris, R. (2001). Span: An energy efficient coordination algorithm for topology maintenance in ad hoc wireless networks. *ACM/IEEE International Conference on Mobile Computing and Networkin* (pp. 85–96).

Colouqueur, T., Phipatanasuphorn, V., Ramanathan, P., & Saluja, K.K. (2003). Sensor deployment strategy for detection of targets traversing a region. *Mobile Networks and Applns., 8*(4), 453-61.

Clouqueur, T., Ramanathan, P., Saluja, K. K., & Wang, K. C. (2001). Value fusion versus decision fusion for fault tolerance in collaborative target detection in sensor networks. In *Proceedings of the Fusion 2001 Conference* (pp. 25-30).

Heo, N. & Varshney, P. K. (2005). Energy-efficient deployment of intelligent mobile sensor networks. *IEEE Trans. on Systems, Man and Cybernetics, 35*(1), 78-92.

Howard, A., Mataric, M. J., & Sukhatme, G. S. (2002). Mobile sensor network deployment using potential fields: A distributed, scalable solution to the area coverage problem. In *Proceedings of the Sixth International Symposium on Distributed Autonomous Robotic System* (pp. 299–308).

Iyengar, S. S., Jayasimha, D. N., & Nadig, D. (1994). A versatile architecture for the distributed sensor integration problem. *IEEE Trans. Computers, 43*(2), 175-185.

Kalpakis, K., Dasgupta, K., & Namjoshi, P. (2003). Efficient algorithms for maximum lifetime data gathering and aggregation in wireless sensor networks. *Computer Networks, 42*(6), 697-716.

Meguerdichian, S., Koushanfar, F., Potkonjak, M., & Srivastava, M. (2001). Coverage problems in wireless ad-hoc sensor networks. In *Proceedings of the IEEE Infocom* (pp. 1380–1387).

Papavassiliou, S., Puliafito, A., Tomarchio, O., & Ye, J. (2002). Mobile agent-based approach for efficient network management and resource allocation: Framework and applications. *IEEE Journal on Selected Areas in Communications, 20*(4), 858-872.

Perrig, A., Szewczyk, R., Tygar, J. D., Wen, V., & Culler, D. E. (2002). SPINS: Security protocols for sensor networks. *Wireless Networks, 8*(5), 521-34.

Raghunathan, V., Schurgers, C., Park, S., & Srivastava, M. B. (2002). Energy aware wireless microsensor networks. *IEEE Signal Processing Magazine, 19*, 40–50.

Stojmenović, I. (2005). *Handbook of sensor networks: Algorithms and architectures.* Wiley-Interscience.

Umezawa, T., Satoh, I., & Anzai, Y. (2002). A mobile agent-based framework for configurable sensor networks. In *Proceedings of the Fourth International Workshop Mobile Agent for Telecommunication Applications* (pp. 128-140).

Younis, O. & Fahmy, S. (2004). HEED: A hybrid, energy-efficient, distributed clustering approach for ad hoc sensor networks. *IEEE Transactions on Mobile Computing, 3*(4), 366-79.

Zhao, F. & Guibas, L. (2004). *Wireless sensor networks: An information processing approach.* Morgan Kaufmann

Zou, Y. & Chakrabarty, K. (2004). Sensor deployment and target localization in distributed sensor networks. *ACM Transactions on Embedded Computing Systems, 3*(1), 61-91.

Chapter IX
Evolutionary Multi-Objective Optimization for DNA Sequence Design

Soo-Yong Shin
Seoul National University, Korea

In-Hee Lee
Seoul National University, Korea

Byoung-Tak Zhang
Seoul National University, Korea

ABSTRACT

Finding reliable and efficient DNA sequences is one of the most important tasks for successful DNA-related experiments such as DNA computing, DNA nano-assembly, DNA microarrays and polymerase chain reaction. Sequence design involves a number of heterogeneous and conflicting design criteria. Also, it is proven as a class of NP problems. These suggest that multi-objective evolutionary algorithms (MOEAs) are actually good candidates for DNA sequence optimization. In addition, the characteristics of MOEAs including simple addition/deletion of objectives and easy incorporation of various existing tools and human knowledge into the final decision process could increase the reliability of final DNA sequence set. In this chapter, we review multi-objective evolutionary approaches to DNA sequence design. In particular, we analyze the performance of ε-multi-objective evolutionary algorithms on three DNA sequence design problems and validate the results by showing superior performance to previous techniques.

INTRODUCTION

The genomic revolution including the Human Genome Project has been producing a huge amount of data in rapid succession, which are too large or complex to solve with traditional methods. Therefore, a variety of techniques have been applied to understand these data. Among them, evolutionary computation has been highlighted as one of the most successful techniques due to its rapid search ability in a very large and complex problem space and reasonable solution quality (Fogel & Corne, 2002).

Recently, researchers have found lots of biological problems naturally having more than one conflicting objective or constraint to satisfy. This multi-objective nature of biological problems and the success of evolutionary computation have encouraged the usage of multi-objective evolutionary algorithms for bioinformatics such as cancer classification (Deb & Reddy, 2003), protein structure prediction (Cutello, Narzisi, & Nicosia, 2006; Ray, Zydallis, & Lamont, 2002), DNA sequence/probe design (Lee, Wu, Shiue, & Liang, 2006; Rachlin, Ding, Cantor, & Kasif, 2005a; Shin, Lee, Kim, & Zhang, 2005a; Shin, Lee, & Zhang, 2006), gene regulatory networks inference (Spieth, Streichert, Speer, & Zell, 2005), peptide binding motifs discovery (Rajapakse, Schmidt, & Brusic, 2006), protein-ligand docking problems (Oduguwa, Tiwari, Fiorentino, & Roy, 2006), and medicine (Lahanas, 2004; Lahanas, Baltas, & Zamboglou, 2003).

Among the various biological problems, we review the multi-objective evolutionary optimization approaches to DNA sequence design in this chapter. The DNA sequence design problem is the most basic and important task for biological applications which require DNA sequences. Therefore, it involves many applications, including DNA microarray design, DNA computing, and DNA nanotechnology. Previous works have found that sequence design involves a number of heterogeneous and conflicting design criteria with many local optima and little gradient information (Shin, 2005). This supports that multi-objective evolutionary algorithms are actually a good approach for DNA sequence optimization.

Here we report on the evaluation results of MOEAs on the three representative DNA sequence design problems: orthogonal DNA sequence design for DNA computing, probe design for DNA microarrays, and primer design for multiplex polymerase chain reaction. We first formulate each problem as a multi-objective optimization task. Then, ε-multi-objective evolutionary algorithm is applied to the chosen problems. Finally, the performance of the evolutionary multi-objective approach is analyzed.

BACKGROUND

In this section, we will briefly introduce the background information for DNA sequence design. First, the abstract criteria for good DNA sequence and their mathematical definitions will be shown. Then, the three chosen target problems such as DNA computing sequence design, microarray probe design, and multiplex PCR primer design will be explained shortly. These applications belong to the most popular DNA sequence optimization problems and cover a wide variety of similar problems.

Criteria of Good DNA Sequence

In biology experiments which handle DNA sequences, the hybridization between a DNA sequence and its base-pairing complementary (also known as Watson-Crick complementary) sequence is the most important factor to retrieve and process the information stored in DNA sequences, since the rest of experimental steps are based on the perfect hybridization. For this reason, we desire a set of DNA sequences should form a stable duplex (double stranded DNA) with their complements. Also, we require crosshybridization (hybridization among noncomplementary sequences) or secondary structures (self-hybridization of single sequence) should be prohibitive or relatively unstable, compared to any perfectly matched duplex formed by a DNA sequence and its complement (see Figure 1).

The basic sequence design criteria could be summarized as in Figure 2 (Shin et al., 2005a; Shin et al., 2006; Lee, Shin, & Zhang, 2007). In general, a set of good DNA sequences should form stable duplex with their complements only, should not have undesirable secondary structures, and should have the similar chemical characteristics.

In the following, we will explain the DNA sequence design criteria in more detail and give mathematical formulations of them. Before going into detail, we will introduce the basic notations first. We denote each DNA sequence as a string from an alphabet $\Lambda_{nb} = \{A, C, G, T\}$, where "A", "C", "G", and "T" denote each nucleotide. Also, an alphabet set consists of each nucleotide with blank (gap) can be defined as $\Lambda = \{A, C, G, T, -\}$, where "–" denotes a blank. Then the set of all DNA sequences including the empty sequence is denoted as Λ_{nb}^*. A set of n sequences with the same length l from Λ_{nb}^l is denoted by Σ, where ith member of Σ is denoted as Σ_i. Let $a, b \in \Lambda$ and x, y $\in \Sigma$. $x_i (1 \leq i \leq l)$ means ith nucleotide from 5'-end (leftmost letter) of sequence x. $\bar{a}$ is the complementary base of a. $|x|$ represents the length of sequence x. A complementary of a sequence $x = x_1...x_l$ is $\bar{x}_l \cdots \bar{x}_1$ and denoted as $\bar{x}$.

The first criterion in Figure 2 forces the set Σ of sequences to form the duplexes with their complements only. For this purpose, two kinds of crosshybridization must be minimized: hybridization between the sequences in the set and hybridization of a sequence in the set with complements of other sequences. Both should be checked, because a sequence usually accompa-

Figure 1. The examples of DNA sequence hybridization. "A" is Adenine, "T" is thymine, "G" is guanine, and "C" is cytosine, which are four basic bases for DNA sequence. 5' or 3' means the direction of DNA sequence. For hybridization, two DNA sequences should be aligned in opposite directions each other. (a) The stable duplex (perfect hybridization) between a target sequence and its complementary sequence. "A-T" and "G-C" form Watson-Crick base-pairing. (b) The crosshybridization between noncomplementary sequences. This duplex is very unstable compared to the duplex in (a). (c) The secondary structure example of DNA sequence, called hairpin loop.

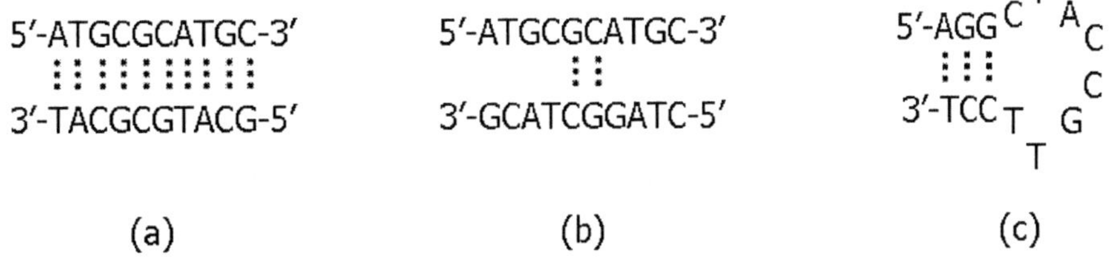

```
5'-ATGCGCATGC-3'          5'-ATGCGCATGC-3'           5'-AGG C T A C
   ::::::::::                 ::         ::               :::      C
3'-TACGCGTACG-5'          3'-GCATCGGATC-5'           3'-TCC T   G
                                                             T

      (a)                        (b)                        (c)
```

Figure 2. Three abstracted basic DNA sequence design criteria

1) Preventing crosshybridization
2) Controlling secondary structures
3) Controlling the chemical characteristics of DNA sequences.

nies its complement in experimental steps and the crosshybridization to either sequence causes erroneous results. The former can be formulated as $f_{H-measure}(\Sigma)$ and the latter as $f_{Similarity}(\Sigma)$.

$$f_{H-measure}(\Sigma) = \sum_i \sum_j H-measure(\Sigma_i, \Sigma_j) \quad (1)$$

where,

$$H-measure(x, y) = \max_{g,i} h(x, shift(y(-)^g y, i))$$

for $0 \leq g \leq l-3$ and $|i| \leq g + l - 1$,

$$h(x, y) = \sum_{i=1}^{l} bp(x_i, y_{l+1-i})$$

$$bp(a, b) = \begin{cases} 1 & a = \bar{b} \\ 0 & \text{otherwise} \end{cases},$$

$$shift(x, i) = \begin{cases} (-)^i x_1 \cdots x_{l-i} & i \geq 0 \\ x_{i+1} \cdots x_l (-)^i & i < 0 \end{cases}.$$

Larger $H-measure(x, y)$ value means more hybridization between x and y can be possible.

$$f_{Similarity}(\Sigma) = \sum_i \sum_{i \neq j} H-measure(\Sigma_i, \bar{\Sigma}_j)$$
$$= \sum_i \sum_{i \neq j} Similarity(\Sigma_i, \Sigma_j), \quad (2)$$

where,

$$Similarity(x, y) = \max_{g,i} s(x, shift(y(-)^g y, i)),$$

for $0 \leq g \leq l-3$ and $|i| \leq g + l - 1$, where,

$$s(x, y) = \sum_{i=1}^{l} eq(x_i, y_i)$$

and

$$eq(a, b) = \begin{cases} 1 & a = b \\ 0 & \text{otherwise} \end{cases}.$$

The last equivalence in equation (2) is from $Similarity(x, y) = H-measure(x, \bar{y})$ due to the direction of DNA sequences and Watson-Crick complementary base pairing ($s(x, y) = h(x, \bar{y})$). Larger $Similarity(x, y)$ value means more resemblance of sequences x and y, or more crosshybridization of a sequence with complement of the other.

The formulations of crosshybridization are only approximations based on string matching. For DNA sequences shorter than 50, more accurate approximation method based on nearest neighbor model is established (SantaLucia, Jr. & Hicks, 2004). This model explains the stability of hybridization between two sequences as free energy change when basepairs are stacked one after another. For example, the stability of hybridization in Figure 1 (a) is explained by successive stacking of stabilizing basepairs: T-A over A-T, G-C over T-A, and so on. Depending on the stacking pairs the overall hybridization can be stabilized or destabilized. The first three stacking pairs in Figure 1 (b) are the examples of destabilizing stacking pairs. The crosshybridization among sequences in the set can be alternatively defined using nearest neighbor model as,

$$f_{FreeEnergy}(\Sigma) = -\sum_i \sum_j FEnergy(\Sigma_i, \Sigma_j), \quad (3)$$

where,

$$FEnergy(x, y) = \min_{i_0 \cdots i_l, j_0 \cdots j_l} deltaG((-)^{i_0} x_1 (-)^{i_1}$$
$$\cdots (-)^{i_{l-1}} x_l (-)^{i_l}, (-)^{j_0} y_1 (-)^{j_1} \cdots (-)^{j_{l-1}} y_l (-)^{j_l}),$$

for $0 \leq i_0 \ldots i_l, j_0 \ldots j_l$, and

$$deltaG(x, y) = \sum_{i=1}^{l-1} fe(x_i, x_{i+1}, y_{l-i+1}, y_{l-i}),$$

where $fe(a_1, a_2, b_2, b_1)$ denotes the approximate free energy when the pair $a_2 - b_1$ is stacked over $a_1 - b_2$ using nearest neighbor model.

Smaller $FEnergy(x, y)$ value means more stable hybridization between x and y. Therefore, $f_{FreeEnergy}(\Sigma)$ is minimized for noninteracting sequence set Σ.

The second criterion checks the undesired secondary structures. The secondary structure can be checked by two factors: self-hybridization and continuous occurrence of the same base. A DNA sequence can self-hybridize by binding onto itself as in Figure 1 (c). The long repeat of the same nucleotide can also disturb the linear structure of DNA sequence. These two factors are formulated as $f_{Hairpin}(\Sigma)$ and $f_{Continuity}(\Sigma)$.

$$f_{Hairpin}(\Sigma) = \sum_i Hairpin(\Sigma_i). \qquad (4)$$

The function *Hairpin(x)* can be defined either by calculating stacking free energy as,

$$Hairpin(x) = - \sum_{p=P_{min}}^{(l-R_{min})/2} \sum_{r=R_{min}}^{l-2p} \sum_{i=0}^{l-2p-r} \sum_{j=1}^{p-1} fe(x_{p+i-j}, x_{p+i-j+1}, x_{p+i+r+j}, x_{p+i+r+j-1}), \qquad (5)$$

or by calculating matching basepairs as,

$$Hairpin(x) = \sum_{p=P_{min}}^{(l-R_{min})/2} \sum_{r=R_{min}}^{l-2p} \sum_{i=1}^{l-2p-r} T\left(\sum_{j=1}^{p} bp(x_{p+i+1-j}, x_{p+i+r+j}), p/2\right), \qquad (6)$$

where P_{min} and R_{min} denote the minimum length of the basepairs and loop in the hairpin and

$$T(i,j) = \begin{cases} i & i > j \\ 0 & \text{otherwise} \end{cases}.$$

Larger *Hairpin(x)* value means higher likelihood to self-hybridize.

$$f_{Continuity}(\Sigma) = \sum_i Continuity(\Sigma_i), \qquad (7)$$

where,

$$Continuity(x) = \sum_{i=0}^{l-C^U} \sum_{a \in \Lambda_{nb}} T\left(\arg\max_{j=C^U}^{l-i}\left[j \times I(x_{i+1} \cdots x_{i+j} = a^j)\right], C^U\right)^2$$

and $I(\bullet)$ is an indicator function. *Continuity(x)* checks if there is longer repeat of the same base than C^U. Large value means the more and longer repeats which can cause the secondary structures.

The last one tries to keep DNA sequences have the similar chemical characteristics for successful and easy experiments. Among the various chemical characteristics of DNA sequences, the melting temperature (Tm, the critical temperature when a sequence and its complement start to hybridize or dehybridize) and GC-ratio (the ratio of guanine and cytosine) are important. Since it is difficult for a set of sequences has the same values of Tm and GC-ratio, biologists usually try to keep their values within a predefined range [TM^L, TM^U] and [GC^L, GC^U]. $Value^L$ and $Value^U$ denote the lower limit and the upper limit of *Value*, respectively. The corresponding formulations are:

$$f_{Tm}(\Sigma) = \sum_i \left|Tm(\Sigma_i) - TM^L\right| I(Tm(\Sigma_i) < TM^L) + \sum_i \left|TM^U - Tm(\Sigma_i)\right| I(Tm(\Sigma_i) > TM^U), \qquad (8)$$

where

$$Tm(x) = \frac{deltaH(x)}{deltaS(x) + R\ln\left(\frac{C_T}{4}\right)},$$

$$deltaH(x) = \sum_{i=1}^{l-1} enthalpy(x_i, x_{i+1}, \bar{x}_{l-i+1}, \bar{x}_{l-i})$$

and

$$deltaS(x) = \sum_{i=1}^{l-1} entropy(x_i, x_{i+1}, \bar{x}_{l-i+1}, \bar{x}_{l-i}).$$

The functions $enthalpy(x_i, x_{i+1}, \bar{x}_{l-i+1}, \bar{x}_{l-i})$ and $entropy(x_i, x_{i+1}, \bar{x}_{l-i+1}, \bar{x}_{l-i})$ correspond to the change of enthalpy and entropy when the basepair $x_{i+1} - \bar{x}_{l-i}$ is stacked over $x_i - \bar{x}_{l-i+1}$ and are approximated by nearest neighbor model.

$$f_{GC}(\Sigma) = \sum_i |GC(\Sigma_i) - GC^L| I(GC(\Sigma_i) < GC^L)$$
$$+ \sum_i |GC^U - GC(\Sigma_i)| I(GC(\Sigma_i) > GC^U), \quad (9)$$

where

$$GC(x) = \frac{\sum_i I(x_i = G) + I(x_i = C)}{l}.$$

However, we have to point out that the above criteria should be chosen carefully and other criteria or constraints could be necessary depending on the purpose of the experiments. For example, though a general DNA computing sequence design has no additional constraint or objective than the criteria, the probe selection has one more constraint that a probe should be a unique subsequence of the target gene. And the multiplex PCR primer selection needs another objective that the number of the different groups of targets should be minimized. The more detailed explanation for each problem will be explained in the following sections.

DNA Computing Sequence Design

DNA computing is an emerging branch of computational models in which biological materials are used as means of computation. Biomolecules such as DNA are used to store information while various enzymes and chemicals are used to manipulate information in molecules. The ability of DNA computers to perform calculation through specific biochemical reactions among different DNA strands by Watson-Crick complementary base-pairing, affords a number of useful properties such as massive parallelism, a huge memory capacity, and biofriendly operations (Garzon & Deaton, 1999; Maley, 1998). It has been applied to various fields: combinatorial optimization, satisfiability problem, logic circuit design, finite state machines, associative memory building, machine learning models, medical diagnosis and building nanostructures (Amos, Paun, Rozenberg, & Salomaa, 2002; Reif, 2002; Shin, 2005).

In DNA computing experiments, information of the problem is encoded in DNA sequences and the operations on information are also implemented by the chemical reactions involving DNA sequences. Therefore, DNA sequences that encode the information should be carefully designed for the successful experiments because the improper encoding may cause the illegal reactions between DNA sequences and lead to the wrong results. Moreover, the DNA computing sequence design was proven to be equivalent as finding maximal independent set of vertices in a graph, which belongs to NP complete problem (Garzon & Deaton, 2004).

The previous works for the DNA computing sequence design can be categorized into information theoretical approach, heuristic approach, dynamic programming, evolutionary methods, and *in vitro* approach. The information theoretical method is based on coding theory with Watson-Crick complementarity as a new feature (Mauri & Ferretti, 2004). The enumerative search method (Hartemink, Gifford, & Khodor, 1999) and the random search method (Penchovsky & Ackermann, 2003) belong to simple local search methods. Another heuristics such as template-map strategy (Arita & Kobayashi, 2002) and directed graph method (Feldkamp, Saghafi, Banzhaf, & Rauhe, 2001) have been also suggested. Marathe, Condon, and Corn (1999) have applied dynamic programming for DNA computing sequence design. As evolutionary methods, simulated annealing (Tanaka, Nakatsugawa, Yamamoto, Shiba, & Ohuchi, 2002) and conventional genetic algorithm (Deaton, Garzon, Murphy, Rose, Franceschetti, & Stevens, 1998; Zhang & Shin, 1998), not multi-objective evolutionary algorithm, were used. Recently, biology-inspired methods have been offered to design DNA sequences: PCR-based protocol for in vitro selection of DNA sequences (Deaton, Chen, Bi, Garzon, Rubin, & Wood, 2002).

Microarray Probe Design

DNA microarrays have been widely used for many research and commercial areas to monitor the expression levels of a large number of genes simultaneously. Usually, short specific complementary subsequences of target genes, called probes, are immobilized on microarray plate and the expression level of gene is estimated from the amount of mRNAs hybridized to its probe. If the chosen probe is specific to its target within allowable mismatches throughout the whole genome, it will combine with its target gene only and the amount of hybridization on the probe will correctly reflect the expression level of the gene. Otherwise, the probe may hybridize to the undesirable targets, which produces a misleading signal. Thus, the specificity of the probes affects the reliability of the microarrays experiments.

In literature, a variety of probe design methods have been suggested reflecting its importance. These microarray probe design tools could be categorized in different ways. From the algorithmic point of view, the previous approaches could be classified into two classes: filter-out approach and machine learning approach. Filter-out methods search for the suitable probe for each gene by scanning throughout the gene and selecting the subsequences satisfying certain criteria only. These methods with various design criteria are widely used since they are simple and fast (Drmanac, Stravropoulos, Labat, Vonau, Hauser, Soares, & Drmanac, 1996; Gordon & Sensen, 2004; Li & Stormo, 2001; Rouillard, Zuker, & Gulari, 2003; Wang & Seed, 2003). Machine learning approaches such as naïve Bayes, decision trees, neural networks, and evolutionary algorithms have also been used (Bourneman, Chrobak, Vedova, Figueroa, & Jiang, 2001; Lee, Kim, & Zhang, 2004b; Tobler, Molla, Nuwaysir, Green, & Shavlik, 2002).

The way of evaluating specificity of probes can be another direction to categorize the previous approaches. There are two probe specificity evaluation approaches: thermodynamic approach and sequence similarity search approach. In thermodynamic approach, the likelihood of the hybridization between two sequences is measured by the amount of the free energy change (SantaLucia, Jr. & Hicks, 2004). If the free energy after hybridization is much smaller than before, the hybridization is highly stable and very much likely to occur. In this approach, the probes are picked to minimize free energy when hybridized to the correct target only and to maximize the free energy when hybridized to other mismatched target sequences (Rouillard et al., 2003; Li & Stormo, 2001). Otherwise, the sequence similarity search methods measure the chance of hybridization between two sequences simply by comparing sequence strings (Flikka, Yadetie, Laegreid, & Jonassen, 2004; Wang & Seed, 2003).

Multiplex PCR Primer Design

A polymerase chain reaction (PCR) is one of the most important and widely used experimental techniques to amplify the amount of a certain DNA molecule at a time. Recently, the multiplex PCR has been proposed to amplify multiple target DNAs simultaneously using a different primer pair for each target DNA. Due to this advantage, multiplex PCR has a wide variety of applications in biology, and is recently spotlighted as a core tool for high throughput single nucleotide polymorphism genotyping (Aquilante, Langaee, Anderson, Zineh, & Fletcher, 2006; Rachlin et al., 2005a).

Though both probe and primer designs try to find the subsequences, they have a big difference. Probe selection is to find one probe per one gene, and does not consider the interactions between probes since they are fixed on the microarray. However, multiplex PCR primer selection tries to find a different primer pair for each target gene and should consider the interactions between primers. If the hybridization between primer pair is more stable than between primer and its target, the target cannot be amplified successfully. Moreover, one should consider the existence of other target genes and their primer pairs in multiplex PCR primer design, because multiple targets are amplified together in one experiment. Therefore, the crosshybridization between primers and nontargets as well as between primers should be avoided.

The previous works can be classified into two types. One is to find a single optimized group by discarding the targets which can not fit to be amplified together (Lee et al., 2006; Rouchka, Khalyfa, & Cooper, 2005; Schoske, Vallone, Ruiberg, & Butler, 2003; Yamada, Soma, & Morishita, 2006). The other is to handle the partitioning of targets into multiple groups (Kaplinski, Andreson, Puurand, & Remm, 2005; Nicodeme & Steyaert, 1997; Rachlin et al., 2005a). From the methodological point of view, most of the previous works have used a deterministic search and only a few evolutionary approaches have been reported (Lee et al., 2006). And, some researchers adopted a multi-objective way to solve this problem (Lee et al., 2007; Rachlin et al., 2005a; Rachlin, Ding, Cantor, & Kasif, 2005b).

ε-MULTI-OBJECTIVE EVOLUTIONARY ALGORITHM

ε-multi-objective evolutionary algorithm (ε-MOEA) is used for all DNA sequence design problems in this chapter, since it has shown better convergence and divergence for the benchmark problems and DNA sequence design problem (Lee, Shin, & Zhang, 2004c; Shin, Lee, & Zhang, 2005b). It is a steady-state genetic algorithm using elite archive and ε-dominance relation (Deb, Mohan, & Mishra, 2003; Deb, Mohan, & Mishra, 2005; Laumanns, Thiele, Deb, & Zitzler, 2002). For general multi-objective evolutionary algorithm (MOEA) concept, readers are referred to Chapter I. In this chapter, we only describe the distinct characteristics of ε-MOEA compared to the general MOEAs.

The most important characteristic of ε-MOEA is the ε-dominance relation. X ε-dominates Y if the difference between X and Y is greater than or equal to a certain amount ε in all objectives and X is strictly better than Y by ε in at least one objective. The mathematical definition in maximization case is

X ε –dominates Y iff
$\forall i \in \{1,..., M\}, f_i(X) \geq f_i(Y) + \varepsilon$
$\exists i \in (1,..., M), f_i(X) > f_i(Y) + \varepsilon$

The ε-dominance is introduced to maintain a representative subset of nondominated individuals by dividing whole search space into many grids whose size is defined by ε. The ε-nondominated set is smaller than the usual nondominated set, for the nondominated solutions which can be ε-dominated by others are removed in ε-nondominated set. Therefore, ε-Pareto set is a subset of the Pareto-optimal set which ε-dominates all Pareto-optimal solutions. And the minimum distance between nearest solutions can be guaranteed. The density of the approximate set can be adjusted by controlling the value of ε (Laumanns et al., 2002). By utilizing the ε-dominance for selecting representative subset of nondominated set and maintaining them in the archive throughout generations, ε-MOEA achieved good convergence and diversity performance (Deb et al., 2003; Laumanns et al., 2002).

The flow of ε-MOEA is shown in Figure 3. At each generation, parents for new offspring are chosen from the population and the archive respectively. One parent from the population is chosen by tournament selection, and the other parent from the archive is selected randomly. Then, an offspring is produced from these parents and evaluated. If any individual in the population is dominated by the offspring, the latter replaces the former. If the offspring ε-dominates one or more members of the archive, it replaces the ε-dominated members. Or, the offspring is added to the archive if no archive member ε-dominates it. Otherwise, the offspring is discarded. Therefore,

Figure 3. The basic flow of ε-MOEA (Adapted from Deb et al., 2003)

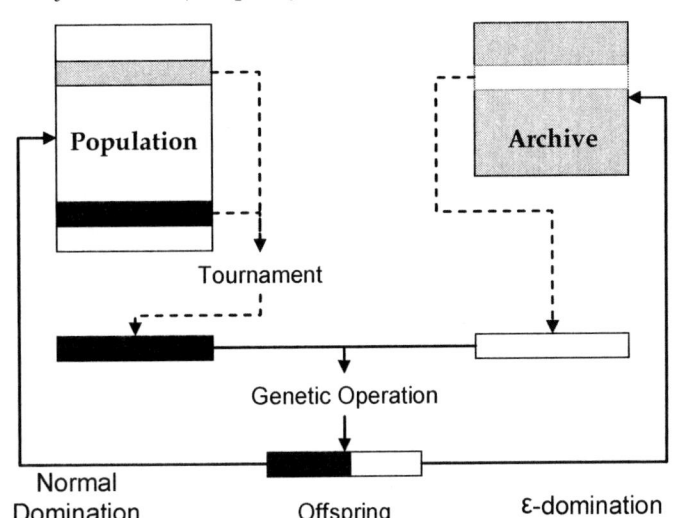

the ε-nondominated individuals are always accepted as a member of the archive. This process is repeated until termination. By this way, the archive grows as the generation passes and is filled with ε-approximated Pareto-optimal solution.

The real implementation of the algorithm for the three problems handled here is modified to reflect the characteristics of the problem. The constraint handling technique is added in the problem of orthogonal DNA sequence design for DNA computing and probe design for microarray. Further, local search and niching method are used in multiplex PCR primer design. However, the main flow of the algorithm is not changed over the applications. The detailed implementation will be explained in the corresponding sections.

DNA SEQUENCE DESIGN FOR DNA COMPUTING

In this section, we will introduce the DNA sequence design problem which needs a set of DNA sequences of the same length. Each sequence in the set corresponds to a different variable or value of the original problem to be solved by DNA computing. From the assumption that every sequence in the set are put in the same reactor and can move freely, there is a chance of every pair of sequences in the set to collide and hybridize. Therefore, we have to consider all of the three criteria in Figure 2.

Based on the analysis of the application, six objective functions such as Similarity, H-measure, Hairpin, Continuity, GC content, and Melting temperature are used as the embodiment of criteria (Shin, 2005). Table 1 summarizes the chosen objective functions.

MULTI-OBJECTIVE FORMULATION OF DNA COMPUTING SEQUENCE DESIGN

For DNA computing sequence design, we define an individual X as a set of DNA sequences of length l from Λ_{nb}^{l}. The ith member of X will be denoted as X_i. As for specific formulation of objectives, equations (1) and (2) are chosen for the crosshybridization prevention criterion, since

Table 1. The objectives to design orthogonal DNA sequences for DNA computing

Objective	Description	Criterion
H-measure	The unexpected hybridization between pair of sequences should be minimized.	Crosshybridization prevention
Similarity	The similarity between sequences should be minimized.	Crosshybridization prevention
Hairpin	The unexpected secondary structure formation should be prohibited.	Secondary structure control
Continuity	The successive occurrence of the same base in a sequence should be minimized.	Secondary structure control
Melting temperature	The melting temperatures should be close to target value.	Chemical feature control
GC content	The G, C portion should be close to target value.	Chemical feature control

the length of the sequences for DNA computing can be very long. From the same reason, equation (7) and equation (4) with equation (6) are chosen for the secondary structure control criterion. The functions which belong to the chemical feature control criterion use equations (8) and (9).

The relationship between objective functions is shown in Figure 4 by analyzing the objective space of each function. The objective space of H-measure and Similarity shows the traditional conflict relationship with local optima. GC content and Similarity also depicts the trade-off relationship. Even though other objectives do not conflict with each other, they are all discontinuous functions with little gradient information to the global optimum (Shin, 2005; Shin et al., 2005a).

From their definitions as well as characteristics, some objectives such as melting temperature and GC content could be naturally regarded as constraints, not objective functions (Shin, 2005). Therefore, the formulation of DNA sequence optimization is a constrained multi-objective optimization task.

Minimize $F(X) = (f_{Continuity}(X), f_{Hairpin}(X), f_{H\_measure}(X), f_{Similarity}(X))$ subject to $g_{TM}(X) = g_{GCcontent}(X) = 0$.

Here, $g_{TM}(X)$ and $g_{GCcontent}(X)$ use the same formula as equations (8) and (9), respectively.

Equations (8) and (9) return zero, when X is feasible (melting temperature and GC content do not exceed the predefined ranges).

Multi-Objective Evolutionary Sequence Optimization

To tackle this task, ε-multi-objective evolutionary algorithm (ε-MOEA) is modified to work within the scope of DNA sequence optimization. Here, constrain-dominance condition is used to handle the constraint functions (Deb, 2001). As summarized in Figure 5, there are three cases in the constrain-dominance relation between two individuals. The constrain-dominance favors the feasible over the infeasible, the individuals with smaller constraint violation among the infeasible, and dominant ones among the feasible. Therefore, the evolution is directed toward dominating individuals in the feasible area.

The detailed procedure of the modified ε-MOEA with constraint handling techniques for DNA computing sequence design is explained in Figure 6. As can be seen in Figure 6, the constraint violation is checked first whenever the archive or population member is to be updated. The ε-dominance or dominance check is performed only when both are feasible. In this way, population and archive are driven towards the feasible and nondominated region. And due to

Figure 4. The scatter plot matrix of similarity, H-measure, continuity, and GC ratio (Shin, 2005). The data are obtained from the complete space of DNA sequence with length 5 ($4^5 = 1024$ sequences).

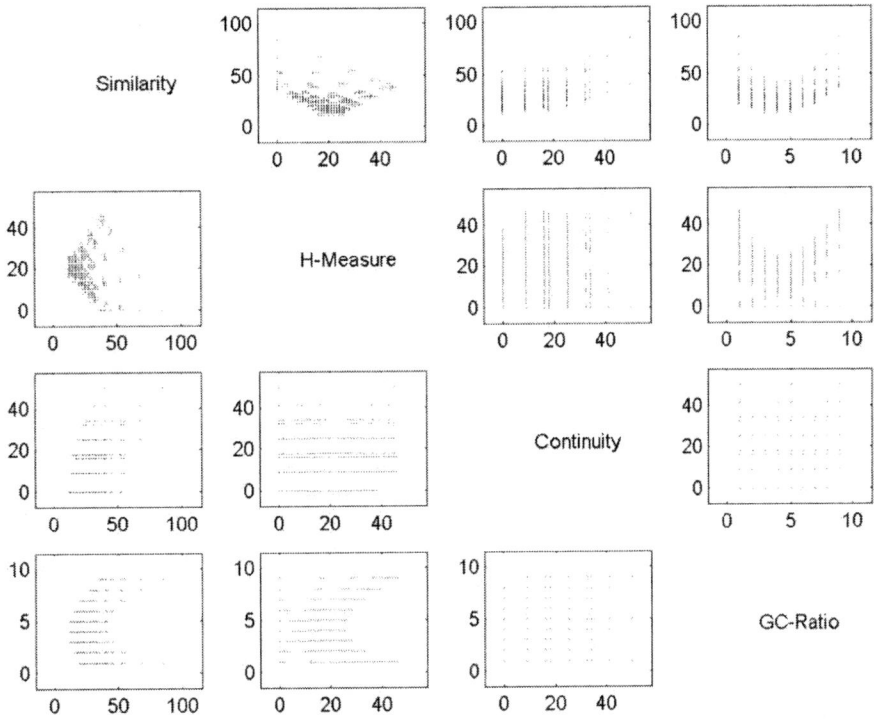

Figure 5. The constrain-dominance condition

Case 1. One individual is feasible and the other is not: the feasible one wins.
Case 2. Both individuals are infeasible: one with the smaller constraint violation wins.
Case 3. Both individuals are feasible: dominant or ε-dominant one wins

the ε-dominance relation, the archive can keep the representative and proper subset of nondominated set found so far.

DNA Computing Sequence Optimization Results

We compared multi-objective evolutionary approach with other approaches such as simple genetic algorithm (Lee, Shin, Park, & Zhang, 2004a) and simulated annealing (Tanaka et al., 2002).

For the parameter setting of ε-MOEA, ε is set to 1, population size is 3,000, maximum generation is 200, crossover rate is 0.9, and mutation rate is 0.01. It is also assumed that the hairpin formation requires at least six base-pairings and a six base loop. The melting temperature is calculated by the nearest neighbor method with 1 M salt concentration and 10 nM DNA concentrations. All these values are decided empirically with biochemical background. The more detailed parameter settings are described in (Shin et al., 2005b).

Figure 6. The pseudocode of ε-MOEA for DNA sequence optimization (Adapted from Shin, 2005)

1	Randomly generate initial population (DNA sequence sets).
2	Sort by domination, and set first front as archive.
3	Generate one new individual by choosing parents from population and archive.
3.1	Choose two individuals from population.
3.2	Choose constrain-dominant individual. If both are feasible and nondominant, choose random one.
3.3	Choose one individual at random from archive.
3.4	Perform crossover and mutation.
4	Update archive.
4.1	Replace individual(s) of larger constraint violation in the archive than the new individual, if the new individual has smaller constraint violation than some archive individual(s).
4.2	Replace ε-dominated individual(s) in the archive with the new individual, if every archive individual and the new individual satisfy the constraint and the new individual ε-dominates any archive individual(s).
4.3	Leave dominating individual, if there are more than one archive members in the same grid.
4.4	Add the new individual, if either the individuals of archive or the new individual do not dominate each other.
5	Update population.
5.1	Replace dominated individual(s) with the new individual.
5.2	Replace randomly selected population member with the new individual, if there is no population member which dominates the new individual.
6	Check termination.

Table 2. Comparison results between simulated annealing and multi-objective approach. Each value represents the corresponding objective function value of the compared individual

Objectives	ε-MOEA	Simulated Annealing (Tanaka et al., 2002)
Similarity	829	905
H-measure	925	994
Hairpin	6	45
Continuity	0	0

And since the previous approaches used single objective methods, they could generate only one best final sequence set. Hence, for comparison, one individual having the least crosshybridization is selected from the archive of one random run of ε-MOEA. The hybridization simulator, NACST/Sim (Shin et al., 2005a) is used to select the appropriate individual.

The performance of MOEA is first compared to that of simulated annealing which is a widely used heuristic. As in the previous simulated annealing approach (Tanaka et al., 2002), 14 DNA sequences were designed using ε-MOEA. As shown in Table 2, the multi-objective evolutionary approach outperforms for all objectives. This implies the sequences optimized by ε-MOEA have much lower probability to hybridize with the nontarget sequences (smaller H-measure value), and to form unexpected secondary structures (smaller Hairpin value). In addition, by considering melting temperature as one of constraints, melting temperature uniformity is better than Tanaka's sequence set.

Next, the sequence set designed to solve 7-traveling salesman problem (7-TSP) by DNA computing (Lee et al., 2004a) was compared to that by ε-MOEA. The target TSP is a seven-node incomplete graph with 24 edges and 5 different weights. At the first trial, the sequence set for 7-TSP was designed using simple genetic algorithm with weighted sum of the objectives as fitness value. And the sequences were successfully

Table 3. Comparison results for 7-TSP between ε-MOEA and GA

Objectives	ε-MOEA	GA (Lee et al., 2004a)
Similarity	174	190
H-measure	206	227
Hairpin	3	9
Continuity	0	34

Table 4. The summary of comparison results of DNA sequence design for 7-TSP between NSGA-II and ε-MOEA

	NSGA-II	ε-MOEA
Convergence	1.63 ± 0.24	0.13 ± 0.11
Diversity	165.72 ± 33.82	202.23 ± 17.41

confirmed by the laboratory experiment (Lee et al., 2004a). Similar to the previous results, ε-MOEA finds more reliable DNA sequence set for all objectives as shown in Table 3. Since the reliability of the objectives has been confirmed by the laboratory experiment, multi-objective evolutionary approach can be regarded that it can find better solution.

To confirm the effectiveness of ε-MOEA in DNA sequence design, it was compared to other MOEA. Among various MOEAs, NSGA-II (Deb, Pratap, Agarwal, & Meyarivan, 2001), which is one of the most widely used and efficient multi-objective evolutionary algorithms without ε-dominance, was chosen for comparison. Here, the convergence and diversity of total nondominated sets obtained from each of the algorithms was compared on 7-TSP, a practical problem of sequence design for DNA computing. Generational distance (Veldhuizen, 1999) and maximum spread (Zitzler, 1998) were used as measures for convergence and diversity, respectively. Unfortunately, the Pareto-optimal front which is required to compute generational distance is not known in DNA sequence design similar to other real-world problems. Thus, 10 nondominated sets from 10 independent runs of ε-MOEA and NSGA-II (5 runs each) were combined. Then, the nondominated set among them was regarded as a putative Pareto-optimal set and generational distance was calculated on this imaginary front. Table 4 shows that ε-MOEA outperformed NSGA-II for both diversity and convergence; 92.1% improvement in convergence and 22% in diversity. The density controlling by ε-dominance and elitist archive can be pointed out as the possible source of ε-MOEA's success (Shin, 2005).

In summary, multi-objective evolutionary approach can generate better or comparative sequences in all objectives than other systems such as single objective genetic algorithm and simulated annealing as shown in Tables 2 and 3. Also, the sequences in Table 3 are proven by its successful application to a wide range of laboratory experiments. The good performance of multi-objective approach can be explained from the fact that the objective space is not distorted unlike in the single-objective approach. In addition, other objectives than those used here can be incorporated for DNA computing sequence design (Brennenman & Condon, 2002). This also confirms the benefits of multi-objective evolutionary algorithms.

PROBE DESIGN FOR OLIGONUCLEOTIDE MICROARRAY

We will introduce multi-objective evolutionary search method for DNA microarray probe design as the second example of DNA sequence design problem. Here, we try to find a set of "subsequences" (probes) of the given set of genes. These probes are fixed on the surface of microarray and the genes are poured onto the surface. In this example, the last criterion in Figure 2 could be less important than the others, and it is excluded during the optimization and used in the final decision-making.

Table 5 summarizes the necessary objectives for the successful microarray probe design. First and second objectives concern the specificity of the probes. And the third objective concerns the secondary structure of a probe, since the secondary structure can disturb the hybridization with its target gene.

Multi-Objective Formulation of Oligonucleotide Microarray Probe Design

We assume the set of target genes $\{t_1,...,t_n\}$ is given *a priori* and an individual X is a set of probes $\{p_1,...,p_n\}$ such that p_i's are substrings of t_i's, respectively. The objective functions in Table 5 are defined as follows:

$$g_{Uniqueness}(X) = \sum_{i \neq j} I(\Lambda^*_{nb} p_i \Lambda^*_{nb} = t_j) \quad (10)$$

$$f_{Specificity}(X) = \sum_{i \neq j} FEnergy(p_i, \bar{t}_j) \quad (11)$$

$$f_{Hairpin}(X) = \sum_i Hairpin(p_i) \text{ with equation (5)}.$$

The first function $g_{Uniqueness}(X)$ calculates how many probes are the subsequences of other nontarget genes. This should be regarded as a fundamental constraint since a probe needs to be designed to detect only one target gene. From its definition, this constraint should be zero. The second function checks the crosshybridization of a probe with nontarget genes. The crosshybridization between probes is not considered, since the probes are fixed on the surface of microarray and cannot move. The nearest neighbor model is used for both $f_{Specificity}(X)$ and $f_{Hairpin}(X)$, because the usual lengths of the probes are shorter than 50. Therefore, the probe design problem is formulated as a constrained multi-objective problem with two minimization objectives and one equality constraint.

Minimize $F(X) = (f_{Specificity}(X), f_{Hairpin}(X))$, subject to $g_{Uniqueness}(X) = 0$.

The scatter plot between specificity and hairpin is shown in Figure 7. The graph is drawn using 4^{20}

Table 5. The objectives for good probe selection

Objective	Description	Criterion
Uniqueness	The probe sequence for each gene should not appear in the other genes except its target gene.	Crosshybridization prevention
Specificity	The probe sequence for each gene should minimize the interaction among nontarget genes.	
Hairpin	The probe sequence for each gene should not have secondary structures such as hairpin.	Secondary structure Control

20-mer DNA sequences and their Watson-Crick complementary combination. These objectives are suitable to be solved by MOEAs.

Multi-Objective Evolutionary Probe Optimization

Since both DNA computing sequence optimization and microarray probe selection are formulated as constrained multi-objective problems in similar way, the same procedure described in Figure 6 can be used again. The difference is that the objective functions in probe selection are calculated by thermodynamic method unlike in DNA computing sequence optimization.

Probe Selection Results

The performance of ε-MOEA in probe selection was tested on two different gene families: 19 Human Papillomavirus (HPV) genes and 52 Arabidopsis Calmodulin (AC) genes. The resulting probes were compared with those from two popular open programs for probe design: OligoArray (Rouillard et al., 2003) and OligoWiz (Wernersson & Nielsen, 2005). In contrast to ε-MOEA, OligoWiz adopted a dynamic programming and OligoArray used a simple filtering methods. However, both programs used thermodynamic method to test crosshybridization.

The parameter settings for ε-MOEA are as follows: the length of each probe is set to 30 nucleotides for HPV and 24 for AC. The crossover and mutation rates are set as 0.9 and 0.01 respectively, and ε is 1 for better convergence. Population size is 50 and maximum generation is 300. The more detailed explanation will be shown in (Shin, Lee, & Zhang, submitted). For each gene family, one representative probe was chosen for comparison based on the number of crosshybridization and melting temperature variation. Additionally, the final decision step is essential for probe design process, since the most promising probe set is necessary to make a microarray.

The probe sets are compared in three evaluation terms: Total Crosshybridization, Gene Similarity, and Tm Variation. "Total Crosshybridization" estimates the possible unexpected hybridizations which should be prohibited in the biological process expected by thermodynamic calculation, "Gene Similarity" shows the number of undesirable sequence similarities by BLAT (Kent, 2002), and "Tm Variation" represents the standard deviation of melting temperature based on nearest neighbor model. First two criteria estimate the reliability of probe set by thermodynamic calcula-

Figure 7. The relationship between specificity and hairpin for probe design

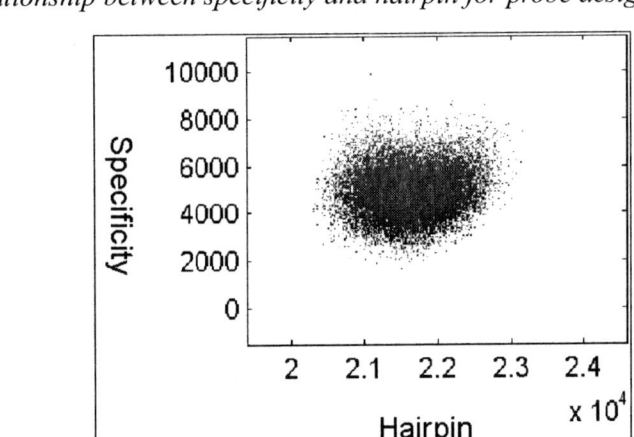

tion and sequence similarity search respectively, and last criterion checks the chemical property control for the easy microarray experiments.

As can be seen in Table 6 and 7, the probe set designed using ε-MOEA shows much smaller tendency of crosshybridization and similarity to gene sequences than the other two programs. OligoArray and OligoWiz have 2 or 3 times higher possibility of crosshybridization than ε-MOEA. In addition, probe set by ε-MOEA does not have similar sequences, which can disturb the correct hybridization, while a few similarities were found in probe set from the other tools. From these, it can be expected that probe set by ε-MOEA produce more accurate experimental results. Unfortunately, ε-MOEA result shows larger variance of melting temperatures than the others. However, it could be explained by the difference of the probe search strategy. In OligoArray and OligoWiz, some candidate probes are removed to get a narrow range of melting temperature and the survived probes get scores according to other criteria, which means the criteria of uniform melting temperature has priority over other criteria. On the other hand, ε-MOEA handles it only as a final decision maker not as an objective.

In summary, there are various benefits of multi-objective approach for probe design. First, evolutionary optimization improves the probe quality drastically in the aspect of total crosshybridization. In addition, it can be further improved by incorporating existing tools for initial population generation. Since the most probe design programs do not require the much computation time, the performance of multi-objective approach can be improved while not increasing execution time. Next, multi-objective evolutionary approach tries to find the optimized combination of probes for

Table 6. The probe design results for Human Papillomavirus. Each column represents the evaluation results from three different criteria. "Total Crosshybridization" represents the number of possible crosshybridization between probes and nontarget genes calculated by NACST/Sim. "Gene Similarity" gives the similarity between probe and nontarget genes using BLAT. "Tm Variation" is the standard deviation of the melting temperatures of the probes.

Evaluation Terms	Human Papillomavirus		
	OligoArray	OligoWiz	ε-MOEA
Total Crosshybridization	268	290	102
Gene Similarity	2	1	0
Tm Variation	2.72	1.27	3.22

Table 7. The probe design results for Arabidopsis Calmodulin family

Evaluation Terms	Arabidopsis Calmodulin		
	OligoArray	OligoWiz	ε-MOEA
Total Crosshybridization	282	368	151
Gene Similarity	1	1	0
Tm Variation	2.57	2.10	4.00

Table 8. The objectives of primer design for multiplex PCR assay

Objective	Description	Criterion
H-measure	The undesirable hybridization between targets and their primers should be minimized.	Crosshybridization prevention
Similarity	The sequence similarity between targets and their primers should be minimized.	
Group	The number of different groups of targets should be minimized.	

the given gene set, not to search the qualifying probes for each gene independently. This also could improve the reliability of whole probe sequences. Third, multi-objective strategy provides the various set of probe combination which can be chosen depending on the target applications.

PRIMER DESIGN FOR MULTIPLEX POLYMERASE CHAIN REACTION

As the last example, we will introduce the multi-objective evolutionary approach to design the primer set for multiplex polymerase chain reaction (PCR) assay. A multiplex PCR assay design is a complex problem which has two main goals. One is to select two sub-sequences of target gene sequence, called primers, specific for each target. Since the multiple targets are amplified in the same tube simultaneously, it is important that the primers for one target do not interact with another targets or primers. The other is to minimize the number of different groups which will be amplified separately. It should be ideal, if all of the target DNAs could be amplified together. However, it is hard to put all compatible targets in the same tube because there is a limitation on the number of targets that can be amplified in one tube to prevent crosshybridization.

Here, the first goal is simplified to assigning primers to each target from a set of primer candidates given *a priori* by another tool. Therefore, the simplified problem would be assigning reliable primers to each target from candidates and grouping targets while minimizing the number of groups.

The objectives for simplified primer design for multiplex PCR assay are explained in Table 8. Among three criteria in Figure 2, the second and third criteria are excluded, since they are already considered in generating primer candidates.

Multi-Objective Formulation of Multiplex PCR Assay

Here, we assume a set of target genes $T = \{t_1,...,t_n\}$ and a set $z_i = \{pr_1^i,...,pr_M^i\}$ of candidate primers for each target t_i are given. M and N mean the number of candidate primers and the maximum number of partitions, respectively. Then an individual X consists of the partition of T, $Pa = \{Pa_1,...,Pa_N\}$, where $Pa_i \subset T$, $Pa_i \cap Pa_j = \phi$ for $i \neq j$, and $\bigcup_i Pa_i = T$, and the primer assignment $A \in z_1 \times \cdots \times z_n$. $A(i)$ denotes the element of z_i assigned to t_i. The objectives in Table 8 can be defined as:

$$f_{H-measure}(X)' = \sum_{i=1}^{N} \sum_{t_j,t_k \in Pa_i, j \neq k}$$
$$\begin{pmatrix} H-measure(A(j),t_k) + H-measure(A(k),t_j) \\ +H-measure(t_i,t_k) + H-measure(A(j),A(k)) \end{pmatrix}$$
(12)

$$f_{Similarity}(X)' = \sum_{i=1}^{N} \sum_{t_j,t_k \in Pa_i, j \neq k}$$
$$\begin{pmatrix} Similarity(A(j),t_k) + Similarity(A(k),t_j) \\ +Similarity(t_i,t_k) + Similarity(A(j),A(k)) \end{pmatrix}$$
(13)

$$f_{Group}(X) = \sum_i I(|Pa_i| \neq 0) \quad (14)$$

$f_{H\ measure}(X)$ and $f_{Similarity}(X)$ are redefined based on equations (1) and (2) to reflect the characteristics of multiplex PCR primer design.

The first and second objectives concern the possible crosshybridization between two primer pairs and their target genes in a group. The last objective is to handle the number of different non-empty partitions. Rachlin et al. (2005b) formulated multiplex PCR assay design as finding cliques in a graph and empirically showed that there is a tradeoff relationship between the specificity of each primer pair to their target and the overall degree of multiplexing (number of partitions).

The mathematical formulation is

Minimize $F(X) = (f_{H\ measure}(X), f_{Similarity}(X), f_{Group}(X))$.

where $X = (Pa, A)$ is an individual.

The more detailed explanation can be found at (Lee et al., 2007).

Hybrid Multi-Objective Evolutionary Design for Multiplex PCR Assay

In this problem, two variable spaces should be searched: primer assignment and target partition. Both spaces were explored by hybrid MOEA. ε-MOEA searches the space of the primer assignment, since H-measure and similarity have the trade-off relationship as described in Section 4. The space of target partition is explored by local search for fast convergence.

The whole procedure for multiplex PCR primer design consists of two steps: selecting primer candidates for each target and hybrid evolutionary search for optimal partition of groups and primer assignments. The first step is done by Primer3 program (Rozen & Skaletsky, 2000). Considering the size of the search space and running time, five candidate primers are selected for each target. The procedure of multi-objective evolutionary search is described in Figure 8.

Compared to the general ε-MOEA procedure, there are three different points in the above search method. The first is the local search operators. Since every candidate primer generated by Primer3 guarantees the minimum level of quality, the change of primers assigned to a target may not result in the drastic change in objective values. Therefore, the local search operators concentrated on target partitioning. Two local search operators such as swapping operators (exchanging two targets between two groups) and migration operator (moving one target to another group) are adopted to explore the space of target partition-

Figure 8. The evolutionary search for multiplex PCR assay design (Adapted from Lee et al., 2007)

1	One parent is chosen at random from the archive and the other parent is chosen from the population by tournament selection.
2	Generate two offsprings by uniform crossover and 1-bit mutation.
3	Apply the local search to offsprings for a predefined number of times.
3.1	Two offsprings are modified through local search operators in random.
3.2	Replace the original offspring with a modified one, if the modified one dominates the original one. If nondominates each other, the modified one replace the original one with probability of 0.5. Otherwise, the modified one is discarded.
4	Update archive.
4.1	The offspring is accepted to the archive if it is in the same front as the archive members or it dominates one or more of them. The dominated archive members are removed.
4.2	If the archive reaches its maximum size, the nearest archive member in objective space is replaced.
5	Update population.
5.1	If the offspring dominates one of population, the dominated member is replaced with the offspring.
5.2	If the offspring and the population do not dominate each other, the nearest population member in variable space is replaced with probability of 0.5.
6	Check termination condition.

ing. Second, the maximum size of the archive is restricted for the practical reason. Last, related to second difference, an explicit niching method is used. The experimental results demonstrate that the ε-domination concept is not enough to keep the size of the archive in reasonable size and the random replacement in the population can lose genetic diversity. Therefore, it tries to keep genetic diversity in the population by selecting the nearest individual to the offspring in variable space as the victim. On the other hand, the distance in objective space is used in archive update to keep diversity among archive members. More explanation can be found at Lee et al. (2007).

Multiplex PCR Assay Selection Results

The multi-objective evolutionary approach was tested on 52 target sequences from Arabidopsis multigene family and compared the results with an open program, MuPlex (Rachlin et al., 2005a). MuPlex used an agent-based multi-objective optimization method which works similar with an evolutionary algorithm.

The size of population and archive are set as 100 and 200, respectively. The maximum generation is set to 100,000 and local search is performed 100 times for each offspring. The crossover rate is 0.9 and mutation rate is 0.01. The maximum number of partition and maximum size of one group are both set to 10. And Primer3 was used with its default setting.

The results are evaluated from three perspectives. First one is the sum of total crosshybridization within a partition to estimate total experimental errors. The crosshybridization is also estimated by NACST/Sim. Second is the number of groups as an estimation of the efficiency of multiplex PCR assay. Last is total number of genes which are partitioned into the groups to check the coverage of partition.

Table 9 shows the only solution obtained from MuPlex and three solutions in the final archive of the single run for fair comparison. ε-MOEA archive solutions in Table 9 show better specificity of primers, which means less possibility of experimental errors that is the most important characteristic for biological sequence design. Table 9 clearly shows the trade-off between primer optimization and partition efficiency. As the number of group increases, the number of total crosshybridization is decreased. However, the small number of group is preferred for the easy experimental setting. Finally, only 47 out of 52 targets are partitioned in MuPlex, since it discards some target if it is hard to find a partition for that target. In contrast, multi-objective evolutionary approach did not discard any target. But, this is dependent on the purpose of the user. In some cases such as high throughput screening, user needs an efficient design, even though the design does not cover every target. However, the coverage can be critical in the other case including clinical assay. For multi-objective approach, this constraint on perfect coverage could be relaxed based on its purpose.

In summary, this section demonstrates the powerful ability of easy addition of fitness functions as well as heuristics into the multi-objective

Table 9. The comparison of designed Multiplex PCR Assay (Adapted from Lee et al., 2007)

Evaluation Term	MuPlex	ε-MOEA 1	ε-MOEA 2	ε-MOEA 3
Total crosshybridization	13719	10915	13269	10683
Number of groups	5	9	8	10
Total number of genes	47	52	52	52

evolutionary computation framework. First, not modifying the general procedure, the additional objective, number of groups, is easily incorporated. Second, the local search operators are added to improve the performance of MOEA. Last, the well-developed biological domain program called Primer3 is used to initial population generation of MOEA. This combination could be important to evolutionary approaches for biological application. Even though the evolutionary process can improve the quality of the solution, many biologists will hesitate to choose the evolutionary methods due to its long computational time compared to the existing filtering methods. Using the existing program to generate initial population of evolutionary methods could be one way to reduce the computation time.

SUMMARY

The problems in the biological domain naturally have diverse objectives and constraints. In addition, some objectives have a traditional trade-off relationship. Therefore, multi-objective evolutionary algorithms (MOEAs) are good candidates for the biological problems. This chapter focuses on a multi-objective evolutionary approach to tackle the DNA sequence design problems, since DNA sequence optimization is one of the basic and important issues for lots of biochemical related experiments.

Among diverse DNA sequence design problems, we chose three representative cases: sequence optimization for DNA computing, microarray probe selection, and multiplex PCR primer selection. The rationale for multiobejctive evolutionary approach is based on the analysis of the given problems. DNA sequence optimization for DNA computing showed the conflicting relationship among fitness objectives with many local optima and little gradient information. These results support that MOEA is actually a good candidate for DNA sequence optimization. Microarray probe selection depicted the similar trade-off relationship with an important constraint. Primer selection for multiplex polymerase chain reaction was also formulated as multi-objective optimization problem. Based on these results, the multi-objective approach was applied to the related DNA sequence design fields.

All these DNA sequence design problems have been solved by ε-multi-objective evolutionary algorithm (ε-MOEA). Even though the specific implementation of algorithm is slightly different based on the characteristics of the given problems, the basic framework is not changed over the problems. The usefulness of MOEA was confirmed experimentally by comparing with other heuristics such as genetic algorithm and simulated annealing, or open programs such as OligoArray, OligoWiz and MuPlex.

Compared to other traditional methods, one advantage of MOEA for biological problems is that the Pareto optimal set allows use of the additional domain knowledge. Biological problems have been investigated over many years, and there exist various well-developed traditional tools. Also, abundant amounts of human experts' knowledge still remain unavailable in the digital computer. The ability of MOEA that can easily add or delete objective functions without changing main procedure can allow all these information as well as other tools to be adopted as final decision step or additional prior knowledge / objectives of multi-objective evolutionary algorithm framework.

FUTURE RESEARCH DIRECTIONS

Future research of multi-objective evolutionary approach for biological problems could be proposed in two directions: the application point and the algorithmic point. First, from the application point of view, the DNA sequence design problem exemplifies a new practical application of multi-objective evolutionary algorithm that demonstrates its usefulness in bioinformatics fields.

This multi-objective evolutionary approach could be used to any kind of DNA applications which need DNA sequences. Other than the applications introduced in this chapter, the medical diagnosis can be possible application area of multi-objective evolutionary DNA sequence optimization with the development of a special kind of DNA strands, aptamers, that can be used to detect the proteins which are expressed by the disease. Or, designing DNA sequences for DNA nano-structures can be another area. Since DNA nanostructure is made by DNA self-assembly, the error-minimized DNA sequences are one of the essential requirements. And, there are still lots of multi-objective optimization problems in biorelated area which can be effectively tackled by MOEA. Some examples are introduced in Section 1. And other examples of multi-objective optimization applications for computational biology are well reviewed in (Handl, 2006).

Another direction of future research is, from the algorithmic point of view, developing the algorithm by reflecting the nature of biological problems. Biological problems have lots of constraints as well as objectives. For example, DNA sequence design problem has several constraints such as melting temperature variation, GC ratio variation, and uniqueness for the whole sequences. In addition, the biochemical processes are not error-free operation; they always have a possibility of errors. Therefore, efficient techniques to handle constraints and uncertainties in biological problems are also necessary.

In addition, though the ability of ε-MOEA was confirmed in this chapter, we also found there is much room for improving the performance of ε-MOEA. For example, the size of the archive often grows very large, since ε-dominance concept is not enough to keep the size of the archive in reasonable size. Though the number of archive members that ε-dominate the population is not infinite theoretically (Laumanns et al., 2002), a limit on the maximum size of the archive is required for the practical reason. And the random replacement in the population can lead to the quick loss of genetic diversity. To handle this problem, explicit niching method with ε-dominance concept will be necessary.

ACKNOWLEDGMENT

This work was supported in part by the National Research Laboratory program of MOST and the Molecular Evolutionary Computing (MEC) project of MOCIE.

REFERENCES

Amos, M., Paun, G., Rozenberg, G., & Salomaa, A. (2002). Topics in the theory of DNA computing. *Theoretical Computer Science, 287,* 3-38.

Aquilante, C. L., Langaee T. Y., Anderson P. L., Zineh, I., & Fletcher, C. V. (2006). Multiplex PCR-pyrosequencing assay for genotyping CYP3A5 polymorphisms. *Clinica Chimica Acta, 372*(102), 195-198.

Arita, M., & Kobayashi, S. (2002). DNA sequence design using templates. *New Generation Computing, 20,* 263-277.

Bourneman, J., Chrobak, M., Vedova, G. D., Figueroa, A., & Jiang, T. (2001). Probe selection algorithms with applications in the analysis of microbial communities. *Bioinformatics, 17*(Supplement 1), 39-48.

Brennenman, A. & Condon, A. (2002). Strand design for biomolecular computation. *Theoretical Computer Science, 287,* 39-58.

Cutello, V., Narzisi, G., & Nicosia, G. (2006). A multi-objective evolutionary approach to the protein structure prediction problem. *Journal of the Royal Society Interface, 3*(6), 139-151.

Deaton, R., Garzon, M., Murphy, R. C., Rose, J. A., Franceschetti, D. R., & Stevens, S. E., Jr.

(1998). Reliability and efficiency of a DNA-based computation. *Physical Review Letters, 80*(2), 417-420.

Deaton, R., Chen, J., Bi, H., Garzon, M., Rubin, H., & Wood, D. H. (2002). A PCR-based protocol for in vitro selection of non-crosshybridizing oligonucleotides. *Lecture notes in computer science* (Vol. 2568, pp. 196-204).

Deb, K. (2001). *Multi-objective optimization using evolutionary algorithms*. John Wiley & Sons.

Deb, K. & Reddy, A. R. (2003). Reliable classification of two-class cancer data using evolutionary algorithms. *Biosystems, 72*(1-2), 111-129.

Deb, K., Pratap, A., Agarwal, S., & Meyarivan, T. (2001). A fast and elitist multiobejctive genetic algorithm: NSGA-II. *IEEE Transactions on Evolutionary Computation, 6*, 182-197.

Deb, K., Mohan, M., & Mishra, S. (2003). Towards a quick computation of well-spread Pareto-optimal solutions. In G. Goos et al. (Eds.), In *Proceedings of the Second International Conference on Evolutionary Multi-Criterion Optimization* (pp. 222-236). Springer-Verlag.

Deb, K., Mohan, M., & Mishra, S. (2005). Evaluating the epsilon-domination based multi-objective evolutionary algorithm for a quick computation of Pareto-optimal solutions. *Evolutionary Computation, 13*(4), 501-525.

Drmanac, S., Stravropoulos, N. A., Labat, I., Vonau, J., Hauser, B., Soares, M. B., & Drmanac, R. (1996). Gene representing cDNA clusters defined by hybridization of 57,419 clones from infant brain libraries with short oligonucleotide probes. *Genomics, 37*, 29-40.

Feldkamp, U., Saghafi, S., Banzhaf, W., & Rauhe, H. (2001). DNASequenceGenerator – A program for the construction of DNA sequences. *Lecture notes in computer science* (Vol. 2340, pp. 179-188).

Flikka, K., Yadetie, F., Laegreid, A., & Jonassen, I. (2004). XHM: A system for detection of potential cross hybridization in DNA microarrays. *BMC Bioinformatics, 5*(117).

Fogel, G. B. & Corne, D. W. (2002). *Evolutionary computation in bioinformatics*. Morgan Kaufmann.

Garzon, M. H. & Deaton, R. J. (1999). Biomolecule computing and programming. *IEEE Transactions on Evolutionary Computation, 3*(3), 236-250.

Garzon, M. H. & Deaton, R. J. (2004). Codeword design and information encoding in DNA ensembles. *Natural Computing, 3*, 253-292.

Gordon, P. M. K. & Sensen, C. W. (2004). Osprey: A comprehensive tool employing novel methods for design of oligonucleotides for DNA sequencing and microarrays. *Nucleic Acid Research, 32*(17), 133.

Handl, J. (2006). *Multi-objective approaches to the data-driven analysis of biological systems*. Unpublished doctoral dissertation, University of Manchester, Manchester, UK.

Hartemink, D. K., Gifford, D. K., & Khodor, J. (1999). Automated constraint-based nucleotide sequence selection for DNA computation. *Biosystems, 52*(1-3), 227-235.

Kaplinski, L., Andreson, P., Puurand, T., & Remm, M. (2005). MultiPLX: Automatic grouping and evaluation PCR assay design. *Bioinformatics, 21*(8), 1701-1702.

Kent, W. J. (2002). BLAT – The BLAST-like alignment tool. *Genome Research, 12*, 656-664.

Lahanas, M., Baltas, D., & Zamboglou, N. (2003). A hybrid evolutionary algorithm for multi-objective anatomy-based dose optimization in high-dose-rate brachytherapy. *Physics in Medicine and Biology, 48*(3), 339-415.

Lahanas, M. (2004). Application of multi-objective evolutionary optimization algorithms in

Medicine. In C. A. Coello Coello & G. B. Lamont (Eds.), *Applications of multi-objective evolutionary algorithms* (pp. 365-391). World Scientific.

Laumanns, M., Thiele, L., Deb, K., & Zitzler, E. (2002). Combining convergence and diversity in evolutionary multi-objective optimization. *Evolutionary Computation, 10*(3), 263-282.

Lee, J. Y., Shin, S.-Y., Park, T. H., & Zhang, B.-T. (2004a). Solving traveling salesman problems with DNA molecules encoding numerical values. *BioSystems, 78*, 39-47.

Lee, I.-H., Kim, S., & Zhang, B.-T. (2004b). Multi-objective evolutionary probe design based on thermodynamic criteria for HPV detection. *Lecture notes in computer science* (Vol. 3157, pp. 742-750).

Lee, I.-H., Shin, S.-Y., & Zhang, B.-T. (2004c). Experimental analysis of ε-multi-objective evolutionary algorithm. In *Proceedings of International Conference on Simulated Evolution and Learning 2004*, SWP-1/127.

Lee, C., Wu, J.-S., Shiue, Y.-L., & Liang, H.-L. (2006). MultiPrimer: Software for multiplex primer design. *Applied Bioinformatics, 5*(2), 99-109.

Lee, I.-H., Shin, S.-Y., & Zhang, B.-T. (2007). Multiplex PCR assay design by hybrid multi-objective evolutionary algorithm. *Lecture notes in computer science* (Vol. 4403, pp. 376-385).

Li, F. & Stormo, G. D. (2001). Selection of optimal DNA oligos for gene expression arrays. *Bioinformatics, 17*, 1067-1076.

Maley, C. C. (1998). DNA computation: Theory, practice, and prospects. *Evolutionary Computation, 6*(3), 201-229.

Marathe, A., Condon, A. E., & Corn, R. M. (1999). On combinatorial DNA word design. In E. Winfree & D. K. Gifford (Eds.), In *Proceedings of 5th International Meeting on DNA Based Computers* (pp. 75-89). AMS-DIMACS Series.

Mauri, G. & Ferretti, C. (2004). Word design for molecular computing: A survey. *Lecture notes in computer science* (Vol. 2943, pp. 32-36).

Nicodeme, P. & Steyaert, J.-M. (1997). Selecting optimal oligonucleotide primers for multiplex PCR. In T. Gaasterland et al. (Eds.), In *Proceedings of the 5th International Conference on Intelligent Systems for Molecular Biology* (pp. 210-213). AAAI.

Oduguwa, A., Tiwari, A., Fiorentino, S., & Roy, R. (2006). Multi-objective optimization of the protein-ligand docking problem in drug discovery. In M. Keijzer et al. (Eds.), In *Proceedings of the 8th Annual Conference on Genetic and Evolutionary Computation* (pp. 1793-1800). ACM Press.

Penchovsky, R. & Ackermann, J. (2003). DNA library design for molecular computation. *Journal of Computational Biology, 10*(2), 215-229.

Rachlin, J., Ding, C., Cantor, C., & Kasif, S. (2005a). MuPlex: Multi-objective multiplex PCR assay design. *Nucleic Acids Research, 33*(web server issue), w544-w547.

Rachlin, J., Ding, C., Cantor, C., & Kasif, S. (2005b). Computational tradeoffs in multiplex PCR assay design for SNP genotyping. *BMC Genomics, 6*(102).

Rajapakse, M., Schmidt, B., & Brusic, V. (2006). Multi-objective evolutionary algorithm for discovering peptide binding motifs. *Lecture notes in computer science* (Vol. 3907, pp. 149-158).

Ray, R. O., Zydallis, J. B., & Lamont, G. B. (2002). Solving the protein structure prediction problem through a multi-objective genetic algorithm. In *Proceedings of IEEE/DARPA International Conference on Computational Nanoscience* (pp. 32-35).

Reif, J. H. (2002). The emergence of the discipline of biomolecular computation in the US. *New Generation Computing, 20*(3), 217-236.

Rouchka, E. C., Khalyfa, A., & Cooper, N. G. F. (2005). MPrime: Efficient large scale multiple primer and oligonucleotide design for customized gene microarrays. *BMC Bioinformatics, 6*(175).

Rouillard, J.-M., Zuker, M., & Gulari, E. (2003). OligoArray 2.0: Design of oligonucleotide probes for DNA micorarrays using a thermodynamic approach. *Nucleic Acids Research, 31*(12), 3057-3062.

Rozen, S. & Skaletsky, H. J. (2000). Primer3 on the www for general users and for biologist programmers. In S. Krawetz & S. Misenser (Eds.), *Bioinformatics and methods and protocols: Methods in molecular biology* (pp. 365-386). Humana Press.

SantaLucia, J., Jr. & Hicks, D. (2004). The thermodynamics of DNA structural motifs. *Annual Review of Biophysics and Biomolecular Structure, 33*, 415-440.

Schoske, R., Vallone, P. M., Ruiberg, C. M., & Butler, J. M. (2003). Multiplex PCR design strategy used for the simultaneous amplification of 10 Y chromosome short tandem repeat (STR) loci. *Analytical and Bioanalytical Chemistry, 375*, 333-343.

Shin, S.-Y. (2005). *Multi-objective evolutionary optimization of DNA sequences for molecular computing.* Unpublished doctoral dissertation, Seoul National University, Seoul, Korea.

Shin, S.-Y., Lee, I.-H., Kim, D., & Zhang, B.-T. (2005a). Multi-objective evolutionary optimization of DNA sequences for reliable DNA computing. *IEEE Transactions on Evolutionary Computation, 9*(2), 143-159.

Shin, S.-Y., Lee, I.-H., & Zhang, B.-T. (2005b). DNA sequence design using ε-multi-objective evolutionary algorithms. *Journal of Korea Information Science Society: Software and Application, 32*(12), 1218-1228.

Shin, S.-Y., Lee, I.-H., & Zhang, B.-T. (2006). Microarray probe design using ε-multi-objective evolutionary algorithms with thermodynamic criteria. *Lecture notes in computer science* (Vol. 3907, pp. 184-195).

Shin, S.-Y., Lee, I.-H., & Zhang, B.-T. (submitted). EvoOligo: Oligonucleotide probe design with multi-objective evolutionary algorithms.

Spieth, C., Streichert, F., Speer, N., & Zell, A. (2005). Multi-objective model optimization for inferring gene regulatory networks. *Lecture notes in computer science* (Vol. 3410, pp. 607-620).

Tanaka, F., Nakatsugawa, M., Yamamoto, M., Shiba, T., & Ohuchi, A. (2002). Towards a general-purpose sequence design system in DNA computing. In X. Yao (Ed.) In *Proceedings of 2002 Congress on Evolutionary Computation* (pp. 73-84). IEEE Press.

Tobler, J. B., Molla, M. N., Nuwaysir, E. F., Green, R. D., & Shavlik, J. W. (2002). Evaluating machine learning approaches for aiding probe selection for gene-expression arrays. *Bioinformatics, 18*, 164-171.

Veldhuizen, D. V. (1999). *Multi-objective evolutionary algorithms: Classification, analyses, and new innovations.* Unpublished doctoral dissertation, Air Force Institute of Technology, Dayton.

Wang, X. & Seed, B. (2003). Selection of oligonucleotide probes for protein coding sequences. *Bioinformatics, 19*(7), 796-802.

Wernersson, R. & Nielsen, H. B. (2005). OligoWiz 2.0 – Integrating sequence feature annotation into the design of microarray probes. *Nucleic Acids Research, 33*(web server issue), W611-W615.

Yamada, T., Soma, H., & Morishita, S. (2006). PrimerStation: A highly specific multiplex genomic PCR primer design server for the human genome. *Nucleic Acid Research, 34*(web server issue), W665-W669.

Zhang, B.-T. & Shin, S.-Y. (1998). Molecular algorithms for efficient and reliable DNA computing. In J. R. Koza et al. (Eds.), In *Proceedings of the Third Annual Conference on Genetic Programming* (pp. 735-742). Morgan Kaufmann.

Zitzler, E. (1998). *Evolutionary algorithms for multi-objective optimization: Methods and applications.* Unpublished doctoral dissertation, Swiss Federal Institute of Technology (ETH), Zuerich, Switzerland.

ADDITIONAL READING

For General Bioinformatics Backgrounds

Baldi, P. & Brunak, S. (2001). *Bioinformatics: The machine learning approach.* The MIT Press.

Baxevanis, A. D. & Francis Ouelette, B. F. (2004). *Bioinformatics : A practical guide to the analysis of genes and proteins.* Wiley-Interscience.

Durbin, R., Eddy, S. R., Krogh, A., & Mitchison, G. (1999). *Biological sequence analysis: Probabilistic models of proteins and nucleic acids.* Cambridge University Press.

Fogel, G. B. & Corne, D. W. (2002). *Evolutionary computation in bioinformatics.* Morgan Kaufmann.

Mount, D. W. (2004). *Bioinformatics: Sequence and genome analysis.* Cold Spring Harbor Laboratory Press.

Tozeren, A. & Byers, S. W. (2003). *New biology for engineers and computer scientists.* Prentice Hall.

For DNA Computing

Adleman, L. M. (1994). Molecular computation of solutions to combinatorial problems. *Science, 266,* 1021-1024.

Adleman, L. M. (1998). Computing with DNA. *Scientific American, 279*(2), 34-41.

Amos, M. (2005). *Theoretical and experimental DNA computation.* Springer-Verlag.

Beneson, Y., Gil, B., Ben-Dor, U., Adar, R., & Shapiro, E. (2004). An autonomous molecular computer for logical control of gene expression. *Nature, 429,* 423-429.

Calude, C. & Paun, G. (2000). *Computing with cells and atoms: An introduction to quantum, DNA and membrane computing.* CRC press.

Macdonald, J., Li, Y., Sutovic, M., Lederman, H., Pendri, K., Lu, W., Andrew, B. L., Stefanovic, D., & Stojanovic, M. N. (2006). Medium scale integration of molecular logic gates in an automaton. *Nano Letters, 6*(11), 2598-2603.

Paun, G., Rozenberg, G., & Salomaa, A. (2006). *DNA computing: New computing paradigms.* Springer-Verlag.

Shapiro, E. & Beneson, Y. (2006). Brining DNA computer to life. *Scientific American, 294*(5), 44-51.

For Probe Selection

He, Z., Wu, L., Li, X., Fields, M. W., & Zhou, J. (2005). Empirical establishment of oligonucleotide probe design criteria. *Applied and Environmental Microbiology, 71*(7), 3753-3760.

Herwig, R., Schmitt, A. O., Steinfath, M., O'Brien, J., Seidel, H., Meier-Ewert, S., Lehrach, H., & Radelof, U. (2000). Information theoretical probe selection for hybridization experiments. *Bioinformatics, 16*(10), 890-898.

Matveeva, O. V., Shabalina, S. A., Memsov, V. A., Tsodikov, A. D., Gesteland, R.F., & Atkins, J. F. (2003). Thermodynamics calculations and statistical correlations for oligo-probes design. *Nucleic Acids Research, 31*(15), 4211-4217.

Wu, C., Carta, R., & Zhang, L. (2005). Sequence dependence of crosshybridization on short oligo microarrays. *Nucleic Acids Research, 33*(9), 84.

Zuker, M. (2003). Mfold web server for nucleic acid folding and hybridization prediction. *Nucleic Acid Research, 31*(13), 3406-3415.

For Primer Selection

Cortez, A. L. L., Carvalho, A. C., Ikuno, A. A., Buerger, K. P., & Vidal-Martins, A. M. C. (2006). Identification of Salmonella spp. Isolates from chicken abattoirs by multiplex-PCR. *Research in Veterinary Science, 81*(3), 340-344.

Liang, H.-L., Lee, C., & Wu. J.-S. (2005). Multiplex PCR primer design for gene family using genetic algorithm. In H.-G. Beyer (Ed.), In *Proceedings of Genetic and Evolutionary Computation Conference 2005* (pp. 67-74). ACM.

Lin, F.-M., Huang, H.-D., Huang, H.-Y., & Horng, J.-T. (2005). Primer design for multiplex PCR using a genetic algorithm. In H.-G. Beyer (Ed.), In *Proceedings of Genetic and Evolutionary Computation Conference 2005* (pp. 475-476). ACM.

Lee, C., Wu, J.-S., Shiue, Y.-L., & Liang, H.-L. (2006). MultiPrimer: Software for multiple primer design. *Applied Bioinformatics, 5*(2), 99-109.

Chapter X
Computational Intelligence to Speed-Up Multi-Objective Design Space Exploration of Embedded Systems

Giuseppe Ascia
Università degli Studi di Catania, Italy

Vincenzo Catania
Università degli Studi di Catania, Italy

Alessandro G. Di Nuovo
Università degli Studi di Catania, Italy

Maurizio Palesi
Università degli Studi di Catania, Italy

Davide Patti
Università degli Studi di Catania, Italy

ABSTRACT

Multi-Objective Evolutionary Algorithms (MOEAs) have received increasing interest in industry, because they have proved to be powerful optimizers. Despite the great success achieved, MOEAs have also encountered many challenges in real-world applications. One of the main difficulties in applying MOEAs is the large number of fitness evaluations (objective calculations) that are often needed before a well acceptable solution can be found. In fact, there are several industrial situations in which both fitness evaluations are computationally expensive and, meanwhile, time available is very low. In this applications efficient strategies to approximate the fitness function have to be adopted, looking for a trade-off between optimization performances and efficiency. This is the case of a complex embedded system design, where it is needed to define an optimal architecture in relation to certain performance indexes respecting strict time-to-market constraints. This activity, known as Design Space Exploration DSE), is still a great challenge for the EDA (Electronic Design Automation) community. One of the most important bottleneck in the overall design flow of a embedded system is due to the simulation. Simulation occurs at every phase of the design flow and it is used to evaluate a system candidate to be implemented. In this chapter we focus on system level design proposing a hybrid computational intelligence approach based on fuzzy approximation to speed up the evaluation of a candidate system. The methodology is applied to a real case study: optimization of the performance and power consumption of an embedded architecture based on a Very Long Instruction Word (VLIW) microprocessor in a mobile multimedia application domain. The results, carried out on a multimedia benchmark suite, are compared, in terms of both performance and efficiency, with other MOGAs strategies to demonstrate the scalability and the accuracy of the proposed approach.

INTRODUCTION

Multi-Objective Evolutionary Algorithms (MOEAs) have received increasing interest in industry, because they have proved to be powerful optimizers. Despite the great success achieved, however, MOEAs have also encountered many challenges in real-world applications. One of the main difficulties in applying MOEAs is the large number of fitness evaluations (objective calculations) that are often needed before an acceptable solution can be found. There are, in fact, several industrial situations in which fitness evaluations are computationally expensive and the time available is very short. In these applications efficient strategies to approximate the fitness function have to be adopted, looking for a trade-off between performance and efficiency. This is the case in designing a complex embedded system, where it is necessary to define an optimal architecture in relation to certain performance indexes while respecting strict time-to-market constraints.

An embedded system is some combination of computer hardware and software, either fixed in capability or programmable, that is specifically designed for a particular kind of application device. Industrial machines, automobiles, medical equipment, cameras, household appliances, airplanes, vending machines, and toys (as well as the more obvious cellular phone and PDA) are among the myriad possible hosts of an embedded system. In fact, the embedded systems market is without doubt of great economic importance nowadays. The global embedded systems market is expected to be worth nearly US$88 billion in 2009, including US$78 billion of hardware and US$3.5 billion of software, according to a Canadian research firm.

For some years now the market has far exceeded that of PC systems. To have an idea of how embedded systems are pervading our daily lives it is sufficient to recall, for example, that there are more than 80 software programs for driving, brakes, petrol control, street finders and air bags installed in the latest car models. As compared with a general-purpose computing system, embedded systems are much more cost sensitive and have strict time-to-market constraints.

The design flow of an embedded system features the combined use of heterogeneous techniques, methodologies and tools with which an architectural template is gradually refined step by step on the basis of functional specifications and system requirements. Each phase in the design flow can be seen as a complex optimization problem which is solved by defining and setting some of the system's free parameters in such a way as to optimize certain performance indexes.

Defining strategies to "tune" parameters so as to establish the optimal configuration for a system is a challenge known as *Design Space Exploration* (DSE). Obviously, it is computationally unfeasible to use an exhaustive exploration strategy. The size of the design space grows as the product of the cardinalities of the variation sets for each parameter. In addition, evaluation of a single system configuration almost always requires the use of simulators or analytical models which are often highly complex. Another problem is that the objectives being optimized are often conflicting. The result of the exploration will therefore not be a single solution but a set of tradeoffs which make up the Pareto set.

These optimization problems are usually tackled by means of processes based on successive cyclic refinements: starting from an initial system configuration, they introduce transformations at each iteration in order to enhance its quality. As in any development process requiring a series of steps towards completion, the presence of cycles is generally a factor which determines its complexity.

From a practical viewpoint, a cycle can be schematized as shown in the shaded part in Figure 1. It comprises four basic components:

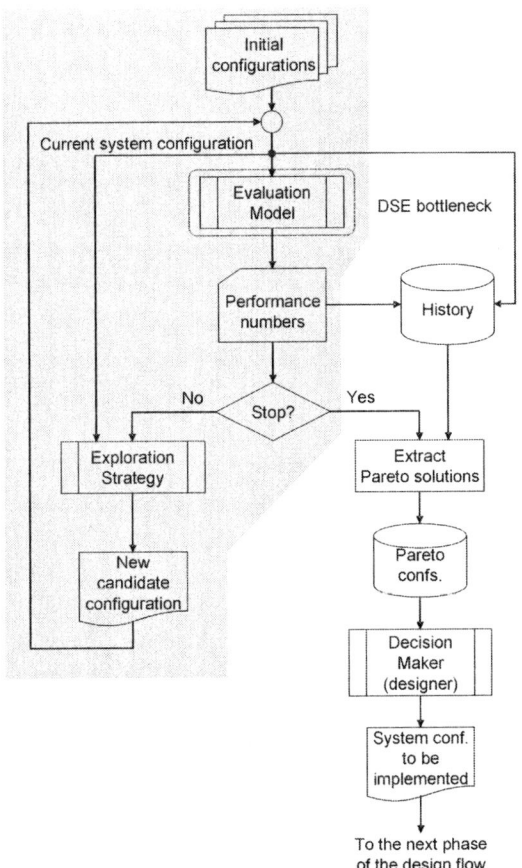

Figure 1. A general design space exploration flow

1. An entry point represented by an initial configuration or set of initial configurations;
2. An evaluation model to measure the validity of a certain configuration;
3. A set of transformations that can be applied to a configuration along with a strategy to apply them (Exploration Strategy);
4. A stop criterion.

DSE is addressed differently according to the level of abstraction involved. In this chapter we will refer to platform based design (Chang, Cooke, Hunt, Martin, McNelly, & Todd, 1999) with particular reference to the use of parameterized platforms (Vahid & Givargis, 2001). A parameterized platform is a pre-designed and preverified system the components of which can be configured by tuning its parameters. In a parameterized platform for digital camera applications, for example, the parameters could be the configuration of the memory subsystem (e.g., cache memory size, associativity, write policies), application-specific parameters such as the pixel width of a jpeg codec, the size and coding schemes of buses and so forth. The objective of a design space exploration strategy is therefore to determine the optimal value for each parameter in order to optimize certain performance indexes (Ascia, Catania, & Palesi, 2004, 2005; Givargis, Vahid, & Henkel, 2002) (in the previous example, these indexes could be energy consumption and computational performance, e.g., shots per second).

Within the DSE flow, the component which most affects the weight of an iteration is the evaluation model. The techniques used to evaluate a design depend heavily on the level of abstraction involved (Buyuksahin & Najm, 2005; Gupta & Najm, 2000b; Najm, 1995; Najm & Nemani, 1998). The use of mathematical models (Ghosh & Givargis, 2004; Liao, Basile, & He, 2002; Gupta & Najm, 2000a), functional simulators (Austin, Larson, & Ernst, 2002; Liao & He, 2001) and hybrid techniques (Ascia, Catania, Palesi, & Patti, 2003; Givargis, Vahid, & Henkel, 2000; Vijaykrishnan, Kandemir, Irwin, Kim, Ye, 2003; Yan, Srikanthan, & Gang, 2006) as system-level evaluation tools is particularly suitable during the initial stages of the design flow. In particular, the use of back-annotated functional simulators to evaluate variables that are typically observable at a lower level of abstraction is highly effective as it yields accurate estimates right from the initial design flow phases. With these simulators it is possible to evaluate complex systems which execute entire applications in an acceptable length of time. Unfortunately their use as evaluation tools in a DSE strategy, which requires evaluation of thousands of system configurations, is confined to small subsystems or simple application kernels.

In this chapter we propose a methodology for efficient, accurate exploration of the design space of a parameterized embedded system. To address the problem of the complexity of the evaluation phase we propose using approximators based on fuzzy systems to evaluate the various components of the models estimating the variables to be optimized. Design space pruning, on the other hand, is achieved by using Pareto-based evolutionary computing techniques which allow multi-objective exploration of the design space.

Although we will discuss a case study involving the design of an embedded system in a multimedia application domain with strict power consumption and computational performance requirements, the methodology presented can easily be extended and is of general applicability.

The rest of the chapter is organized as follows. The next section outlines some of the main contributions to DSE proposed in the literature. A formal statement of the problem is given in Section 3. Section 4 is a general description of the DSE approach called MOEA+Fuzzy because it integrates a MOEA with a Fuzzy approximation system. Section 5 presents the simulation framework and the quality measures we used to assess and compare the performances of the MOEA+Fuzzy. In Section 6 the methodology is applied to a real case study and evaluated in terms of both efficiency and accuracy. In Section 7 new research directions are presented. Finally, Section 8 summarizes the chapter.

BACKGROUND

Design space exploration (DSE) is a key issue in embedded system design. In this paper we focus on efficient and accurate DSE of parameterized System-on-a-Chip (SoC) platforms. Precisely, we consider a *configure-and-execute* design paradigm (Givargis, 2002) in which, a highly parameterized pre-designed platform is configured, by means of parameters tuning, according to the application (or set of applications) it will have to execute.

In this section we first review some of the most relevant contributions in DSE presented in literature. It will be shown that a common practice consists in minimizing the number of system configurations being visited. However, as the dimension of the design space increases, and the applications to be mapped on the platform become more and more complex, the evaluation of a single system configuration becomes the real DSE bottleneck. A complementary approach is based on minimizing the computational effort needed to evaluate a system configuration. Based on this, a set of relevant contributions aimed at building an approximated model of the system which can be analyzed with a lower effort as compared to the original system, are also reviewed in this section. Finally, we close the section summarizing the main contribution of this work.

Design Space Exploration Approaches

The main objective of a design space exploration strategy is to minimize the exploration time while guaranteeing good quality solutions. Most of the contributions to the problem of design space exploration to be found in the literature focus on defining strategies for pruning the design space so as to minimize the number of configurations to visit. One exact technique proposed by Givargis et al. (2000) is based on a dependence analysis between parameters. The basic idea is to cluster dependent parameters and then carry out an exhaustive exploration within these clusters. If the size of these clusters increases too much due to great dependency between the parameters, however, the approach becomes a purely exhaustive search, with a consequent loss of efficiency. To deal with these problems several approximate approaches have been proposed which further reduce the exploration space but give no guarantee that the solutions found will be optimal. Fornaciari, Sciuto, Silvano, and Zaccaria (2002) uses sensitivity analysis to reduce the design space to be explored from the product of the cardinalities of the sets of variation of the parameters to their sum. However, the approach has been presented as a mono-objective approach in which multiple optimizing objectives are merged together by means of agregation functions.

Another approximate approach was proposed by Ascia et al. (2004, 2005) where they proposed a strategy based on evolutionary algorithms for exploration of the configuration space of a parameterized SoC architecture, based on a Reduced Instruction Set Computing (RISC) processor (Ascia et al., 2004) and a Very Long Instruction Word (VLIW) processor (Ascia et al., 2005), to determine an accurate approximation of the power/performance Pareto-surface.

In Hekstra, Hei, Bingley, and Sijstermans (1999) the authors present an approach to restrict the search to promising regions of the design space. Investigation of the structure of the Pareto-optimal set of design points, for example using a hierarchical composition of subcomponent exploration and filtering was addressed in Abraham, Rau, and Schreiber (2000) and Szymanek, Catthoor, and Kuchcinski (2004). A technique that explicitly models the design space, uses an appropriate abstraction, derives a formal characterization by symbolic techniques and uses pruning techniques is presented in Neema, Sztipanovits, and Karsai (2002).

Fast Evaluation through Approximated Models

A different approach for reducing the overall exploration time is minimize the time required to evaluate the system configurations being visited. The use of an analytical model to speed up evaluation of a system configuration is presented in Ghosh and Givargis (2004). Although the approach is not general (it is fully customized to design space exploration of a memory hierarchy) the authors show that it is possible to compute cache parameters satisfying certain performance criteria without performing simulations or exhaustive exploration.

Statistical simulation is used in Eeckhout, Nussbaum, Smith, and Bosschere (2003) to enable quick and accurate design decisions in the early stages of computer design, at the processor and system levels. It complements detailed but slower architectural simulations, reducing total design time and cost. A recent approach

(Eyerman, Eeckhout, & Bosschere, 2006) uses statistical simulation to speed up the evaluation of configurations by a multi-objective evolutionary algorithm. However, neither of the previous approaches are general; they were developed for and are applicable to specific cases.

Coupling Efficient Exploration with Fast System Evaluation

The previously discussed techniques can be combined to tackle the DSE problem. That is, an efficient optimization algorithm is used to guide the exploration of the design space, and an approximated model of the system is used to evaluate the system configurations being visited. This approach, known as *Multidisciplinary Design Optimization* emphasizes the interaction between modeling and optimization. One of the most spread approaches uses evolutionary algorithms as optimization technique.

Broadening the scope to applications not directly connected with the design of an embedded system, the proposals to speedup the evaluation of a single configuration to be found in the literature can be grouped into two main categories: the first comprises methods which use a predefined model that completely replaces the original fitness function (Redmond & Parker, 1996) the second category comprises algorithms that evolve the model on-line during the evolution of the evolutionary algorithm, parsimoniously evaluating the original function (Jin, Olhofer, & Sendhoff, 2002). The second category can be further subdivided into algorithms that use fixed control during evolution (Grierson & Pak, 1993; Jin, Olhofer, & Sendhoff, 2000) and those that use adaptive control (Nair & Keane, 1998). The most popular models for fitness approximation are polynomials (often known as response surface methodology), the kringing model, whereby Gaussian process models are parameterized by maximum likelihood estimation, most popular in the design and analysis of computer experiments, and artificial neural networks. Details of these models are to be found in (Jin, 2005).

In the case of multiple objective evolutionary algorithms, a few recent papers have begun to investigate the use of models to approximate fitness evaluations. The study in (Nain & Deb, 2002) proposes the use of a neural network approximation combined with the NSGA-II algorithm. Some speedup is observed as compared with using the original exact fitness function alone, but the study is limited to a single, curve-fitting problem. In Gaspar-Cunha and Vieira (2004) an inverse neural network is used to map back from a desired point in the objective space (beyond the current Pareto surface) to an estimate of the decision parameters that would achieve it. The test function results presented look particularly promising, though fairly long runs (of 20,000 evaluations) are considered. An algorithm that can give good results with a small number of expensive evaluations is Binary Multiple Single Objective Pareto Sampling (Bin_MSOPS) (Hughes, 2003a, 2003b), which uses a binary search tree to divide up the decision space, and tries to sample from the largest empty regions near fit solutions. Bin_MSOPS converges quite quickly and is good in the 1,000–10,000 evaluations range. A recent multi-objective evolutionary algorithm, called ParEGO (Knowles, 2006), was devised to obtain an efficient approximation of the Pareto-optimal set with a budget of a few hundred evaluations. The ParEGO algorithm begins with solutions in a latin hypercube and updates a Gaussian process surrogate model of the search landscape after every function evaluation, which it uses to estimate the solution with the largest expected improvement. The effectiveness of these two algorithms is compared in (Knowles & Hughes, 2005).

Contribution

As has been highlighted in the introductory section of this work, the system evaluation through system-level simulators can be infeasible in practical cases. To the best of our knowledge, there are no contribution proposed in literature about the efficient and accurate design space exploration of embedded systems which tackle the problem on both the fronts of minimizing the number of system configurations being visited and reducing the computational effort needed to evaluate the visited system configurations through the use of approximated models. Unfortunately, all the approaches reviewed in the previous subsection, do not guarantee satisfactory results with problems characterized by a broad input space of integer variables which are typical of embedded computer systems.

In this chapter we propose a methodology for efficient, accurate exploration of the design space of a parameterized embedded system. Design space pruning is achieved by using Pareto-based evolutionary computing techniques which allow multi-objective exploration of the design space. On the other hand to address the problem of the complexity of the evaluation phase we propose using approximators based on fuzzy systems to evaluate the various components of the models estimating the variables to be optimized.

The capabilities of fuzzy systems as universal function approximators have been systematically investigated. We recall, for example, some recent works (Landajo, Río, & Pérez, 2001; Zeng & Singh, 1996; Zeng, Zhang, & Xu, 2000) where the authors demonstrated that a fuzzy system was capable of approximating any real function to arbitrary accuracy and they proved that fuzzy systems perform better than neural networks without an expensive learning process. In this work we use a fuzzy system based on hierarchical rules, whose characteristics as a universal approximator were investigated in Zeng and Keane (2005).

FORMULATION OF THE PROBLEM

Although the methodology we propose is applied to and evaluated on a specific case study (the optimization of a highly parameterized VLIW-based SoC platform), it is widely applicable. For this reason, in this section we will provide a general formulation of Design Space Exploration (DSE) problem.

Let S be a parameterized system with n parameters. The generic parameter p_i, $i \in \{1,2,...,n\}$ can take any value in the set V_i. A *configuration* **c** of the system S is a n-tuple $<v_1,v_2,...,v_n>$ in which $v_i \in V_i$ is the value fixed for the parameter p_i. The *configuration space* (or *design space*) of S [which we will indicate as $C(S)$] is the complete range of possible configurations [$C(S) = V_1 \times V_2 \times ... \times V_n$]. Naturally not all the configurations of $C(S)$ can really be mapped on S. We will call the set of configurations that can be physically mapped on S the *feasible configuration space* of S [and indicate it as $C^*(S)$].

Let m be the number of objectives to be optimized (e.g., power, cost, performance, etc.). An *evaluation function* $E: C^*(S) \times \mathcal{B} \to R^m$ is a function that associates each feasible configuration of S with an m-tuple of values corresponding to the objectives to be optimized when any application belonging to the set of benchmarks $\mathcal{B}$ is executed.

Given a system S, an application $b \in \mathcal{B}$ and two configurations **c'**, **c''** $\in C^*(S)$, **c'** is said to *dominate* (or *eclipse*) **c''**, and is indicated as **c'** $\succ$ **c''**, if given **o'**=$E($**c'**$,b)$ and **o''**=$E($**c''**$,b)$ it results that **o'**$\leq$**o''** and **o'**$\neq$**o''**. Where vector comparisons are interpreted component-wise and are true only if all of the individual comparisons are true ($o_i'\leq o_i''$ $i=1,2,...,m$).

The *Pareto-optimal set* of S for the application b is the set:

$$P(S,b) = \{\mathbf{c} \in C^*(S) : \mathbf{c'} \in C^*(S), \mathbf{c'} \succ \mathbf{c}\}$$

that is, the set of configurations $\mathbf{c} \in C^*(S)$ not dominated by any other configuration. Pareto-optimal configurations are configurations belonging to the Pareto-optimal set and the *Pareto-optimal front* is the image of the Pareto-optimal configurations, that is, the set:

$$P_F(S,b) = \{\mathbf{o}:\mathbf{o} = E(\mathbf{c},b), \mathbf{c} \in P(S,b)\}$$

The aim of the chapter is to define a DSE strategy that will give a good approximation of the Pareto-optimal front for a system S and an application b, simulating as few configurations as possible.

THE MOGA+FUZZY APPROACH TO SPEED-UP DESIGN SPACE EXPLORATION

It has been shown in Ascia, Catania, and Palesi (2004, 2005) how the use of Evolutionary Algorithms (EAs) to tackle the problem of DSE gives optimal solutions in terms of both accuracy and efficiency as compared with the state of the art in exploration algorithms. Unfortunately, EA exploration may still be expensive when a single simulation (i.e., the evaluation of a single system configuration) requires a long compilation and/or execution time.

For the sake of example, referring to the computer system architecture considered in this chapter (which will be described in Section 5), Table 1 reports the computational effort needed for the evaluation (i.e., simulation) of just a single system configuration for several media and digital signal processing application benchmarks. By a little multiplication we can notice that a few thousands of simulations (just a drop in the immense ocean of feasible configurations) could last from a day to weeks!

The primary goal of this work was to create a new approach which could run as few simulations as possible without affecting the good performance of the EA approach. For this reason we developed an intelligent EA approach which has the ability to avoid the simulation of configurations that it foresees to be not good enough to belong the Pareto-set and to give them fitness values according to a fast estimation of the objectives. This feature was implemented using a Fuzzy System (FS) to approximate the unknown function from configuration space to objective space. The approach could be briefly described as follows: the EA evolves normally; in the meanwhile the FS learns from simulations until it becomes expert and reliable. From this moment on the EA stops launching simulations and uses the FS to estimate the objectives. Only if the estimated objective values are good enough to enter the Pareto-set

Table 1. Evaluation time for a simulation (compilation + execution) for several multimedia benchmarks on a Pentium IV Xeon 2.8 GHz Linux Workstation

Benchmark	Description	Input size (KB)	Evaluation time (s)
wave	Audio Wavefront computation	625	5.4
fir	FIR filter	64	9.1
g721-enc	CCITT G.711, G.721 and G.723 voice compressions	8	25.9
gsm-dec	European GSM 06.10 full-rate speech transcoding	16	122.4
ieee810	IEEE-1180 reference inverse DCT	16	37.5
jpeg-codec	jpeg image compression and decompression	32	33.2
mpeg2-enc	MPEG-2 video bitstream encoding	400	245.1
mpeg2-dec	MPEG-2 video bitstream decoding	400	143.7
adpcm-enc	Adaptive Differential Pulse Code Modulation speech encoding	295	22.6
adpcm-dec	Adaptive Differential Pulse Code Modulation speech decoding	16	20.2

will the associated configuration be simulated. It should be pointed out, however, that a "good" configuration might be erroneously discharged due to the approximation and estimation error. At any rate, this does barely affect the overall quality of the solution found as will be shown in Section 6.

We chose a fuzzy rule-based system as an approximator above all because it has cheap additional computational time requirements for the learning process, which are negligible as compared with simulation time. A further advantage of the system of fuzzy rules is that these rules can be easily interpreted by the designer. The rules obtained can thus be used for detailed analysis of the dynamics of the system.

The basic idea of our methodology is depicted in Figure 2. The qualitative graph shows the exploration time versus the number of system configurations evaluated. If we consider a constant simulation time, the exploration time grows linearly with the number of system configurations to be visited. The basic idea is to use an approximator which learns during the initial phase of the exploration (training phase). When the approximator becomes reliable, the simulator engine is turned off and the exploration continues by using the approximator in place of the simulator. Since the evaluation of a system configuration carried out by a simulator is generally much more time consuming as compared to the evaluation carried out by the approximator, the saving in terms of computation time increase with the number of system configurations to be explored.

More in detail, Figure 3 shows the flow chart of the operations performed. In the training phase the approximator is not reliable and the system configurations are evaluated by means of a simulator which represents the bottleneck of the DSE. The actual results are then used to train the approximator. This cycle continues until the approximator becomes reliable. From that point on, the system configurations are evaluated by the approximator. If the approximated results are predicted to belong the Pareto set, the simulation is performed. This avoids the insertion in the Pareto set of nonPareto system configurations.

The reliability condition is essential in this flow. It assures that the approximator is reliable and that it can be used in place of the simulator. The reliability test can be performed in several way as follows:

Figure 2. Saving in exploration time achieved by using the proposed approach

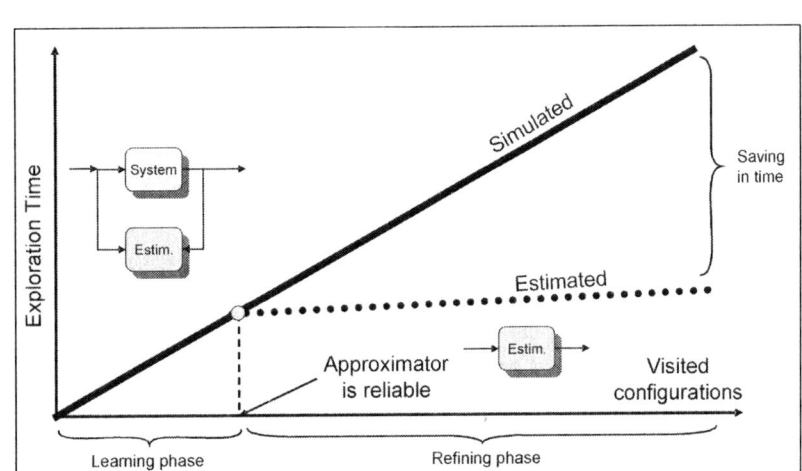

Figure 3. Flow chart of the proposed methodology

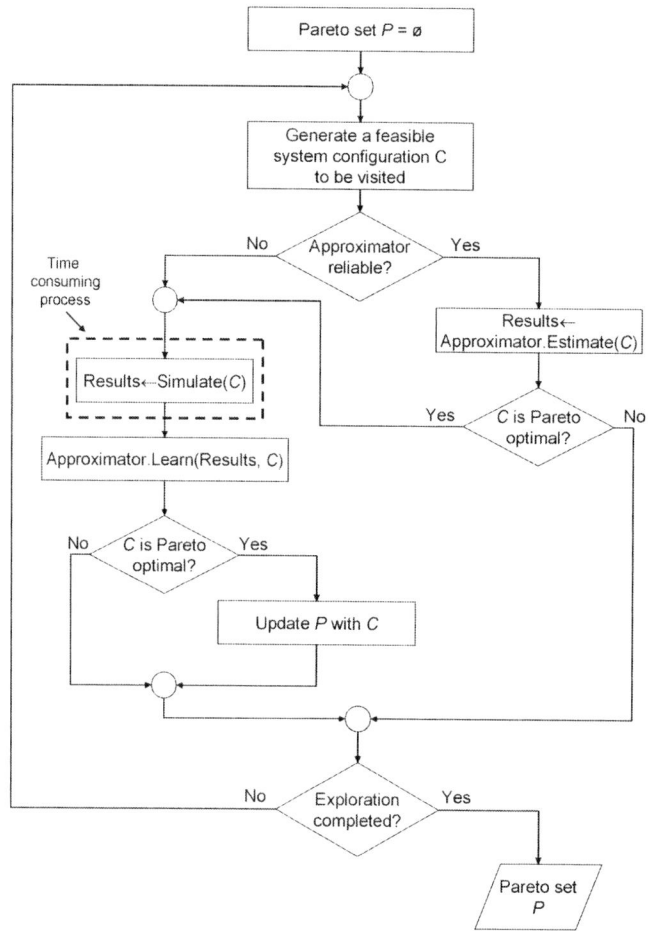

1. The approximator is considered to be reliable after a given number of samples have been presented. In this case the duration of the training phase is constant and user defined.
2. During the training phase the difference between the actual system output and the predicted (approximated) system output is evaluated. If this difference (error) is below a user defined threshold, the approximator is considered to be reliable.
3. The reliability test is performed using a combination of criteria 1 and 2. That is, during the training phase the difference between the actual system output and the predicted (approximated) system output is evaluated. If this difference (error) is below a user defined threshold and a minimum number of samples have been presented, the approximator is considered to be reliable.

The first test is suitable only when the function to approximate is known a priori, so it is possible to preset the number of samples needed by the approximator before the EA exploration starts. In our application the function is obviously not known, so the second test appear to be more suitable. However the design space is wide, for this reason we expect that the error measure oscillates for early evaluations and it will be reliable only when a representative set of system configurations were visited, that is, a minimum number of configurations were evaluated. So only the third test meets our requirements.

MULTI-OBJECTIVE EVOLUTIONARY ALGORITHM

Multi-objective optimization is an area in which evolutionary algorithms have achieved great success. Most real-world problems involve several objectives (or criteria) to be optimized simultaneously, but a single, perfect solution seldom exists for a multi-objective problem. Due to the conflicting nature of the objectives, often only compromise solutions may exist, where improvement in some objectives must always be traded-off against degradation in other objectives. Such solutions are called Pareto-optimal solutions, and there may be many of them for any given problem.

For this work we chose SPEA2 (Zitzler, Laumanns, & Thiele, 2001), which is very effective in sampling from along the entire Pareto-optimal surface and distributing the solutions generated over the trade-off surface. SPEA2 is an elitist multi-objective evolutionary algorithm which incorporates a fine-grained fitness assignment strategy, a density estimation technique, and an enhanced archive truncation method.

The representation of a system configuration can be mapped on a chromosome whose genes define the parameters of the system. The chromosome of the EA will then be defined with as many genes as the number of free parameters and each gene will be coded according to the set of values it can take. For instance Figure 4 shows our reference parameterized architectures, which will be presented in Section 5 and its mapping on the chromosome.

For each objective to be optimized it is necessary to define the respective measurement functions. These functions, which we will call *objective functions*, frequently represent cost functions to be minimized. (e.g., area, power, delay, etc.).

Figure 4. From system to chromosome

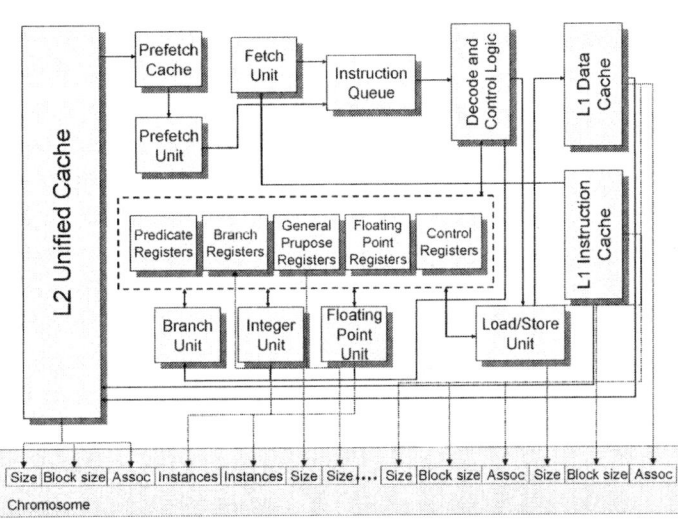

Crossover (recombination) and mutation operators produce the offspring. In our specific case, the mutation operator randomly modifies the value of a parameter chosen at random. The crossover between two configuration exchanges the value of two parameters chosen at random. Application of these operators may generate nonvalid configurations (i.e., ones that cannot be mapped on the system). Although it is possible to define the operators in such a way that they will always give feasible configurations, or to define recovery functions, these have not been taken into consideration in the chapter. Any unfeasible configurations are filtered by the feasible function. A feasible function assigns a generic configuration c belonging to the configuration space C a value of *true* if it is feasible and *false* if c cannot be mapped onto the parameterized system.

The stop criterion used in our experiments was a prefixed number either of fitness evaluations or of generations.

FUZZY FUNCTION APPROXIMATION

In our work we use a k-level Hierarchical Fuzzy System (HFS), that has been demonstrated to be an universal approximator (Zeng & Keane, 2005). The HFS is generated as a cascade of single fuzzy submodel. Each fuzzy sub-system is used to model a particular component of the embedded system. In this hierarchical fuzzy system the output of the fuzzy subsystem at level $l-1$ are used as inputs of the fuzzy subsystem at level l. This hierarchical decomposition of the system allows us to reduce drastically the complexity of the estimation problem with the additional effect of improving estimation accuracy. Single fuzzy systems are generated with a method is based on the well-known Wang and Mendel method (Wang & Mendel, 1992), which consists of five steps:

- **Step 1:** Divides the input and output space of the given numerical data into fuzzy regions;
- **Step 2:** Generates fuzzy rules from the given data;
- **Step 3:** Assigns a degree to each of the generated rules for the purpose of resolving conflicts among them (rule with higher degree wins);
- **Step 4:** Creates a combined fuzzy rule base based on both the generated rules and, if there were any, linguistic rules previously provided by human experts;
- **Step 5:** Determines a mapping from the input space to the output space based on the combined fuzzy rule base using a defuzzifying procedure.

From Step 1 to 5 it is evident that this method is simple and straightforward, in the sense that it is a one-pass buildup procedure that does not require time-consuming training.

In our implementation the output space could not be divided in Step 1, because we had no information about boundaries. For this reason we used Takagi-Sugeno (1985) fuzzy rules, which have as consequents a real number associated with all the M outputs:

IF x_1 is S_1 AND x_2 is S_2 AND ... AND x_N is S_N
 THEN $y_1 = s_1, y_2 = s_2, ..., y_M = s_M$

where S_i are the fuzzy sets associated with the N inputs.

The number of input fuzzy regions should be chosen carefully according to the problem being addressed. In fact, higher is the number of fuzzy regions, higher will be the number of rules, higher will be the time required to insert a new rule and to compute the output values. In this application it is to be set to guarantee the maximum approximation precision of the system, the approximation precision will increase as the number of fuzzy regions grows until a saturation point is reached. This saturation point coincides with the dimensionality of the search space, that is the maximum granularity available. After this saturation point adding fuzzy regions will have the only effect to slow down the system.

In this work the fuzzy rules were generated from data as follows: for each of the N inputs (x_i) the fuzzy set S_i with the greatest degree of truth out of those belonging to the term set of the i-th input is selected. After constructing the set of antecedents the consequent values y_j equal to the values of the outputs are associated. The rule is then assigned a degree equal to the product of the N highest degrees of truth associated with the fuzzy sets chosen S_i.

Let us assume that we are given a set of two input - one output data pairs: $(x_1,x_2;y)$, and a total of four fuzzy sets (respectively Low_1, $High_1$ and Low_2, $High_2$) associated with the two inputs. Let us also assume that has a degree of 0.8 in $High_1$ and 0.2 in $High_2$, and has a degree of 0.4 in Low_1 and 0.6 in Low_2, y = 10. As can be seen from Figure 5, the fuzzy sets with the highest degree of truth are $High_1$ and Low_2, so the rule generated would be:

if x_1 is $High_1$ and x_2 is Low_2 then y=10. The rule degree is $0.8 \times 0.6 = 0.48$.

The rules generated in this way are "AND" rules, that is,, rules in which the condition of the IF part must be met simultaneously in order for the result of the THEN part to occur. For the problem considered in this chapter, that is, generating fuzzy rules from numerical data, only "AND" rules are required since the antecedents are different components of a single input vector.

Steps 2 to 4 are iterated with the EA: after every evaluation a fuzzy rule is created and inserted into the rule base, according to its degree in case of conflicts. More specifically, if the rule base already contains a rule with the same antecedents, the degrees associated with the existing rule are compared with that of the new rule and the one with the highest degree wins. For example consider an other input/output vector where x_1 has a degree of 0.9 in $High_1$ and 0.7 in Low_2, y = 8. As can be seen from Figure 5, the fuzzy sets with the highest degree of truth are $High_1$ and Low_2, so the rule generated would have the same antecedents of the previous rule but different consequent. The rule with the highest degree wins (in our example it is the second rule with a degree of 0.63 against 0.48).

The defuzzifying procedure chosen for Step 5 was, as suggested in (Wang & Mendel, 1992), the weighted sum of the values estimated by the K rules (y_j) with degree of truth (m_j) of the pattern to be estimated as weight:

Figure 5. Fuzzy rule generation example

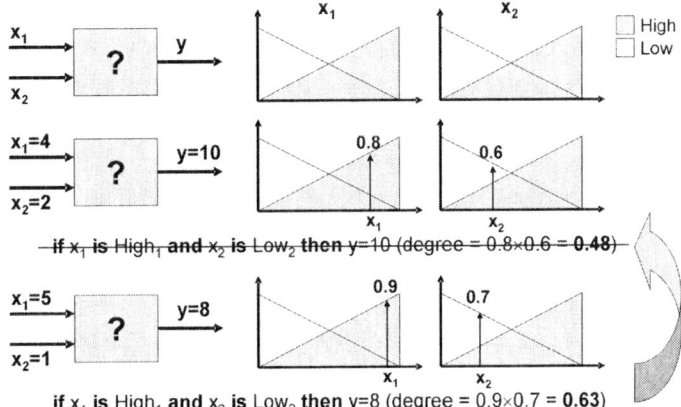

$$\dot{y} = \frac{\sum_{i=1}^{K} m_i y_i}{\sum_{i=1}^{K} m_i} \quad (1)$$

For the sake of example let us consider a fuzzy estimation system composed by the fuzzy sets in Figure 6 and the following rule base:

if x_1 is $HIGH_1$ and x_2 is $HIGH_1$ then $y=5$
if x_1 is $HIGH_1$ and x_2 is LOW_2 then $y=8$
if x_1 is LOW_1 and x_2 is $HIGH_2$ then $y=4$
if x_1 is LOW_1 and x_2 is LOW_2 then $y=3$

Using this fuzzy estimation system we can approximate the output from any couple of inputs. For example consider $x_1 = 2$ and $x_2 = 4$ as input pair, as can be seen graphically in Figure 6, this pair has 0.6, 0.3, 0.2 and 0.8 degree of truth with respectively LOW_1, $HIGH_1$, LOW_2 and $HIGH_2$. Applying (1) we have that the approximated objective value (y) is, (see Box 1).

In our implementation the defuzzifying procedure and the shape of the fuzzy sets were chosen a priori. This choice proved to be effective as well as a more intelligent implementation which could embed a selection procedure to choose the best defuzzifying function and shape to use online. The advantage of our implementation is a lesser complexity of the algorithm and a faster convergence without appreciable losses in accuracy as will be shown in the rest of the chapter.

SIMULATION FRAMEWORK AND QUALITY MEASURES

In this section we present the simulation framework used to evaluate the objectives to be optimized, and the quality measures used to assess different approaches.

Parameterized System Architecture

Architectures based on Very Long Instruction Word (VLIW) processors (Fisher, 1983) are emerging in the domain of modern, increasingly complex embedded multimedia applications, given their capacity to exploit high levels of performance while maintaining a reasonable trade-off between hardware complexity, cost and power consumption. A VLIW architecture, like a superscalar architecture, allows several instructions to be issued in a single clock cycle, with the aim of obtaining a good degree of Instruction Level Parallelism (ILP). But the feature which distinguishes the VLIW approach from other multiple issue architectures is that the compiler is exclusively responsible for the correct parallel scheduling of instructions. The hardware, in fact, only carries out a plan of execution that is statically established in the compilation phase. A plan of execution consist of a sequence of very long instructions, where a very long instruction consists of a set of instructions that can be issued in the same clock cycle.

The decision as to which and how many operations can be executed in parallel obviously depends

Box 1.

$$\dot{y}(x_1, x_2) = \frac{5 \times (0.3 \times 0.8) + 8 \times (0.3 \times 0.2) + 4 \times (0.6 \times 0.8) + 3 \times (0.6 \times 0.2)}{(0.3 \times 0.8) + (0.3 \times 0.2) + (0.6 \times 0.8) + (0.6 \times 0.2)} = 4.4$$

on the availability of hardware resources. For this reason several features of the hardware, such as the number of functional units and their relative latencies, have to be "architecturally visible", in such a way that the compiler can schedule the instructions correctly. Shifting the complexity from the processor control unit to the compiler considerably simplifies design of the hardware and the scalability of the architecture. It is preferable to modify and test the code of a compiler than to modify and simulate complex hardware control structures. In addition, the cost of modifying a compiler can be spread over several instances of a processor, whereas the addition of new control hardware has to be replicated in each instance.

These advantages presuppose the presence of a compiler which, on the basis of the hardware configuration, schedules instructions in such a way as to achieve optimal utilization of the functional units available.

Simulation Flow

To evaluate and compare the performance indexes of different architectures for a specific application, one needs to simulate the architecture running the code of the application. When the architecture is based on a VLIW processor this is impossible without a compiler because it has to schedule instructions. In addition, to make architectural exploration possible both the compiler and the simulator have to be retargetable. Trimaran (http://www.trimaran.org/) provides these tools and thus represents the pillar central to Ascia, Catania, Palesi, and Patti (2003), which is a framework that not only allows us to evaluate any instance of a platform in terms of area, performance and power, exploiting the state of the art in estimation approaches at a high level of abstraction, but also implements various techniques for exploration of the design space. The EPIC-Explorer platform, which can be freely downloaded from the Internet (Patti & Palesi, 2003), allows the designer to evaluate any application written in C and compiled for any instance of the platform. For this reason it is an excellent testbed for comparison between different design space exploration algorithms.

The tunable parameters of the architecture can be classified in three main categories:

- *Register files.* Each register file is parameterized with respect to the number of registers

Figure 6. Simulation flow

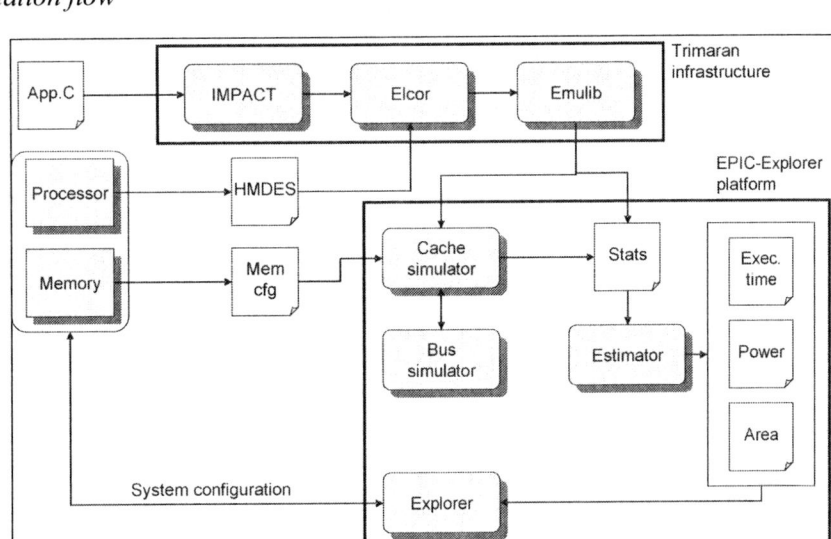

it contains. These include a set of general purpose registers (GPR) comprising 32-bit registers for integers with or without sign; FPR registers comprising 64-bit registers for floating point values (with single and double precision); Predicate registers (PR) comprising 1-bit registers used to store the Boolean values of instructions using predication; and BTR registers comprising 64-bit registers containing information about possible future branches.
- *The functional units.* Four different types of functional units are available: integer, floating point, memory and branch. Here parametrization regards the number of instances for each unit.
- *The memory sub-system.* Each of the three caches, level 1 data cache, level 1 instruction cache, and level 2 unified cache, is independently specified with the following parameters: size, block size and associativity.

Each of these parameters can be assigned a value from a finite set of values. A complete assignment of values to all the parameters is a configuration. A complete collection of all possible configurations is the configuration space, (also known as the design space). A configuration of the system generates an instance that is simulated and evaluated for a specific application according to the scheme depicted in Figure 7. The application written in C is first compiled. Trimaran uses the IMPACT compiler system as its front-end. This front-end performs ANSI C parsing, code profiling, classical code optimizations and block formation. The code produced, together with the High Level Machine Description Facility (HMDES) machine specification, represents the Elcor input. The HMDES is the machine description language used in Trimaran. This language describes a processor architecture from the compiler's point of view. Elcor is Trimaran's back-end for the HPL-PD architecture

and is parameterized by the machine description facility to a large extent. It performs three tasks: code selection and scheduling, register allocation, and machine dependent code optimizations. The Trimaran framework also consists of a simulator which is used to generate various statistics such as compute cycles, total number of operations, etc. In order to consider the impact of the memory hierarchy, a cache simulator has been added to the platform.

Together with the configuration of the system, the statistics produced by simulation contain all the information needed to apply the area, performance and power consumption estimation models. The results obtained by these models are the input for the exploration block. This block implements an optimization algorithm, the aim of which is to modify the parameters of the configuration so as to minimize the three cost functions (area, execution time and power dissipation).

The performance statistics produced by the simulator are expressed in clock cycles. To evaluate the execution time it is sufficient to multiply the number of clock cycles by the clock period. This was set to 200MHz, which is long enough to access cache memory in one single clock cycle.

The Hierarchical Fuzzy Model

The estimation block of the framework consists of a Hierarchy of Fuzzy Systems that models the embedded system shown in Figure 7. This system is formed by three levels: the processor level, the L1 cache memory level, and the L2 cache memory level. A FS at level l uses as inputs the outputs of the FS at level $l-1$. For example, the FS used to estimate misses and hits in the first-level instruction cache uses as inputs the number of integer operations, float operations and branch operations estimated by the processor level FS as well as the cache configuration (size, block size and associativity). The knowledge base was defined on the basis of experience gained from an extensive series of tests. We verified that a

Figure 7. A block scheme of the Hierarchical Fuzzy System used. SoC components (Proc, L1D$, L1I$ and L2U$) are modeled with a MIMO Fuzzy System, which is connected with others following the SoC hierarchy.

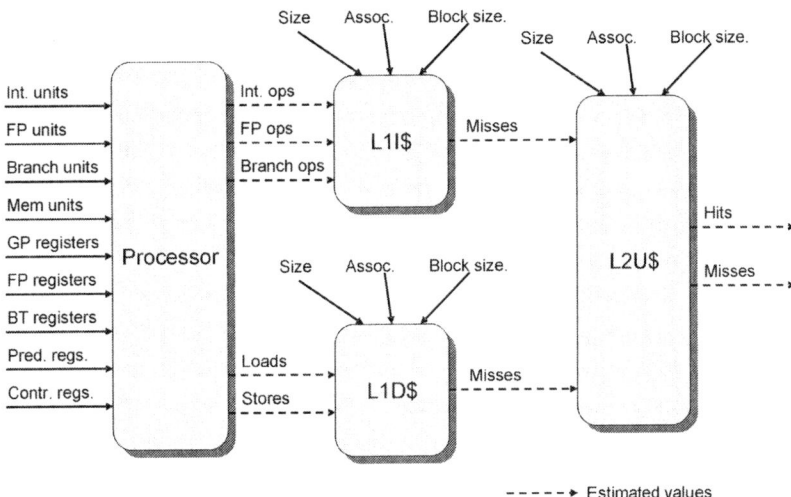

fuzzy system with a few thousands rules takes milliseconds to approximate the objectives, which is some orders of magnitude less than the time required for simulation. We therefore chose to use the maximum granularity, that is we chose to describe each input variable with as many membership functions (fuzzy sets) as the number of values available to that input variable. The number of fuzzy sets used to describe the input variables, that are also output variables of a previous level, was fixed to 9, because the number of values available is unknown a priori. The shape chosen for the sets was Gaussian intersecting at a degree of 0.5.

Assessment of Pareto Set Approximations

It is difficult to define appropriate quality measures for Pareto set approximations, and as a consequence graphical plots were until recently used to compare the outcomes of MOEAs. Nevertheless quality measures are necessary in order to compare the outcomes of multi-objective optimizers in a quantitative manner. Several quality measures have been proposed in the literature in recent years, an analysis and review of these is to be found in Zitzler, Thiele, Laumanns, Fonseca, and daFonseca (2003).

In this work we follow the guidelines suggested in Knowles, Thiele, and Zitzler (2006). The quality measures we considered most suitable for our context are the followings:

1. *Hypervolume*, This is a widely-used index, that measures the hypervolume of that portion of the objective space that is weakly dominated by the Pareto set to be evaluated. In order to measure this index the objective space must be bounded- if it is not, then a bounding reference point that is (at least weakly) dominated by all points should be used. In this work we define as bounding point the one which has coordinates in the objective space equal to the highest values obtained. Higher quality corresponds to smaller values.

2. *Pareto Dominance*, the value this index takes is equal to the ratio between the total number of points in Pareto set *P* that are also present in a reference Pareto set *R* (i.e., it is the number of nondominated points by the other Pareto set). In this case a higher value obviously corresponds to a better Pareto set. Using the same reference Pareto set, it is possible to compare quantitatively results from different algorithms.
3. *Distance*, this index explains how close a Pareto set (*P*) is to a reference set (*R*). We define the average and maximum distance index as follows:

$$dist_{average} = \sum_{\forall \mathbf{x}_i \in P} \min_{\forall \mathbf{y}_j \in R}(d(\mathbf{x}_i, \mathbf{y}_j))$$

$$dist_{max} = \max_{\forall \mathbf{x}_i \in P}(\min_{\forall \mathbf{y}_j \in R}(d(\mathbf{x}_i, \mathbf{y}_j)))$$

where $\mathbf{x}_i$ and $\mathbf{y}_j$ are vectors whose size is equal to the number of objectives M and $d(\cdot,\cdot)$ is the Euclidean distance. The lower the value of this index, the more similar the two Pareto sets are. For example a high value of maximum distance suggest that some reference points are not well approximated, and consequently an high value of average distance tells us that an entire region of the reference Pareto is missing in the approximated set.

A standard, linear normalization procedure was applied to allow the different objectives to contribute approximately equally to index values.

If the Pareto-optimal set is not available, we used the following approach to obtain a reference Pareto-set: first, we combined all approximations sets generated by the algorithms under consideration, and then the dominated objective vectors are removed from this union. At last, the remaining points, which are not dominated by any of the approximations sets, form the reference set. The advantage of this approach is that the reference set weakly dominates all approximation sets under consideration.

For the analysis of multiple runs, we compute the quality measures of each individual run, and report the mean and the standard deviation of these. Since the distribution of the algorithms we compare are not necessarily normal, we use two nonparametric tests to indicate if there is a statistically significant difference between distributions: the Mann-Whitney rank-sum test to compare two distributions and Kruskal-Wallis test respectively for more than two distributions (Gibbons, 1985).

EXPERIMENTS AND RESULTS

In this section we evaluate the proposed approach on two systems based on a Very Long Instruction Word (VLIW) microprocessor. The first one is based on a commercial available VLIW microprocessor core from STMicroelectronics, the LX/ST200 (Fisher, Faraboschi, Brown, Desoli, & Homewood, 2000), targeted for multimedia applications. The second one is a completely customizable (parameterized) VLIW architecture. The decision to conduct the analysis using two different case studies was made so as to evaluate how the proposed approach scales as the complexity of the system increases. As will be described in the following subsections, the design space of the LX/ST200 system is much smaller than that of the completely customizable VLIW. The limited size of the design space in the first case will thus allow us to evaluate the approach and compare it with an exhaustive exploration.

In this research we compare our approach with SPEA2 (MOEA), ParEGO and Bin_MSOPS, the pseudo-codes of these algorithms are in Appendix. The parameters of the ParEGO and Bin_MSOPS algorithms were those used in (Knowles & Hughes, 2005). Parameters of the MOEA are as follows: The internal and external population for the evolutionary algorithm were set as comprising 30 individuals, using a crossover probability of 0.8 and a mutation probability of 0.1. These values were set following the indications given in Ascia et al. (2004), where the convergence times and accuracy of the results were evaluated with various crossover and mutation probabilities. The approximation error in MOEA+Fuzzy is calculated in a window of 20 evaluations for the objectives, and the reliability threshold was set to 5% of the Euclidean distance between the real point (individuated by the simulation results) and the approximate one in the objective space. The minimum number of evaluations, before which consider the error test to assess the reliability of the fuzzy approximator, was set to 90. Both thresholds were chosen after extensive series of experiments with computationally inexpensive test functions.

A Case Study: Application Specific Cache Customization

To evaluate the accuracy of the approach we considered the problem of exploring the design space of a system comprising the STMicroelectronics LX/ST200 VLIW processor and a parameterized 2-level memory hierarchy. This choice was made because the size of the design space and the time required to evaluate a configuration for this architecture are sufficiently small as to make an exhaustive exploration computationally feasible. The 2-level memory hierarchy consists of a separated first level instruction and data cache and a unified second-level cache. The parameter space along with the size of the design space to be explored is reported in Table 2.

Table 3 summarizes the exploration results for gsm-decode application. The evaluation of a single system configuration running gsm-decoding application requires about 2 minutes to be executed by an instrumented LX/ST200 instruction set simulator[1] on a Pentium IV Xeon 2.8GHz workstation. The following exploration strategies were compared:

- Exhaustive exploration in which each feasible configuration of the design space was evaluated.
- The approach proposed in Ascia et al. (2005) which uses SPEA2 as the optimization algorithm (MOEA).
- The approach proposed in this chapter, which uses SPEA2 as the optimization algorithm and fuzzy systems as approximation models (MOEA+Fuzzy).

For each approach the Table 3 reports the total number of configurations simulated and the values of the performance indexes discussed in Section 5.4. For the approaches using EAs, the reported values are averaged over 100 runs. As can be observed in Table 3, the number of configurations simulated during exhaustive exploration is lower than the size of the design space. This is due to the fact that some of the configurations (about 10%) are unfeasible. ParEGO results are not present, because it is not suitable with numbers of iterations larger than very few hundreds (Knowles, 2006).

Table 2. Design space for the LX/ST200 based system

Parameter	Parameter space
L1D cache size	2KB,4KB...,128KB
L1D cache block size	16B,32B,64B
L1D cache associativity	1,2
L1I cache size	2KB,4KB...,128KB
L1I cache block size	16B,32B,64B
L1I cache associativity	1,2
L2U cache size	128KB,...,512KB
L2U cache block size	32B,64B,128B
L2U cache associativity	2,4,8
Space size	47,628

Table 3. Exhaustive, MOEA and MOEA+Fuzzy explorations comparisons

Approach	Simulations	Total time	Pareto-optimal points discovered (%)	Hypervolume	Average Distance (%)	Max Distance (%)
Exhaustive	43416	2 months	100.00%	52.61	0.0000	0.0000
MOEA	5219.2	1 week	100.00%	52.61	0.0000	0.0000
MOEA+Fuzzy	749.5	1 day	90.76%	52.60	0.0098	0.1895
Bin_MSOPS	8614.2	1.5 weeks	12.31%	48.21	0.4297	2.4539

Table 4. Random search, SPEA2 (MOEA), MOEA+Fuzzy, ParEGO and Bin_MSOPS comparisons on a budget of 250 simulations

Approach	Hypervolume (%)	Distance (%)		Pareto Dominance* (%)
		average	maximum	
Random search	29.30 (1.44)	4.25 (0.30)	9.93 (0.75)	0.33 (0.11)
MOEA	50.54 (0.32)	0.21 (0.08)	0.83 (0.53)	13.85 (4.43)
MOEA+Fuzzy	**52.30 (0.09)**	**0.06 (0.02)**	**0.41 (0.22)**	**46.15 (1.45)**
ParEGO	35.60 (0.37)	3.14 (0.09)	7.66 (0.57)	0.51 (0.23)
Bin_MSOPS	34.55 (1.12)	4.30 (0.29)	14.05 (2.16)	0.77 (0.42)

* In this case Pareto Dominance index assesses the Pareto-optimal points discovered.

In this case study the Pareto-optimal set is available, so it is the reference set for all comparisons reported in this subsection. The results are represented in tables using the mean and standard deviation (the latter in brackets) of the performance indexes.

With the MOEA approach all points of the Pareto-optimal set are obtained after about 250 generations, visiting on average slightly over 5,000 configurations. From Table 3 it can be seen that the MOEA+Fuzzy approach, which converges after about 250 generations like the MOEA approach, offers a great saving in the time required for exploration at the average cost of 10% of the Pareto-optimal points. Considering hypervolume and distance, we see that the Pareto set obtained by the MOEA+Fuzzy approach is highly representative of the complete set, so the missing points can be considered negligible.

Table 4 gives the results (hypervolume and distance between approximated Paretos and the Pareto-optimal set) obtained on a budget of 250 evaluations by a random search, MOEA, MOEA+Fuzzy and the ParEGO and Bin_MSOPS algorithms. The Pareto-set obtained by MOEA+Fuzzy after just 250 evaluations is very close to the Pareto-optimal set (average distance is 0.06%) and little less than 50% of the Pareto-optimal points were already discovered. All the indexes calculated in the experiment with 250 evaluations confirm a significant improvement in quality by MOEA when the fuzzy approximation system is used. As expected, the results obtained by ParEGO and Bin_MSOPS confirm that both the algorithms are not suitable to tackle DSE problems. The main reason for the low quality of the solutions found is mainly related to the integer nature of the input parameter space along with the rough-

Figure 8. Box plot for hypervolume (a); Hypervolume evolution (b)

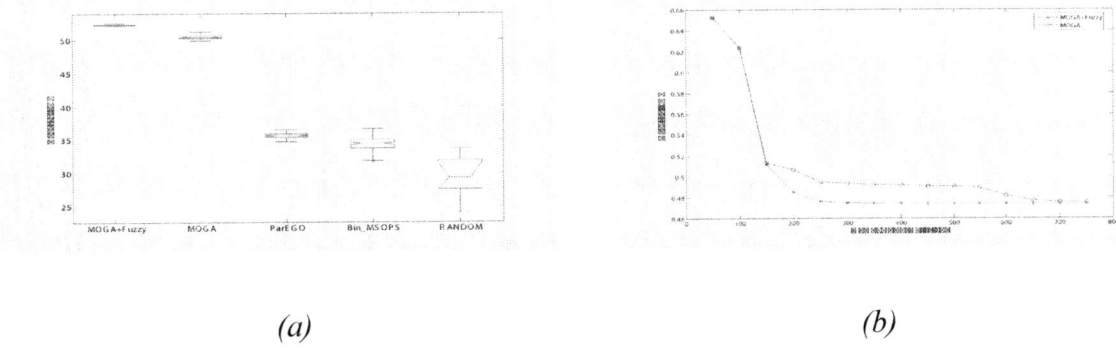

(a) *(b)*

ness and sharpness of the fitness landscape which characterize such kind of systems. This is also confirmed by the Kruskal-Wallis test where the results found by Bin_MSOPS algorithm are not so significant as compared to pseudo-random search (it is clearly visible in Figure 8(a) that reports box plots for hypervolume distributions). This result is due to the roughness of the functions to approximate, which are nonlinear.

Figure 8(b) shows the trend of the hypervolume for MOEA and MOEA+Fuzzy as the number of simulations increases. As can be seen, the MOEA and MOEA+Fuzzy approaches proceed equally until the approximator becomes reliable. At this point MOEA+Fuzzy decidedly speeds up after a few generations, which are equivalent to a few tens of evaluations, and converges after a few hundred simulation. MOEA is slower to converge: only after about a thousand simulations it is able to produce a better Pareto set than the one found by MOEA+Fuzzy.

Figure 9 shows the objective space for all configurations simulated by exhaustive exploration (light grey), by MOEA (dark grey) and by MOEA+Fuzzy (black). Each configuration simulated gives a pair of objective values (i.e., results), which are used as coordinates for the points depicted in Figure 9. As can be seen, the configurations explored by the MOEA+Fuzzy approach are distributed with greater density around the Pareto optimal set. Numerically this concept is explained by the average distance of all points from the Pareto optimal set, that is 3.72% for MOEA+Fuzzy (the maximum distance is 52.41%) against 5.31% (the maximum distance is 64.16%) of MOEA. This confirms that the MOGA+Fuzzy is capable to identify less promising configurations and it avoids to waste time to simulate them.

An interesting feature of the proposed approach is the possibility to build an interpretable fuzzy system that the designer can use to study more in-depth the system. Interpretability means that human beings are able to understand the fuzzy system behavior by inspecting the rule base (Mikut, Jäkel, & Gröll, 2005). As an example, we show a human understandable set of fuzzy rules, extracted from the approximator generated by our MOEA+Fuzzy approach after the exploration described in this section. To this end, we considered the execution time as the variable to be characterized. To make the fuzzy system interpretable we firstly divided the output space in five classes into which the possible configurations can be equally subdivided. The classes defined are as follows: FAST (*time*), QUICK (*time*), MEDIUM (*time*), SLOW (*time*), TURTLE (*time*). Then we applied a rule reduction approach for Takagi-Sugeno fuzzy systems (Taniguchi, Tanaka, Ohtake, & Wang,

Figure 9. Results of all configurations simulated with Exhaustive (light grey), MOEA (dark grey), MOEA+Fuzzy (black) approaches. Each configuration simulated gives a pair of objective values (i.e., results), which are the coordinates of the points in this figure.

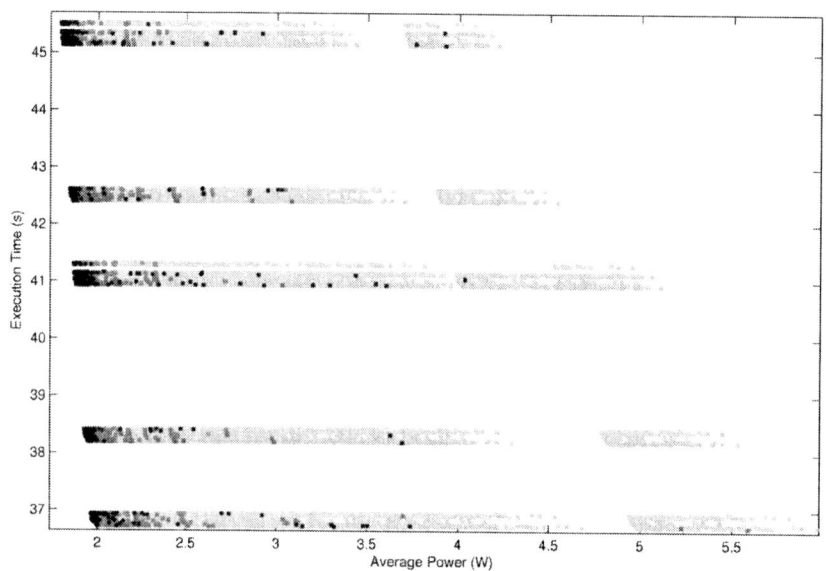

Figure 10. The knowledge base along with the set of rules

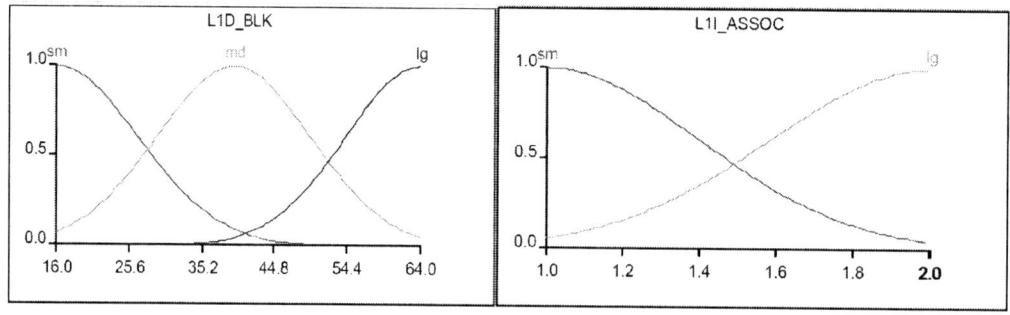

if L1D-BLK is *small* **and** L1I-ASSOC is *small* **then** FAST
if L1D-BLK is *medium* **and** L1I-ASSOC is *small* **then** QUICK
if L1D-BLK is *large* **and** L1I-ASSOC is *small* **then** MEDIUM
if L1D-BLK is *small* **and** L1I-ASSOC is *large* **then** MEDIUM
if L1D-BLK is *medium* **and** L1I-ASSOC is *large* **then** SLOW
if L1D-BLK is *large* **and** L1I-ASSOC is *large* **then** TURTLE

2001). Thanks to these operations it is possible to eliminate seven parameters and simplify drastically the rule base: the number of rules is reduced to six but they are still able to classify with 100% accuracy all the possible 43,416 configurations in the five groups. The knowledge base along with the set of rules is shown in Figure 10.

It should be pointed out that in our approach the fuzzy system is designed to achieve the best accuracy possible, for this reason it is not possible to generate an interpretable fuzzy system, because interpretability and accuracy are two conflicting objectives. However a rule reduction strategy can be always applied, and it is computationally inexpensive compared with the whole exploration.

DSE of a Parameterized VLIW-Based Embedded System

In this subsection we present a comparison between the performance of MOEA, ParEGO and our MOEA+Fuzzy approach. Bin_MSOPS was not considered because it does not work well with larger decision spaces. In this study we repeated the execution of the algorithms 10 times using different random seeds.

The 18 input parameters, along with the size of the design space for the parameterized VLIW based system architecture being studied, are reported in Table 5. As can be seen from Table 5, the size of the configuration space is such as to be able to explore all the configurations in a 365-day year a simulation needs to last about 3 ms, a value which is several orders of magnitude away from the values in Table 1. A whole human lifetime would not, in fact, be long enough to obtain complete results for an exhaustive exploration of any of the existing benchmarks, even using the most powerful workstation currently available. Even if we use High Performance Computing systems, they will be extremely expensive (in terms of money) and will still require a long time.

Essentially DSE must identify some suitable configurations, among the enormous space in Table 4, for in-depth studies at lower design levels. DSE is a crucial high-level design procedure, so even a less efficient decision in this phase could doom the entire design process to failure. However, a well-known market law says that the first product to appear wins over late-comers and, more interestingly, it can be sold at the highest price. So it is preferable for DSE not to be time-consuming. For this reason it is not necessary to discover all the Pareto-optimal configurations, but only some of them and/or some very good quality approximations. Keeping this in mind, we decided to carry out two different tests to compare the performance of our approach with that of others. The first test was performed on a budget of 250 evaluations, because we consider it to be a good milestone in DSE. Even in the case of the most time-consuming benchmark, in fact, 250 evaluations take about 8 hours (i.e., it is possible to leave a workstation to explore overnight and to have the results the next morning). In the

Table 5. Design space of the parameterized VLIW based system architecture

Parameter	Parameter space
Integer Units	1,2,3,4,5,6
Float Units	1,2,3,4,5,6
Memory Units	1,2,3,4
Branch Units	1,2,3,4
GPR/FPR	16,32,64,128
PR/CR	32,64,128
BTR	8,12,16
L1D/I cache size	1KB,2KB,...,128KB
L1D/I cache block size	32B,64B,128B
L1D/I cache associativity	1,2,4
L2U cache size	32KB,64KB,...,512KB
L2U cache block size	64B,128B,256B
L2U cache associativity	2,4,8,16
Design Space size	$7.739 \cdot 10^{10}$

Table 6. Pareto Dominance, a comparison between ParEGO, SPEA2 (MOEA) and MOEA+Fuzzy on a budget of 250 simulations

Benchmark	Pareto Dominance* (%) mean (standard deviation)		
	ParEGO	MOEA	MOEA+Fuzzy
wave	2.10 (3.42)	19.93 (11.17)	**77.97 (10.62)**
fir	7.18 (3.60)	23.73 (10.98)	**69.09 (11.76)**
adpcm-encode	2.99 (2.35)	13.30 (8.66)	**83.71 (9.26)**
adpcm-decode	0.00 (0.00)	13.65 (6.40)	**86.35 (6.40)**
g721-encode	21.67 (7.46)	31.69 (16.94)	**46.65 (18.52)**
ieee810	1.55 (1.22)	14.42 (6.15)	**84.03 (7.96)**
jpeg-codec	3.48 (2.45)	19.58 (16.13)	**76.94 (17.67)**
mpeg2-encode	12.33 (5.92)	35.46 (6.04)	**52.22 (6.65)**
mpeg2-decode	18.63 (7.81)	45.21 (5.93)	**36.16 (5.71)**

* In this case, unlike the others, in building the reference Pareto sets we considered the sets obtained by all the approaches after 250 evaluations.

Table 7. Hypervolume, a comparison between ParEGO, SPEA2 (MOEA) and MOEA+Fuzzy on a budget of 250 simulations

Benchmark	Hypervolume (%) mean (standard deviation)			Best algorithm according to Kruskal-Wallis test*
	ParEGO	MOEA	MOEA+Fuzzy	
wave	37.21 (8.36)	53.72 (2.93)	**65.07 (1.54)**	MOEA+Fuzzy wins
fir	51.25 (8.45)	57.88 (3.89)	**61.20 (1.51)**	MOEA & MOEA+Fuzzy win
adpcm-encode	55.49 (3.24)	62.66 (2.63)	**67.85 (0.85)**	MOEA+Fuzzy wins
adpcm-decode	25.36 (4.84)	43.26 (5.64)	**54.70 (4.49)**	MOEA+Fuzzy wins
g721-encode	63.37 (1.14)	66.61 (1.26)	**66.89 (0.21)**	MOEA & MOEA+Fuzzy win
ieee810	48.27 (4.11)	51.12 (3.13)	**61.71 (2.95)**	MOEA+Fuzzy wins
jpeg-codec	61.35 (9.18)	74.49 (1.84)	**76.82 (2.33)**	MOEA & MOEA+Fuzzy win
mpeg2-encode	56.15 (5.70)	66.81 (2.98)	**70.86 (1.25)**	MOEA+Fuzzy wins
mpeg2-decode	80.30 (0.73)	80.19 (0.54)	**80.86 (1.24)**	none

* An algorithm "wins" when its results are better than others with statistical significance level α at 1%.

second test we compared the Pareto sets obtained after 100 generations to assess performance and quality when longer runs are possible.

The results are represented in tables using the mean and standard deviation (the latter in brackets) of the performance indexes obtained from the compared algorithms (columns) in the nine benchmarks (rows).

In the first test on 250 evaluations we focused only on quality of results, and the research

Table 8. Efficiency comparison between SPEA2 (MOEA) and MOEA+Fuzzy Pareto sets after 100 generations

Benchmark	Number of simulations mean (standard deviation)		Simulations saving (%)	Time saving (hh:mm)
	MOEA	MOEA+Fuzzy		
wave	2682.0 (8.76)	797.0 (63.64)	70.28	2:50
fir	2743.0 (9.69)	902.0 (24.04)	67.77	4:39
adpcm-encode	2702.3 (16.15)	875.5 (41.72)	67.60	11:28
adpcm-decode	2677.5 (26.63)	863.0 (74.95)	67.77	10:11
g721-encode	2659.7 (10.53)	835.6 (103.94)	68.57	13:07
ieee810	2717.5 (20.07)	949.3 (38.89)	65.06	18:25
jpeg-codec	2694.3 (54.79)	947.5 (7.77)	64.83	16:07
mpeg2-encode	2701.1 (13.76)	995.4 (30.29)	63.15	116:09
mpeg2-decode	2708.0 (14.44)	999.1 (33.86)	63.10	68:13
Average	2701.1 (31.50)	904.6 (87.78)	66.51	------

proved that the proposed MOEA+Fuzzy approach outperforms the competitors in terms of both hypervolume and Pareto dominance indexes. In fact MOEA+Fuzzy comes out top in eight out of nine benchmarks in the Pareto dominance index comparison, as shown in Table 6.

The hypervolume comparison, Table 7, shows that MOEA+Fuzzy is significantly better than other algorithms in five out of nine test cases, and it obtains the best result in the remaining four cases. Considering the two indexes, we can see that MOEA+Fuzzy always discovers a good number of high-quality points over the Pareto front, which is the most important feature in DSE. Looking at the index values and Figure 12, we can also state that even though MOEA discovers more Pareto reference points than MOEA+Fuzzy in the mpeg2-dec benchmark, the quality of the Pareto set obtained by the latter is better because hypervolume index has the highest value. This is the only case in which ParEGO performs as well as the others.

In the second test, time requirements were also taken into account, and results were assessed as a trade-off between performance and the length of time required.

As regards the efficiency of the proposed approach, Table 8 gives the number of configurations simulated by the two approaches and presents a comparison between the MOEA and MOEA+Fuzzy Pareto sets obtained after 100 generations. Comparisons exhibit an average 66% saving on exploration time, which may mean several hours or almost a day depending on the benchmark (from about 3 hours for wave to 5 days for mpeg2-encode).

Table 9, that reports hypervolume and Pareto distance obtained by MOEA and MOEA+Fuzzy after 100 generations, shows that MOEA+Fuzzy yields a similar result to that of the approach based on MOEA. The consideration that the Pareto sets obtained are equal, as can be seen graphically in Figure 13, is numerically justified by the short distance between the two sets and the statisti-

Table 9. Accuracy comparison between SPEA2 (MOEA) and MOEA+Fuzzy Pareto sets after 100 generations

Benchmark	Hypervolume % mean (standard deviation)		Mann-Withney test significance level α at 1%	Pareto Distance %, mean (standard deviation)			
				MOEA		MOEA+Fuzzy	
	MOEA	MOEA+Fuzzy		average	max	average	max
wave	83.00 (0.25)	81.86 (0.87)	yes	0.1198 (0.0422)	1.8996 (1.0422)	0.2543 (0.0313)	1.0826 (0.0493)
fir	67.82 (0.45)	67.39 (0.12)	no	0.2059 (0.1762)	7.7688 (10.0664)	0.2940 (0.0711)	1.6639 (0.7087)
adpcm-encode	75.11 (0.14)	74.71 (0.49)	yes	0.1878 (0.2188)	10.2360 (18.9680)	0.2269 (0.0802)	2.6574 (0.8783)
adpcm-decode	63.38 (0.30)	63.01 (0.25)	no	1.0318 (0.7189)	10.6251 (6.7781)	1.7091 (0.4637)	17.1550 (10.9834)
g721-encode	79.02 (0.32)	77.09 (1.31)	yes	0.6367 (0.0675)	7.0375 (1.7207)	1.4560 (0.1729)	32.8320 (23.5490)
ieee810	75.22 (0.85)	74.84 (1.05)	no	0.3830 (0.1303)	8.6368 (4.2494)	0.5633 (0.2674)	7.5960 (1.1332)
jpeg-codec	86.61 (0.10)	84.11 (0.42)	yes	0.3542 (0.0894)	11.8634 (9.8378)	0.8724 (0.4674)	6.2673 (0.2829)
mpeg2-encode	79.31 (0.88)	78.82 (1.01)	no	0.6964 (0.2567)	9.6398 (6.4279)	1.0460 (0.4914)	4.3445 (1.6066)
mpeg2-decode	90.12 (1.33)	90.04 (1.13)	no	0.9105 (0.6510)	11.4480 (1.9849)	1.2196 (0.8439)	4.8435 (2.6586)
Average	0.00* (0.58)	-0.86* (1.10)	yes	0.5029 (0.4885)	8.7950 (7.8971)	0.8492 (0.6547)	8.7984 (11.8153)

* To make the distributions comparable, results from different benchmarks were translated in such a way that the mean value obtained by MOEA was equal to zero.

Table 10. Average approximation performances of the fuzzy systems built by MOEA+Fuzzy, after 100 generations, tested a random unknown set of 10,000 configurations

Benchmark						
	fir	adpcm-enc	adpcm-dec	mpeg2-dec	ieee810	g721-enc
Average Time (millisecs)						
- Learn*	1.81	1.14	1.15	1.29	1.81	1.05
- Estimate	3.71	2.33	2.35	2.43	3.70	2.28
Average Error (%) in Whole Random Set (all 10,000 configurations) and its Pareto Set						
Whole Set						
- Avg Power	7.27	8.69	7.64	9.55	7.28	8.01
- Exec Time	6.81	9.00	7.66	10.33	6.66	6.93
Pareto Set						
- Avg Power	1.26	1.43	1.21	2.55	2.00	1.77
- Exec Time	2.32	2.67	2.27	3.33	1.52	2.55

* Learning time is the time required to insert a new rule into the Fuzzy System.

Figure 11. mpeg2-decode: *Pareto sets and attainment surfaces obtained by MOEA, MOEA+Fuzzy and ParEGO on a budget of 250 evaluations*

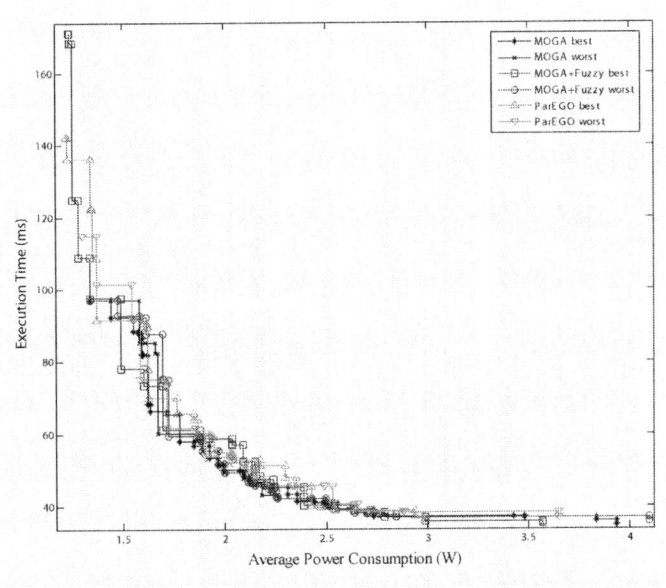

Figure 12. jpeg: *MOEA and the MOEA+Fuzzy attainment surfaces obtained after 100 generations*

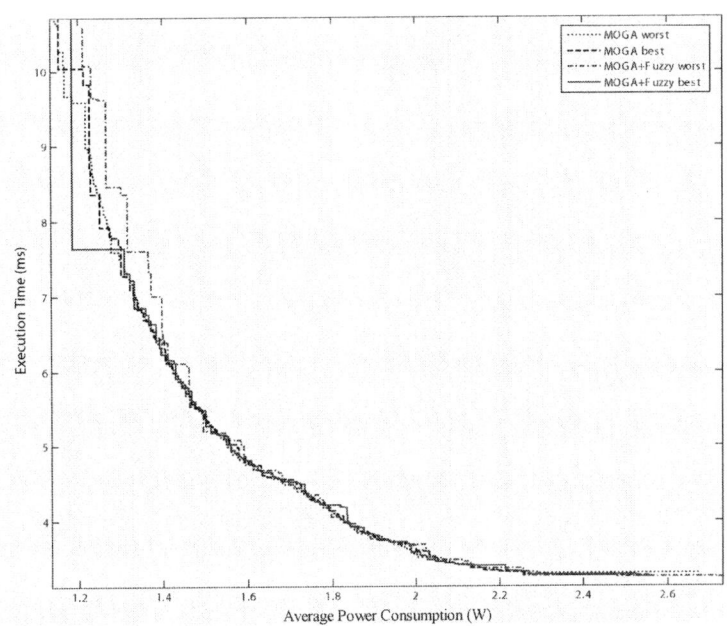

cal equality between the hypervolumes. We can observe that the hypervolume indexes are very close in all the benchmarks and that the average maximum distance between the reference Pareto sets and the MOEA+Fuzzy Pareto sets is 8.7984%, an excellent result compared with the 8.795% obtained by MOEA.

Summarizing results reported in Tables 8 and 9 although MOEA requires three times more evaluations in five benchmarks, its results are not significantly better than MOEA+Fuzzy, that is, we still have a significant probability of getting a better result by using the proposed MOEA+Fuzzy approach and saving 2/3 of the time required by the MOEA approach. This means that for DSE purposes the Pareto sets obtained by the two approaches are the same and obviously MOEA+Fuzzy is preferable because it is 3 times faster. Another consideration is the Pareto approximation quality gain registered by MOEA+Fuzzy when a larger number of evaluations are performed. In fact, comparing the hypervolume results in Tables 6 and 7 we can see that the index has a gain of about 10%. We can also state that the improvement is well distributed along the Pareto front. In fact, 90% of the Pareto points obtained after 100 generations are different (i.e., new configurations) from those obtained with 250 evaluations.

At the end of the evolution the fuzzy system is able to approximate any system configuration. To evaluate its accuracy Table 10 gives the estimation errors for the fuzzy system obtained after 100 generations on a random set of configurations different than those used in the learning phase. Table 10 shows also the time needed for an estimate in a Pentium IV 2.8 GHz workstation: despite the great number of rules it is several orders of magnitude shorter than that of a simulation and the degree of accuracy in estimating the objectives is still high.

FUTURE RESEARCH DIRECTIONS

The use of approximated models within EA-based optimization methods proved to be beneficial whenever dealing with problems which need computationally expensive objective evaluations. New directions are the so called Multidisciplinary design optimization which emphasizes the interaction between modeling and optimization. Although an EA in the presented approach is involved in modeling part, the interaction between EAs and could be strenghtened. Further developments of our work may involve the use of acquired knowledge to create a set of generic linguistic rules to speed up the learning phase, providing an aid for designers and a basis for teaching. An other interesting research direction could be the use of a hierarchy of Artificial Neural Networks to model the embedded system components. Finally, it is interesting the application of the approximation technique by means of a fuzzy system to the other design space exploration approaches as well, with a view to speeding them up.

CONCLUSION

In this chapter we have presented an approach to speed up the evolutionary design of application-specific embedded systems by means of fuzzy approximation. The methodology uses a MOEA for heuristic exploration of the design space and a fuzzy system to evaluate the candidate system configurations to be visited. Our methodology works in two phases: firstly all configurations are evaluated using computationally expensive simulations and their results are used to train the fuzzy system until it becomes reliable; in the second phase the accuracy of the fuzzy system is refined using results obtained by simulating promising configurations. Although the methodology was applied to the design of an embedded architecture based on a Very Long Instruction Word (VLIW) microprocessor in a mobile multimedia application domain, it is of general applicability. Two case studies were considered: in the first one we deal with the optimization of a 2-level memory hierarchy in a commercial processor; in the second one we designed the whole processor. The experiments, carried out on a multimedia benchmark suite demonstrated the scalability and accuracy of the proposed approach in comparison with other related MOEA approaches.

REFERENCES

Abraham, S. G., Rau, B. R., & Schreiber, R. (2000, July). *Fast design space exploration through validity and quality filtering of subsystem designs* (Tech. Rep. No. HPL-2000-98). HP Laboratories Palo Alto.

Ascia, G., Catania, V., & Palesi, M. (2004, August). A GA based design space exploration framework for parameterized system-on-a-chip platforms. *IEEE Transactions on Evolutionary Computation, 8*(4), 329–346.

Ascia, G., Catania, V., & Palesi, M. (2005, April). A multi-objective genetic approach for system-level exploration in parameterized systems-on-a-chip. *IEEE Transactions on Computer-Aided Design of Integrated Circuits and Systems, 24*(4), 635–645.

Ascia, G., Catania, V., Palesi, M., & Patti, D. (2003, October 3–4). EPIC-Explorer: A parameterized VLIW-based platform framework for design space exploration. In *First workshop on embedded systems for real-time multimedia (ESTIMEDIA)* (pp. 65–72). Newport Beach, California.

Austin, T., Larson, E., & Ernst, D. (2002, February). SimpleScalar: An infrastructure for computer system modeling. *IEEE Computer, 35*(2), 59–67.

Buyuksahin, K. M. & Najm, F. N. (2005, July). Early power estimation for VLSI circuits. *IEEE Transactions on Computer-Aided Design, 24*(7), 1076–1088.

Carpenter, W. & Barthelemy, J.-F. (1994). *A comparison of polynomial approximation and artificial neural nets as response surface* (Tech. Rep. 92 – 2247). AIAA.

Chang, H., Cooke, L., Hunt, M., Martin, G., McNelly, A., & Todd, L. (1999). *Surviving the SOC revolution a guide to platform-based design.* Kluwer Academic Publishers.

Eeckhout, L., Nussbaum, S., Smith, J. E., & Bosschere, K. D. (2003, September-October). Statistical simulation: Adding efficiency to the computer designer's toolbox. *IEEE Micro, 23*(5), 26–38.

Eyerman, S., Eeckhout, L., & Bosschere, K. D. (2006). Efficient design space exploration of high performance embedded outof-order processors. In *Date '06: Proceedings of the conference on design, automation and test in europe* (pp. 351–356).

Fisher, J. A. (1983, June). Very long instruction word architectures and the ELI512. In *Tenth annual international symposium on computer architecture* (pp. 140–150).

Fisher, J. A., Faraboschi, P., Brown, G., Desoli, G., & Homewood, F. (2000, June). LX: A technology platform for customizable VLIW embedded processing. In *International symposium on computer architecture* (pp. 203–213).

Fornaciari, W., Sciuto, D., Silvano, C., & Zaccaria, V. (2002). A sensitivity-based design space exploration methodology for embedded systems. *Design Automation for Embedded Systems, 7,* 7–33.

Gaspar-Cunha, A. & Vieira, A. S. (2004, August). A hybrid multi-objective evolutionary algorithm using an inverse neural network. In *Hybrid metaheuristics, workshop at ECAI 2004.*

Gaweda, A. & Zurada, J. (2001, July 16-19). Equivalence between neural networks and fuzzy systems. In *Proceedings of international joint conference on neural networks* (p. 1334-1339).

Ghosh, A. & Givargis, T. (2004, October). Cache optimization for embedded processor cores: An analytical approach. *ACM Transactions on Design Automation of Electronic Systems, 9*(4), 419–440.

Gibbons, J. D. (1985). *Nonparametric statistical inference* (2nd ed.). M. Dekker.

Givargis, T., Vahid, F., & Henkel, J. (2000). A hybrid approach for core-based system-level power modeling. In *Asia and South Pacific Design Automation Conference*.

Givargis, T., Vahid, F., & Henkel, J. (2002, August). System-level exploration for Pareto-optimal configurations in parameterized System-on-a-Chip. *IEEE Transactions on Very Large Scale Integration Systems, 10*(2), 416–422.

Grierson, D. & Pak, W. (1993). Optimal sizing, geometrical and topological design using genetic algorithms. *Journal of Structured Optimization, 6*, 151–159.

Gupta, S. & Najm, F. N. (2000a, July). *Analytical models for RTL power estimation of combinational and sequential circuits*.

Gupta, S. & Najm, F. N. (2000b, February). Power modeling for high-level power estimation. *IEEE Transactions on Very Large Scale Integration Systems, 8*(1), 18–29.

Hekstra, G., Hei, D. L., Bingley, P., & Sijstermans, F. (1999, October 10–13). TriMedia CPU64 design space exploration. In *International conference on computer design* (pp. 599–606). Austin Texas.

Hughes, E. (2003a, April). Multi-objective binary search optimization. In *Lecture notes on computer science*. In *Proceedings of Second International Conference on Evolutionary Multi-Criterion Optimization* (pp. 102–117).

Hughes, E. (2003b, December). Multiple single objective pareto sampling. In *Proceedings of IEEE Congress on Evolutionary Computation, 2003* (Vol. 4, pp. 2678–2684).

Jiang, R., & Sun, C. (1993). Functional equivalence between radial basis function networks and fuzzy inference systems. *IEEE Transactions on Neural Networks, 4*, 156-159.

Jin, Y. (2005). A comprehensive survey of fitness approximation in evolutionary computation. *Soft Computing Journal, 9*, 3–12.

Jin, R., Chen, W., & Simpsons, T. (2000). *Comparative studies of metamodeling techniques under multiple modeling criteria* (Tech. Rep. No. 2000 – 4801). AIAA.

Jin, Y., Olhofer, M., & Sendhoff, B. (2000). On evolutionary optimization with approximate fitness functions. In *Proceedings of genetic and evolutionary computation conference* (pp. 786–793).

Jin, Y., Olhofer, M., & Sendhoff, B. (2002). A framework for evolutionary optimization with approximate fitness function. *IEEE Transactions on Evolutionary Computation, 6*(5), 481–494.

Knowles, J. (2006, February). ParEGO: A hybrid algorithm with on-line landscape approximation for expensive multi-objective optimization problems. *IEEE Transactions on Evolutionary Computation, 10*(1), 50–66.

Knowles, J. & Hughes, E. J. (2005, March). Multi-objective optimization on a budget of 250 evaluations. *Lecture notes on computer science.* In *Proceedings of Third International Conference on Evolutionary Multi-Criterion Optimization* (Vol. 3410, p. 176-190).

Knowles, J. D., Thiele, L., & Zitzler, E. (2006, February). *A tutorial on the performance assessment of stochastive multi-objective optimizers* (Tech. Rep. No. 214). ETH Zurich, Swiss: Computer Engineering and Networks Laboratory.

Landajo, M., Río, M. J., & Pérez, R. (2001, April). A note on smooth approximation capabilities of fuzzy systems. *IEEE Transactions on Fuzzy Systems, 9*, 229–236.

Liao, W., Basile, J., & He, L. (2002, November). Leakage power modeling and reduction with data retention. In *IEEE/ACM International Conference on Computer-Aided Design*.

Liao, W. & He, L. (2001, September). Power modeling and reduction of VLIW processors. In *International Conference on Parallel Architectures and Compilation Techniques* (pp. 81–88).

Mikut, R., Jäkel, J., & Gröll, L. (2005). Interpretability issues in data-based learning of fuzzy systems. *Fuzzy Sets and Systems, 150*, 179–197.

Nain, P. & Deb, K. (2002). *A computationally effective multi-objective search and optimization technique using coarse-to-fine grain modeling* (Tech. Rep. No. Kangal 2002005). Kanpur, India: IITK.

Nair, P. & Keane, A. (1998). Combining approximation concepts with genetic algorithm-based structural optimization procedures. In *Proceeding of 39th AIAA/AASME/ASCE/AHS/ASC Structures, Structural Dynamics and Materials Conference* (p. 1741-1751).

Najm, F. N. (1995, January). A survey of power estimation techniques in VLSI circuits. *IEEE Transactions on Very Large Scale Integration Systems, 2*(4), 446–455.

Najm, F. N. & Nemani, M. (1998). Delay estimation VLSI circuits from a high-level view. In *Conference on Design Automation Conference* (pp. 591–594).

Neema, S., Sztipanovits, J., & Karsai, G. (2002, June). *Design-space construction and exploration in platform-based design* (Tech. Rep. No. ISIS-02-301). Institute for Software Integrated Systems Vanderbilt University Nashville Tennessee.

Patti, D. & Palesi, M. (2003, July). *EPIC-Explorer*. Retrieved February 11, 2008, http://epic-explorer.sourceforge.net/

Ratle, A. (1999). Optimal sampling stategies for learning a fitness model. In *Proceedings of 1999 congress on evolutionary computation* (Vol. 3, p. 2078-2085). Washington, DC.

Redmond, J. & Parker, G. (1996, August). Actuator placement based on reachable set optimization for expected disturbance. *Journal of Optimization Theory and Applications, 90*(2), 279–300.

Sami, M., Sciuto, D., Silvano, C., & Zaccaria, V. (2000). Power exploration for embedded VLIW architectures. In *IEEE/ACM International Conference on Computer Aided Design* (pp. 498–503). San Jose, California: IEEE Press.

Simpsons, T., Mauery, T., Korte, J., & Mistree, F. (1998). *Comparison of response surface and kringing models for multidisciplinary design optimization* (Tech. Rep. No. 98 – 4755). AIAA.

Szymanek, R., Catthoor, F., & Kuchcinski, K. (2004). Time-energy design space exploration for multi-layer memory architectures. In *Design, Automation and Test in Europe* (pp. 181–190).

Takagi, T. & Sugeno, M. (1985). Fuzzy identification of systems and its application to modeling and control. *IEEE Transaction on System, Man and Cybernetics, 15*, 116–132.

Taniguchi, T., Tanaka, K., Ohtake, H., & Wang, H. O. (2001). Model construction, rule reduction, and robust compensation for generalized form of Takagi-Sugeno fuzzy systems. *IEEE Transactions on Fuzzy Systems, 9*(4), 525–538.

Vahid, F. & Givargis, T. (2001, March). Platform tuning for embedded systems design. *IEEE Computer, 34*(3), 112–114.

Vijaykrishnan, N., Kandemir, M., Irwin, M. J., Kim, H. S., Ye, W., (2003, January). Evaluating integrated hardwaresoftware optimizations using a unified energy estimation framework. *IEEE Transactions on Computers, 52*(1), 59–73.

Wang, L.-X. & Mendel, J. M. (1992). Generating fuzzy rules by learning from examples. *IEEE Transactions on System, Man and Cybernetics, 22*, 1414–1427.

Yan, L., Srikanthan, T., & Gang, N. (2006). Area and delay estimation for FPGA implementation of coarse-grained reconfigurable architectures. In *ACM SIGPLAN/SIGBED Conference on Language, Compilers and Tool Support for Embedded Systems* (pp. 182–188).

Zeng, K., Zhang, N.-Y., & Xu, W.-L. (2000, December). A comparative study on sufficient conditions for takagi-sugeno fuzzy systems as universal approximators. *IEEE Transactions on Fuzzy Systems, 8*(6), 773–778.

Zeng, X.-J. & Keane, J. A. (2005, October). Approximation capabilities of hierarchical fuzzy systems. *IEEE Transactions on Fuzzy Systems, 13*(5), 659–672.

Zeng, X.-J. & Singh, M. G. (1996, February). Approximation accuracy analisys of fuzzy systems as function approximators. *IEEE Transactions on Fuzzy Systems, 4*, 44–63.

Zitzler, E., Laumanns, M., & Thiele, L. (2001, September). SPEA2: Improving the performance of the strength pareto evolutionary algorithm. In *EUROGEN 2001 Evolutionary Methods for Design, Optimization and Control with Applications to Industrial Problems* (pp. 95–100). Athens, Greece.

Zitzler, E., Thiele, L., Laumanns, M., Fonseca, C. M., & daFonseca, V. G. (2003, April). Performance assessment of multi-objective optimizers: An analysis and review. *IEEE Transactions on Evolutionary Computation, 7*(2), 117–132.

ADDITIONAL READINGS

Berger, A. S. (2001). *Embedded systems design: An introduction to processes, tools and techniques.* CMP Books.

Coello Coello, Carlos A., Van Veldhuizen, D. A., & Lamont, G. B. (2002, March). *Evolutionary algorithms for solving multi-objective problems.* New York: Kluwer Academic Publishers.

Cordón, O., del Jesus, M. J., & Herrera, F. (1999). *Evolutionary approaches to the learning of fuzzy rule-Based classification systems.* In L.C. Jain (Ed.), *Evolution of enginnering and information systems and their spplications* (pp. 107-160). CRC Press.

Cordón, O., Herrera, F., Hoffmann, F., & Magdalena, L. (2001, July). GENETIC FUZZY SYSTEMS evolutionary tuning and learning of fuzzy knowledge bases. *Advances in fuzzy systems - Applications and theory* (Vol. 19, pp. 462). World Scientific

Deb, K. (2001). *Multi-objective optimization using evolutionary algorithms.* Chichester, UK: John Wiley & Sons.

Dick, R. P. & Jha, N. K. (1998, Oct.). Mogac: A multi-objective genetic algorithm for hardware-software cosynthesis of distributed embedded systems. *IEEE Transactions on Computer-Aided Design of Integrated Circuits and Systems, 17* (10), 920-935.

Eisenring, L. T. & Zitzler, E. (2000, April). Conflicting criteria in embedded system design. *IEEE Design & Test of Computers, 17* (2), 51-59.

Emmerich, M. T., Giannakoglou, K. C., & Naujoks, B. (2006, August). Single- and multi-objective evolutionary optimization assisted by gaussian random field metamodels. *IEEE Transactions on Evolutionary Computation, 10*(4), 421–439.

Erbas, G. (2006). *System-level modeling and design space exploration for multiprocessor em-*

bedded system-on-chip architectures. Amsterdam University Press.

Ganssle, J. (1999). *The art of designing embedded systems*. Newnes.

Grun, A. N. & Dutt, N. D. (2007). *Memory architecture exploration for programmable embedded systems*. Springer.

Goldberg, D. E. (2000). *A meditation on the computational intelligence and its future* (Tech. Rep. No. Illigal 2000019). Illinois Genetic Algorithms Laboratory, University of Illinois at Urbana-Champaign.

Henkel, J. & Li, Y. (2002, August). Avalanche: An environment for design space exploration and optimization of low-power embedded systems. *IEEE Transactions on Very Large Scale Integration (VLSI) Systems, 10* (4), 45-468.

Jin, Y. (Ed.) (2006). *Multi-objective machine learning*. Berlin: Springer.

Klein, R. M. (2007). *Performance measurement and optimization for embedded systems designs*. Newnes.

Marwedel, P. (2004). *Embedded system design*. Springer.

Noergaard, T. (2005). *Embedded systems architecture: A comprehensive guide for engineers and programmers*. Newnes.

Panda, A. N. & Dutt, N. D (1998). *Memory issues in embedded systems-on-chip: Optimizations and exploration*. Springer.

Paenke, I., Branke, J., & Jin, Y. (2006, August). Efficient search for robust solutions by means of evolutionary algorithms and fitness approximation. *IEEE Transactions on Evolutionary Computation, 10*(4), 405–420.

Pimentel, C. E. & Polstra, S. (2006, February). A systematic approach to exploring embedded system architectures at multiple abstraction levels. *IEEE Transactions on Computers, 55* (2), 99-112.

Poloni, C. & Pediroda, V. (1998). GA coupled with computationally expensive simulations: Tools to improve efficiency. In D. Quagliarella, J. Périaux, C. Poloni, & G. Winter (Eds.), *Genetic algorithms and evolution strategies in engineering and computer science. Recent advances and industrial applications* (pp. 267-288). Chichester, UK: John Wiley & Sons.

Sakawa, M. (2002). *Genetic algorithms and fuzzy multi-objective optimization*. Boston: Kluwer Academic Publishers.

Sangiovanni-Vincentelli, A. & Martin, G. (2001, Nov.-Dec.). Platform-based design and software design methodology for embedded systems. *IEEE Design & Test of Computers, 18* (6), 23-33.

Schmitz, B. M. & Eles, P. (2004). *System-level design techniques for energy-efficient embedded systems*. Springer.

Tabbara, A. T. & Sangiovanni-Vincentelli, A. L. (1998). *Function/architecture optimization and co-design of embedded systems*. Springer.

Vahid, F. & Givargis, T. D. (2001). *Embedded system design: A unified hardware/software introduction*. Wiley.

Wattanapongsakorn, N. & Levitan, S. P. (2004, Sept.). Reliability optimization models for embedded systems with multiple applications. *IEEE Transactions on Reliability, 53* (3), 406-416.

ENDNOTE

[1] The LX/ST200 instruction-set simulator has been instrumented with an instruction-level power model which allows to estimate the average power dissipation with an accuracy of 5% as compared with a gate level power analysis (Sami, Sciuto, Silvano, & Zaccaria, 2000).

APPENDIX: ALGORITHMS PSEUDO-CODE

Algorithm 1. SPEA2 Pseudo-Code

1: Initialize population P (internal population) at random
2: Create empty external set E (external population)
3: **while** Stop condition is false **do**
4:    Compute fitness of each individual in P and E
5:    Copy all nondominated individuals in P and E to E
6:    Use the truncation operator to remove elements from E when the capacity has been exceeded
7:    If the capacity of E has not been exceeded then use dominated individuals in P to fill E
8:    Perform binary tournament selection with replacement to filll the mating pool
9:    Apply crossover and mutation to the mating pool
10: **end while**

Algorithm 2. ParEGO Pseudo-Code

1: **procedure** PAREGO(f, d, k, s)
2:   xpop[ ] ← LATINHYPERCUBE(d) /* Initialize using procedure: line 15 */
3:   **for** each i in 1 to 11d − 1 **do**
4:     ypop[i] ← EVALUATE(xpop[i], f) /* See line 36 */
5:   **end for**
6:   **while** not finished **do**
7:     λ ← NEWLAMBDA(k, s) /* See line 19 */
8:     model ← DACE(xpop[ ], ypop[ ], λ) /* See line 22 */
9:     xnew ← EVOLALG(model, xpop[ ]) /* See line 28 */
10:     xpop[ ] ← xpop[ ] ∪ {xnew}
11:     ynew ← EVALUATE(xnew, f)
12:     ypop[ ] ← ypop[ ] ∪ {ynew}
13:   **end while**
14: **end procedure**
15: **procedure** LATINHYPERCUBE(d)
16:   divide each dimension of search space into 11d − 1 'rows' of equal width
17:   **return** 11d − 1 vectors x such that no two share the same 'row' in any dimension
18: **end procedure**
19: **procedure** NEWLAMBDA(k, s)
20:   **return** a k-dimensional scalarizing weight vector chosen uniformly at random from amongst all those defined by the equation $\Lambda = \{\lambda = (\lambda_1, \lambda_2, \ldots, \lambda_k) \mid \sum_{j=1}^{k} \lambda_j = 1 \wedge \forall j, \lambda_j = l/s, l \in 0..s\}$,
21: **end procedure**
22: **procedure** DACE(xpop[ ], ypop[ ], λ)
23:   compute the scalar fitness fλ of every cost vector in ypop[ ], using equation 2
24:   choose a subset of the population based on the computed scalar fitness values
25:   maximize the likelihood of the DACE model for the chosen population subset
26:   **return** the parameters of the maximum likelihood DACE model
27: **end procedure**
28: **procedure** EVOLALG(model, xpop[ ])
29:   initialize a temporary population of solution vectors, some as mutants of xpop[ ] and others purely randomly
30:   **while** set number of evaluations not exceeded **do**

31:    evaluate the expected improvement of solutions using the model
32:    select, recombine and mutate to form new population
33: **end while**
34: **return** best evolved solution
35: **end procedure**
36: **procedure** EVALUATE(x, f)
37:    call the expensive evaluation function f with the solution vector x
38: **return** true cost vector y of solution x
39: **end procedure**

Chapter XI
Walking with EMO:
Multi-Objective Robotics for Evolving Two, Four, and Six-Legged Locomotion

Jason Teo
Universiti Malaysia Sabah, Malaysia

Lynnie D. Neri
Universiti Malaysia Sabah, Malaysia

Minh H. Nguyen
University of New South Wales, Australia

Hussein A. Abbass
University of New South Wales, Australia

ABSTRACT

This chapter will demonstrate the various robotics applications that can be achieved using evolutionary multi-objective optimization (EMO) techniques. The main objective of this chapter is to demonstrate practical ways of generating simple legged locomotion for simulated robots with two, four and six legs using EMO. The operational performance as well as complexities of the resulting evolved Pareto solutions that act as controllers for these robots will then be analyzed. Additionally, the operational dynamics of these evolved Pareto controllers in noisy and uncertain environments, limb dynamics and effects of using a different underlying EMO algorithm will also be discussed.

INTRODUCTION

Although multi-objective optimization (MO) and evolutionary multi-objective optimization (EMO) techniques have been used successfully in numerous engineering and scientific applications (Coello Coello, van Veldhuizen, & Lamont, 2002; Deb, 2001) there is much less work that applies these techniques to robotics. Being a highly complex endeavor, the automatic generation of robots with multiple distinct and useful behavioral as well as morphological characteristics can be highly beneficial. One possible way of achieving this is through the use of EMO techniques, which can automatically synthesize robots with multiple distinct characteristics in a single evolutionary run (Teo & Abbass, 2004). For an introduction to EMO techniques, the reader may refer to Chapter 1.

In this chapter, we will attempt to demonstrate the various robotics applications that can be achieved using EMO techniques. The main objective is to demonstrate practical means of generating simple legged locomotion for simulated robots with two, four and six legs using EMO and then presenting the operational performance as well as complexities of the resulting evolved Pareto solutions that act as controllers for these robots. The use of simulated robotics should not be discounted here as it has been recently shown that the use of simulation in evolutionary robotics is particularly beneficial in the training phase of automatic behavior generation in real physical robots (Walker, Garrett, & Wilson, 2003). Furthermore, we will provide additional discussions on the operational dynamics of these evolved Pareto controllers in noisy and uncertain environments, limb dynamics as well as effects of using a different underlying EMO algorithm on the Pareto evolutionary optimization process.

The remainder of this chapter is divided into five main sections, namely, the (1) previous studies on MO and robotics (Section 2), (2) the artificial evolution and virtual simulation setup (Section 3), (3) application of EMO to the automatic generation of legged locomotion in a biped, quadruped and hexapod (Section 4), (4) operational and limb dynamics analysis using the quadruped (Section 5), and (5 comparison of two different EMO algorithms for driving the Pareto evolutionary optimization process for generating locomotion controllers using the quadruped (Section 6). More specifically, the technical contributions are organized as follows:

- Presentation of the EMO algorithm for the automatic evolution of artificial neural network controllers (ANNs) that maximize horizontal locomotion as one objective and minimize controller complexity as another objective is given in Section 4.1;
- Presentation and discussion of results for the evolved Pareto controllers for autonomous locomotion of simulated robots with two, four and six legs is given in Section 4.2;
- Empirical comparison of the evolved complexities for the bipedal, quadrupedal and hexapedal robots using an EMO approach is given in Section 4.2
- Analysis of the operational dynamics under noisy conditions is given in Section 5.1;
- Analysis of the operational dynamics beyond the evolutionary window is given in Section 5.2;
- Qnalysis of the evolved limb dynamics is given in Section 5.3;
- Empirical comparison of different EMO algorithms for evolving Pareto locomotion controllers is given in Section 6.1.

PREVIOUS WORKS ON EVOLUTIONARY ROBOTICS AND MULTI-OBJECTIVE OPTIMIZATION

Evolutionary robotics is defined to be the synthesis of autonomous robots using artificial evolutionary methods (Nolfi & Floreano, 2000). An early review of this field of research is given by Mataric and Cliff (1996) where the majority of studies focused mainly on the evolution of control structures. A more recent overview highlights the move of evolutionary robotics into evolving both the control and morphology of robots where the interplay between brain and body is considered to be a crucial factor in the successful synthesis of autonomous robots (Nolfi & Floreano, 2002). Another recent review was conducted by Walker et al. (2003) covering both simulated and physical evolutionary robotics. A thorough treatment of the field can be found in the seminal textbook written by Nolfi and Floreano (2000) on this subject. A more recent text by Wang, Tan, and Chew (2006) covers algorithmic implementations of genetic algorithms applied to evolvable hardware, FPGA-based autonomous robots as well as humanoid robots involving evolution of bipedal gaits. Also, a very recent paper presents some interesting perspectives from a developmental point of view when analyzing the results of an evolutionary robotics experiment (Nelson & Grant, 2006).

MO has been used to generate action selection modules in a behavior-based robotics experiment (Pirjanian, 1998; 2000). However, this study utilized conventional mathematical optimization methods and did not make use of an evolutionary optimization approach. EMO was used for a robotics design problem but this experiment involved only a nonautonomous subject in the form of an attached robotic manipulator arm (Coello Coello, Christiansen, & Aguirre, 1998). EMO was also used in another robotics application although it was used for optimizing the physical configurations of modular robotic components rather than for the generation of autonomous robotic controllers (Leger, 1999). There have been a number of other studies involving the use of some form of EMO for the design of attached robotic manipulator arms (Coello Coello et al. 2002). Evolutionary methods have been used to solve autonomous navigational problems with multiple objectives but only for 2D mobile agents in simulation (Dozier, McCullough, Homaifar, Tunstel, & Moore, 1998; Gacogne, 1997; 1999; Kim & Hallam, 2002).

A limited study using EMO methods for generating bipedal gaits in simulation for an abstract two-legged robot has also been reported (Lee & Lee, 2004). An EMO algorithm has also been used to tune fuzzy controllers for a forklift docking maneuvering problem (Lucas, Martinez-Barbera, & Jimenez, 2005). A recent series of studies (Barlow & Oh, 2006; Barlow, Oh, & Grant, 2004; Oh & Barlow, 2004) have also demonstrated in simulation that a multi-objective genetic programming (GP) system can be successfully applied to the evolution of controllers for unmanned aerial vehicles (UAVs), although it was interesting to note that the multi-objective evolutionary system required an enormous amount of computational power to evolve the controllers (Beowulf cluster with 92 Pentium 4 machines). These controllers were later shown to be transferable to a mobile wheeled robot by reconstructing the UAV's task environment using a mobile robot platform as a precursor to full transference from simulated to real-world UAVs (Barlow & Oh, 2005).

As can be seen, there is a serious lack of literature available in terms of applying EMO for the generation of autonomous robot behavior. Furthermore, the limited studies that are available focused only on highly restricted movements in 2D. Only very recently has a comprehensive study been reported in the literature on the use of EMO for automatic generation of legged locomotion controllers in a fully continuous 3D environment (Teo & Abbass, 2004). In this chapter, we will not only demonstrate the use of EMO for evolving an autonomous, embodied and situated quadruped in a fully continuous 3D environment but also for bipeds and hexapods. This will represent a first comprehensive report on the application of EMO for the automatic generation of two, four and six-legged locomotion, including an empirical comparison of the related evolved complexities across the three inherently different robot morphologies. Moreover, this chapter will also contain new results on the operational and limb dynamics as well as the effects of using different EMO algorithms for multi-objective robotics.

ATIFICIAL EVOLUTION AND VIRTUAL SIMULATION SETUP

Physics Engine

The accurate modeling of the simulation environment plays a crucial part in producing virtual embodied organisms that move and behave realistically in 3D. A dynamic rather than kinematic approach is paramount in allowing effective artificial evolution to occur (Taylor & Massey, 2001). Physical properties such as forces, torques, inertia, friction, restitution and damping need to be incorporated into the artificial evolutionary system. To this end, the Vortex physics engine (CM Labs, 2007) was employed to generate the physically realistic artificial creature and its simulation environment. Vortex is a physics-based simulation toolkit consisting of a set of C++ routines for robust rigid-body dynamics, collision detection, contact creation, and collision response. However, as Vortex is a constraint-based simulation, it suffers from increasingly higher computational requirements as the number of simulated joints connecting objects together in the world increases. As such, the design of the artificial creature and its world are kept relatively simple in order to maintain a reasonable run time, especially when conducting the evolutionary experiments.

Simulated Robot Morphologies

Four different robot morphologies were simulated in this study (Figure 1): (1) a biped with two legs and a length-wise torso orientation, (2) a biped with two legs and a breadth-wise torso orientation, (3) a quadruped with four legs, (4) a hexapod with six legs. The torsos of the bipeds and quadruped are connected to the upper leg limbs using hinge joints (one degree of freedom) and the upper limbs are connected to the lower limbs using hinge joints as well. The hexapod has a torso which is connected to its legs using insect hip joints. Each insect hip joint consists of two hinges, making it a joint with two degrees of freedom: one to control the back-and-forth swinging and another for the lifting of the leg. Each leg has an upper limb connected to a lower limb by a hinge joint. The hinges are actuated by motors whose target velocities are determined through the outputs of the ANN controller. The inputs to

Figure 1. Screen capture of the 1. biped with length-wise torso orientation (top left), 2. biped with breadth-wise torso orientation (top right), 3. quadruped (bottom left), 4. hexapod (bottom right) simulated robots

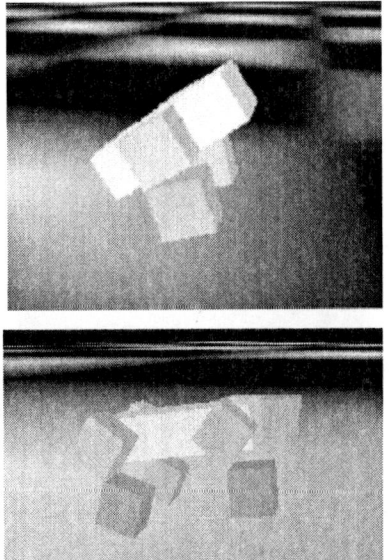
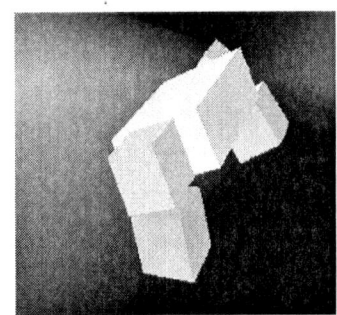
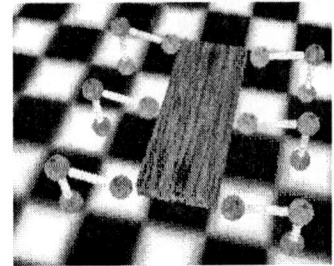

the controller consist of touch sensors located on the lower limbs and joint angle sensor present in every hinge joint.

Table 1 presents a comparison of the main features of the different simulated robot morphologies. It would appear that the biped has a much simpler design compared quadruped and hexapod, and similarly, the quadruped to the hexapod. However, this is only a subjective observation from a human designer's perspective. It remains to be seen whether this view will hold when we compare the complexities of these four different robot morphologies from the controller's and behavior's perspectives (see Section 4.2).

Evolutionary Objectives

The Pareto-frontier of our evolutionary runs are obtained from optimizing two conflicting objectives: (1) maximizing horizontal locomotion distance of the artificial creature denoted as fitness function f_1, and (2) minimizing the number of hidden units used in the ANN that act as the creature's controller denoted as fitness function f_2. The formulations of the optimization problem are given below:

$$\text{Maximize } f_1 = d(\vec{g}) \quad (1)$$

$$\text{Minimize } f_2 = \sum_{i=0}^{H} h_i \quad (2)$$

where $d(g)$ represents the horizontal distance achieved by a simulated robot as controlled by the ANN represented in the genotype $\vec{g}$, and h_i represents if the ith hidden node is active ($h_i = 1$) or not ($h_i = 0$) in the hidden layer of the ANN with H representing the maximum allowable number of nodes in the hidden layer.

The Evolutionary Neural Network Algorithm and Controller

An ANN may be described as a directed graph: $G(N,\omega,\psi)$, where N is a set of nodes, ω denotes the connections between the nodes, and ψ represents the learning rule which enables the strengths of inter-neuron connections to be automatically adjusted. A node receives its inputs from an external source or from other nodes in the network. The node undertakes some processing on its inputs and sends the result as its output. The activation, a, is calculated as a weighted sum of the inputs to the node in addition to a constant value called the bias. The processing function of a node, σ, is called the activation function. In this work, the activation function is taken to be the sigmoidal function, hence applying σ to a gives $\sigma(a) = \dfrac{1}{1+e^{-Da}}$, where D represents the functions steepness, which is set to a value of 1 here.

The ANN architecture used in this study is a fully connected feed-forward network with recurrent connections on the hidden units as well as direct input-output connections. Recurrent connections were included to allow the creature's controller to learn time-dependent dynamics of

Table 1. A comparison of the simulated bipeds, quadruped and hexapod robot's morphological characteristics

Morphological Characteristic	Biped	Quadruped	Hexapod
No. of legs	2	4	6
Degrees of freedom	4	8	24
No. of sensors	6	12	24
No. of motors	4	8	18

the system. Direct input-output connections were also included in the controller's architecture to allow for direct sensor-motor mappings to evolve that do not require hidden layer transformations. Bias is incorporated in the calculation of the activation of the hidden as well as output layers. A diagrammatic representation of part of the ANN architecture is illustrated in Figure 2.

Traditionally ANNs are trained using learning algorithms such as *back-propagation* (BP) (Rumelhart, Hinton, & Williams, 1986) to determine the connection weights between nodes. However such methods are gradient-based techniques which usually suffer from the inability to escape from local minima when attempting to optimize the connection weights. To overcome this problem, evolutionary approaches have been proposed as an alternative method for optimizing the connection weights. ANNs evolved via this method are thus referred to as evolutionary ANNs (EANNs). In the literature, research into EANNs usually involves one of three approaches: (1) evolving the weights of the network (Belew, McInerney, & Schraudolph, 1992; Fogel, Fogel, & Porto, 1990), (2) evolving the architecture (Kitano, 1990; Miller, Todd, & Hegde, 1989), or (3) evolving both simultaneously (Angeline, Saunders, & Pollack, 1994; Koza & Rice, 1991). For a thorough review of EANNs, refer to the comprehensive survey conducted by (Yao, 1999). In this work, both the weights and the architecture of the ANN controller are evolved, which will be described the in the following section.

Genotype Representation

Let I be the number of inputs, H the number of hidden units, and O the number of outputs. The genotype is a class with an $(I+H)\times(H+O)$ dimension matrix $\vec{\Omega}$, an H dimension vector $\vec{\rho}$, δ as the crossover rate and η as the mutation rate. Our chromosome is a class that contains one matrix $\vec{\Omega}$ and one vector $\vec{\rho}$. The matrix $\vec{\Omega}$ is of dimension $(I+H)\times(H+O)$. Each element $\omega_{ij} \in \vec{\Omega}$, is the weight connecting unit i with unit j, where $i=0,\ldots,(I-1)$ is the input unit i, $i=I,\ldots,(I+H-1)$ is the hidden unit $(i-I)$, $j=0,\ldots,(H-1)$ is the hidden unit j, and $j=H,\ldots,(H+O-1)$ is the output unit $(j-H)$.

The vector $\vec{\rho}$ is of dimension H, where $h_i \in \vec{\rho}$ is a binary value used to indicate if the ith hidden unit of h is active in the ANN or not. As such, it works as a switch to turn a hidden unit on or off. The sum, $\sum_{i=0}^{H} h_i$, represents the number of active hidden units in a network, where H is the maximum number of hidden units. The use of $\vec{\rho}$ allows a hidden node to evolve even if it is not

Figure 2. Neural network architecture

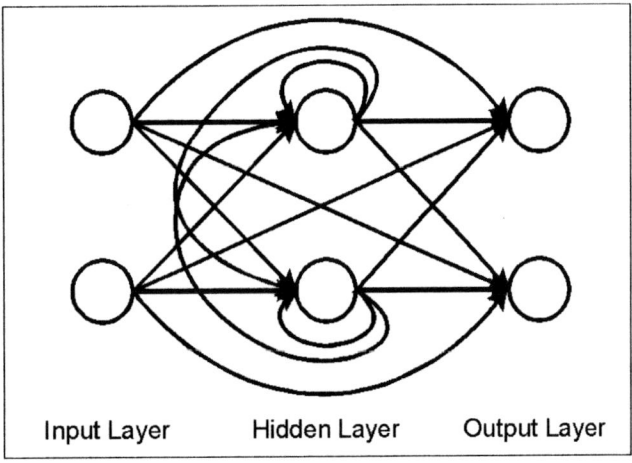

active during certain periods of the evolutionary optimization process.

The chromosome has two additional components when the crossover and mutation rates are also subjected to evolutionary optimization and self-adapted in the algorithms. These additional elements are the crossover rate δ and the mutation rate η. The addition of these last two elements to the genotype representation allows simultaneous training of the weights in the network and selecting a subset of hidden units as well as allowing for the self-adaptation of crossover and mutation rates during optimization.

A direct encoding method was chosen to represent these variables in the genotype as an easy-to-implement and simple-to-understand encoding scheme. Other more complex direct as well as indirect encoding schemes such as those involving developmental mechanisms may prove to be useful and represent possible future work extending from this investigation. A summary of the variables used in the chromosome to represent the artificial creature's genotype is listed in Table 2. The mapping of the chromosome into the ANN is depicted in Figure 3.

Table 2. Description of the variables used in the chromosome to represent the artificial creature's genotype

Variable	Representing	Value Type	Value Range
$\vec{\Omega}$	ANN Connection Weights	Real	$]-\infty,+\infty[$
$\vec{\rho}$	Status of Hidden Units	Discrete	$\{0,1\}$
δ	Crossover Rate	Real	$[0,1]$
η	Mutation Rate	Real	$[0,1]$

Figure 3. A diagram illustrating the mapping from a chromosome to an ANN controller

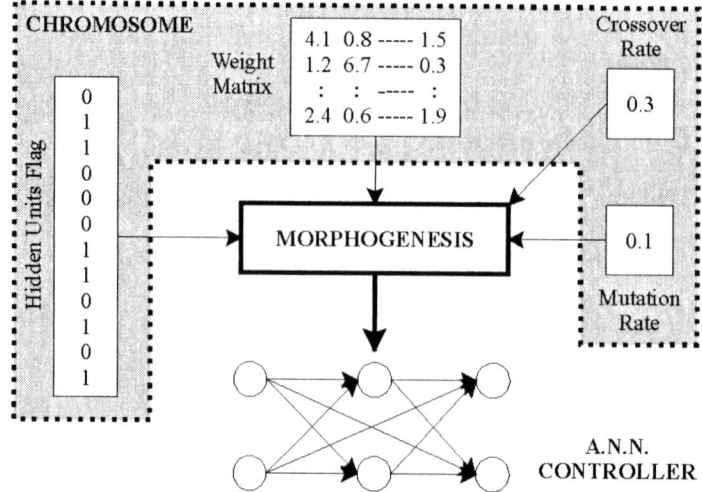

EMO-BASED GENERATION OF 2, 4 AND 6-LEGGED LOCOMOTION

We used the SPANN (Self-adaptive Pareto Artificial Neural Network) algorithm (Abbass, 2003) to drive the artificial evolutionary process, which is a Pareto evolutionary multi-objective optimization algorithm based on the *Differential Evolution* algorithm (Storn & Price, 1995) that self-adapts the crossover and mutation rates. SPANN allows for the simultaneous optimization of the connection weights and hidden layer architecture of evolved ANNs. In this work, we propose a modified version of SPANN for controller evolution which we denote as SPANN-R. There are two major differences between SPANN and SPANN-R. Firstly, in SPANN, back-propagation is used for local search, while in SPANN-R it is not. Secondly, the truncation repair function used in SPANN for evolving the crossover and mutation rates, although useful for the data-mining task, was found to cause premature convergence of these rates to the lower boundary of 0 in our problem. Consequently, the evolutionary process would also prematurely stagnate due to the lack of crossover and mutation during reproduction. Hence a new repair function is proposed in SPANN-R to overcome this problem, which is described in the following section.

SPANN-R Algorithm for Multi-Objective Evolution of Robotic Controllers

The pseudocode for the SPANN-R algorithm is as follows:

1. Create a random initial population of potential solutions. The elements of the weight matrix $\vec{\Omega}$ are assigned random values according to a Gaussian distribution $N(0,1)$. The elements of the binary vector $\vec{\rho}$ are assigned the value 1 with probability 0.5 based on a randomly generated number according to a uniform distribution between [0,1]; otherwise 0. The crossover rate δ and mutation rate η are assigned random values according to a uniform distribution between [0,1].
2. Repeat
   a. Evaluate the individuals in the population and label those who are nondominated.
   b. If the number of nondominated individuals is less than 3 repeat the following until the number of nondominated individuals is greater than or equal to 3:
      i. Find a nondominated solution among those who are not labelled.
      ii. Label the solution as nondominated.
   c. Delete all dominated solutions from the population.
   d. Repeat
      i. Select at random an individual as the main parent α_1, and two individuals, α_2, α_3 as supporting parents.
      ii. Select at random a variable z from $\vec{\Omega}$.
      iii. **Crossover:** With some probability

$Uniform(0,1) < \delta^{\alpha_1}$ or if $\omega_{xy} = z$, do

$$\omega_{xy}^{child} \leftarrow \omega_{xy}^{\alpha_1} + N(0,1)(\omega_{xy}^{\alpha_2} - \omega_{xy}^{\alpha_3}) \quad (3)$$

$$h_i^{child} \leftarrow \begin{cases} 1 & if \ (h_i^{\alpha_1} + N(0,1)(h_i^{\alpha_2} - h_i^{\alpha_3})) \geq 0.5 \\ 0 & otherwise \end{cases} \quad (4)$$

$$\delta^{child} \leftarrow \delta^{\alpha_1} + N(0,1)(\delta^{\alpha_2} - \delta^{\alpha_3}) \quad (5)$$

$$\eta^{child} \leftarrow \eta^{\alpha_1} + N(0,1)(\eta^{\alpha_2} - \eta^{\alpha_3}) \qquad (6)$$

otherwise

$$\omega_{xy}^{child} \leftarrow \omega_{xy}^{\alpha_1} \qquad (7)$$

$$h_i^{child} \leftarrow h_i^{\alpha_1} \qquad (8)$$

$$\delta^{child} \leftarrow \delta^{\alpha_1} \qquad (9)$$

$$\eta^{child} \leftarrow \eta^{\alpha_1} \qquad (10)$$

where each variable in the main parent is perturbed by adding to it a ratio, $F \in N(0,1)$, of the difference between the two values of this variable in the two supporting parents. At least one variable in $\bar{\Omega}$ must be changed. If δ or η are not in [0,1], repair by adding (if <0) or subtracting (if >1) a random number between [0,1] until δ and η are in [0,1].

iv. **Mutation:** With some probability $Uniform(0,1) < \eta^{\alpha_1}$, do

$$\omega_{xy}^{child} \leftarrow \omega_{xy}^{child} + N(0, \eta^{\alpha_1}) \qquad (11)$$

$$h_i^{child} \leftarrow \begin{cases} 1 & \text{if } h_{timesteps}^{child} = 0 \\ 0 & \text{otherwise} \end{cases} \qquad (12)$$

$$\delta^{child} \leftarrow N(0,1) \qquad (13)$$

$$\eta^{child} \leftarrow N(0,1) \qquad (14)$$

Until the population size is M
Until maximum number of generations is reached.

The first round of labeling (**step 2a**) finds nondominated solutions in the first generation which may number less than 3. The reproduction process in SPANN-R requires at least 3 individuals to create offspring for the next generation. As such, if the number of nondominated solutions is less than 3 (**step 2b**), a second round of labeling is carried out among the nondominated solutions of the next Pareto-front (**step 2bi**). The random variable z (**step 2dii**) is used to ensure that at least one element in the weight matrix Ω is changed during the reproduction process, which is guaranteed by the condition $\omega_{xy} = z$ (**step 2diii**).

Experimental Setup

In this first set of experiments, 10 evolutionary runs were conducted using SPANN-R for each of the three different robot morphologies respectively, which are the biped, quadruped and hexapod. The two distinct objectives to be optimized as explained earlier were (1) maximization of the locomotion distance achieved denoted as fitness function and (2) minimization of the usage of hidden units in the ANN controller denoted as fitness function. The resulting solutions thus form a set of Pareto optimal solutions that trade-off between locomotion distance achieved and size of the ANN's hidden layer. The evolutionary parameters were set as follows in all experiments: 1000 generations, 30 individuals, maximum of 15 hidden units and 500 timesteps. One timestep in the simulation corresponds to an elapsed time of 0.02 seconds in real time.

First, we present all the Pareto optimal solutions found from applying the SPANN-R EMO algorithm over the 10 runs for generating locomotion behavior for the biped as well as a table which summarizes the global Pareto optimal solutions over the 10 runs. Then we present the results obtained for the quadruped followed by the hexapod in a similar fashion. Finally, we compare the between the evolved controller complexities of the different simulated robot morphologies in the last subsection.

Evolved Pareto Controllers for Two-Legged Locomotion

The evolved Pareto controllers for the two different biped morphologies are plotted in Figures 4 and 5 from each of the 10 evolutionary runs. For the biped with the length-wise torso, the solutions appeared to be highly clustered around a locomotion distance of between 8 and 11 with the majority of ANNs having 5 or less number of hidden units. On the other hand, the solutions for the breadth-wise biped were less clustered and had a wider spread of solutions that achieved locomotion distances of between 8 and 16. Again, most of the Pareto controllers had less than 5 hidden units with the exception of two runs which had up to six, which were similar to the length-wise biped.

Table 3 lists the global Pareto solutions for the two different biped robots. Although the length-wise biped had one more global Pareto solution that the breadth-wise biped, the overall locomotion achieved was more successful in the breadth-wise biped. All the solutions of the length-wise biped were dominated the breath-wise biped, so it can be concluded that under the simulated conditions of this experiment, it was easier to evolve bipedal locomotion using a breadth-wise orientation than a length-wise orientation of the torso. It is also interesting to note that larger ANNs found it difficult to compete with the smaller-sized controllers, which shows that 5 to 6 units in the hidden layer was sufficient for the bipedal to have successful locomotion. Another interesting point to note is that controllers with no hidden units that are controllers with direct input-output connections could also generate rather successful locomotion behavior.

Evolved Pareto Controllers for Four-Legged Locomotion

The Pareto-fronts achieved at the last generation for each of the 10 runs are plotted in Figure 6. It

Figure 4. Pareto-frontiers of controllers obtained from 10 runs for the biped with length-wise torso. X-axis: Locomotion distance, Y-axis: No. of hidden units

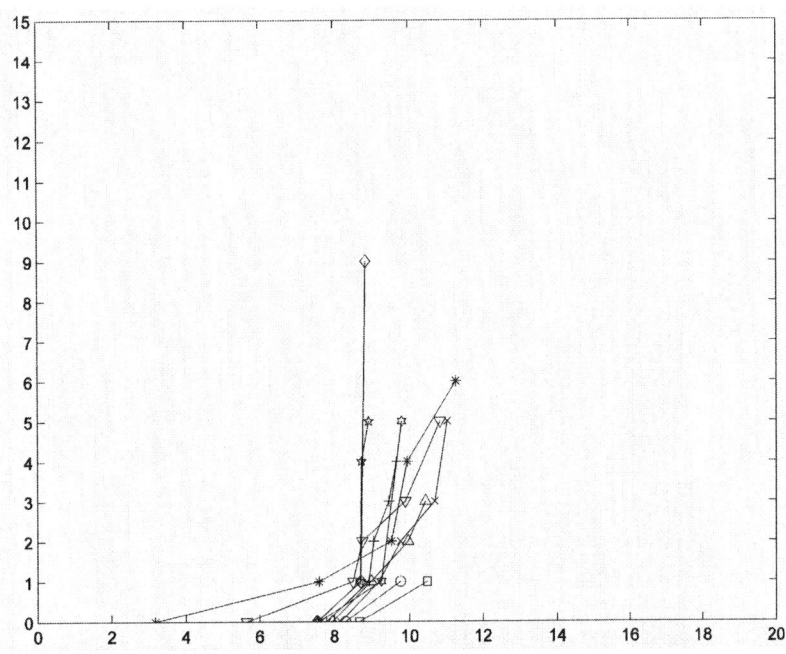

Figure 5. Pareto-frontiers of controllers obtained from 10 runs for the biped with breadth-wise torso. X-axis: Locomotion distance, Y-axis: No. of hidden units

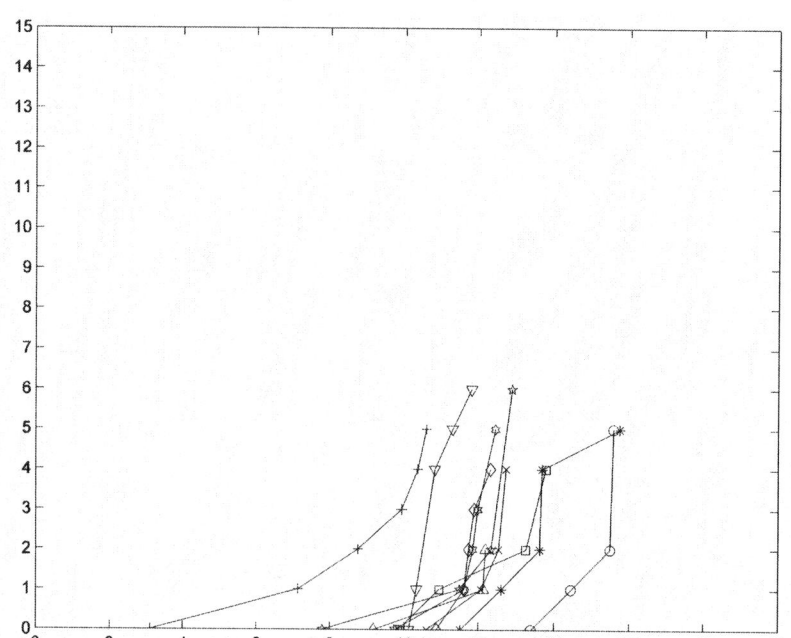

Table 3. Comparison of number of hidden units used and locomotion distance for global Pareto optimal controllers obtained using the SPANN-R algorithm over 10 independent runs for the biped with both length-wise (top) and breadth-wise (bottom) torso orientation

Torso Orientation	No. of Hidden Units	Locomotion Distance
Length-Wise	0	8.6756
	1	10.4819
	3	10.6918
	5	11.0339
	6	11.2686
Breadth-Wise	0	13.3918
	1	14.4495
	2	14.4495
	5	15.7481

can be noticed that a variety of solutions in terms of controller size and locomotion capability was obtained in the majority of the evolutionary runs. The solutions on the Pareto-frontier comprised of controllers ranging between 0 and 9 hidden units with the majority using less than 5 hidden units in the ANN. This is an indication that larger networks did not offer significant advantages in terms of generating better locomotion capabilities compared to smaller networks. The locomotion

Figure 6. Pareto-frontiers of controllers obtained from 10 runs for the quadruped. X-axis: Locomotion distance, Y-axis: No. of hidden units

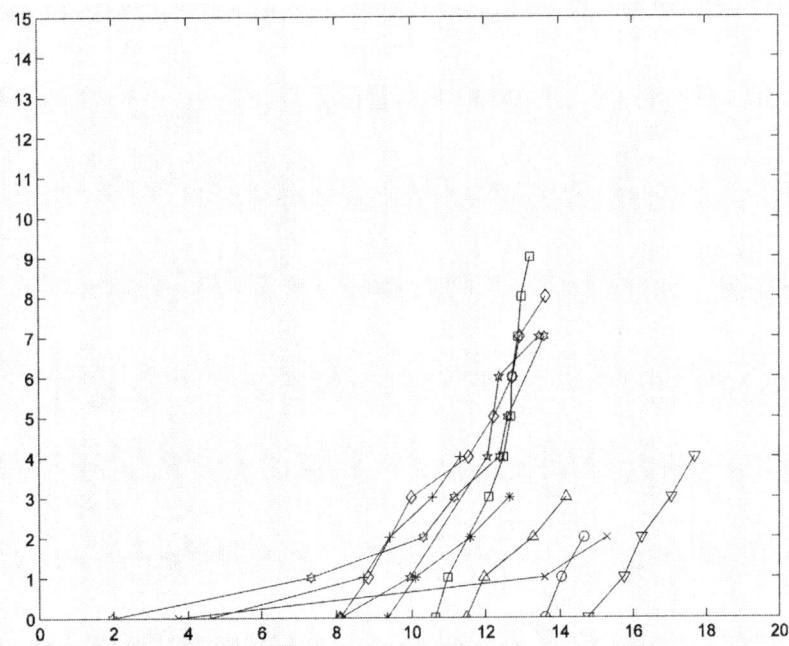

Table 4. Comparison of number of hidden units used and locomotion distance for global Pareto optimal controllers obtained using the SPANN-R algorithm over 10 independent runs for the quadruped

No. of Hidden Units	Locomotion Distance
0	14.7730
1	15.7506
2	16.2295
3	17.0663
4	17.6994

achieved ranged between 2 up to almost 15. It is interesting to note that controllers with direct input-output connections (i.e., solutions on the Pareto front with 0 hidden units) could achieve sufficiently good locomotion capabilities without requiring a hidden layer. The ability of such *pure reactive* agents for solving complex sensory-motor coordination tasks have previously been reported in wheeled robots (Lund & Hallam, 1997; Nolfi, 2002; Pasemann, Steinmetz, Hulse, & Lara, 2001). These direct connections between the input and output layers also appeared to have generated Pareto optimal networks with smaller sizes in a large majority of the runs. This may be due to the fact that the direct input-output connections are already providing a good mechanism for basic locomotion, thus requiring only a few extra hidden units to further improve on this basic locomotion.

Figure 7. Pareto-frontiers of controllers obtained from 10 runs for the hexapod. X-axis: Locomotion distance, Y-axis: No. of hidden units

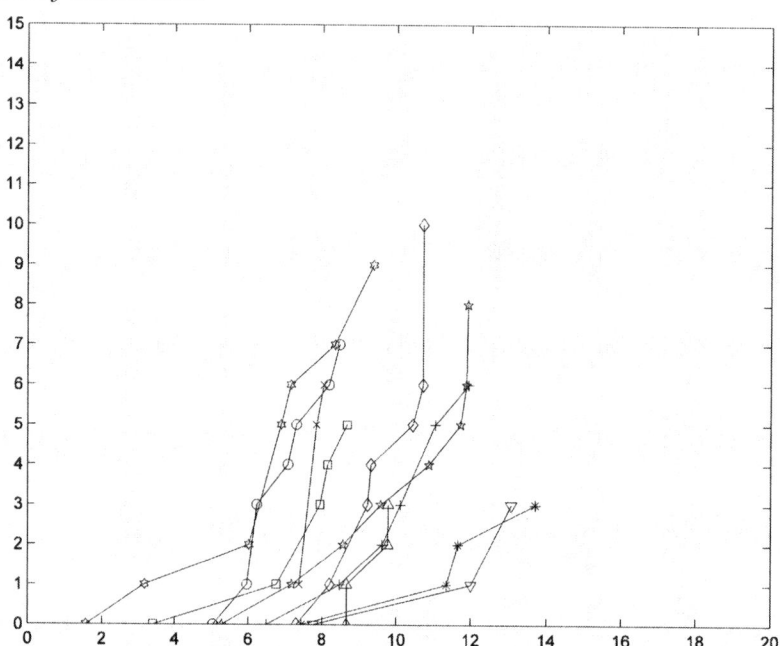

Table 5. Comparison of number of hidden units used and locomotion distance for global Pareto optimal controllers obtained using the SPANN-R algorithm over 10 independent runs for the hexapod

No. of Hidden Units	Locomotion Distance
0	8.6772
1	12.0020
3	13.7040

Table 4 lists the global Pareto optimal solutions found by SPANN-R over the 10 runs. It is interesting to note that by allowing direct input-output connections, controllers which did not use the hidden layer at all (0 hidden units) could generate a sufficiently good locomotion ability, moving the creature up to a distance of 14.7-14.8 units. This is empirical proof that perceptron-like controllers, which rely only on input-to-output connections without any internal nodes, are sufficient for generating simple locomotion in a four-legged artificial creature. As such, robots that are only required to perform simple tasks can be evolved as purely reactive agents, which would dramatically simplify the process of synthesizing successful robot controllers.

Evolved Pareto Controllers for Six-Legged Locomotion

Similar to the quadruped, there was a range of values obtained in terms of the final Pareto controllers obtained from the EMO process as shown in Figure 7. The locomotion distances ranged from just under 2 to almost 14 while the number of hidden units used in the ANN ranged from 0 to 10. These results are similar to what was obtained with the quadruped but were slightly inferior both in terms of the locomotion distances achieved as well as the number of hidden units used. In general, in can also be seen from the individual Pareto curves that the evolved hexapod controllers required the use of more hidden units to achieve locomotion compared to the quadruped, where only four runs evolved nondominated solutions that used 5 or more hidden units compared to seven runs in the hexapod.

In terms of the overall global Pareto controllers obtained over the 10 runs, only three solutions remain nondominated as compared to five obtained using the quadruped. Furthermore, the locomotion distances achieved were all lower compared to the quadruped. This suggests that it was a harder task to evolve six-legged locomotion compared to four-legged locomotion. A more objective comparison in this vein is given in the next section where the resulting Pareto solutions are used as a complexity measure when comparing the evolved behavior against the different morphologies. However, it is interesting to note again that direct input-output connections were sufficient for generating a reasonable amount of locomotion as achieved by the controller with 0 hidden units.

Complexity Comparison Between Bipedal, Quadrupedal and Hexapedal Controllers

The locomotion distances achieved by the different Pareto solutions will provide a common ground where locomotion competency can be used to compare different behaviors and morphologies. It will provide a set of ANNs with the smallest hidden layer capable of achieving a variety of locomotion competencies. The structural definition of the evolved ANNs can now be used as a measure of complexity for the different creature behaviors and morphologies.

Figure 8 plots the global Pareto-front for both the two bipeds, quadruped and hexapod. As such, we are comparing four different Pareto-fronts that characterize the complexities of four different robot morphologies. From the graph, it is clear that it was hardest to evolve successful locomotion for the biped with length-wise torso orientation compared to all the other morphologies since all of its solutions are dominated by the other robot morphologies except the Pareto solution with no hidden units, which is very similar to the hexapod. It also provides an interesting view when it is seen that the hexapod was also quite a difficult morphology to evolve locomotion, and in fact was completed dominated by the solutions found for the biped with breadth-wise torso orientation. So although the hexapod had pre-designed static stability, the requirement for coordination and synchronization between six legs very likely outweighed the requirement for the biped to generate sufficient stability. This was also probably assisted by the help of the change in the torso orientation from length-wise to breadth-wise in the biped, which reduced the complexity of the biped morphology. Lastly, the quadruped morphology appeared to be the least complex in terms automatically evolving locomotion since its Pareto solutions completely dominated all other morphologies. This is logical since the quadruped, similar to the hexapod, had built-in static stability from its design, unlike the biped which had to learn how to balance itself through the operations of the controller, but unlike the hexapod, the coordination and synchronization between four legs was much simpler than six legs.

In short, by analyzing the outcomes of the Pareto evolution, interesting comparisons and conjectures can be offered regarding the complexities of evolving locomotion for the different simulated robot morphologies.

Figure 8. Global Pareto-front of controllers obtained from 10 runs for all robot morphologies. X-axis: Locomotion distance, Y-axis: No. of hidden units

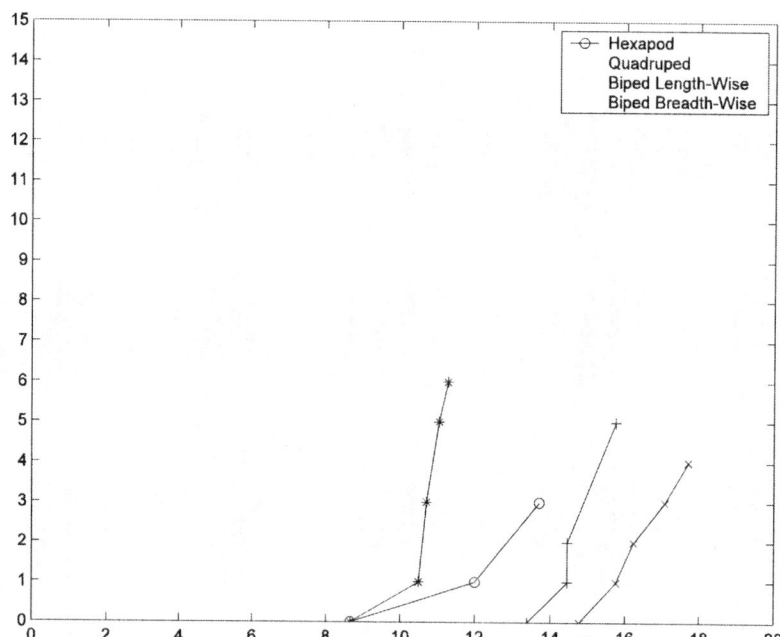

OPERATIONAL AND LIMB DYNAMICS

In this section, we investigate the operational dynamics of the overall best evolved controller of the quadruped obtained using the SPANN-R algorithm under the effects of noise as well as performance beyond the evolutionary window of 500 timesteps. This is followed by a thorough analysis of the limb dynamics in the last subsection.

Operational Dynamics under Noisy Conditions

Seven different levels of noise were applied to the joint angle sensors, touch sensors and outputs to the actuators individually as well as in combination for all three elements. Random noise levels ranging from 1% to 50% of the individual ranges of values for these sensors and actuators (see Section 3.2) were applied.

Table 6 lists the average and standard deviation of locomotion distances achieved by the overall best locomotion controller from SPANN-R with varying levels of noise applied to the sensors and actuators of the artificial creature. The performance of the controller degraded monotonically in all cases as the level of noise was increased from 1% to 50%, except for 50% noise in the joint angle sensor. At the lowest level of noise of 1%, the least significantly affected component was the touch sensor which still achieved on average 81.1% of the original locomotion distance. However, as the noise level was increased, the touch sensors

Table 6. Comparison of average locomotion distance achieved over 10 runs by overall best controller evolved for locomotion distance using the SPANN-R algorithm with varying noise levels in the sensors and actuators

Noise Level	f_1 with Noise in Joint Angle Sensors ± SD	f_1 with Noise in Touch Sensors ± SD	f_1 with Noise in Actuators ± SD	f_1 with Noise in All Sensors and Actuators ± SD
1%	13.4402 ± 1.7281	14.3599 ± 0.9073	13.8640 ± 0.9970	13.8147 ± 1.2219
5%	13.2121 ± 2.0271	12.5348 ± 1.0275	13.2310 ± 0.7213	11.2828 ± 0.8163
10%	11.8406 ± 1.2960	10.6214 ± 1.3914	12.9669 ± 1.2229	9.5492 ± 0.5552
20%	8.7969 ± 0.8017	6.3701 ± 1.9298	10.8933 ± 2.5271	4.8763 ± 0.4763
30%	6.8828 ± 0.4429	3.5598 ± 1.2999	8.8441 ± 1.9260	2.6185 ± 1.0707
40%	6.6890 ± 0.6028	1.6049 ± 1.1109	6.7339 ± 1.7209	1.2486 ± 0.6111
50%	6.7256 ± 0.9367	1.3050 ± 1.0950	3.7132 ± 1.9092	1.2153 ± 0.4210

seemed to be most affected by the presence of noise. In all cases where noise ranging from 5% to 50% was applied to the individual components, the lowest average locomotion distance was obtained when there was the presence of noise in the touch sensors. When noise was introduced to all sensors and actuators of the artificial creature in combination, the performance was lower than in all cases where noise was applied to each individual component except for 1% noise in the joint angle sensors. A visual inspection of the artificial creature in simulation with 10% random noise added to the sensors and actuators both individually and in combination revealed that the major characteristics of the locomotion behavior was still present, such as the backwards oriented walk and general movement of the limbs. Therefore, the evolved controller was still able to perform reasonably well with low levels of noise present in the sensors and actuators of the artificial creature.

Operational Dynamics Beyond the Evolutionary Window

A top-down view of the artificial creature's path as controlled using the overall best ANN evolved for locomotion distance is plotted in Figure 9 for the actual period between 1–500th timestep where the fitness of the controller is being evaluated. The X- and Z-planes are defined to be the horizontal axes within the Vortex simulator. The Y-plane in Vortex actually refers to the vertical plane, which is not of interest here. A second graph of the artificial creature's path for the period between the 501–1000th timestep is plotted in Figure 10 to observe the locomotion behavior beyond the actual fitness evaluation window used during evolution. Although the path taken was not exactly a straight line, it did however maximize the horizontal distance moved fairly well. It begins from the origin at coordinates (0,0) and after 500 timesteps ends approximately at coordinates (-6.9, -16.5). This emergent behavior is interesting in that although the initial setup has the creature's forward orientation as being in the positive coordinate areas of the X-Plane and Z-Plane, the evolved locomotion behavior was in fact a backward oriented walk if the initial positioning of the creature is taken as the reference frame. Visualization of the other global Pareto solutions revealed similar orientations for the evolved locomotion behaviors. This can be explained by the fact that all the global Pareto solutions were actually obtained from one run using a particular seed. Across the global Pareto solutions obtained with other architectures using

Figure 9. Path taken by artificial creature as controlled by overall best ANN evolved for locomotion distance using the SPANN-R algorithm for the 1–500th timestep

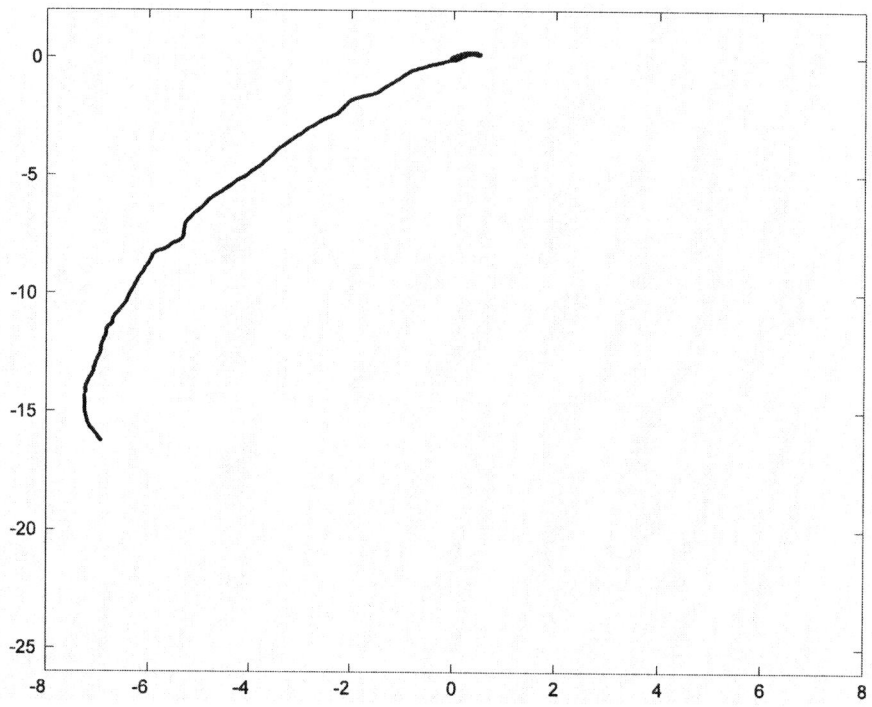

Figure 10. Path taken by artificial creature as controlled by overall best ANN evolved for locomotion distance using the SPANN-R algorithm for the 501–1000th timestep

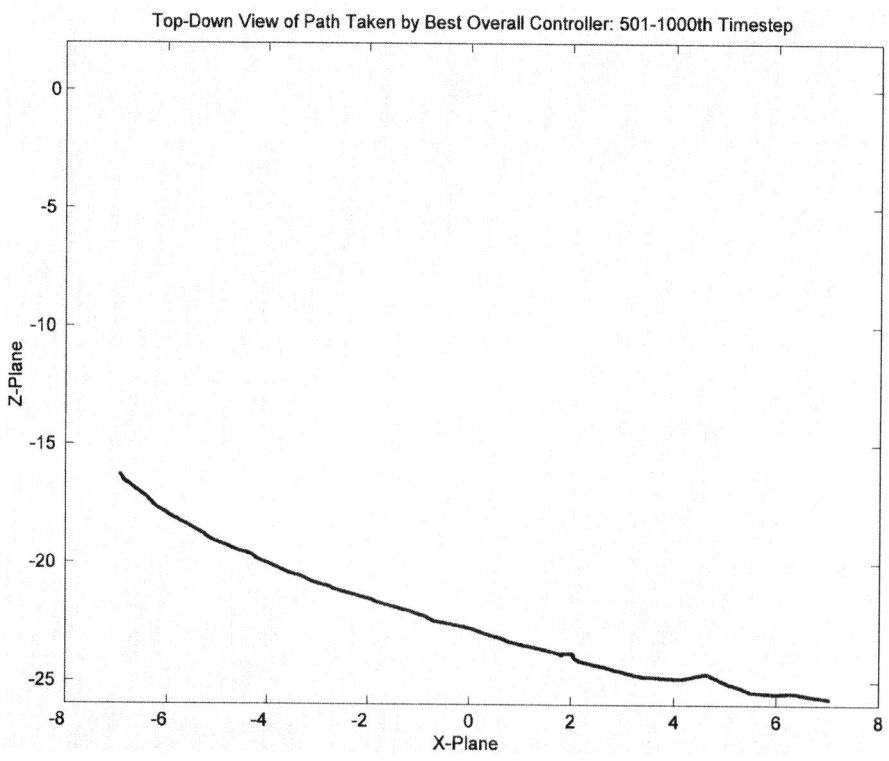

SPANN-R, the majority of the evolved controllers produced movement in the forward direction rather than this backwards movement. The design of the creature's limbs and in particular how the joint constraints were set up allowed for both forwards and backwards oriented walks to be evolved. Note that the initial movement seen in the other direction from coordinates (0,0) to approximately (0.5,0) occurred during the standing up phase of the creature's locomotion. Once the creature stood up, it then started the backward oriented walk to achieve the maximal horizontal distance moved.

Towards the end of the walk, the path could be seen to start curving back towards the X-Plane. The continuation of this peculiar behavior beyond 500 timesteps as controlled by this evolved ANN can be seen in the plot of the path in Figure 10. Nonetheless, the creature was still able to walk in a fairly straight line thereby achieving a reasonably maximal locomotion distance during the next 500 timesteps. If the path of the creature is considered over the entire 1-1000th timestep, what this analysis shows is that the operational dynamics of the evolved behavior during the period which the controller was actually evolved to perform can be quite different to the operational dynamics when used beyond its evolutionary design period. This phenomenon has been highlighted in another study which states that the use of biologically-inspired solutions in engineering problems may be problematic because unexpected and sometimes unwanted results or behaviors might arise (Ronald & Sipper, 2001). Hence it is essential to test evolved solutions thoroughly even beyond the evolutionary window to be sure that the desired behavior is still performing within reasonable parameters.

Limb Dynamics

The outputs generated from the operation of the overall best controller evolved for locomotion distance to Actuators y_1 - y_8 are plotted in Figure 11. In all except one of the outputs, sine-like wave signals were generated by the evolved ANN to the motors in the respective limb actuators. This is consistent with the evolved walking behavior which is cyclic in nature.

It is also interesting to note that the signals generated were quite distinctive over time as near maximal outputs of either 0 and 1 at the peaks and troughs of the cycle were being generated by the ANN. This behavior is close to the optimal control strategy known as "Bang-Bang Controls", which take their values on the extreme points (in our case, 0 and 1) (Macki & Strauss, 1982). In terms of the single output which generated a totally flat signal of practically 0 magnitude over time (Figure 11.7), this indicated the presence of a passively controlled lower limb, which obtained its swinging motion from the movement of the attached upper limb. A visual inspection of the creature in simulation confirmed that this limb did in fact exhibit some dynamical behavior during locomotion. This suggests that the evolutionary

Table 7. Correlation coefficients for neural network outputs between the upper and lower limbs of each leg

Limbs	Correlation Coefficient
Upper and Lower Back Left	0.9410
Upper and Lower Front Left	-0.9648
Upper and Lower Back Right	0.0376
Upper and Lower Front Right	-0.9998

Figure 11. The outputs from the overall best evolved ANN controller to Actuators 1-8. X-axis: Timestep, Y-axis: Neural network output

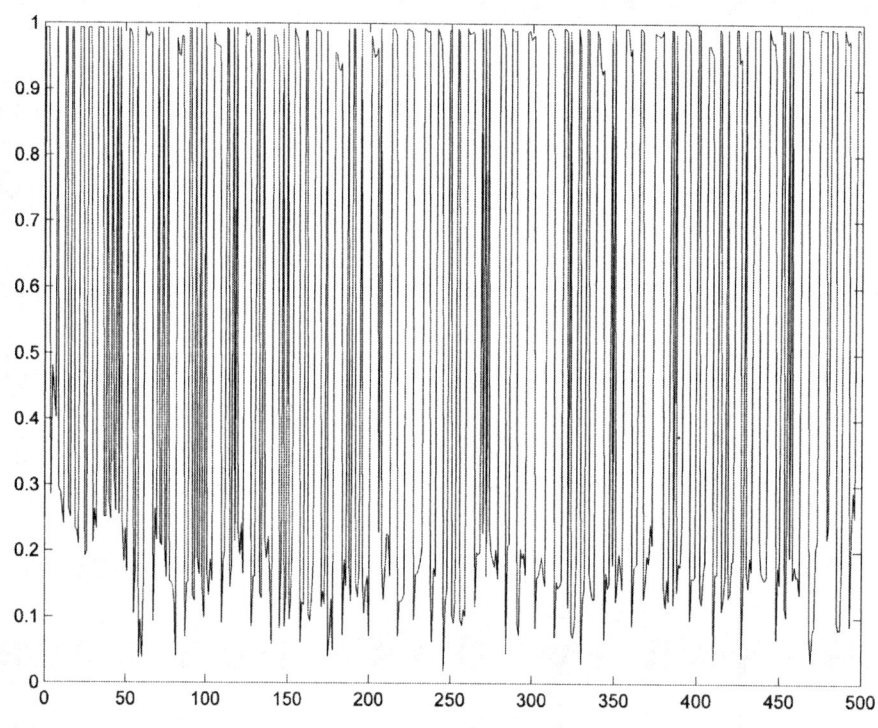

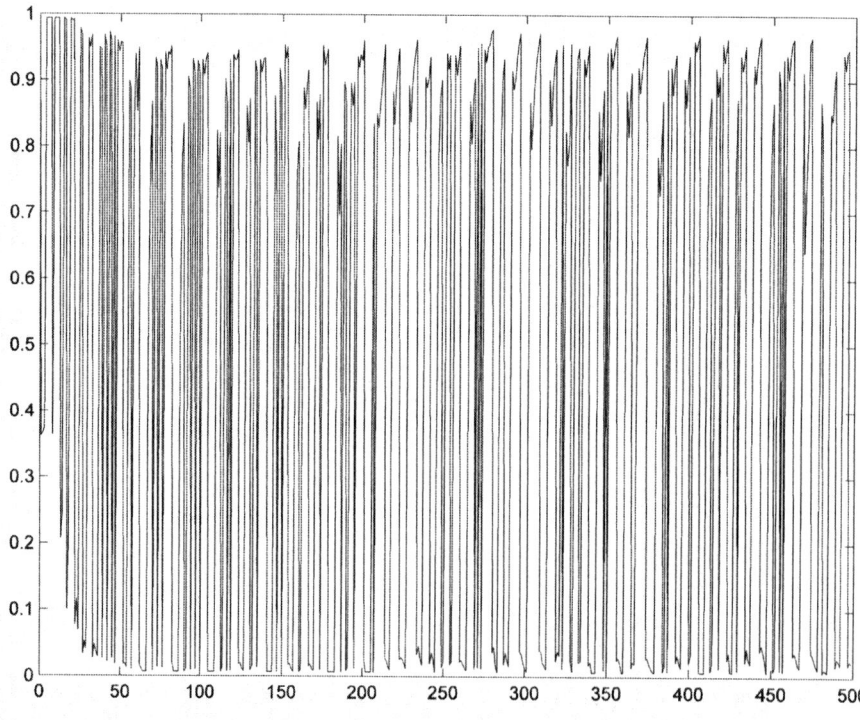

continued on following page

Figure 11. continued

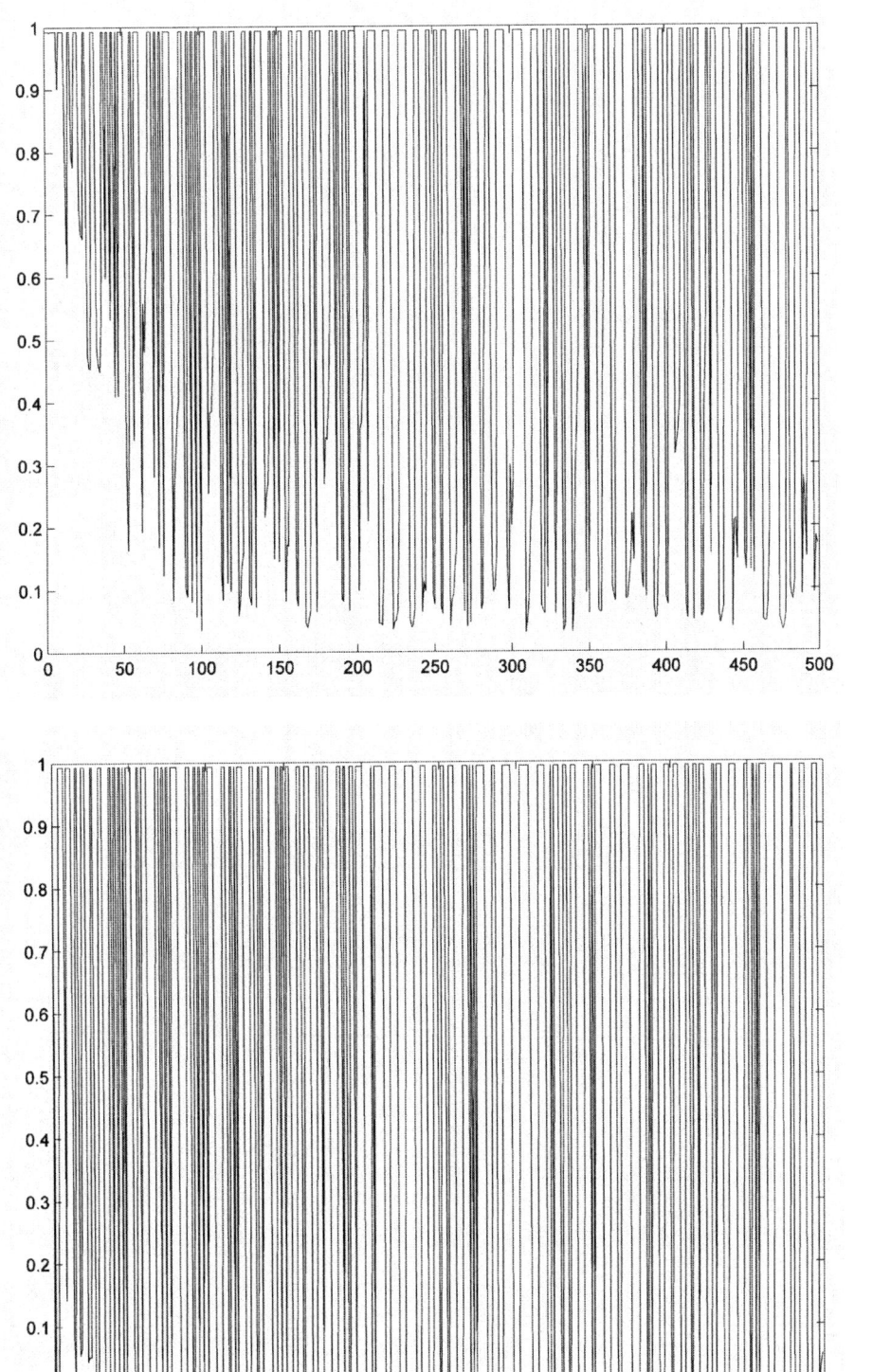

continued on following page

Figure 11. continued

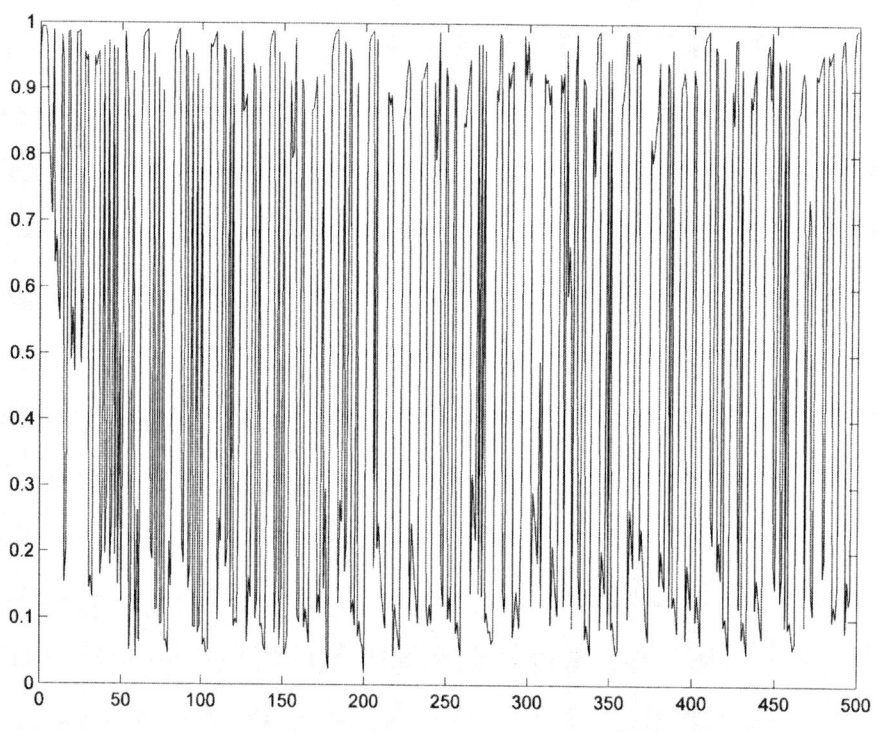

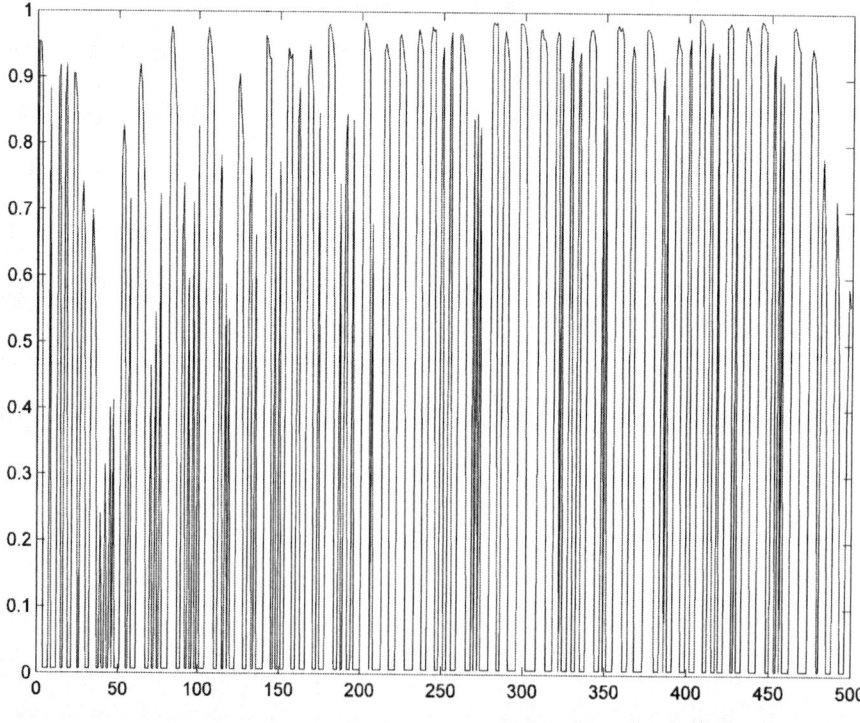

continued on following page

Figure 11. continued

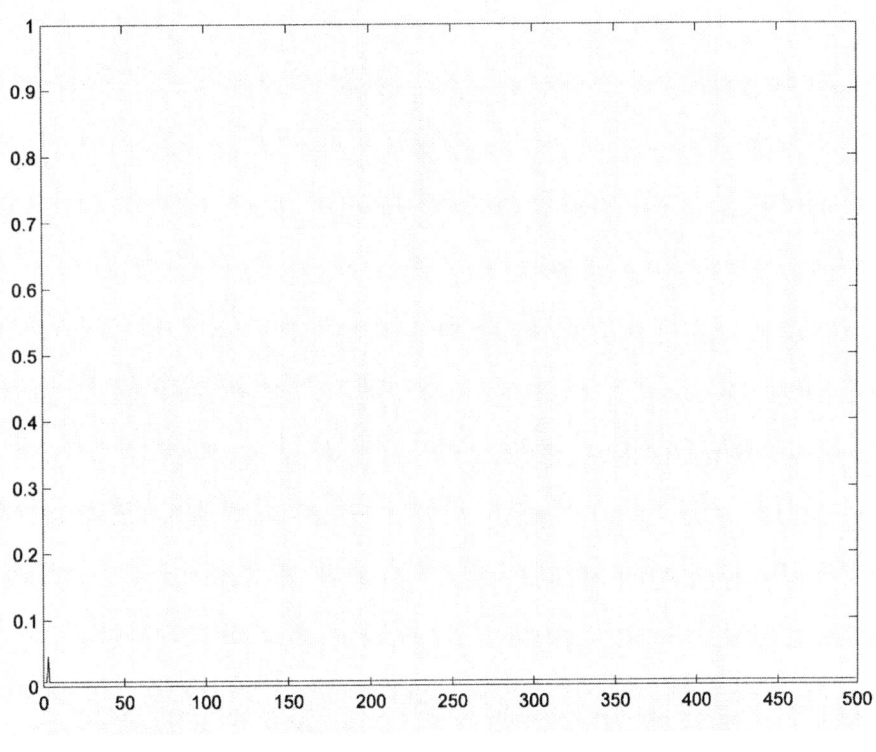

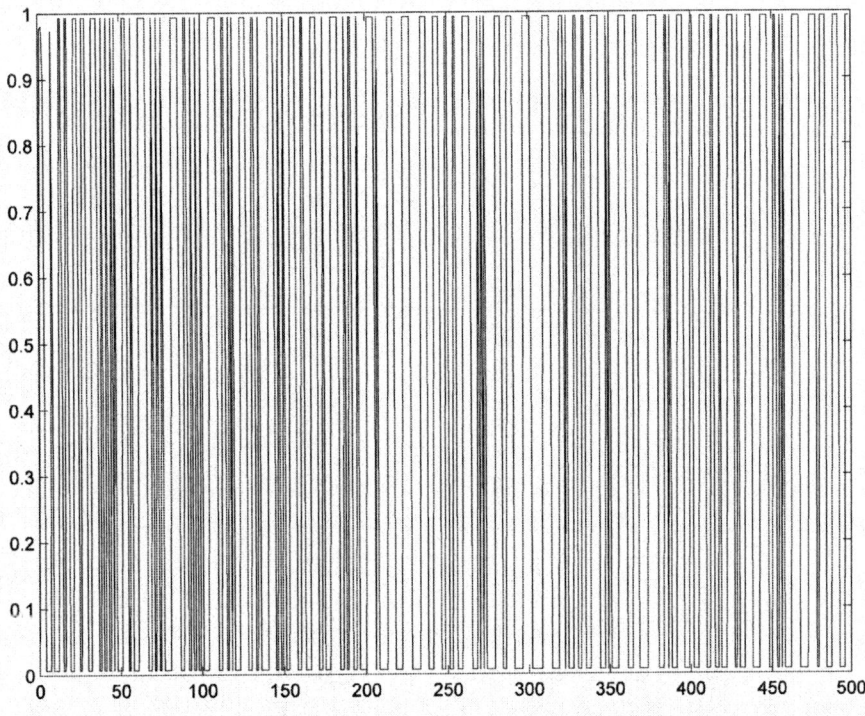

search found a simpler control solution through the use of a passive dynamic limb (McGeer, 1990).

Another interesting dynamical behavior that emerged from the outputs of the ANN is that the component limbs in all of the legs learnt to coordinate and synchronize their movements within each leg, with the exception of the leg containing the passive dynamic limb. This is evidenced by the very high correlation between the upper and lower limbs of the back left, front left and front right legs as shown in Table 7. For a legged gait with good locomotion capabilities, the constituent components in each leg would be expected to function as a cohesive unit in order for each leg to generate useful movements for locomotion. The outputs to the individual limb actuators for the back left leg have evolved to be almost entirely in-phase, as evidenced by the very high positive correlation coefficient (0.9410). On the other hand, the outputs to the individual limb actuators for the front left and front right legs have evolved to be almost entirely out-of-phase, as evidenced by the very high negative correlation coefficients (-0.9648 & -0.9998). This shows that the neural network controller has learnt to coordinate and synchronize between the limbs of each leg, thereby allowing for successful locomotion to occur.

EMPIRICAL COMPARISON OF DIFFERENT EMO ALGORITHMS

To conclude our verification of SPANN-R as a beneficial Pareto EMO algorithm, we compare its results against one of the current state-of-the-art Pareto EMO algorithms called the Non-Dominated Sorting Genetic Algorithm II (NSGA-II) (Deb, Agrawal, Pratab, & Meyarivan, 2000) using the quadruped morphology. NSGA-II is an elitist Pareto EMO algorithm which utilizes an explicit-diversity preserving mechanism. It also employs a nondominated sorting procedure to identify the different layers of the Pareto fronts from both the parent and offspring populations, after which a crowding distance operator is used as the tournament selection operator. Our objective here is simply to verify that the solutions obtained using SPANN-R are comparable to those obtained using a well-known and well-tested Pareto EMO algorithm and not to determine which Pareto EMO algorithm is better for evolving locomotion controllers as this is beyond the scope of this work. The NSGA-II algorithm was obtained from the authors' Web site (KanGAL, 2003) and used as a benchmark algorithm without any modification to the NSGA-II algorithm.

SPANN-R vs. NSGA-II for Pareto Evolution of Locomotion Controllers

The same ANN architecture was again used in this set of experiments and all other parameters remained the same: 1000 generations, 30 individuals, 500 timesteps and 10 repeated runs. NSGA-II requires a number of other parameters to be set by the user including the crossover and mutation rates which are nonself-adaptive. Recently, the authors of NSGA-II conducted a comprehensive comparative study of NSGA-II against other EMO algorithms, which were reported in (Deb, Agrawal, Pratab, & Meyarivan, 2002). Hence, in the first setup, these user-defined parameters were set according to those used in the above-mentioned comparative study as follows: crossover rate 90%, mutation rate for real-coded variables 0.1553% (representing the reciprocal of the number of real-coded variables), and mutation rate for binary-coded variables 6.6667% (representing the reciprocal of the number of binary-coded variables), distribution index for crossover operator 20, distribution index for mutation operator 20, and single-point crossover. The remaining setups are defined later in the following paragraphs.

Table 8 lists the best Pareto solutions for locomotion distance obtained using the NSGA-II algorithm and compares them against those obtained using the SPANN-R algorithm. The best solutions obtained using the first setup for

Table 8. Comparison of best locomotion distance for Pareto solutions obtained over 10 independent runs using the SPANN-R and NSGA-II algorithms. Setup 1: c = 90%, m(r) = 0.1553%, m(b) = 6.6667%. Setup 2: c=50%, m(r) = 50%, m(b) = 50%. Setup 3: c=50%, m(r) = 90%, m(b) = 90%. Setup 4: c = 90%, m(r) = 50%, m(b) = 50%. c = crossover rate, m(r) = mutation rate for real-coded variables; m(b) = mutation rate for binary-coded variables

Algorithm	Overall Best Locomotion Distance	Average Best Locomotion Distance ± Standard Deviation	t-statistic (against SPANN-R)	No. of Hidden Units
SPANN-R	17.6994	13.9626 ± 1.7033	-	4.9 ± 2.6
NSGA-II Setup 1	15.5452	11.7421 ± 2.0497	(3.78)	0 ± 0
NSGA-II Setup 2	18.3941	16.2022 ± 1.5860	2.85	6.8 ± 2.3
NSGA-II Setup 3	20.4144	17.8635 ± 1.9744	4.54	8.4 ± 2.1
NSGA-II Setup 4	20.9806	16.2667 ± 2.1868	2.54	7.7 ± 1.7

NSGA-II produced controllers that used no hidden units in all 10 runs. The overall best locomotion distance achieved was lower than that obtained using SPANN-R. The very small mutation rate used in this setup most probably caused the evolutionary search to prematurely converge to local optima centered around controllers which did not use any hidden units. A t-test showed that the results obtained using NSGA-II were significantly worse than SPANN-R at the $\alpha=0.01$ significance level for this setup. Also, the overall best controller from SPANN-R achieved over 2 units of distance more than the overall best controller obtained from this setup of NSGA-II (representing a decrease of 12.2% compared to the overall best locomotion distance achieved by SPANN-R).

To overcome the inferior results obtained using the setup reported in (Deb et al., 2002), a second experiment utilizing the best combination of crossover and mutation rates obtained from the hand-tuned EMO was conducted. This second setup used crossover and mutation rates of 50% with all other parameters unchanged. Much better results were obtained in this second setup, where the overall best controller in terms of locomotion achieved a higher distance than that obtained using SPANN-R by just under 0.7 units (representing a 3.9% improvement over the best locomotion distance achieved by SPANN-R). A t-test showed that the solutions obtained using NSGA-II with the second setup were significantly better than those obtained using SPANN-R at the $\alpha=0.05$ significance level.

Since these results suggest that a high mutation rate may improve the performance of NSGA-II, we carried out a third experiment using a setup with an even higher mutation rate of 90% while maintaining the crossover rate at 50%. However, a t-test comparing the results from this third setup against the second setup for NSGA-II showed no significant improvements. To test whether a higher crossover rate would yield better results, a fourth experiment was conducted using a setup with crossover rate of 90% and maintaining the mutation rate at 50%. Again, a t-test showed no significant improvements in the results obtained with the fourth setup compared to the second setup of NSGA-II. The solutions obtained with third and fourth setup for NSGA-II were significantly better than those obtained with SPANN-R at the $\alpha=0.01$ and $\alpha=0.05$ levels respectively. The best solutions obtained from the third setup of NSGA-II used an average of 8.4 hidden units, which is almost double the number used by the best solutions obtained using SPANN-R, while the fourth setup used an average of 7.7 hidden units.

Figure 12. Pareto-front of solutions obtained for 10 runs using the NSGA-II algorithm for Setup 1 - 4

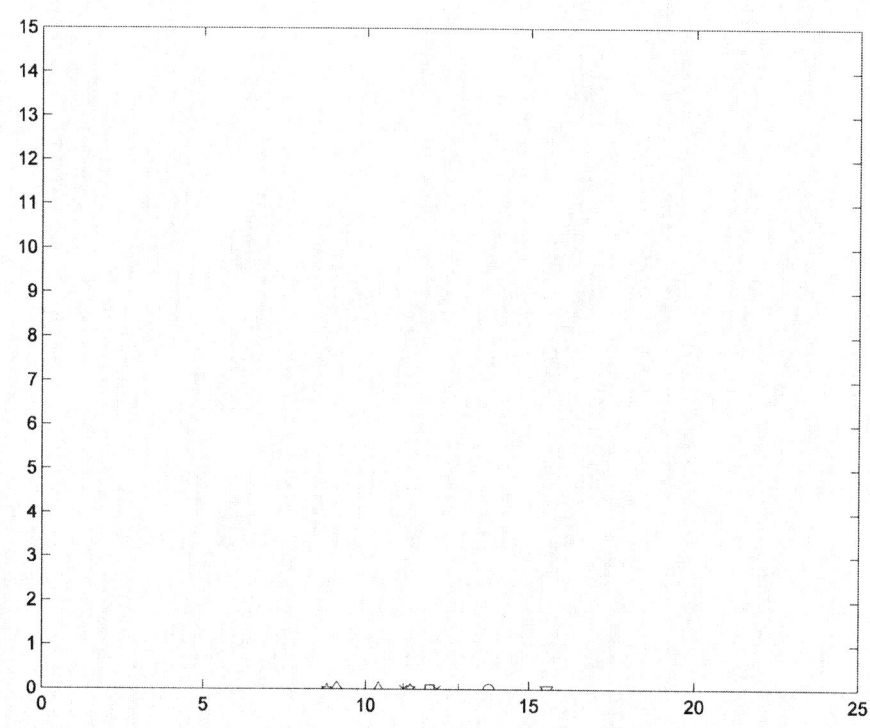

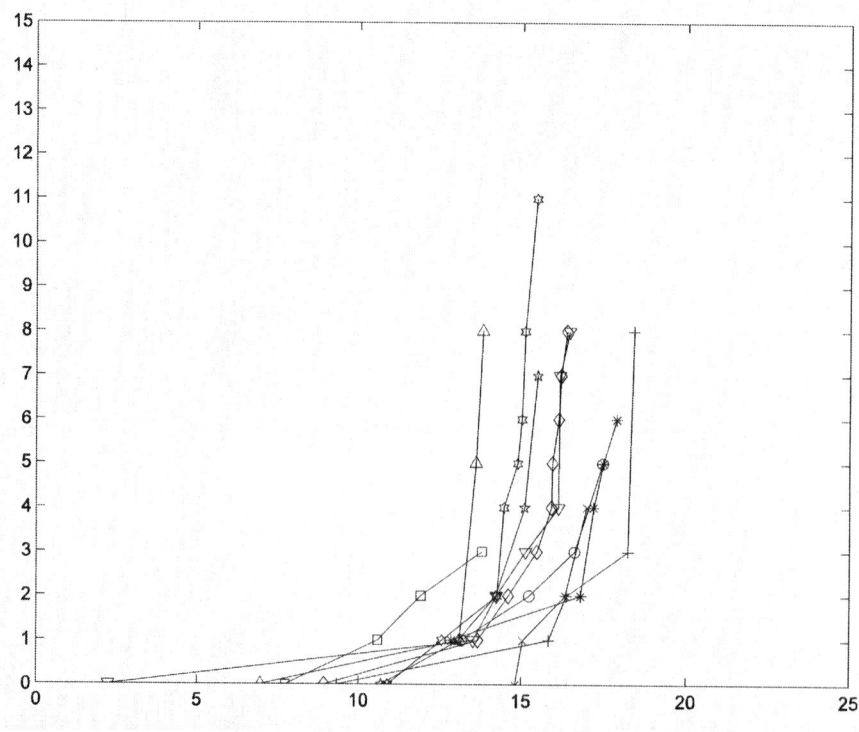

continued on following page

Walking with EMO

Figure 12. continued

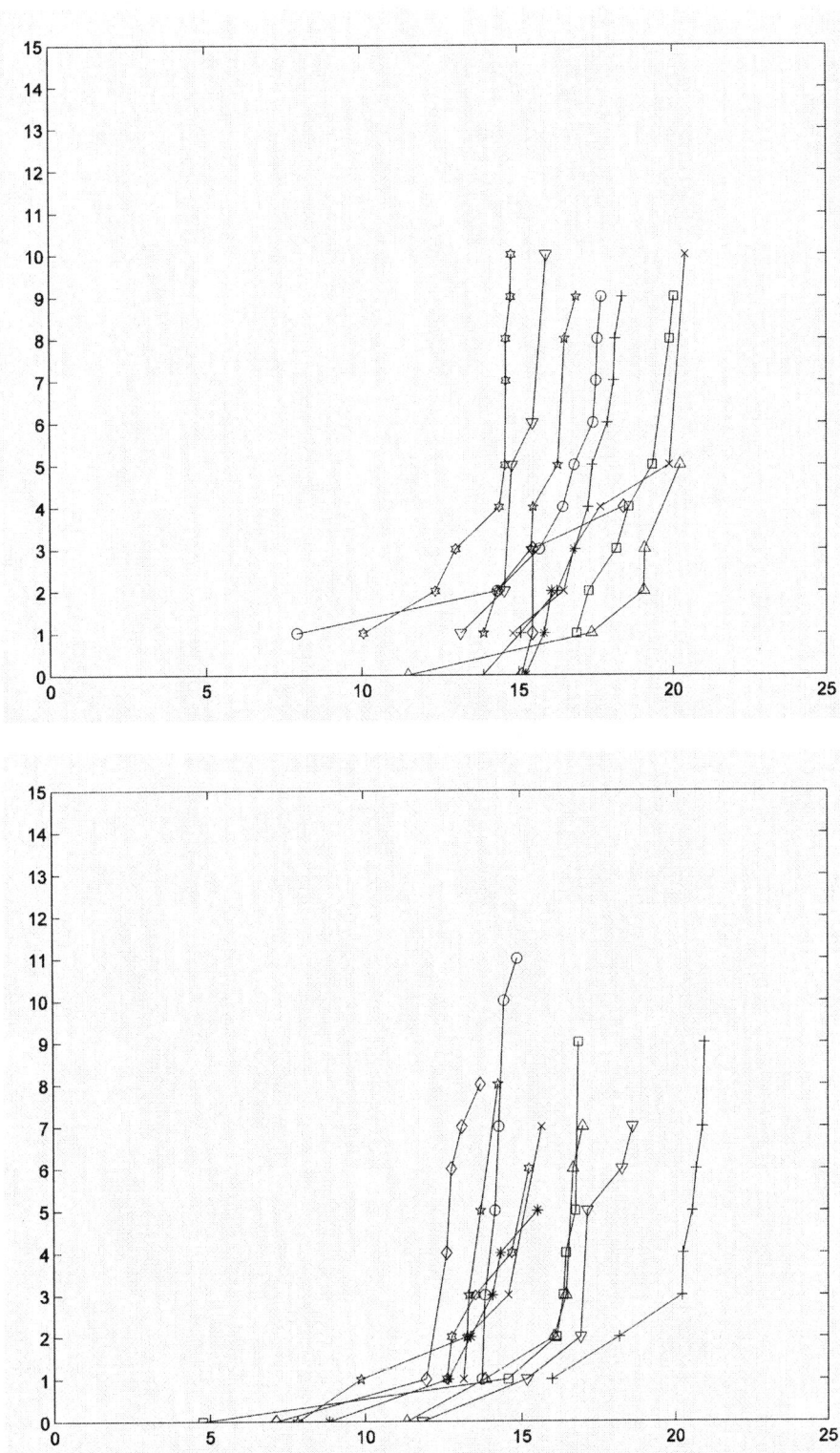

The Pareto-frontiers obtained over the 10 runs of NSGA-II for the four setups are depicted in Figure 12. The first setup only produced controllers that did not make use of any hidden units in the ANN controller as can be seen in Figure 12.1. All runs converged to solutions that did not require any hidden layer transformation resulting in purely reactive controllers being generated. In comparison, the second, third and fourth setups which used much higher mutation rates all produced a much greater variety of controllers as shown by the Pareto-fronts plotted in Figures 12.2, 12.3 and 12.4 respectively.

Figure 13 plots the global Pareto-front of SPANN-R and NSGA-II. It can be seen that the Pareto-front generated through 10 runs of SPANN-R is comparable though dominated by the Pareto-front generated through 40 runs of NSGA-II (10 runs each in Setup 1–4). The solution with 0 hidden units of the NSGA-II global Pareto-front was contributed from the first setup of NSGA-II while the remaining 8 other solutions on the global Pareto-front were contributed from the other three setups.

In summary, although at first glance it appeared that the use of a different EMO algorithm in NSGA-II resulted in far inferior solutions than SPANN-R, a proper tuning of the parameters showed that it could similarly produce highly successful locomotion controllers for the simulated robot. However, it also shows that there is a trade-off between obtaining better locomotion controllers using NSGA-II at the cost of incurring greater computational expense to find the optimal parameter settings. It is clear that the performance of NSGA-II is also sensitive to the parameters used. Nonetheless, this experiment does show that different underlying EMO algorithms can be used for evolutionary multi-objective robotics.

Figure 13. Global Pareto-front of controllers obtained using the SPANN-R and NSGA-II algorithms. X-axis: Locomotion distance, Y-axis: No. of hidden units

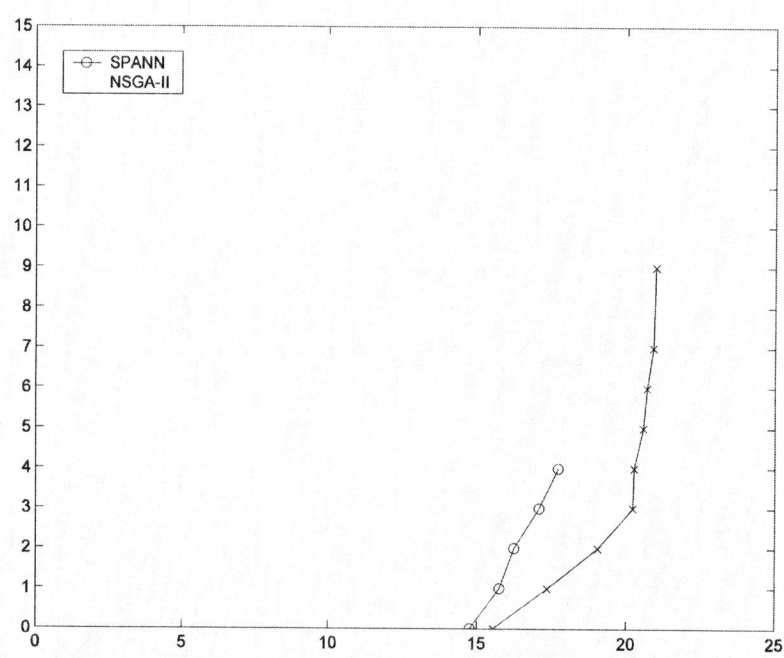

CONCLUSION

We have demonstrated in this chapter the viability of the Pareto EMO approach for the automatic generation of locomotion behavior for two, four and six-legged locomotion using physically-accurate simulations of bipedal, quadrupedal and hexapedal robots. The main advantage of utilizing and EMO approach over conventional single-objective EAs for evolutionary robotics is clear—a single evolutionary run with EMO can generate a set of controllers that satisfy multiple objectives. Furthermore, we have demonstrated that the operational dynamics of the evolved controllers are robust under the influence of noise and are able to function beyond the evolutionary window. An analysis has also been provided to show that the evolved limb dynamics are near optimal and even the natural emergence of a passively-controlled limb. Finally, a simple comparison was made between our Differential Evolution-based EMO algorithm, SPANN-R against a more established EMO, NSGA-II that shows that the evolutionary multi-objective robotics approach is extendable to any EMO algorithm as the baseline algorithm.

FUTURE RESEARCH DIRECTIONS

An immediate extension to this body of work is to extend the experimentation of the SPANN-R algorithm, and the Pareto EMO approach in general, to the evolution of controllers and even morphologies of real physical robots. This would provide some valuable insights into the practicality of multi-objective evolutionary robotics such the actual real time required to complete one robotic evolutionary optimization process and how to decide which of the Pareto optimal controllers would actually be used in the real task environment. Such can extension can now be easily realized using relatively simple-to-program and cheap commercial-off-the-shelf robots such as Cyberbotics' e-puck (Cyberbotics, 2007), LEGO Mindstorms NXT (LEGO, 2007) and Kyosho's Manoi AT-01 (Kyosho, 2007).

The power of a Pareto EMO approach lies in the flexibility and ease of incorporating new objectives and elements into the artificial evolutionary process. Hence, the inclusion of elements such as compactness of genetic material in EAs that utilize variable length chromosomes or other more elaborate developmental encodings as a distinct and separate objective on top of the primary objective will not only provide useful ways of improving the efficiency of the EA but may possibly also provide interesting insights into why vastly different genome lengths are found in biological organisms. Since evolutionary robotics is widely regarded as one of the important components of artificial life research, other elements that will be fruitful to investigate as separate evolutionary objectives from an artificial life perspective include phylogenetic diversity, number of body parts/joints and physical energy consumption to name but a few.

Moreover, the SPANN-R algorithm can be beneficial in evolving controllers not only for legged robots but also wheeled and other forms of physical robots. Again, the multi-objectivity of the artificial evolution can easily incorporate additional engineering factors such as noise and stress tolerance into the optimization process. It will also be interesting to expand the SPANN-R algorithm to allow for fully and freely evolvable robotic forms that are not based on any underlying body plan and evolved from very basic structures, perhaps even at the atomic level. This can have far-reaching implications on the evolution of minimal controllers and morphologies of recyclable micro-machines that can be created with nanotechnology and evolvable hardware. The fully automated design, fabrication and re-use cycle of such evolvable systems would then truly constitute a form of artificial life.

REFERENCES

Abbass, H. A. (2003). Speeding up back-propagation using multi-objective evolutionary algorithms. *Neural Computation, 15*(11), 2705–2726.

Angeline, P. J., Saunders, G. M., & Pollack, J. B. (1994). An evolutionary algorithm that constructs recurrent neural networks. *IEEE Transactions on Neural Networks, 5*(1), 54–65.

Barlow, G. J. & Oh, C. K. (2005). Transference of evolved unmanned aerial vehicle controllers to a wheeled mobile robot. In *2005 IEEE International Conference on Robots & Automation (ICRA 2005)* (pp. 2087-2092). Piscataway, NJ: IEEE Press.

Barlow, G. J. & Oh, C. K. (2006). Robustness analysis of genetic programming controllers for unmanned aerial vehicles. In *2006 ACM Genetic & Evolutionary Computation Conference (GECCO 2006)* (pp. 135-142). New York: ACM Press.

Barlow, G. J., Oh, C. K. & Grant, E. (2004). Incremental evolution of autonomous controllers for unmanned aerial vehicles using multi-objective genetic programming. In *2004 IEEE International Conference on Systems, Man & Cybernetics* (pp. 689-694). Piscataway, NJ: IEEE Press.

Belew, R. K., McInerney, J. & Schraudolph, N. N. (1992). Evolving networks: Using the genetic algorithm with connectionist learning. In C. G. Langton, C. Taylor, J. D. Farmer, & S. Rasmussen (Eds.), *Artificial Life II: Proceedings of the Second International Workshop on the Synthesis & Simulation of Living Systems* (pp. 511–547). Redwood City, CA: Addison-Wesley.

CM Labs. (2007). Retrieved February 12, 2008, from http://www.cm-labs.com/software/vortex/

Coello Coello, C. A., Christiansen, A. D., & Aguirre, A. H. (1998). Using a new GA-based multi-objective optimization technique for the design of robot arms. *Robotica, 16*, 401–414.

Coello Coello, C. A., van Veldhuizen, D. A. & Lamont, G. B. (2002). *Evolutionary algorithms for solving multi-objective problems.* New York: Kluwer Academic.

Cyberbotics. (2007). Retrieved February 12, 2008, from http://www.cyberbotics.com/products/robots/e-puck.html

Deb, K. (2001). *Multi-objective optimization using evolutionary algorithms.* Chicester, UK: John Wiley & Sons.

Deb, K., Agrawal, S., Pratab, A., & Meyarivan, T. (2000). A fast elitist non-dominated sorting genetic algorithm for multi-objective optimization: NSGA-II. In M. Schoenauer, K. Deb, G. Rudolph, X. Yao, E. Lutton, J. J. Merelo, & H.-P. Schwefel (Eds.), In *Proceedings of the Parallel Problem Solving from Nature VI Conference (PPSN VI)* (pp. 849–858). Berlin: Springer-Verlag.

Deb, K., Agrawal, S., Pratab, A., & Meyarivan, T. (2002). A fast & elitist multi-objective genetic algorithm: NSGA-II. *IEEE Transactions on Evolutionary Computation, 6*(2), 182–197.

Dozier, G., McCullough, S., Homaifar, A., Tunstel, E., & Moore, L. (1998). Multi-objective evolutionary path planning via fuzzy tournament selection. In *Proceedings of the IEEE International Conference on Evolutionary Computation (ICEC'98)* (pp. 684–689). Piscataway, NJ: IEEE Press.

Fogel, D. B., Fogel, L. J., & Porto, V. W. (1990). Evolving neural networks. *Biological Cybernetics, 63*(6), 487–493.

Gacogne, L. (1997). Research of Pareto set by genetic algorithm, application to multicriteria optimization of fuzzy controller. In *Proceedings of the 5th European Congress on Intelligent Techniques & Soft Computing (EUFIT'97)* (pp. 837–845), Aachen, Germany.

Gacogne, L. (1999). Multiple objective optimization of fuzzy rules for obstacles avoiding by an evolution algorithm with adaptative operators. In

Proceedings of the Fifth International Mendel Conference on Soft Computing (Mendel'99) (pp. 236–242), Brno, Czech Republic.

KanGAL. (2003). *NSGA-II source code (real & binary-coded + constraint handling)*. Retrieved February 12, 2008, from http://www.iitk.ac.in/kangal/code/nsga2code.tar

Kyosho. (2007). Retrieved February 12, 2008, from http://www.kyosho.com/jpn/products/robot/index.html

Kim, D. E. & Hallam, J. (2002). An evolutionary approach to quantify internal states needed for the Woods problem. In B. Hallam, D. Floreano, G. Hayes, J. Hallam, & J.A. Meyer (Eds.), *From Animals to Animats 7: Proceedings of the Seventh International Conference on the Simulation of Adaptive Behavior (SAB2002)* (pp. 312–322). Cambridge, MA: MIT Press.

Kitano, H. (1990). Designing neural networks using genetic algorithms with graph generation system. *Complex Systems, 4*(4), 461–476.

Koza, J. R. & Rice, J. P. (1991). Genetic generation of both the weights & architecture for a neural network. In *Proceedings of the 1991 International Joint Conference on Neural Networks: Vol. 2* (pp. 397–404). Piscataway, NJ: IEEE Press.

Lee, J. Y. & Lee, J. J. (2004). Multi-objective walking trajectories generation for a biped robot. In *Proceedings of the IEEE/RSJ International Conference on Intelligent Robots & Systems (IROS 2004)* (pp. 3853-3858), Sendai, Japan.

Leger, P. C. (1999). *Automated synthesis & optimization of robot configurations: An evolutionary approach*. Unpublished doctoral dissertation, Carnegie Mellon University, Pennsylvania.

LEGO. (2007). Retrieved February 12, 2008, from http://mindstorms.lego.com/

Lucas, J. M., Martinez-Barbera, H., & Jimenez, F. (2005). Multi-objective evolutionary fuzzy modeling for the docking maneuver of an automated guided vehicle. In *2005 IEEE International Conference on Systems, Man & Cybernetics* (pp. 2757-2762). Piscataway, NJ: IEEE Press.

Lund, H. H. & Hallam, J. (1997). Evolving sufficient robot controllers. In *Proceedings of the 4th IEEE International Conference on Evolutionary Computation* (pp. 495–499). Piscataway, NJ: IEEE Press.

Macki, J. & Strauss, A. (1982). *Introduction to optimal control theory*. New York: Springer-Verlag.

Mataric, M. & Cliff, D. (1996). Challenges in evolving controllers for physical robots. *Robotics & Autonomous Systems, 19*, 67-83.

McGeer, T. (1990). Passive dynamic walking. *International Journal of Robotics Research, 9*(2), 62–82.

Miller, G. F., Todd, P. M., & Hegde, S. U. (1989). Designing neural networks using genetic algorithms. In J.D. Schaffer (Ed.), In *Proceedings of the Third International Conference on Genetic Algorithms* (pp. 379–384). San Mateo, CA: Morgan Kaufmann.

Nelson, A. L. & Grant, E. (2006). Developmental analysis in evolutionary robotics. In *2006 IEEE Mountain Workshop on Adaptive & Learning Systems* (pp. 201-206). Pistacaway, NJ: IEEE Press.

Nolfi, S. & Floreano, D. (2000). *Evolutionary robotics: The biology, intelligence & technology of self-organizing machines*. Cambridge, MA: MIT Press/Bradford Books.

Nolfi, S. (2002). Power & limits of reactive agents. *Neurocomputing, 42*, 119–145.

Oh, C. K. & Barlow, G. J. (2004). Autonomous controller design for unmanned aerial vehicles using multi-objective genetic programming. In *2004 IEEE Congress on Evolutionary Compu-*

taton (CEC 2004) (pp. 1538-1545). Piscataway, NJ: IEEE Press.

Pasemann, F., Steinmetz, U., Hulse, M., & Lara, B. (2001). Evolving brain structure for robot control. In J. Mira & A. Prieto (Eds.), In *Proceedings of the International Work-Conference on Artificial & Natural Neural Networks (IWANN'2001): Vol. 2* (pp. 410–417). Berlin: Springer-Verlag.

Pirjanian, P. (1998). Multiple objective action selection in behavior-based control. In *Proceedings of the 6th Symposium for Intelligent Robotic Systems* (pp. 83–92), Edinburgh, UK.

Pirjanian, P. (2000). Multiple objective behavior-based control. *Robotics & Autonomous Systems, 31*(1-2), 53–60.

Ronald, E. M. A. & Sipper, M. (2001). Surprise versus unsurprise: Implications of emergence in robotics. *Robotics & Autonomous Systems, 37*, 19–24.

Rumelhart, D. E., Hinton, G. E., & Williams, R. J. (1986). Learning internal representations by error propagation. In D.E. Rumelhart & J.L McClelland (Eds.), *Parallel Distributed Processing: Vol. 1* (pp. 381–362). Cambridge, MA: MIT Press.

Storn, R. & Price, K. V. (1995). *Differential evolution: A simple & efficient adaptive scheme for global optimization over continuous spaces* (Tech. Rep. No. TR-95-012). Berkeley: International Computer Science Institute.

Taylor, T. & Massey, C. (2001). Recent developments in the evolution of morphologies & controllers for physically simulated creatures. *Artificial Life, 7*(1), 77–87.

Teo, J. & Abbass, H. A. (2004). Automatic generation of controllers for embodied legged organisms: A Pareto evolutionary multi-objective approach. *Evolutionary Computation, 12*(3), 355–394.

Walker, J., Garrett, S., & Wilson, M. (2003). Evolving controllers for real robots: A survey of the literature. *Adaptive Behavior, 11*(3), 179–203.

Wang, L .F., Tan, K. C., & Chew, C. M. (2006). *Evolutionary robotics: From algorithms to implementations.* Singapore: World Scientific Publishing.

Yao, X. (1999). Evolving artificial neural networks. In *Proceedings of the IEEE, 87*(9), 1426–1447.

ADDITIONAL READINGS

Multi-Objective Robotics

Proceedings of the IEEE/RSJ 2006 workshop on Multi-Objectie Robotics (IROS-MOR 2006). A. Moshaiov (ed). Beijing, China. The is the first ever workshop organized for multi-objective robotics & was recently held as part of the 2006 International Conference on Intelligent Robots & Systems (IROS 2006). The following papers that were presented represent a first attempt at collecting together some relevant & recent works on multi-objective robotics:

Benjamin, M. R. (2006). Multi-objective helming with interval programming on autonomous marine vehicles. In *Proceedings of the IEEE/RSJ 2006 Workshop on Multi-Objectie Robotics (IROS-MOR 2006),* Beijing China.

Moshaiov, A. & Avigad, G. (2006). The extended concept-based multi-objective path planning. In *Proceedings of the IEEE/RSJ 2006 workshop on Multi-Objectie Robotics (IROS-MOR 2006),* Beijing China.

Cajals, A., Amat, J., & de la Fuente, C. P. (2006). Study & optimization of a multi-arm workstation for laparoscopic telesurgery. In *Proceedings of the IEEE/RSJ 2006 workshop on Multi-Objectie Robotics (IROS-MOR 2006),* Beijing China.

Takahashi, Y., Kawamata, T., & Asada, M. (2006). Learning utility for behavior acquisition & intention inference of other agent. In *Proceedings of* the *IEEE/RSJ 2006 workshop on Multi-Objectie Robotics (IROS-MOR 2006)*, Beijing China.

Calvo, R. & Romero, R.A.F. (2006). Multi-objective reinforcement learning for autonomous navigation robots. In *Proceedings of the IEEE/RSJ 2006 workshop on Multi-Objectie Robotics (IROS-MOR 2006)*, Beijing China.

Evolutionary Algorithms

Back, T., Fogel, D.B., & Z. Michalewicz (1997). *Handbook of evolutionary computation*. Bristol, PA: Institute of Physics Publishing.

Eiben, A. E. & Smith, J. E. (2003). *Introduction to evolutionary computing*. Berlin: Springer.

Fogel, D. B. (2006). *Evolutionary computation: Toward a new philosophy of machine intelligence* (3rd ed). Pistacaway, NJ: IEEE Press/Wiley Interscience.

de Jong, K. A. (2006). *Evolutionary computation*. Cambridge, MA: MIT Press.

Evolutionary Computation. MIT Press. http://www.mitpressjournals.org/loi/evco

IEEE Transactions on Evolutionary Computation. IEEE Press. http://ieeexplore.ieee.org/xpl/RecentIssue.jsp? punumber=4235

Evolutionary Multi-Objective Optimization

Coello Coello, C. A., van Veldhuizen, D.A., & Lamont, G.B. (2002). *Evolutionary algorithms for solving multi-objective problems*. New York: Kluwer Academic.

Coello Coello, C.A. & G.B. Lamont (eds). 2004. *Applications of Multi-Objective Evolutionary Algorithms*. Singapore: World Scientific.

Deb, K. 2001. *Multi-objective Optimization using Evolutionary Algorithms*. John Wiley & Sons, Chicester, UK.

Tan, K.C., E.F. Khor & T.H. Lee. 2005. *Multi-objective Evolutionary Algorithms & Applications*. Berlin: Springer.

Evolutionary Robotics

Nolfi, S. & Floreano, D. (2000). *Evolutionary robotics: The biology, intelligence & technology of self-organizing machines*. Cambridge, MA: MIT Press/Bradford Books.

Wang L. F., Tan, K. C., & Chew, C. M. (2006). *Evolutionary robotics: From algorithms to implementations*. Singapore: World Scientific Publishing.

Walker, J., Garrett, S., & Wilson, M. (2003). Evolving controllers for real robots: A survey of the literature. *Adaptive Behavior, 11*(3), 179–203.

Adaptive Behavior. Sage Publications. http://adb.sagepub.com/

Artificial Life. MIT Press. http://www.mitpressjournals.org/loi/artl

Genetic Programming & Evolvable Machines. Springer. http://www.springerlink.com/content/1573-7632/

IEEE Transactions on Systems, Man & Cybernetics – Part B. IEEE Press. http://ieeexplore.ieee.org/xpl/RecentIssue.jsp? punumber=3477

Physics-Based Simulators

Havok Complete by Havok. http://www.havok.com/content/view/19/32/

Open Dynamics Engine (ODE) by Russell Smith. http://www.ode.org/

Vortex by CM Labs. http://www.cm-labs.com/software/vortex/

Webots by Cyberbotics. http://www.cyberbotics.com/products/webots/download.html

Conferences of Interest

ACM Genetic & Evolutionary Computation Conference (GECCO).

IEEE International Conference on Systems, Man & Cybernetics (SMC).

IEEE Congress on Evolutionary Computation (CEC).

IEEE International Conference on Robotics & Automation (ICRA).

IEEE Symposium Series on Computation Intelligence (SSCI).

IEEE/RSJ International Conference on Intelligent Robots & Systems (IROS).

International Conference on the Simulation of Adaptive Behavior (SAB).

International Conference on Simulation & Synthesis of Living systems (ALIFE).

International Conference on Evolutionary Multi-criterion Optimization (EMO).

International Conference on Informatics in Control, Automation & Robotics (ICINCO).

International Conference on Parallel Problem-Solving from Nature (PPSN).

Chapter XII
Evolutionary Multi-Objective Optimization in Energy Conversion Systems:
From Component Detail to System Configuration

Andrea Toffolo
University of Padova, Italy

ABSTRACT

The research field on energy conversion systems presents a large variety of multi-objective optimization problems that can be solved taking full advantage of the features of evolutionary algorithms. In fact, design and operation of energy systems can be considered in several different perspectives (e.g., performance, efficiency, costs, environmental aspects). This results in a number of objective functions that should be simultaneously optimized, and the knowledge of the Pareto optimal set of solutions is of fundamental importance to the decision maker. This chapter proposes a brief survey of typical applications at different levels, ranging from the design of component detail to the challenge about the synthesis of the configuration of complex energy conversion systems. For sake of simplicity, the proposed examples are grouped into three main categories: design of components/component details, design of overall energy system, operation of energy systems. Each multi-objective optimization problem is presented with a short background and some details about the formulation. Future research directions in the field of energy systems are also discussed at the end of the chapter.

INTRODUCTION

Multi-objective evolutionary algorithms have a multiform spectrum of applications in the research field about energy systems. This chapter is an attempt to give an organized picture of the formulation and solution of multi-objective optimization problems in this field. The subject ranges from the design of component detail zooming out to various aspects about the design and operation of the whole system. Many applications of single-objective evolutionary algorithms have been proposed in the literature as well. They can be easily, and profitably, extended to multi-objective optimization problems by taking into account some other important objectives that have been neglected or incorporated in the considered single-objective function using weighting factors.

A short background of each topic is provided and some of the most recent and significant examples of applications are discussed, analyzing the context and the formulation of each problem. Some details are also provided about the codification of the decision variables, the evaluation of the objective functions, the multi-objective evolutionary algorithms used for the search of the Pareto optimal set and the most interesting features of the obtained results.

DESIGN OF COMPONENT DETAILS

Energy conversion systems feature a large variety of components performing different tasks, which usually involve the exchange or transformation of energy through operating fluids. When the focus is limited to a single component, several objectives related to the main process that takes place in the component can be considered to formulate multi-objective optimization problems. The nature of these objectives primarily involves energetic and economic aspects of the process, although several other objectives can be taken into account as well.

The main objective that is often considered in the formulation of optimization problems is a measure of the efficiency at which component task is performed. In a fan, for instance, the main component task is to transform the mechanical energy supplied by the rotation of impeller blades into a total pressure rise for the air that flows through the machine. The efficiency of this energy conversion process (the ratio between the desired output and the required input) cannot be 100% due to the aerodynamic and volumetric losses inside fan impeller and diffuser.

Two-objective optimization problems of particular interest can be set up when task performance index is taken into account as the second objective, since performance and efficiency are usually conflicting objectives. In the example of the fan, the two objectives would be the maximization of the air total pressure rise (task performance index) and the maximization of the efficiency of the conversion of impeller mechanical energy.

Other objectives that may be considered are the maximization of secondary task performance indexes (e.g., fan discharge static pressure in order to overcome the pressure losses in air ducts), the minimization of detrimental side effects (e.g., fan noise emissions) and the minimization of component or component detail sizes (e.g., the radial and/or axial room required by the fan unit). The minimization of costs (manufacturing, purchase, operating costs) obviously deserves, as always, a special place among the objectives that can be taken into account.

Multi-objective design optimization of components or component details can be exploited for an extremely wide spectrum of applications. Three examples are given in the following, about axial compressor blades, heat exchangers and horizontal-axis wind turbine rotors.

Optimization of Aerofoil Shape for Axial Compressor Blades

Axial turbomachinery design essentially deals with the definition of the geometrical parameters of a series of succeeding blade cascades, a problem in which the definition of blade section geometry plays a key role. In compressor cascades, the shape of blade profile is particularly critical because the flow (relative flow in rotating cascades and absolute flow in stationary cascades) decelerates in the blade channels (Figure 1). On the suction side, the adverse pressure gradient after peak velocity location may lead to flow separation,

Figure 1. Aerofoil shape and incidence angle affect flow deceleration, and therefore the pressure rise and total pressure losses

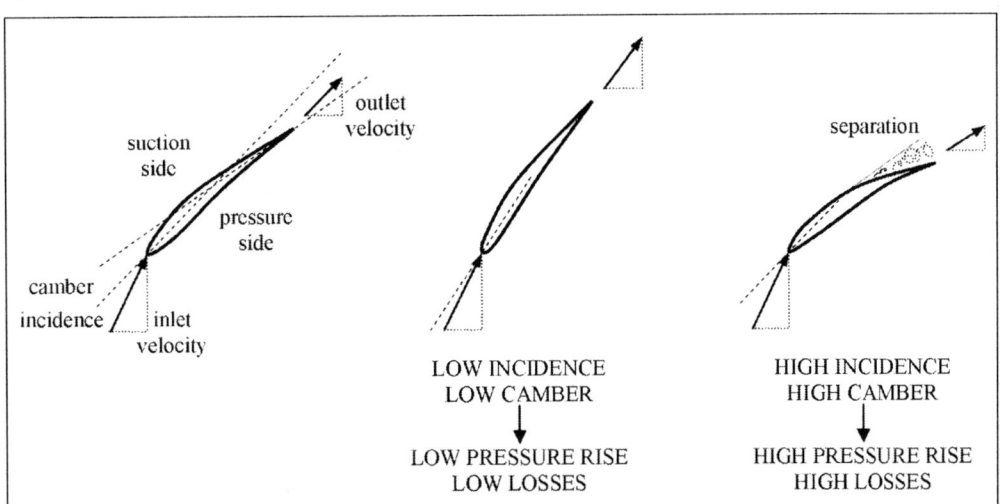

significantly penalizing the efficiency of the energy transfer from the dynamic head (relative or absolute, according to the type of motion) to operating fluid pressure. On the other hand, for a given cascade solidity, a higher amount of this energy transfer, and therefore a higher-pressure rise across the cascade, could be only obtained with a higher blade aerodynamic loading. The latter implies a greater pressure difference between pressure and suction sides, which can be achieved by more cambered aerofoils or by increasing the incidence angle for a given inlet flow angle, and results in a stronger adverse pressure gradient on the suction side.

Thus, the profile of an optimal cascade has to satisfy two conflicting design objectives. The first is the maximum pressure rise, in order to reduce the number of compression stages required to reach the desired overall pressure rise, minimizing the number of cascades to be manufactured and therefore costs as well. The second is the minimum total pressure loss (i.e., maximum energy transfer efficiency) in order to reduce the mechanical work required to obtain the desired overall pressure rise. These objectives are evaluated in the design operating condition only, yet another essential design issue deals with off-design operation. In fact, the performance of an optimal trade-off solution determined for the design conditions may decay abruptly and become unacceptable even for small variations of flow incidence angle. For example, the design angle of attack is too close to its stall value when cambered profiles are used at high inlet flow angles in order to achieve a high pressure rise due to the large flow turning angle. Therefore, some constraints must be applied to guarantee that optimal cascades will operate adequately within a given range of incidence angles centred on the design condition.

In the proposed example (Benini & Toffolo, 2002a) the shape of the profile is almost completely free (i.e., it does not rely on constrained camber or thickness distributions) and is parameterized using two Bezier curves (one for the suction side and the other for the pressure side). Bezier curves have proved to be flexible tools that are suitable to represent with few parameters the complex shapes of geometrical objects or mathematical functions. In general, the shape of a Bezier curve is defined by the coordinates of $n+1$ control points (x_i, y_i), and its analytical expression is:

$$\begin{Bmatrix} x(t) \\ y(t) \end{Bmatrix} = \sum_{i=0}^{n} \frac{n!}{i!(n-i)!} t^i (1-t)^{n-i} \begin{Bmatrix} x_i \\ y_i \end{Bmatrix} \qquad (1)$$

where $t \in [0,1]$ is the nondimensional parameter of the curve which starts in (x_0, y_0) and ends in (x_n, y_n). In this example, seven control points for each curve are used ($n=6$), but, if the abscissas of the control points x_i are fixed, only ten parameters (five ordinates for each curve, y_1 to y_5) are actually required to define the shape of the two sides between fixed leading and trailing edge points. Figure 2 shows an example of this parameterization of aerofoil geometry. Note that the abscissas x_1 and x_5 are set equal to x_0 and x_6, respectively, to describe leading and trailing edge curvature.

Decision variables. Decision variables of the optimization problem are the ten free ordinates of the Bezier control points plus the design incidence angle that defines the stagger angle of the profile for a given angle of the inlet velocity. The other quantities that are required to define cascade geometry and inlet flow features under design operating condition (cascade solidity, profile chord, inlet flow angle, inlet Mach and Reynolds numbers) are all fixed.

Objective Functions. The first of the two objective functions is the nondimensional pressure ratio PR (to be maximized) defined as

$$PR = \frac{p_2}{p_1} \qquad (2)$$

where p_2 is the averaged outlet static pressure and p_1 is the inlet static pressure. The second objective function is the total pressure loss coefficient ω (to be minimized) defined as

$$\omega = \frac{\Delta p_0}{p_{01} - p_1} \qquad (3)$$

that is the ratio between the total pressure losses in the cascade Δp_0 and the (fixed) inlet kinetic energy expressed in terms of difference between inlet total (p_{01}) and static pressures. The quantities required to evaluate the objective functions are determined using a computational fluid dynamic (CFD) tool that solves compressible viscous flows over arbitrary quasi-three-dimensional cascades of aerofoils, using a zonal approach that couples the viscous flow inside the boundary layer and the equivalent inviscid flow that is postulated outside a displacement streamline comprising the boundary layer.

Constraints. A constraint on total pressure losses is also imposed to ensure an adequate margin for off-design operation. Following the operating range definition for a compressor cascade in terms of interval of incidence angles, the total pressure loss coefficient must be less than

Figure 2. Aerofoil shape parameterization using Bezier curves

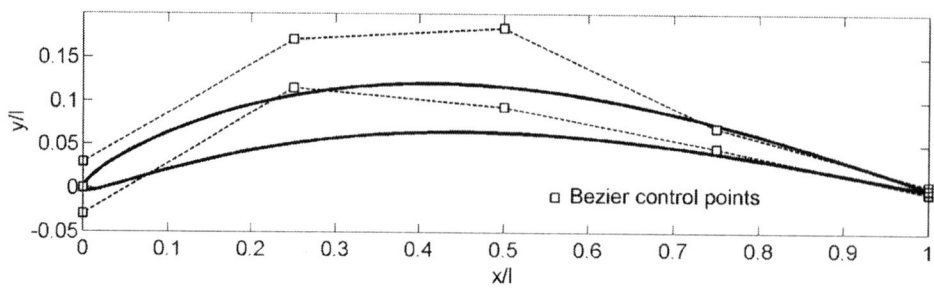

two times its design condition value in a range of ±5deg from the design incidence angle. This constraint is verified by repeating the numerical simulations for the same cascade geometry at different inlet velocity angles, so that the total pressure loss coefficient is sampled at ±2.5deg and ±5deg from the design incidence angle.

Methodology. The multi-objective evolutionary algorithm used to search for the optimal solutions is the Genetic Diversity Evolutionary Algorithm (GDEA), developed by Toffolo and Benini (2003). In this algorithm, a further step is performed after the Pareto ranking of the solutions according to the objectives of the optimization problem. In this step the maximizations of Pareto rank and genetic diversity of each solution are considered as meta-objectives of the search process, and the solutions are ranked again according to these two metaobjectives using the criterion of Pareto dominance. Only the best solution of this further ranking is finally passed to the next generation.

A real-value representation is used for the decision variables. Parent individuals for the mating pool are selected with a uniform probability among the population. The crossover operator simply calculates the mean of the two parental vectors of decision variables and then adds a random variation in a random direction, so that, in the search space, the offspring point falls within a hypersphere centred on the middle point between the points of the two parents. This crossover operator is used to generate all the offspring individuals. The mutation operator is then applied with a probability of 2% and simply replaces one value at random in the vector of the decision variables with a random value. A population of 100 individuals is used and the algorithm is stopped after 200 generations.

Results. An example of the resulting set of the optimized profiles for a given design condition is shown in Figure 3, in which aerofoils from the well-known family of NACA 65-series are considered as reference. In particular, NACA 65-8-10, 65-12-10 and 65-15-10 profiles show lower efficiency (pressure ratio being equal) than individuals A, B and C, whereas they achieve a lower pressure rise (total pressure losses being

Figure 3. The Pareto front of the optimized profiles compared with the objective function values of NACA 65 profiles

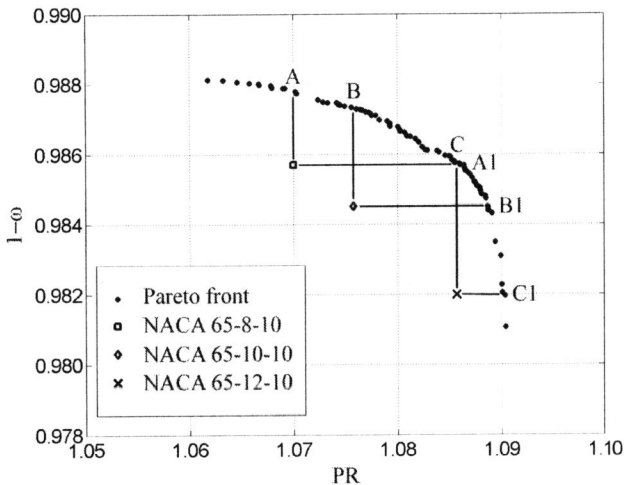

equal) than individuals A1, B1 and C1. A detailed comparison among shapes and design/off-design performance is presented in Figures 3 and 4 for the aerofoils NACA 65-8-10, A and A1. The pressure ratio of high-pressure-rise optimal profiles is superior than that of NACA profiles in most of the operating range, and the total pressure loss distribution as a function of incidence angle is similar but generally shifted towards higher angles of attack. On the other hand, the lower boundary layer and wake losses of the high-efficiency optimal profiles result in lower total pressure losses with respect to those of NACA profiles, whereas the trend of pressure ratio as a function of incidence angle is steeper.

Figure 4. Comparison among the shapes of the NACA 65 and the optimized profiles

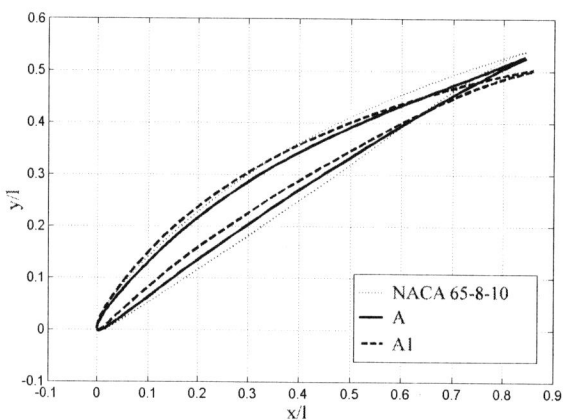

Figure 5. Off-design performance of the NACA 65 profile and of the optimized profiles

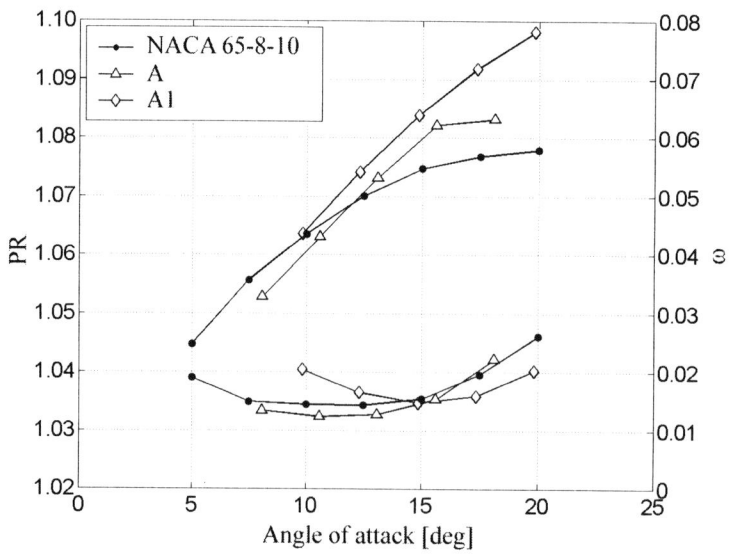

Optimal Design of Heat Exchangers

The design of heat exchangers involves the coupling of fluid- and thermodynamic phenomena. For given inlet temperatures of the hot and cold fluids, heat transfer essentially depends on the exchange area and on the heat transfer coefficient, which in turn depends on fluid velocity and flow regime. On the other hand, the higher friction on a larger exchange area, a higher velocity and a turbulent flow regime are all factors that make the pressure drop increase.

Thus, an optimal geometrical configuration has to achieve the maximization of heat transfer in a constrained space (or, equivalently, maximum unit compactness for a given heat transfer) and the minimization of pressure losses for the operating fluids on both sides.

A typical example of shape optimization in heat exchanger design is presented in Hilbert, Janiga, Baron, and Thévenin (2006).

Decision variables. The blade-shaped symmetric profile of a tube section for a tube bank heat exchanger (Figure 6) is parameterized using the four Cartesian coordinates of the two intermediate points P_1 and P_2 of a nonuniform rational basic spline (NURBS). The coordinates (x_1,y_1) and (x_2,y_2) are the only decision variables of the problem, the other parameters of the geometrical configuration (profile chord and the distances D_1 and D_2 between the profiles) being fixed. The boundary conditions of domain analyzed, that is, velocity and temperature of the inlet air flow (v_{inlet} and T_{inlet}), profile wall temperature (T_{wall}) and outlet pressure (p_{outlet}), are fixed as well.

Objective functions. Two objective functions are considered, the pressure drop Δp (to be minimized) and the temperature rise ΔT (to be maximized) of the air flow that crosses the hot tube:

$$\Delta p = p_{inlet} - p_{outlet} \quad [Pa]$$
$$\Delta T = T_{outlet} - T_{inlet} \quad [K] \quad (4)$$

Inlet pressure p_{inlet} and outlet temperature T_{outlet} are evaluated using a commercial CFD code. The numerical simulations are performed in parallel on several PCs to speed up computational time.

Methodology. The multi-objective genetic algorithm used to search for the optimal solutions is based on the floating-point representation of the decision variables and on the old-fashioned approach proposed by Fonseca and Fleming (1993) for Pareto ranking. When a new generation is created, an individual of the previous generation

Figure 6. A scheme of the geometry of the tube bank heat exchanger considered in Hilbert et al. (2006)

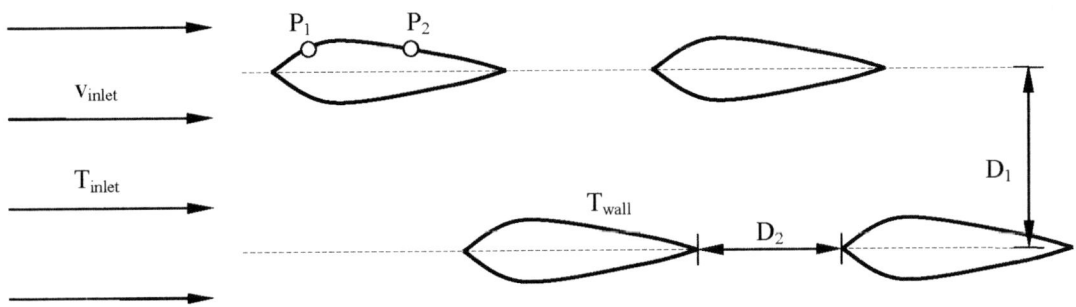

participates in the reproduction process with a probability that is determined by a fitness value depending on its Pareto rank. The lower is the rank, defined as the number of individuals dominating the considered individual, the higher is the probability of being selected for the mating pool. The new population is then generated from the mating pool using three genetic operators: "survival" (one of the two parents is cloned) with a probability of 50%, "average" (the offspring vector of decision variables is exactly the average of the parental vectors) with a probability of 33.33%, and "crossover" (the components of the offspring vector are taken from either one of the parental vectors) with a probability of 16.67%. The mutation operator is finally applied to all the vector components of the offspring generated by the survival and crossover operators. The magnitude of the random variations introduced by the mutation operator is progressively reduced during the search process. At each generation, the nondominated individuals are also stored in an elite set only for archiving purpose.

Results. The results of a population of 30 individuals after 20 generations show that different kind of shapes belong to the Pareto front, with maximum profile thickness facing either the inflow or the outflow (Figure 7).

Foli, Okabe, Olhofer, Jin, and Sendhoff (2006) present another example about the exchange surface that separates the alternate hot and cold flows in the channels of a micro heat exchanger.

Decision variables. Channel height and length are fixed, and the shape of the constant thickness separator between two adjacent channels is defined by a NURBS with ten control points (Figure 8). The coordinates of these control points are the decision variables of the optimization problems. Inlet pressures, temperatures and flow rates are fixed for both the hot and the cold flows.

Objective functions. A commercial CFD code evaluates the two objective functions that are the sum of pressure drops Δp in the hot and cold channels (to be minimized) and the transferred heat Q (to be maximized):

$$f_1 = \Delta p_{hot} + \Delta p_{cold} \quad [Pa]$$
$$f_2 = Q = \dot{m}_{hot} c_{p,hot} \Delta T_{hot} = \dot{m}_{cold} c_{p,cold} \Delta T_{cold} \quad [W]$$
(5)

where $\dot{m}$ are the mass flow rates (fixed), c_p are the specific heats at constant pressure and ΔT are the temperature changes of the hot and cold flows.

Methodology. The optimization process is performed by the well-known NSGA-II (Deb, Pratap, Agarval, & Meyarivan, 2002). Real parameter values are binary encoded (20 bits per value) and standard one-point crossover and bit-flip mutation operators are applied with a probability of 90% and 5%, respectively. The search process is performed with a population of 100 individuals evolved for 500 generations.

Results. All the solutions belonging to the Pareto front show a similar geometry with a low periodicity, although the parameterization allows to consider much more complex shapes due to the high number of control points used to describe a curve.

Figure 7. The shape of the optimized profiles for the tube bank heat exchanger as both temperature rise and pressure drop increase

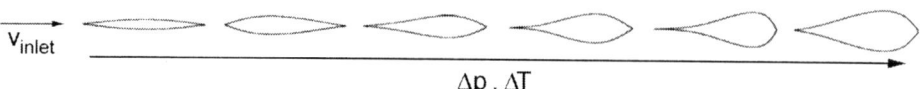

Figure 8. Two different geometries of the exchange surface that can be described by the parameterization chosen in Foli et al. (2006) (a) a low periodicity shape, (b) a high periodicity shape

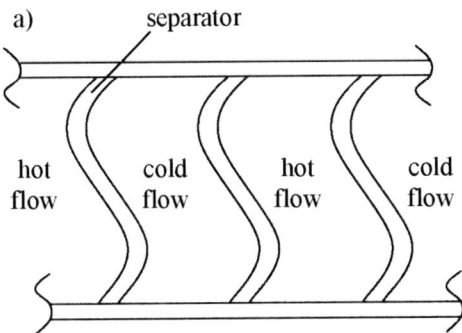
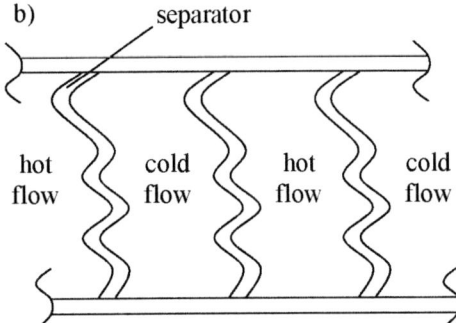

Design of Optimal Rotors for Horizontal-Axis Wind Turbines

The issues involved in the design of optimal rotors for horizontal-axis wind turbines (HAWTs) are quite different from those involved in the design of traditional turbomachinery. In fact, HAWT aerodynamics is very complex, and design criteria cannot be simplified to a matter of trade-offs between aerofoil performance and efficiency at the design wind speed for a given annular section of the rotor. The main feature of the primary energy source, that is, wind kinetic energy, is its extreme variability, so the HAWT operates at its maximum efficiency or at its maximum power only in a small fraction of the total hours per year. Thus, rotor performance has to be evaluated along the entire characteristic curve of power output vs. wind speed, from cut-in to cut-out speed. The merit figure used to express overall rotor aerodynamic performance is the annual energy production (AEP) in kilowatt-hours per year. It is the integral of power output over time during one year and can be evaluated only for a given site according to the specific frequency distribution of wind speed. In fact, it is equal to the integral over wind speed U of the product of the power output P as a function of U and the site-specific frequency distribution $prob(U)$ in hours per year (see Figure 9):

$$AEP = \int_{1\,year} P(t)dt = \int_0^\infty P(U)prob(U)dU \; [kWh/y]$$

(6)

On the other hand, the other fundamental merit figure to evaluate a wind turbine design is the cost of energy (COE), which is expressed in money per unit of energy output. In fact, the COE is the ratio between total (investment plus operation and maintenance) HAWT costs and the AEP. The COE is strongly dependent on rotor design as well, since turbine costs show a roughly linear relationship with blade weight. Therefore, the design of HAWT rotors features a challenging conflict between the amount of energy output and the cost at which this energy is made available.

The proposed example (Benini & Toffolo, 2002b) presents a two-objective optimization problem for the design of a fixed-pitch stall-regulated HAWT rotor.

Decision variables. The parameterization of rotor geometry is based on the free distributions of aerofoil chord length c and twist angle γ_c along blade span, whereas the aerofoil shapes to be used at different radii r are fixed (NACA 63-2-21, 63-2-18 and 63-2-15 are chosen as root, primary and tip aerofoils, respectively). The free distributions are described as functions of blade nondimensional radius using Bezier curves with four control points. The number of blades and rotor tilt and coning angles are instead fixed design parameters. The decision variables of the optimization problem are blade hub/tip ratio, the twelve control point coordinates of the two Bezier curves defining chord length and twist angle (the four ordinates and the two intermediate abscissas per free distribution, see Figure 10) and tip peripheral speed, which is used to determine rotor radius according to the fixed maximum power output. Blade weight is evaluated using a fixed nondimensional shell thickness distribution along blade span, referred to the maximum shell thickness at blade root. To determine the latter, the stresses at blade root due to aerodynamic loads and centrifugal force are calculated, and then the maximum allowable stress condition for the material (fiberglass) is imposed with a safety factor.

Constraints. Two constraints are imposed at any blade section to ensure the feasibility of the optimal solution. The first is an aerodynamic constraint related to the axial induction factor: it checks that axial velocity is decelerated but not halted or inverted downstream the rotor. The second is a geometrical constraint verifying that profile thickness, which is proportional to chord length, is more than two times shell thickness.

Objective functions. The two objective functions considered in the optimization problem are AEP density, that is, the ratio of AEP to the square of rotor radius R, to be maximized, and the COE, to be minimized. AEP density is chosen as a design objective because it is related to the overall AEP of a wind farm installed in a site of given area. In fact, the number of HAWTs that can be fitted in a given area is inversely proportional to the square of rotor radius, since the distances in the grid of the HAWT towers are proportional to rotor radius. On the other hand, if the AEP of a single rotor were chosen as an objective, the search would be driven towards large rotors featuring very thin, and possibly unfeasible, blades (in fact, the larger the radius, the more wind energy is intercepted and can be converted into power). The other objective

Figure 9. The two curves that are required for the evaluation of HAWT annual energy production: the characteristic curve P(U) and site-specific frequency distribution of wind speed prob(U)

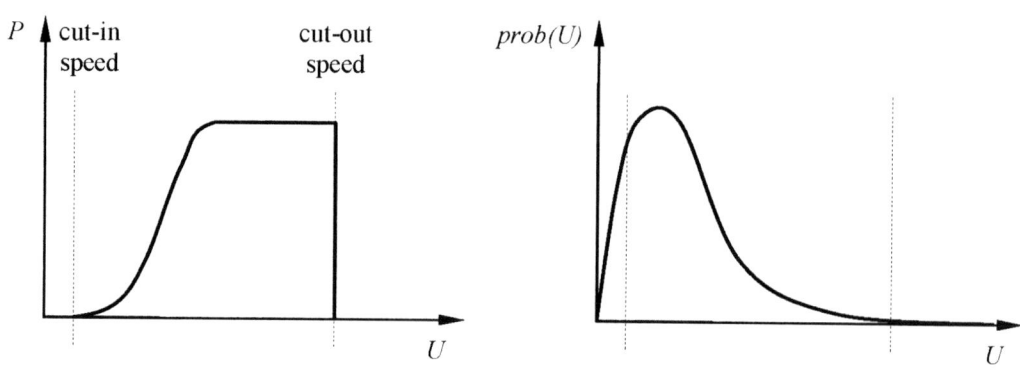

Figure 10. Parameterization of the nondimensional chord distribution and twist angle distribution using Bezier curve with four control points

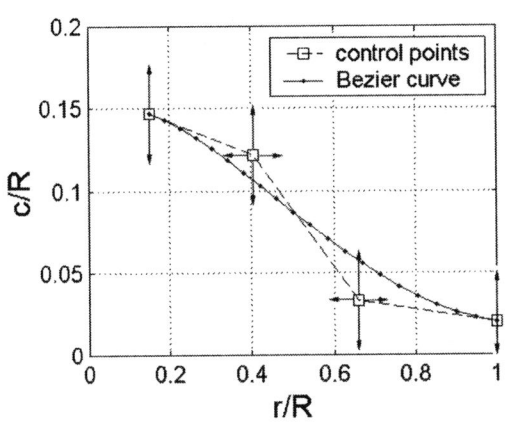
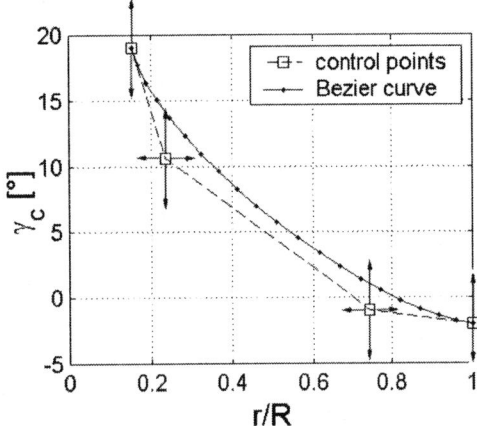

function is determined according to a cost model that defines the COE as follows:

$$COE = \frac{TC + BOS}{AEP} FCR + O\&M \ [\$/kWh] \quad (7)$$

where turbine costs (TC) are proportional to blade weight, the balance of station (BOS) is proportional to the maximum power output and FCR is the fixed charge rate. Operation and maintenance costs are considered proportional to the energy output and therefore only the proportionality constant O&M appears in the COE formula.

The solution of rotor aerodynamics, which is required to evaluate the objective functions, is obtained using an analytical model based on blade element theory. The variations of axial and tangential velocity components as well as the aerodynamic forces acting on blade sections are evaluated at all radii and for the entire range of wind speeds, from cut-in to cut-out speed.

Methodology. The multi-objective evolutionary algorithm used to search for the optimal trade-offs among the objectives is the GDEA (Toffolo & Benini, 2003), in which a real-value representation is used for the decision variables. The settings used for the selection, crossover and mutation operators are the same described in the previous example of the multi-objective optimization of aerofoil shape for axial compressor blades. The algorithm is run for 150 generations with a population of 100 individuals.

Results. The Pareto fronts found for three different rated powers (600kW, 800kW and 1MW) are shown in Figure 11. The objective function values for some commercial wind turbines, calculated using public knowledge design specifications and AEP performance, are shown for comparison in the same figure with filled markers. It is apparent that the position of commercial wind turbines, usually featuring large rotors, is very close to the minimum COE. On the other hand, for high AEP densities, rotor radius decreases while blade weight tends to increase. In fact, the distributions of chord length and twist angles for the individuals labelled as T1 to T4 on the Pareto front (Figure 12) show that higher AEP densities are obtained using larger chords and higher incidence angles. Blade weight and turbine cost are thus higher for a relatively lower AEP of the single rotor, so the COE tends to grow rapidly.

Figure 11. The Pareto fronts for three different rated powers and detail of the comparison with some commercial HAWTs

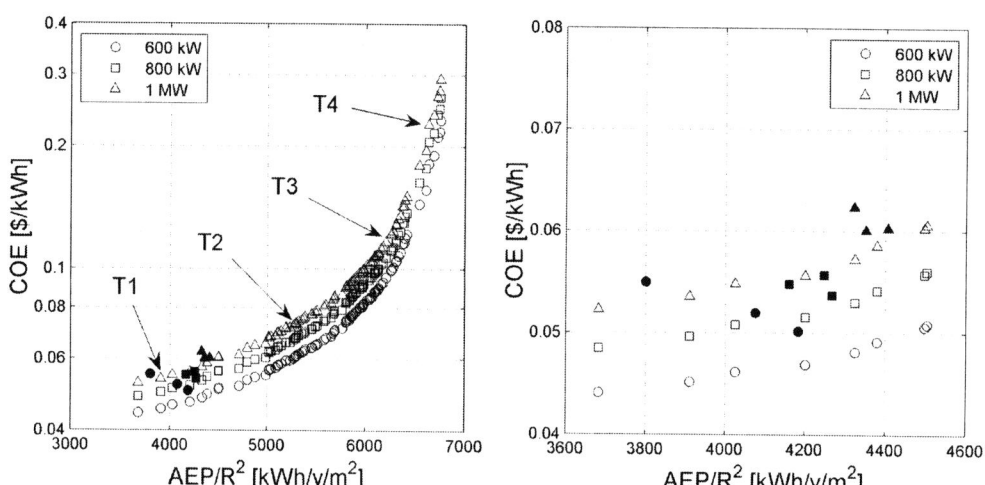

Figure 12. Nondimensional chord and twist angle distributions for different optimized rotors along the Pareto front

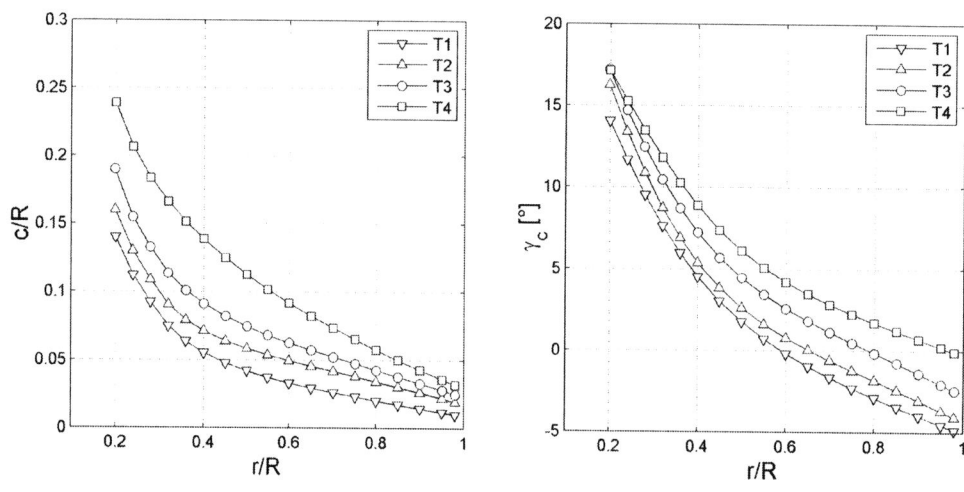

DESIGN OF ENERGY SYSTEMS

The design of energy systems involves the definition of system structure and the determination of the design parameters of a given system structure. Many objectives of different nature can be considered in the design process. The most common ones fall within three main categories: thermodynamic (e.g., maximum efficiency, minimum fuel consumption), economic (e.g., minimum cost per unit of time, maximum profit per unit of production) and environmental (e.g., limited emissions, minimum environmental impact). Several analyses in the literature suggest incorporating the thermodynamic and the environmental objectives in a single overall economic objective function by expressing resource consumption and pollution damage in terms of monetary costs. This is equivalent to build a weighted single objective function in which resource and pollution unit costs are the weighting factors. However, these factors are subject to change unpredictably according to market fluctuations and environmental policies. Therefore, the knowledge of best trade-offs among the objectives allows the decision maker to choose from the entire set of optimal design solutions, whereas the single-objective approach with weighting factors provides just one of them.

The examples that are discussed in the following sections are related to the optimization of system design parameters, the synthesis of heat exchanger networks, the synthesis of complex energy systems and the optimization of district heating networks.

Optimization of System Design Parameters

The optimization of system design parameters is the least complex of the application fields presented in this Section. In fact, when system structure is already defined, the formulation of the optimization problem is a quite straightforward task. The CGAM problem (Valero, Lozano, Serra, Tsatsaronis, Pisa, & Frangopoulos, 1994) represents a paradigmatic case, in which the design parameters of a cogeneration plant are to be optimized (Figure 13). The plant is made up of a regenerative gas turbine and a heat recovery steam generator (HRSG), and satisfies fixed demands of electrical energy (30MW) and steam (14kg/s at 20bar). In the original formulation of the CGAM problem, four different thermoeconomic methodologies were applied to search for the minimum total cost rate, considering a single objective function in which fuel (i.e., operating) and investment cost rates are summed up. This objective function is often referred to as a linear combination of an energetic and an economic objective function, because fuel cost rate directly depends on fuel consumption, and therefore on the exergetic efficiency for a given energy system output. Actually, this relationship does not alter the nature of the objective function, which simply accounts for the money to be spent and so merely expresses an economic objective.

A really two-objective (exergetic and economic) formulation of the CGAM problem is presented in Toffolo and Lazzaretto (2002). The difference about the nature of the results obtained with the original thermoeconomic formulation and the two-objective one is shown graphically in Figure 14. The thermoeconomic objective function guides the search towards the economic minimum only, whereas the Pareto front of the best trade-off solutions between the energetic and the economic objectives allows enlarging the perspective to optimal solutions that feature higher exergetic efficiency at the expense of a reasonable increase of total cost rate.

Decision variables. The design parameters that are considered as decision variables of the optimization problem are:

- The compressor pressure ratio $PR_{cp}=p_2/p_1$
- Turbine inlet temperature T_4
- Compressor isentropic efficiency $\eta_{cp,is}$
- Turbine isentropic efficiency $\eta_{gt,is}$
- air preheater effectiveness $\varepsilon_{ap}=(T_3-T_2)/(T_5-T_2)$

Ambient conditions, the properties of all fluids (air, fuel, combustion gases and steam) and plant products are instead fixed.

Constraints. Feasibility constraints are imposed to ensure that heat transfer occurs between viable temperature profiles in the air preheater and in the HRSG. See Exhibit A.

A minimum temperature limit is also set for the exhaust gases.

HRSG $T_7 > 378.15K$

Objective functions. The two objectives are the maximization of exergetic efficiency ζ, which is the ratio between the exergy flow rates in plant products and the fuel exergy flow rate:

$$\zeta = \frac{\dot{W} + \dot{m}_{steam}(e_9 - e_8)}{\dot{m}_{fuel} e_{fuel}} \qquad (8)$$

and the minimization of total cost rate, which is the sum of the fuel cost rate and the capital investment, operation and maintenance cost rate $\dot{Z}$ for each of the components:

$$\dot{C}_{total} = \dot{C}_{fuel} + \sum_i \dot{Z}_i \quad [\$/s] \qquad (9)$$

The quantities required to evaluate the objective function are obtained using a numerical model in which the equations of the thermodynamic and

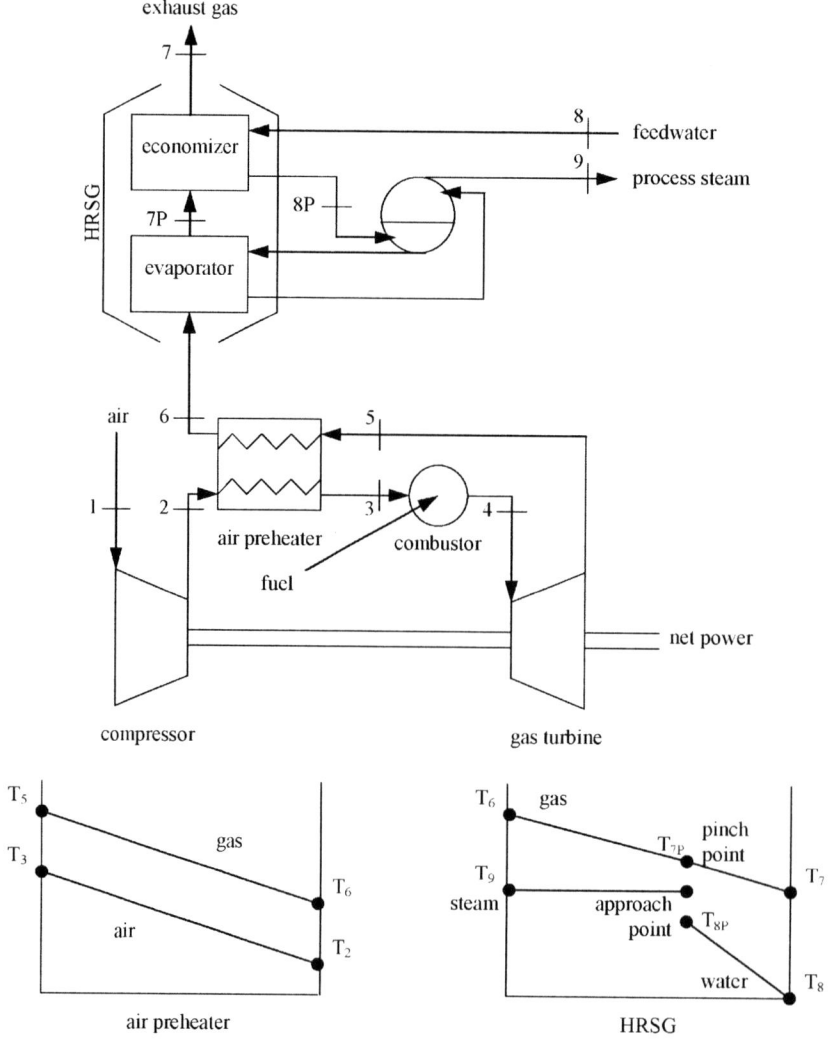

Figure 13. Flow diagram of the CGAM cogeneration plant and temperature profiles in the heat transfer devices

economic models of the cogeneration plant are implemented. In particular, the equations of the economic model are solved after all the thermodynamic quantities are known, because component purchase costs are expressed as functions of the design values of the main thermodynamic parameters, according to statistical correlations (cost laws) obtained on real data series.

Methodology. The evolutionary algorithm used to find the optimal solutions is the GDEA (Toffolo & Benini, 2003) with a real-value representation of the decision variables. The settings used for the selection, crossover and mutation operators are the same described above in the example of the multi-objective optimization of aerofoil shape for axial compressor blades. The algorithm is run for 500 generations with a population of 200 individuals.

Results. The Pareto front of the optimal solutions (Figure 15) show that a two point improvement of the exergetic efficiency corresponds to a slight increase of total cost rate (+5%). A sensitivity analysis is also performed to assess the influence of the unit cost of fuel (i.e., the proportion between fuel and investment cost within the economic objective). The results in Figure 16 show that the choice of an optimal solution that differs from the economic minimum may be strategically more interesting in a scenario featuring increasing unit costs of fuel.

The formulation of the CGAM optimization problem is extended to a third environmental objective in Lazzaretto and Toffolo (2004). It is worth noting that this approach radically differs from imposing constraints on the emission levels tolerated by the regulations in force, and from adding penalty terms related to the amount of released pollutants to a global cost function. The nature of the enviromental objective has its own dignity and derives from the intrinsic undesirable outcomes of the energy conversion process (e.g., toxic emissions, thermal pollution, solid wastes), which are all to be minimized. An

Figure 14. Comparison between the thermoeconomic and the two-objective formulations of the CGAM optimization problem

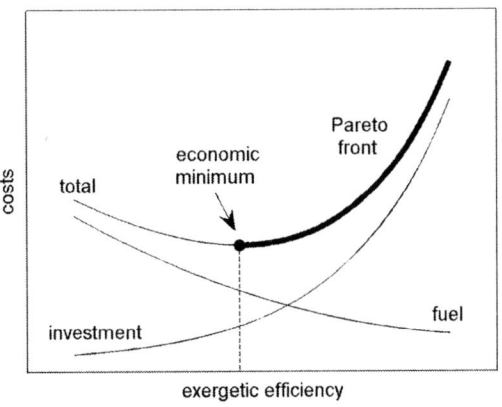

Exhibit A.

Air preheater	$T_5 > T_3$	$T_6 > T_2$	
HRSG	$\Delta T_P = T_{7P} - T_9 > 0$	$T_6 \geq T_9 + \Delta T_P$	$T_7 \geq T_9 + \Delta T_P$

347

environmental objective function can be built by weighting the "environmental impact" of each considered pollutant emission according to its degree of harmfulness. In the proposed example, the environmental impact is expressed in monetary terms, using the unit damage costs as weighting coefficients that multiply the pollutant mass flow rates. If these pollution costs are actually to be paid, the economic objective function has to be modified accordingly to include them.

Decision variables. Due to the increased complexity of the search process, the number of decision variables is limited to three (compressor pressure ratio, turbine inlet temperature and air preheater effectiveness). The isentropic efficiencies of both compressor and gas turbine are assigned a fixed value.

Constraints. The same constraints of the two-objective optimization problem are imposed.

Objective functions. The same objective functions of the two-objective optimization problem are considered: the maximization of exergetic efficiency (equation (8)) and the minimization of total cost rate (equation (9)). A third environmental objective function is added, taking into account the environmental impact of two pollutants (CO_2 production and NO_x emissions) according to their unit damage costs:

$$\dot{C}_{env} = c_{CO_2} \dot{m}_{CO_2} + c_{NO_x} \dot{m}_{NO_x} \; [\$/s] \qquad (10)$$

The mass flow rate of NO_x emissions is evaluated using a simple environmental model, based on semi-analytical correlations, that is added to the thermodynamic and economic models.

Methodology. The same evolutionary algorithm of the two-objective optimization problem is used with the same settings and the same representation of the decision variables. The popula-

Figure 15. The Pareto front and the Pareto optimal set of the two-objective formulation of the CGAM problem

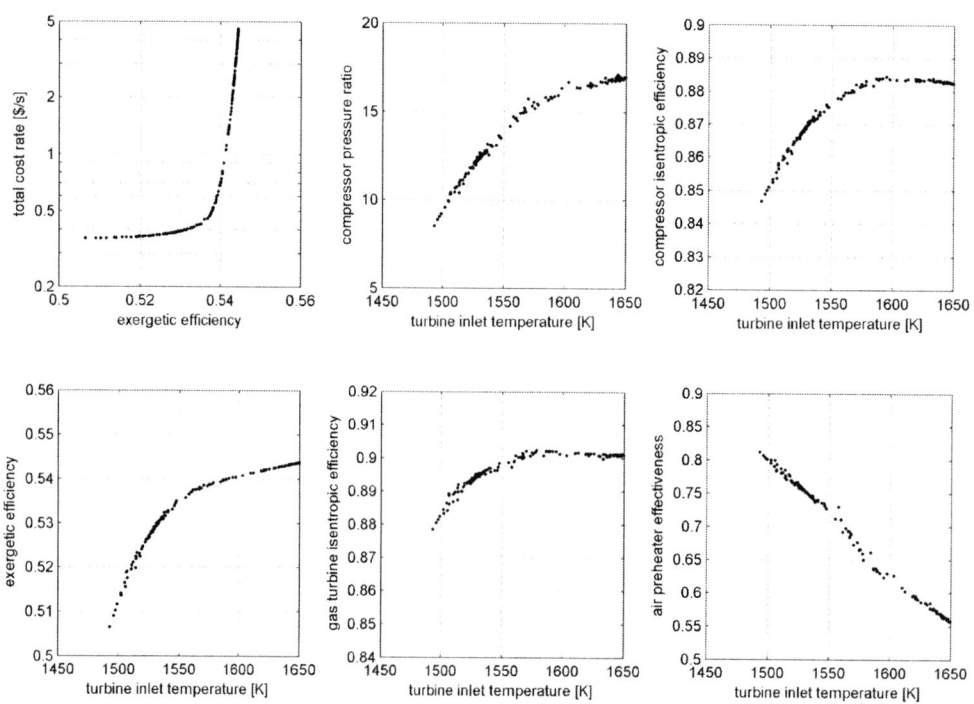

tion is now much larger (2000 individuals) and is evolved for 100 generations.

Results. The Pareto optimal set and the projections of the Pareto front on the planes defined by considering two objective functions at a time are presented in Figure 17, and a three dimensional representation of the Pareto front is shown in Figure 18. A further enlarged perspective on the optimal solutions is now available to the designer, who has to carefully consider the steep increase in the environmental impact objective associated with the solutions near the economic minimum.

Optimal Synthesis of Heat Exchanger Networks

The optimal synthesis of heat exchanger networks (HENs) is a typical example of the class of prob-

Figure 16. The influence of the unit cost of fuel on the Pareto front of the two-objective formulation of the CGAM problem

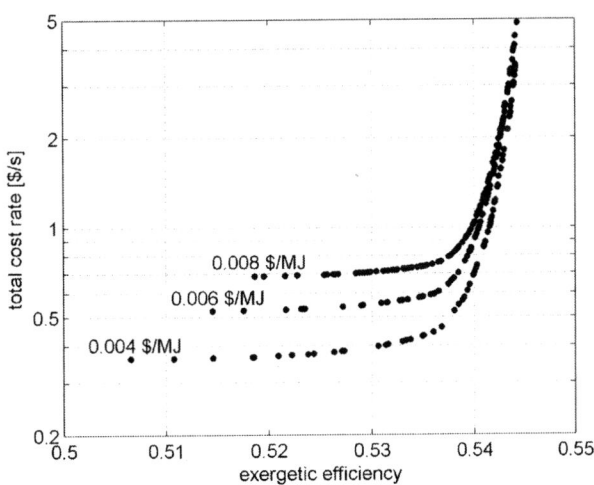

Figure 17. Projections of the Pareto front of the three-objective formulation of the CGAM problem (square = minimum total cost rate, triangle = maximum exergetic efficiency, circle = minimum environmental impact)

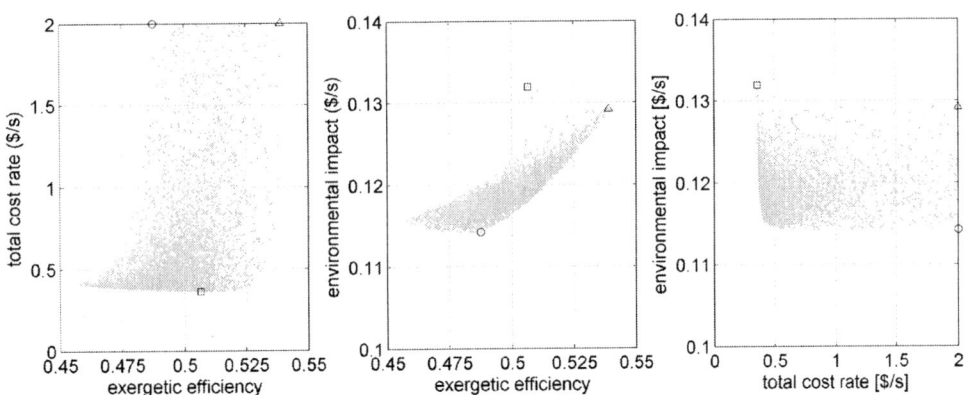

Figure 18. A three-dimensional representation of the Pareto front of the three-objective formulation of the CGAM problem

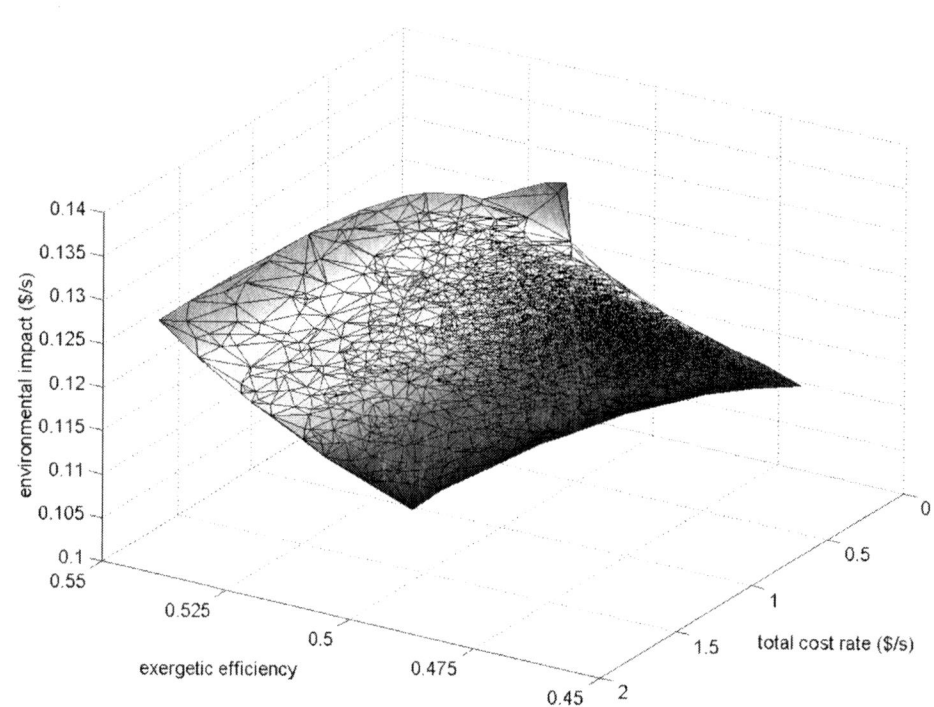

lems in which system topology plays a distinctive role. In fact, thermal energy may be transferred from hot to cold streams in many different ways, according to the number of heat exchangers, their sequence along the streams, the amount of heat transferred by each exchanger and the amount supplied/received by external utilities (Figure 19). Further levels of complexity are introduced if the possibility of splitting a stream (and then remixing its branches) at arbitrary locations is taken into account as well. Thus, the main difficulty related to considering HEN topology as a design variable concerns its representation.

Decision variables. Different techniques are used in the literature to provide a univocal mathematical description of HEN topology by means of a list of real and integer or boolean decision variables that can be handled by an optimization algorithm. Perhaps, the easiest technique involves the so-called "superstructure", a super-topology that should be as general as possible in order to comprise all the combinations of system layouts/flowsheets. The superstructure for a given problem is determined a priori, and the solutions considered for that problem are the possible simplifications of the superstructure only. However, in the case of HENs, it is apparent that any criterion cannot be exhaustive in representing all the feasible solutions (i.e., it is impossible to establish in advance the features of any arbitrary topology), and this may result in the exclusion of significant sets of solutions. Graph representation technique allows the coding of more arbitrary HEN structures, in which nodes correspond to network components (splitters, mixers, heat exchangers, stream inputs and output, external utilities) and edges correspond

Figure 19. Example of a HEN with two hot and two cold streams. One of the cold streams needs an external hot utility (HU) and one of the hot streams needs an external cold utility (CU)

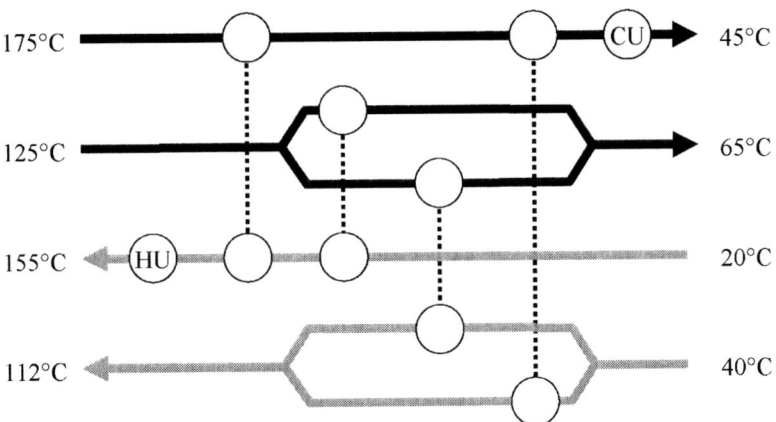

to physical links. The choice of HEN representation also exerts a strong influence on the genetic operators of the evolutionary algorithm, that is, on how pieces of information from two solutions may be recombined or on how a random mutation may affect a solution. Real variables are generally used to represent node temperatures or enthalpy flows, whereas integer or Boolean variables are used to represent alternatives about HEN topology. Each solution may also be represented by a list of variable length of these variables.

Objective functions. The multi-objective optimization problems that can be formulated about HEN synthesis are usually oriented to two main objectives. The first is the maximization of network energy recovery, an energetic objective that measures the level of integration among the streams and is equivalent to the minimization of external utility consumption. For instance, this could be expressed as

$$\min \sum_{i=1}^{Nh} \dot{Q}_{u,i} + \sum_{j=1}^{Nc} \dot{Q}_{u,j} \; [MW] \quad (11)$$

where Nh is the number of the hot streams, Nc is the number of cold streams and $\dot{Q}_u$ is the absolute value of thermal energy flow required by the considered stream from or to the external utility. The second is the economic objective (minimization of costs) that depends on the number of heat exchangers, their exchange surfaces and the costs related to the thermal energy flows from or to the external utilities. It could be expressed as:

$$\min \sum_{i=1}^{Nh} c_h \dot{Q}_{u,i} + \sum_{j=1}^{Nc} c_c \dot{Q}_{u,j} + \sum_{k=1}^{Nex} \dot{Z}_h(A_k) \; [\$/s]$$

(12)

where c_h and c_c are the unit cost of the hot and cold external utilities in \$/MJ, Nex is the number of heat exchangers in the network, and $\dot{Z}$ is the cost rate of the k-th heat exchanger that depends on its area A_k.

Constraints. Several constraints must be imposed to ensure the physical and technological feasibility of the heat transfer (e.g., heat cannot be transferred from a lower temperature to a higher temperature, and the hot and cold composite curves must not intersect). Some heuristic guidelines, such as pinch technology rules, can also be used to simplify the optimization task.

As to the author's knowledge, examples of either multi-objective or evolutionary optimization problems about HEN synthesis can be found in the literature, whereas problems with both features do not appear. However, they could be easily derived from those examples by using a different optimization algorithm or by adding a second objective to the problem formulation.

Optimal Synthesis and Parameter Design of Complex Energy Systems

Optimal synthesis and parameter design of complex energy systems may feature, as already mentioned, objectives of energetic, economic and environmental nature. Problem formulation is again almost completely governed by the definition of system topology, but it features an additional difficulty with respect to the problem discussed in the previous section. In fact, the structure of complex energy conversion systems is not made of just one sort of components, as heat exchangers in HENs, but it may involve and integrate a large variety of components, processes and technologies. On one side, this dramatically increases the number of potential combinations among components and their connections that are to be explored. On the other side, only few connections are physically feasible or, in general, make sense between some kinds of components. In any case, the combinatorial nature of the problem results in an explosive number of theoretically possible configurations as soon as the number of elementary devices grows. Thus, the main and still open problem is again related to the representation and codification of all possible system configurations.

Lazzaretto and Toffolo (2006) propose a method that is based on the remark that the number of actual energy system configurations is not high, most of them being based on few elementary cycles. The synthesis of a configuration can be therefore considered as a composition of one or more thermodynamic cycles, involving one or more working fluids, into a single flowsheet.

Decision variables. Each cycle is represented as the fixed sequence of its four main components, which operate the fundamental transformations of a thermodynamic cycle: compression, heat exchange with a high temperature source, expansion and heat exchange with a low temperature source. The variables describing a cycle are:

- An integer for the substance used as operating fluid (e.g., air/gas, steam/water, ammonia, CO_2, etc.),
- Two real values for low and high pressure levels,
- Two real values for hot and cold source temperatures,
- Other real values for component design parameters.
- A flag associated with each transformation to identify the common transformations shared by different cycles.

Secondary components, such as saturators and mixers, are introduced (yet not codified in the genotype of the solution) to join the streams belonging to different cycles. The mixed stream then undergoes the common transformation, and finally it is branched out in other secondary (not coded) components, such as separators, condensers and splitters. Staged compression or expansion is a natural outcome when common transformations do not start or end at the same pressure levels, and therefore does not require codification.

The insertion of heat exchangers in the structure of the energy system is treated in a special way. Heat transfer may occur between any couple of subsequent components, except for where it is apparently pointless (i.e., between the cold source and the compressor, and between the hot source and the turbine). Thus, a list of the possible positions for heat exchanger insertion can be inferred from the sequence of fundamental and secondary components, without the need of being coded. A real variable codifies the expected temperature change across a heat transfer device, which is equivalent to a virtual interruption of the link between subsequent components and results in a hot flow to be cooled or a cold flow to be heated.

The key feature of this representation is the simplification of the overall problem of system configuration synthesis: the subproblem of the internal heat transfer is isolated and the overall system structure is divided in two parts. The first part, which can be referred to as the "basic system configuration", includes the fundamental and secondary components, and is the subject of the main optimization process. The second part is a sort of "black-box" in which all the internal heat transfers occur independently of the HEN that realizes them. The structure of this HEN is then defined in a sublevel of the optimization process. An example of the suggested decomposition of system topology is shown in Figure 20 for a combined-cycle power plant with two pressure levels. Unfortunately, the cited work is only devoted to the optimization of the design parameters of a given basic system configuration, and this promising representation is not fully applied to the optimization of the synthesis of the overall system.

Another method for coding system topology is the definition of a superstructure, as already mentioned about HEN synthesis. However, such method relies on the assumption that a superstructure (i.e., the most general topology that comprises all the possible topologies) really exists and that the designer is able to define it. This implies that an absolute criterion should exist to generate it, but usually the guidelines that are followed are implicitly based on designer's experience. As a consequence, the complexity of the proposed superstructures is highly subjective.

Design of Optimized District Heating Networks

The distributed generation of electricity, heating and cooling is considered one of the viable options to reduce fossil fuels consumption and CO_2 emissions. This could be achieved with the installation of district polygeneration energy systems, which meet the demand of several users/buildings and

Figure 20. Representation of the topology of a combined-cycle power plant with two pressure levels according to Lazzaretto and Toffolo (2006)

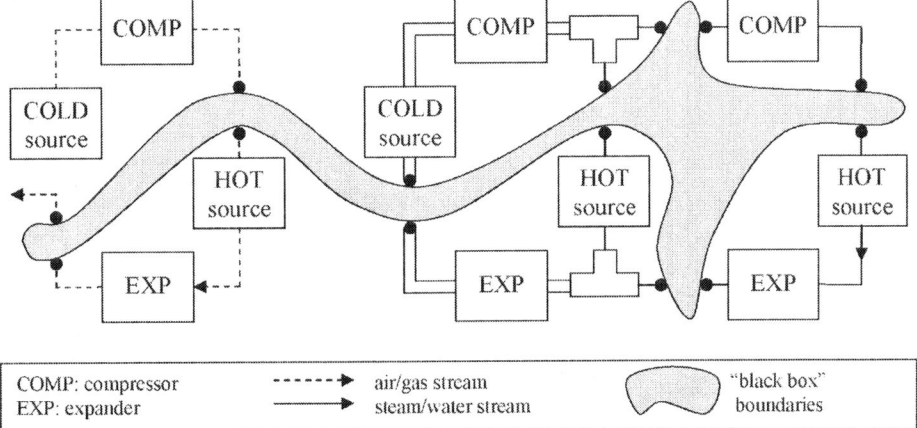

are efficiently managed by professional personnel. Among the facilities of polygeneration systems, the district heating network provides the distribution of thermal energy to a group of end users within a given area. The design of these networks concerns the topology and the sizing of the pipes that connect the energy conversion devices to the users. A further degree of complexity may be introduced if the location and the technology of the energy conversion devices (e.g., heat pumps, cogenerative gas turbines, fuel cells, boilers) is to be defined as well (Figure 21). In this case, a two-objective optimization problem can be set up to minimize both CO_2 emissions from the energy conversion devices that are required to meet given electrical and thermal demands, and the investment and operation costs of energy conversion devices and piping network. The nature of the problem is highly combinatorial. In fact, it must take into account the combinations of the types of energy conversion devices and their sizes, as well as the combinations of the network nodes in which the devices are placed and the piping topologies that connect all the served buildings. Moreover, lots of constraints of different kind must be applied to obtain feasible solutions.

Weber, Maréchal, and Favrat (2006) present the preliminary results of an optimization problem that is very similar to the one formulated above. The scope of the work is to show how a district energy system and its heating network could be designed and optimized to serve an existing quarter in Geneva, Switzerland.

Decision variables. A list of the possible technologies that can be used as energy conversion devices in the buildings is decided in advance. An integer variable codifies the type of the energy conversion device in a building and a real variable codifies its size, so there are two decision variables for each building. The consumption profiles for the different energy services in each building are fixed.

Constraints. The spatial constraints consider that the district energy system and its heating network has to serve existing buildings with a road layout, parts of already existing piping network, specific soil quality and so forth. Other constraints on the available diameters of manufactured pipes or on specific regulations must be taken into account as well.

Objective functions. The first of the two objectives that are considered in this multi-objective optimization problem is the minimization of CO_2 emissions. This is an energetic/environmental objective, because in the devices that are operated with natural gas CO_2 emissions are directly

Figure 21. Two different topologies for a district heating network serving the same group of buildings: a) a network with one gas turbine (GT) only, b) a network with a solid-oxide fuel cell (SOFC) and a heat pump (HP)

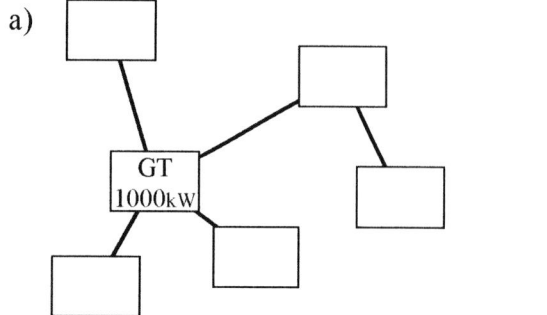
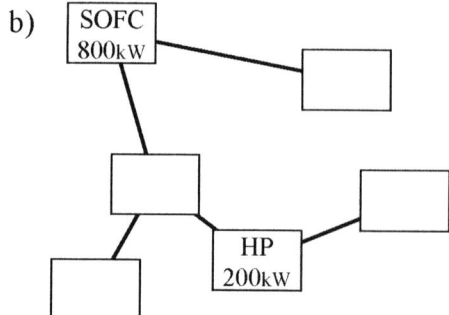

related to fuel consumption. The second objective is the minimization of the overall total costs (investment plus operation) of both the energy conversion devices and the piping network.

Methodology. Two different levels are considered in the optimization process and are implemented using a hybrid strategy. A master evolutionary algorithm governs the overall two-objective search. In order to calculate the values of the two objective functions for a solution, the information codified in its decision variables is passed to a slave nonevolutionary algorithm that optimizes piping network topology with one objective only, that is the minimization of costs.

The multi-objective evolutionary algorithm used as the master algorithm of the process is the MOO by Leyland (2002), which has the following main features:

- It has a queue-based architecture for an easy parallelization of objective function evaluations;
- The probability of using recombination/mutation operators depends on their ability in generating "successful" offspring and is evolved during the search process;
- Nondominated sorting is used for Pareto ranking;
- It is extremely elitist, since it does not use an external elite set, but a single population that contains only the current best individuals;
- Individuals are grouped using fuzzy c-means clustering to preserve diversity and to deal with discontinuous Pareto fronts;
- A tail-preservation ranking is used to ensure that the extreme points of the Pareto front are not removed from the population when the current number of nondominated individuals exceeds population size.

Results. The Pareto front is discontinuous, and the optimal solutions within each cluster feature the same or similar combinations of number and types of energy conversion devices.

OPERATION OF ENERGY SYSTEMS

The optimization of energy system operation determines how to manage an existing system under given external conditions. Different system operating points can be obtained acting on loads, control system set-points and component specific features (e.g., variable geometry, by-pass valves, etc.) in order to satisfy a specified set of objectives. The main categories of objectives are the same as in design optimization, that is, energetic, economic and environmental. However, if investments cost are ignored and only operation costs are taken into account, some objectives may assume multiple meanings. For example, in the case of a power plant with fixed output, fuel consumption can be considered as both an energetic and an economic objective.

An example of the optimized operation of a control system is given in the following, but a special application related to system operation is also worth being mentioned: the diagnosis of a malfunctioning operating condition with fuzzy expert systems.

Optimized Operation of a Control System

The control system of an energy system is designed to react to the variation of the external environment, such as user demand, resource availability or simply atmospheric conditions, in order to maintain satisfactory operation according to some predefined criteria.

The proposed example (Nassif, Kajl, & Sabourin, 2005) presents the case of a heating, ventilating and air conditioning (HVAC) system serving the rooms of a campus building (Figure 22). The scope of the work is to implement a real-time and online optimized supervisory control strategy that governs system-operating point on the basis of the measured outdoor conditions and the internal zones requirements determined by a load prediction tool.

Decision variables. The decision variables of the optimization problem are:

- Supply duct static pressure,
- Supply air temperature,
- Chilled water supply temperature,
- The actual internal zone temperatures in the 70 rooms served by the HVAC system.

Objective functions. The criteria that define optimal system operation are minimum energy consumption (i.e., minimum operating costs) and maximum thermal comfort. Energy consumption is determined by the sum of the powers absorbed by the fan and the chiller unit. Thermal comfort is evaluated as a function of an index predicting the mean response of a large group of people according to the ASHRAE thermal sensation scale. Objective function values are calculated using a simplified analytical model of the variable air volume HVAC system, which requires decision variables, outdoor conditions and predicted loads as inputs.

Methodology. The multi-objective evolutionary algorithm used in this application is the NSGA II (Deb et al., 2002). The probability of the crossover operator (simulated binary crossover) is 90% and the probability of the mutation operator is 4%. A population of 50 individuals is evolved for 100 generations to obtain the Pareto optimal solutions.

Results. An automated selection tool is used to choose the control system set points among the optimized solutions, according to the marginal energy consumption required to increase thermal comfort. The authors report that the optimized control strategy allows cutting energy demand by nearly 20%.

Diagnosis of Malfunction with Fuzzy Expert Systems

The diagnosis of energy systems studies the causes and the consequences of the anomalies occurring during system operation. The main objectives of a diagnostic procedure are:

- The detection of a malfunctioning condition due to the arising of an operation anomaly;
- The identification of the causes of malfunctions;
- The quantification of the detrimental effects.

The most difficult task is definitely the location of malfunction causes. In fact, when an operation anomaly arises, it does not affect the working point of just one component (or process), but induced effects are spread throughout the system by the interaction among components that share the same mass and energy streams and by

Figure 22. Schematic diagram of the HVAC system considered in Nassif et al. (2005)

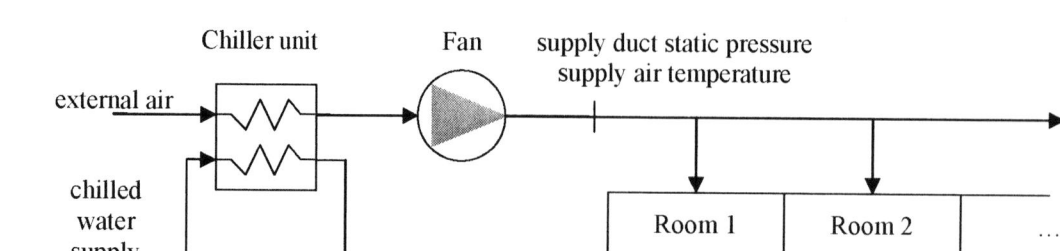

the intervention of the control system. The latter introduces additional loops involving pieces of information and physical quantities, and acts to restore the set points related to load adjustment or to avoid the crossing of dangerous operating limits. The final outcome of physical/control system interactions and loops is that the origin of the true operation anomaly is masked by the induced malfunctions.

Fuzzy logic-based expert systems are among the several artificial intelligence techniques that have been applied to the problem of locating the causes of malfunctions. The features of a fuzzy expert system can be exploited in a diagnostic procedure that performs the following steps:

- The data acquisition system measures some thermodynamic quantities (pressure, temperatures, mass flow rates etc.) of the actual operating conditions;
- The measured quantities are compared to the corresponding quantities of the expected "healthy" operating condition, which is determined by a model of the system under the same external conditions (e.g., ambient pressure and temperature, fuel quality and load adjustment set-points);
- The deltas on the measured quantities are used as inputs to the set of fuzzy rules that is stored in the knowledge base of the expert system. Each rule refers to a fault mode that is likely to have occurred if the input deltas match the pattern defined by the antecedents of that rule. Fuzzy-logic based rules are use to deal with the noise that is due to the measurement accuracy of the data acquisition system.
- If some of the rules are triggered by the input data, they notify the corresponding component/sensor fault modes; otherwise, if none of the rules is triggered, all components and sensors are believed not to be affected by any operation anomaly.

The knowledge base of the expert system usually codifies human expertise in a set of rules that are able to recognize the causes of malfunctions from the pattern of the induced effects.

Instead, in Lazzaretto and Toffolo (2007) a multi-objective evolutionary algorithm searches for the optimal sets of rules according to two conflicting objectives. The first is, of course, to maximize the exactness of the set of rules, that is the number of correct predictions on a given list of test operating conditions, and the second is to minimize its complexity. The diagnostic procedure is applied to a real test case (a two-shaft gas turbine used as the gas section of a combined-cycle cogeneration plant) in which the expert system has to recognize the effects of six component faults and one sensor fault at different loads.

Decision variables. In order to facilitate the codification of the list of rule antecedents and consequents, the rules are expressed using the following general form:

IF *delta1* IS *attribute1*
AND *delta2* IS *attribute2*
AND ...
THEN *fault_mode_k* IS *active*

where the possible attributes of the input deltas are "negative", "null" or "positive". Thus, a rule can be represented by a vector of $ni+1$ integers, where ni is the number of inputs. The first ni elements codify the attributes associated with the input deltas (if an element is zero, the corresponding delta is not considered as an antecedent of the rule), and the last element codifies the fault mode in the consequent. For instance, if the attributes "negative", "null" or "positive" correspond to the integers 1, 2 and 3, respectively, the vector [1 0 2 1 3] codifies the following rule:

IF *delta1* is *negative*
AND *delta3* IS *null*
AND *delta4* IS *negative*
THEN *fault_mode_3* IS *active*

Figure 23. The genetic operators used in Lazzaretto and Toffolo (2007) to generate the offspring

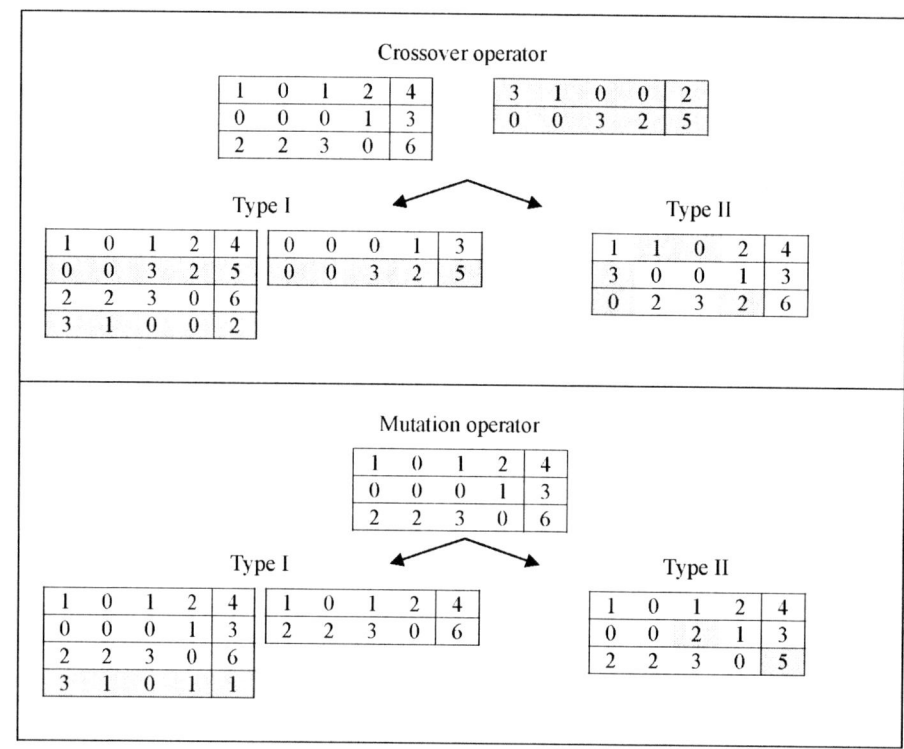

Figure 24. The Pareto front of the optimized sets of fuzzy rules for the diagnosis of malfunctioning operating conditions with expert systems

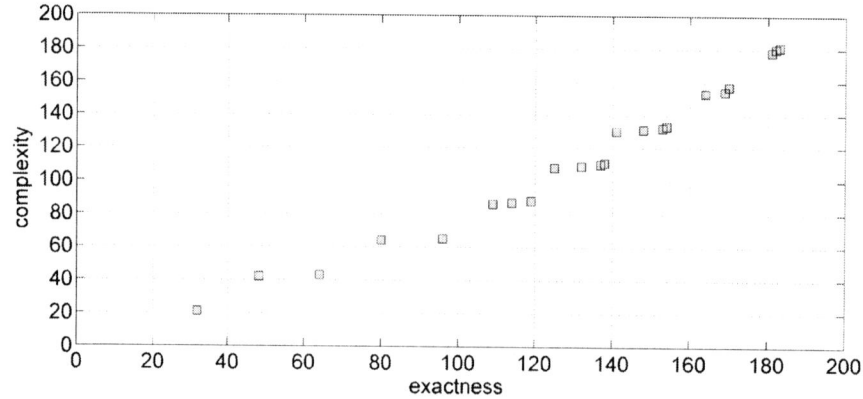

Since the knowledge base of an expert system does not have a fixed number of rules, each individual is codified as a set of a variable number of such vectors.

Objective functions. The first objective is to maximize the exactness of the set of rules. This objective function is evaluated by comparing the predictions obtained on a list of test operating conditions with the corresponding known fault modes. The higher the number of correct predictions, the higher the exactness score. A mild penalization is also assigned if a wrong fault is detected in a malfunctioning operating condition, and a strong penalization is assigned if a fault is detected in a healthy operating condition. The other objective is to minimize the complexity of the set of rules. This is determined as a linear combination of the number of rules N and the overall number of antecedents NA:

$$\text{complexity} = a \cdot N + b \cdot NA \tag{13}$$

where the coefficients a and b are 20 and 1, respectively.

Methodology. The GDEA by Toffolo and Benini (2003) is used to search for the optimal solutions. In this case, the genetic operators act on sets of vectors of the parent solutions to generate new sets from the already existing ones (Figure 23). Two types of crossover operators are used: the first one randomly copies some of the vectors from the two parental sets in the offspring, whereas the second recombines the integers of two sets of vectors into a new set. The probability of the two types is 50% each (all the offspring are generated using a crossover operator). Then two types of mutation operators are applied to the offspring population, both with a probability of 2%: the first adds/deletes one rule vector, whereas the other alters some of the integers in a set of vectors.

Results. The Pareto front shown in Figure 24 is obtained with a population of 200 individuals evolved for 500 generations. The maximum attainable exactness score (224 in the proposed example) is not reached because the induced effects of some of the fault modes are very similar. On the other hand, eight rules and about twenty antecedents are sufficient to obtain the maximum exactness score (183).

CONCLUSION

At the end of this brief and inevitably limited survey of applications, the reader should have become aware of the potential of evolutionary multi-objective optimization techniques in the research field of energy systems.

Because of the wide spectrum of objectives that can be considered, different perspectives of the design and operation of energy systems and their components can be analyzed, and evolutionary multi-objective optimization, aiming at the knowledge of the Pareto optimal set of solutions, is the key tool for the decision maker in order to take into account several of these perspectives at once. Moreover, the results presented in this chapter show that the complexity of the objective function landscapes, the configurations of which are nearly impossible to be predicted in advance, makes it difficult to apply profitably traditional optimization methods.

FUTURE RESEARCH DIRECTIONS

As it has been shown in this chapter, evolutionary techniques for multi-objective optimization are already fully exploited in the design of components (or component details) and in the search for the optimal design parameters of energy systems with a given configuration. In these cases, future efforts should be devoted to the enhancement of multi-objective evolutionary algorithms in order to improve their capability in:

- Maintaining the genetic diversity within the population with reliable diversity preserving mechanisms;
- Handling (i.e., updating, selecting and storing) the high number of nondominated solutions that are required to cover effectively and uniformly the entire Pareto front when more than two objectives are considered.

In the author's opinion, future research in the field of the multi-objective optimization of energy systems should be focused on two main directions.

The first deals with the representation of energy systems topologies. This is an obstacle that is still limiting the applications of traditional and evolutionary techniques to the optimization of energy systems. However, evolutionary techniques have an advantage over the traditional ones, since the toughest challenge is perhaps the ability to deal with systems of arbitrary complexity. The latter imply that the number of decision variables depends on system topology (i.e., a genome of variable length is required) and that a highly combinatorial search space has to be explored, in which only some topologies with particular values of their parameters are actually meaningful (or just feasible).

The other main direction of future research is related to the development of evolutionary algorithms that are able to deal with this kind of representation. Many aspects of the algorithm are involved in this task:

- The genetic operators, the random nature of which should be hybridized with some heuristics in order not to generate and evaluate a large number of useless solutions;
- The diversity preserving mechanism, which is often based on a measure of the "distance" among the solutions (in the case of a variable length genome, the definition of a "distance" in the decision variable space is not straightforward);
- The selection of the nondominated individuals that are passed to the next generation, since the algorithm has to deal with discontinuous Pareto fronts, in which each cluster is formed by a specific topology that may be very different from those forming the adjacent clusters.

These guidelines should allow exhaustively exploration, efficiently and successfully the enormous search spaces that have to be faced in the optimization problems about energy systems.

ACKNOWLEDGMENT

The author wishes to thank Professor Andrea Lazzaretto for the helpful discussions and his useful suggestions.

REFERENCES

Benini, E., & Toffolo A. (2002a). Development of high-performance airfoils for axial flow compressors using evolutionary computation. *Journal of Propulsion and Power, 18*(3), 544-554.

Benini, E., & Toffolo, A. (2002b). Optimal design of horizontal-axis wind turbines using blade-element theory and evolutionary computation. *Journal of Solar Energy Engineering, 124*(4), 357-363.

Deb, K., Pratap, A., Agarval, S., & Meyarivan, T. A. (2002). Fast and elitist multi-objective genetic algorithm: NSGA-II. *IEEE Transactions on Evolutionary Computing, 6*(2), 182–197.

Foli, K., Okabe, T., Olhofer, M., Jin, Y., & Sendhoff, B. (2006). Optimization of micro heat exchanger: CFD, analytical approach and multi-objective evolutionary algorithms. *International Journal of Heat and Mass Transfer, 49*(5-6), 1090-1099.

Fonseca, C. M., & Fleming, P. J. (1993). Genetic algorithms for multi-objective optimization: formulation, discussion and generalization. In S. Forest (Ed.), In *Genetic Algorithms: Proceedings of the Fifth International Conference* (pp. 416–423). San Mateo, CA: Morgan Kaufmann.

Hilbert, R., Janiga, G., Baron, R., & Thévenin, D. (2006). Multi-objective shape optimization of a heat exchanger using parallel genetic algorithms. *International Journal of Heat and Mass Transfer, 49*(15-16), 2567–2577.

Lazzaretto, A., & Toffolo, A. (2004). Energy, economy and environment as objectives in multi-criterion optimization of thermal systems design. *Energy, 29*(8), 1139-1157.

Lazzaretto, A., & Toffolo, A. (2006), On the synthesis of thermal systems: a method to determine optimal heat transfer interactions. In C. A. Frangopoulos, C. D. Rakopoulos, G. Tsatsaronis (Eds.), In *Proceedings of ECOS06: Vol. 1* (pp. 493-501).

Lazzaretto, A., & Toffolo, A. (2007), Energy system diagnosis by a fuzzy expert system with genetically evolved rules. In A. Mirandola, O. Arnas, A. Lazzaretto (Eds.), In *Proceedings of ECOS07: Vol. 1* (pp. 311-318).

Leyland, G. B. (2002). *Multi-objective optimisation applied to industrial energy problems*. Unpublished doctoral thesis 2572, Swiss Federal Institute of Technology, Lausanne.

Nassif, N., Kajl, S., & Sabourin, R. (2005). Evolutionary algorithms for multi-objective optimization in HVAC system control strategy. *International Journal of Heating, Ventilating, Air-Conditioning and Refrigerating Research (ASHRAE), 11*(3), 459-486.

Toffolo, A., & Benini, E. (2003). Genetic diversity as an objective in multi-objective evolutionary algorithms. *Evolutionary Computation, 11*(2), 151-167.

Toffolo, A., & Lazzaretto, A. (2002). Evolutionary algorithms for multi-objective energetic and economic optimization in thermal system design. *Energy, 27*(6), 549-567.

Valero, A., Lozano, M. A., Serra, L., Tsatsaronis, G., Pisa, J., Frangopoulos, C. A., & von Spakovsky, M. R. (1994). CGAM problem: Definition and conventional solution. *Energy, 19*(3), 279-286.

Weber, C., Maréchal, F., & Favrat, D. (2006, August). *Network synthesis for district heating with multiple heat plants*. Paper presented at PRES06, Prague, Czech Republic.

ADDITIONAL READINGS

About Component Design

Benini, E. (2004). Three-dimensional multi-objective design optimization of a transonic compressor rotor. *Journal of Propulsion and Power, 20*(3), 559-565.

Büche, D., Stoll, P., Dornberger, R., & Koumoutsakos, P. (2002). Multi-objective evolutionary algorithm for the optimization of noisy combustion processes. *IEEE Transactions on Systems, Man, and Cybernetics—Part C: Applications and Reviews, 32*(4), 460-473.

Degrez, G., Periaux, J., & Sefrioui, M. (Eds.). (in press). *Evolutionary design optimization methods in aeronautical and turbomachinery engineering*. New York: John Wiley & Sons.

Enomoto, Y., Kurosawa, S., & Suzuki, T. (2006). Design optimization of a high specific speed Francis turbine runner using multi-objective genetic algorithm. In J. Kurokawa (Ed.), In *Proceedings of the 23rd IAHR Symposium on Hydraulic Machinery and Systems* (paper IAHR 303).

Gonzalez, M., Moral, R., Martin, T., Sahoo, D., Dulikravich, G., & Jelisavcic, N. (2006). Multi-objective design optimization of topology and performance of branching networks of cooling passages. In *Proceedings of the ASME Fourth International Conference on Nanochannels, Microchannels and Minichannels* (paper ASME ICNMM2006-96151).

Hampsey, M. (2002). *Multi-objective evolutionary optimisation of small wind turbine blades*. Unpublished doctoral thesis, Department of Mechanical Engineering, University of Newcastle, UK.

Kumar, A., Keane, A. J., Nair, P. B., & Shahpar, S. (2006). Robust design of compressor fan blades against erosion. *Journal of Mechanical Design, 128*(4), 864-873.

Lian, Y., & Liou, M.-S. (2005). Multi-objective optimization of transonic compressor blade using evolutionary algorithm. *Journal of Propulsion and Power, 21*(6), 979-987.

Martin, T. J., & Dulikravich, G. S. (2002). Analysis and multidisciplinary optimization of internal coolant networks in turbine blades. *Journal of Propulsion and Power, 18*(4), 896-906.

Oyama, A., & Liou, M.-S. (2002) Multi-objective optimization of a multi-stage compressor using evolutionary algorithm. In *Proceedings of the 38th AIAA/ASME/SAE/ASEE Joint Propulsion Conference & Exhibit* (paper AIAA 2002-3535).

Sasaki, D., Keane, A. J., & Shahpar, S. (2006). Multi-objective evolutionary optimization of a compressor stage using a grid-enabled environment. In *Proceedings of the 44th AIAA Aerospace Sciences Meeting and Exhibit* (paper AIAA 2006-340).

Tarafder, A., Lee, B. C. S., Ray, A. K., & Rangaiah, G. P. (2005). Multi-objective optimization of an industrial ethylene reactor using a nondominated sorting genetic algorithm. *Industrial & Engineering Chemical Research, 44*(1), 124-141

Voß, C., Aulich, M., Kaplan, B., & Nicke, E. (2006) Automated multi-objective optimisation in axial compressor blade design. In *Proceedings of ASME Turbo Expo 2006* (paper ASME GT2006-90420).

About Energy System Design

Bernal-Agustin, J. L., Dufo-Lopez, R., & Rivas-Ascaso, D. M. (2006). Design of isolated hybrid systems minimizing costs and pollutant emissions. *Renewable Energy, 31*(14), 2227–2244.

Bonataki, E. T., & Giannakoglou, K. C. (2005). Preliminary design of optimal combined cycle power plants through evolutionary algorithms. In R. Schilling, W. Haase, J. Periaux, H. Baier, G. Bugeda (Eds.), *Evolutionary and Deterministic Methods for Design, Optimization and Control with Applications to Industrial and Societal Problems (EUROGEN 2005)*.

Bürer, M., Favrat, D., Tanaka, K., & Yamada, K. (2003). Multi-criteria optimization of a district cogeneration plant integrating a solid oxide fuel cell - Gas turbine combined cycle, heat pumps and chillers. *Energy, 28*(6), 497-518.

Godat, J., & Maréchal, F. (2003). Optimization of a fuel cell system using process integration techniques. *Journal of Power Sources, 118*(1-2), 411-423.

Hu, X., Wang, Z., & Liao, L. (2004). Multi-objective optimization of HEV fuel economy and emissions using evolutionary computation. *SAE SP-1856* (pp. 117-128). Warrendale, PA: SAE International.

Li, H., Bürer, M., Zhi-Ping, S., Favrat, D., & Maréchal, F. (2004). Green heating system: Characteristics and illustration with the multi-criteria optimization of an integrated energy system. *Energy, 29*(2), 225-244.

Li, H., Maréchal, F., Bürer, M., & Favrat, D. (2006). Multi-objective optimization of an advanced combined cycle power plant including CO_2 separation options. *Energy, 31*(15), 3117–3134.

Maréchal, F., Favrat, D., Palazzi, F., & Godat, J. (2005). Thermo-economic modelling and optimisation of fuel cell systems. *Fuel Cells- From Fundamentals to Systems, 5*(1), 5-24.

Pelet, X., Favrat, D., & Leyland, G. (2005) Multi-objective optimisation of integrated energy systems for remote communities considering economics and CO_2 emissions. *International Journal of Thermal Sciences, 44*(12), 1180–1189.

Rajesh, J. K., Gupta S. K., Rangaiah, G. P., & Ray, A. K. (2001). Multi-objective optimization of industrial hydrogen plants. *Chemical Engineering Science, 56*(3), 999-1010.

Roosen, P., Uhlenbruck, S., & Lucas, K. (2003). Pareto optimization of a combined cycle power system as a decision support tool for trading off investment vs. operating costs. *International Journal of Thermal Sciences, 42*(6), 553–560.

Valdes, M., Duran, M. D., & Rovira, A. (2003). Thermoeconomic optimization of combined cycle gas turbine power plants using genetic algorithms. *Applied Thermal Engineering, 23*(17), 2169–2182.

Weber, C., Maréchal, F., Favrat, D., & Kraines, S. (2005). Optimization of a SOFC-based decentralized polygeneration system for providing energy services in an office-building in Tokyo. *Applied Thermal Engineering, 26*(13), 1409-1419.

About Energy System Operation

Barán, B., von Lücken, C., & Sotelo, A. (2005). Multi-objective pump scheduling optimisation using evolutionary strategies. *Advances in Engineering Software, 36*(1), 39-47.

Chipperfield, A. J., & Fleming, P. J. (1996). Multi-objective gas turbine engine controller design using genetic algorithms. *IEEE Transactions on Industrial Electronics, 43*(5), 583-587.

Garduno-Ramirez, R., & Lee, K. Y. (2001). Multi-objective optimal power plant operation through coordinate control with pressure set point scheduling. *IEEE Transaction on Energy Conversion, 16*(2), 115-122.

Nandasana, A. D., Ray, A. K., & Gupta, S. K. (2003). Dynamic model of an industrial steam reformer and its use for multi-objective optimization. *Industrial & Engineering Chemical Research, 42*(17), 4028-4042.

Chapter XIII
Evolutionary Multi-Objective Optimization for Assignment Problems*

Mark P. Kleeman
Air Force Institute of Technology, USA

Gary B. Lamont
Air Force Institute of Technology, USA

ABSTRACT

Assignment problems are used throughout many research disciplines. Most assignment problems in the literature have focused on solving a single objective. This chapter focuses on assignment problems that have multiple objectives that need to be satisfied. In particular, this chapter looks at how multi-objective evolutionary algorithms have been used to solve some of these problems. Additionally, this chapter examines many of the operators that have been utilized to solve assignment problems and discusses some of the advantages and disadvantages of using specific operators.

INTRODUCTION

The application of multi-objective evolutionary algorithms (MOEAs) to solving multi-objective assignment problems has been quite successful and continues to make strides towards solving more complex real-world problems of this type. This chapter is devoted to a wide spectrum of such multi-objective assignment problems that indicate MOEA competitive or improved results over other approaches. In discussing various MOEA applications to multi-objective assignment categories, the specific problem domain is exhibited and the selected MOEA structure illuminated. Experimental results are summarized and the impact of the various MOEA operators and parameters on the results discussed. The intent is to provide insight for selection of MOEA operators and parameters values for a new variation of a multi-objective assignment problem. Multi-objective assignment problem categories addressed range from extended classical NP-Complete and personnel management problems to causality assignment and frequency assignment problems. Contemporary references provide extended details of the various MOEA applications to multi-objective assignment problems. For a discussion on assignment problems in general and their mathematical derivation, see the books by West (2001) and Garey (1979).

Specific multi-objective assignment problems are presented in Section II along with a brief discussion of the MOEA application. The assignment problem examples include the linear gate assignment problem, the multi-objective quadratic assignment problem, the airman assignment problem, causality assignment problem fixed channel assignment problem, frequency assignment problem, multilevel generalized assignment problem, and resource allocation problem. The characteristics of these assignment problems range from linear to nonlinear fitness functions with limited constraints to a multitude of constraints. Assignment problem representations, MOEA operators and their appropriate selection for assignment problems are discussed in Section III. Representations can be fixed or variable with classical and extended crossover and mutation methods discussed.

MULTI-OBJECTIVE ASSIGNMENT PROBLEMS

Researchers have used many different types of algorithms and heuristics to solve a wide variety of assignment problems. The generic assignment problem is in reality a maximum weighting matching problem in a weighted bipartite graph. In general, it can be described as assigning a number of agents to a number of tasks while minimizing the total assignment cost. Single objective variations include the linear fitness assignment problem, the quadratic assignment problem, the bottleneck assignment problem, and others with linear and nonlinear constraints. The precise variety of assignment problems is reflected in different mathematical models. Techniques for solving these single objective assignment problems include the Hungarian algorithm, the simplex algorithm, Tabu search, simulated annealing, and genetic algorithms. Instead of aggregating a multi-objective assignment problem into a single objective model, we attempt to address the multi-objective model directly and focus on the use of MOEAs.

This chapter focuses on multi-objective assignment problems with two or more competing objectives that have been solved using a variety of evolutionary algorithms. However, some aggregated fitness as well as multiple fitness functions are discussed via a variety of applications. Each subsection presents a different type of multi-objective assignment problem and briefly describes the problem domain and the algorithm used. The experimental results are also summarized. Mathematical models reflecting the exact mathematical structure of an assignment problem are found in the associated references. Such models are very useful in generating computational software and should be understood, but they are not presented in this chapter since the focus is on MOEA evaluation. The intent is to generalize in the following sections the various algorithmic approaches and operators and thus provide insight as to appropriate selection of MOEA operators within the specific problem domain.

Linear Gate Assignment Problem

The linear gate assignment problem (LGAP) is related to logic gate matrix layout and programmable logic arrays folding. The problem concerns the assignment of a set of circuit elements in a sequence on circuit board in order to minimize the layout area. The objectives of this problem are to arrange a set of circuit nodes in such a way that it minimizes both the layout area and the cost based on the amount of metal is needed to cover the nets. This multi-objective assignment problem has its importance in very large scale integration (VLSI) design.

Figure 1 shows an example of two different gate matrices with the same 7 nets (nets are gates that are interconnected). In the example on the left, the gates are labeled 1 through 9 and placed in chronological order while the example on the right rearranges the gate order. In order to connect all the necessary gates for a net, it is necessary to cross gates that are not part of the net. To compute the number of tracks to cover all the nets, an aggregation of all the overlapping nets can be done. This number is an important factor in determining the cost of VLSI circuits, so the smaller the number, the lower the cost. In Figure 1, the example on the left shows a gate matrix with 7 tracks, one for each net since, since all the nets overlap. But the example on the right shows only 6 tracks because the gates are arranged in such a way that some of the nets can be combined on a single track.

In addition to tracks, there is also the cost to connect the gates. This cost symbolizes the amount of metal necessary cover the nets. In Figure 1, the example on the left generates a total metal length of 42 while the example on the right generates a length of only 31. So in both cost instances, the example on the right is a better design with respect to cost.

This problem was solved by de Oliveira et al. (2001) using the constructive genetic algorithm (CGA). The CGA is different from more traditional GAs in that it evaluates schemata directly. This type of method is typically called an explicit building block method. The CGA has two phases, the constructive phase and the optimal phase. The constructive phase builds a population of quality solutions by finding well-adapted schemata and structures. The optimal phase is conducted concurrently with the constructive phase and evaluates the schemata and structures in a common way. The population size of the CGA varies. It starts at

Figure 1. Examples of two different gate matrices and the effect that moving gate interconnection points has on the total metal length needed to complete the nets

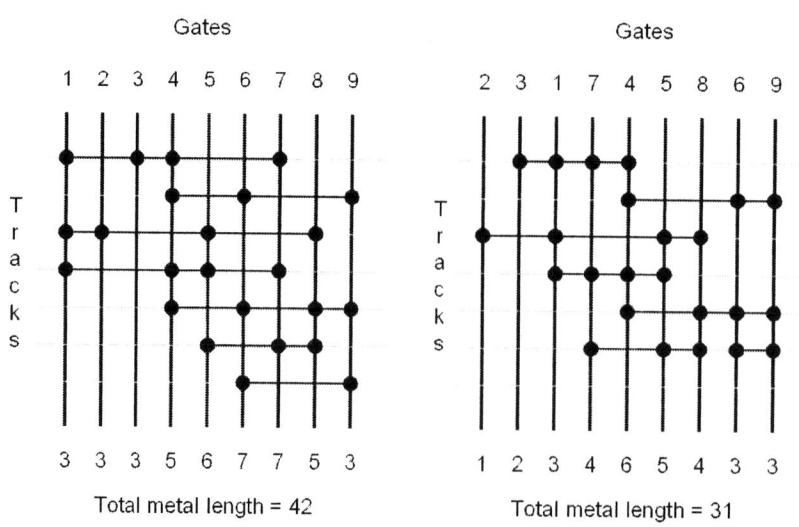

a size of zero and at a given population time, the size grows based on parameter α. As schemata are created, they are ranked for survivability. For this problem, the two objectives are combined via a weighting factor. The algorithm was compared with the microcanonical optimization approach (MCO). The CGA was able to find the same results as the MCO, but it was able to do it faster.

Multi-Objective Quadratic Assignment Problem

The generalized multi-objective quadratic assignment problem category (mQAP) was formulated by Knowles and Corne (2002; 2003) who provide a Webs site of associated benchmarks. Kleeman, Day, and Lamont (Day, Kleeman, & Lamont, 2003; Kleeman, 2004; Kleeman, Day, & Lamont, 2004) solved a range of these problems using the multi-objective messy genetic algorithm (MOMGA-II). The mQAP is a multi-objective version of the QAP. The QAP has n facilities and n locations. Each location has a specified distance between it and the other locations and each facility has a predetermined flow to all the other facilities. These are typically stored as matrices. The goal is to assign each facility to a location in such a way as to minimize the total flow between facilities by attempting to put facilities that have high flow values in locations close to one another. The mQAP is similar to this except there are multiple competing flows from each facility to optimize. Figure 2 shows an example of a four facility/location mQAP with two competing flows. Note that each location is a fixed distance from the others and the facilities are placed in a location. The flows, which are facility based, have different values. In Figure 2, thicker lines represent larger flow values. In order to minimize this problem, the facilities should be place in locations such that the larger flow values travel a smaller distance to reach their destinations.

The MOMGA-II is an explicit building block MOEA used for the mQAP. It differs from most

Figure 2. Example of the mQAP with four facilities, four locations, and two flows

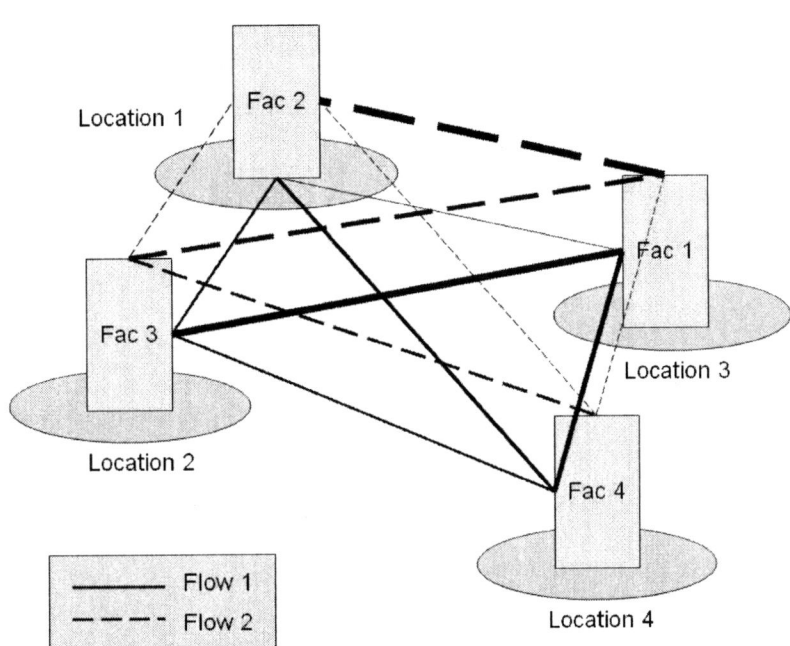

other MOEAs in the way it builds solutions. Most MOEAs attempt to find good solutions by combining two highly fit parents in an effort to create a more fit child. Implicitly, they are trying to combine the good building blocks (or good traits) from one parent with the good building blocks from the other. The MOMGA-II builds solutions through explicitly finding these good building blocks. The algorithm has a variable chromosome length because it allows for over specification of alleles (two values can be assigned to one location in the chromosome). The algorithm uses a type of crossover operator called cut-and-splice, which selects random cut points from each, the parents and then typically splices them with the other parent to create the children. The mutation operator used is bit-flip mutation. The algorithm was able to find good mQAP results. It is suggested that larger building block sizes are typically found on the outer extremities of the Pareto front for mQAPs making it more difficult to find the nondominated extremities. A later but quite similar MOEA approach to the multi-objective assignment problem is found in (Garrett & Dasgupta, 2006).

Airman Assignment Problem

This airman assignment problem is a constrained assignment problem (Kleeman & Lamont, 2007) that attempts to find the best match of Air Force personnel with the jobs available. In this problem, each Air Force member has a rank, job specialty, security clearance level and other similar characteristics that are compared to the requirements of each job available. This problem is similar to the single objective sailor assignment problem (Garrett, Vannucci, Silva, Dasgupta, & Simien, 2005; Holder 2005; Kelemen, Kozma, & Liang, 2002; Liang, Lin, & Kelemen, 2002, Lewis, Lewis, & White, 2004), but it is tailored more for the air force assignment system and for more than one objective. For this problem, there are typically more jobs than there are members to fill them.

Each job has a set of hard and soft constraints. The hard constraints cannot be broken while the soft constraints can be broken but a user defined penalty is added to the fitness function. The ultimate goal is to meet the needs of the Air Force while at the same time keeping the person happy. The two objective functions that attempt to quantify these are costs to move the personnel and the assignment penalties applied for nonideal assignments (assignments that broke soft constraints and incurred penalties).

Kleeman and Lamont (2006; 2007) used an MOEA to solve the airman assignment problem. The MOEA used to solve this problem was the nondominated sorting genetic algorithm – II (NSGA-II) by Deb (Deb, Agarwal, Pratap, & Meyarivan, 2000; Deb, Pratap, Agarwal, & Meyarivan, 2002). The MOEA is a Pareto based algorithm that ranks individuals based on whether they are nondominated, dominated by only one individual, and so on. The next generation is selected based on the lowest rankings. Individuals are stratified based on a crowding operator, which favors individuals that are spread out from its neighbors. Tournament selection is used to select parents. The crossover operator is the standard two-point crossover. The mutation operator randomly changes a selected allele to another integer. The algorithm was able to find good solutions for small instances of the problem. Larger instances should determine how well the problem and algorithm scale empirically.

Causality Assignment Problem

Wong, Bigras, and Khayati (2002) used an MOEA to solve a causality multi-objective assignment problem. Causality assignment is an important task when doing physical modeling and simulation via bond graphs. This approach to determining input and output sets considered as components with multiport devices. Then each device is interconnected and the analysis of the system is done to gain information about the input and output sets. This approach corresponds to the use of a bond graph. The goal of a bond graph is to represent a dynamic system by means of basic multiport devices and their interconnections by bonds. The devices exchange and modulate power through their bonds. With a bond graph, causality assignment is used to partition bond variables into input and output sets. It establishes the cause and effect relationships between the factors of power. There are four types of causal constraints in bond graphs:

- **Mandatory causality:** Only one of the two port variables are allowed to be the output.
- **Preferred causality:** For storage elements, such as capacitors or inductors, there can be time derivative or time integral causality.
- **Constrained causality:** Causal constraints occur when the causality of one port imposes causality on other ports.
- **Indifferent causality:** This means there are no causal constraints.

The Pareto Archived Evolution Strategy (PAES) (Knowles & Corne, 1999; Knowles & Corne, 2000) was the specific MOEA selected. The PAES algorithm is a (1+1)-ES that maintains an external archive of the best nondominated solutions. The archive is partitioned into hypercubes in order to help maintain diversity. The MOEA uses only the mutation operator and does not use a crossover operator. The problem has four objective functions to minimize. These objective functions are the number of causal violations for each multiport of the bond graph. The algorithm was able to find a variety of good nondominated solutions.

Fixed Channel Assignment Problem

Jin, Wu, Horng, and Tsai (2001) used an MOEA to solve the fixed channel assignment problem. The fixed channel assignment (FCA) problem is derived from the channel assignment problem. For this problem, the channels are permanently allocated to each cell. This is different from the dynamic channel assignment (DCA) problem, where all channels are available for every cell and are allocated dynamically upon request. The DCA typically provides better performance, but under heavy traffic loads, the FCA performs better. So this problem's goal is particularly focused on finding solutions where heavy traffic load is expected.

The problem objectives are to minimize the number of blocked calls and to minimize the amount of interference. The authors use a weighting or aggregate scheme to combine these two objectives into a single objective in order to be solved with a single objective genetic algorithm. The chromosome is a fixed length matrix where each row element represents a frequency and each column represents a cell. The crossover operator used is essentially uniform crossover, where two parents are chosen and allele values are chosen from each parent in a random fashion. The mutation operator (called local search in the paper) does a series of pairwise swaps in the chromosome. The swaps continue until there are no improvements after a user-defined number of swaps. Results indicate that the cost function reflects the quality of different assignments and also shows that the algorithm does improve the solution quality.

Frequency Assignment Problems

Weicker, Szabo, Weicker, and Widmayer (2003) designed a large complex cellular network. One objective involves the determination of where to place the base station transmitters in order to provide strong radio signals for the area and keep the deployment costs low. Another major objective is the allocation of frequency channels to the cells in such a way that interference is low. Weicker proposes a new method for positioning base station transmitters in a mobile phone network and assigning frequencies to the transmitters. Two separate optimization steps, one for the base station transmitter location problem and one for the frequency assignment problem, must be taken into account. By integrating these two problems, better solutions are possible than solving them independently.

The problem then is to minimize two objectives: cost and interference. The problem is NP-hard. In order to make the MOEA more efficient, problem specific knowledge is incorporated into the operators. The chromosome used is a variable length chromosome that defines each base station. Nine different mutation operators are used in order to include both problem knowledge and the ability to search the entire search space. The crossover operator is designed to generate children in a region close to the parents. These are discussed in further detail in Section 3. The MOEA created for this problem is called the steady state evolutionary algorithm with Pareto tournaments (stEAPT). The results suggest a strong influence on the choice of selection method on the utility of the problem-specific crossover operator. This approach led to a significant and improved difference in the solution quality.

Cotta and Troya (2001) applied heuristic-based evolutionary algorithms to the Frequency Assignment Problem (FAP) which comprises a number of optimization NP-hard problems. FAPs consist of finding an assignment of a set of frequencies to a set of emitters fulfilling some specific constraints (e.g., avoiding interference between closely located emitters). The proliferation of cellular phone networks and local television stations supports the practical interest in FAPs. There exist two central constraints in a FAP that must be satisfied: the number of frequencies assigned to an emitter must be equal to the number of frequencies the emitter demands, and these frequencies must not interfere with frequencies assigned to other emitters. Moreover, the space of possible solutions must be high enough to allow the existence of feasible FAP solutions.

The authors provide a precise definition of a generic FAP approach; in particular they formally define three formal elements; a characterization of problem instances, a characterization of problem solutions, and quality measures. The authors define two different quality measures or objectives. The first one is the *frequency span*, the maximum separation between assigned frequencies. The other measure is the *assignment size*, the number of different frequencies assigned to all the emitters. The researchers state that the optimal solution with respect to the first quality measure is the one that satisfies the problem constraints within the smallest frequency interval. Note that the authors approach is based upon a single objective model. But, this could easily be changed to a multi-objective problem.

The authors propose a direct search in feasible space, and an indirect search via permutation decoders that uses specifically designed evolutionary operators. The direct search in feasible space is a form of the set-covering problem. This approach leads to a combinatoric problem and thus, it is necessary to introduce some exogenous information—heuristics in a new algorithmic formulation called indirect search via permutation decoders—a form of the coloring problem. Given this new method, the authors compare two separate heuristics with each integrated with a genetic algorithm (GA). Two decoder heuristic variants are: First-Available-Emitter (FAE) local search heuristic and the First-Available-Frequency (FAF) FAE local search heuristic. Both are appropriate to introduce problem-specific knowledge in the statistical GA search process.

The obtained results were conclusive, with respect to the pecking order of the heuristic operators, in that FX (frequency crossover) performs better than EX (emitter crossover) or EFX (emitter-frequency crossover). Optimal solutions are found for three of the problem instances where the test suite is composed of eight 21-emitter FAP instances. It is shown that, despite the apparent emitter/frequency symmetry of the problem, manipulating partial frequency assignments is more adequate that manipulating partial emitter assignments. This insight holds for FAF and FAE heuristics that are used as decoders in the permutation-based GA. Future FAP efforts should develop additional heuristics based upon the landscape, as well as addressing different variants of FAPs as benchmarks. The expanded GA effort should focus on a multi-objective model using a variety of MOEAs for comparison.

Multilevel Generalized Assignment Problem

Hajri-Gabouj (2003) considers a task-operator-machine assignment problem. This assignment problem is common in the clothing industry where a given design pattern has a number of stitching tasks that have to be accomplished by operators who have access to a set of machines. The amount of time to execute a task is dependent upon the operator's individual proficiency, so they vary depending upon the operator. Each task requires a specific machine and only one operator. The machines can perform multiple tasks, but they are assigned to only one operator. An operator can be assigned multiple tasks, but the number of machines required for these tasks must equal one and the operator is assigned to at most, one machine. Resources are saved by limiting the number of operators and machines that are needed to accomplish the tasks. Since the tasks are dependent and have a predefined ordering, a communication link is needed when successive tasks are assigned to different operators.

The problem has three objectives. The objectives are to minimize the total execution time, to come as close as possible to a perfect load balance among the operators and not to exceed neither predefined interoperator communication costs nor a prefixed number of resources. Note that the third objective is in reality a set of constraints. In essence, the multi-objective problem is mapped to an aggregated single objective problem using a penalty function for the constraints which then is a classical assignment problem with constraints. Note that each process may have predecessor constraints and that each operator is assigned to one machine. The fuzzy aspect of the problem domain relates to industrial environments where personnel frequently change and manufacturing systems need to be flexible with real-time critical decision making. The author develops and applies a fuzzy genetic multi-objective optimization algorithm (FGMOA) to solve a multilevel generalized assignment problem encountered in the clothing industry, but based upon an aggregated objective function. The FGMOA is a hybridization of fuzzy logic and genetic algorithms for solving the aggregated model of weighted objectives. The relaxation of the mathematical model is accomplished by employing fuzzy logic according to a generalized objective scaling process.

The FGMOA is able to represent the best trade off between conflicting and/or incommensurable objectives in a reasonable amount of computation time. It also finds satisfactory solutions despite the changes that alter the search landscape relating to decisions and the changing personnel environment such as the operator departure or performance improvement. Further research should apply the FGMOA to more complex problems that have more than two efficiency levels and use benchmark examples for flexible job-shop scheduling problems.

Resource Allocation Problem

Datta, Deb, and Fonseca (2007) addresses two resource allocation or assignment problems (RAPs) that are highly constrained. The application of a MOEA to these two combinatoric optimization provides insight to real-world stochastic methods. Generic The problems are a university resource scheduling problem and a land-use management problem, similar problems, yet diverse.

The first problem is a classical university scheduling problem (spatial and temporal) involving classes, teachers and students in classrooms. Specifically, the two objectives are: (1) minimize the average number of weekly free-time slots between two classes of a student, (2) maximize the weekly average span of time-slots of classes for each teacher. Regarding constraints, they include: (a) a student should only have one class at a time, (b) the teacher should only have one class at a time, (c) a room should only be booked for one class at a time, (d) a course should only have one class a day (could be more), (e) because of class size, assigned room should have sufficient sitting capacity, and (f) possible constraint on time of offering (evening course). To computationally solve this RAP, the authors construct an extended version of the NSGA-II with unique operators on a specific chromosome representation: a two-dimensional matrix where each column is a time slot (gene) and a row represents a room from a resource list. This representation permits a specialized crossover operator for valid resource allocation. Two parents only generate a random feasible portion of the first offspring by checking constraints as each portion is placed in the offspring. The second feasible offspring is generated by another crossover heuristic approach using the two parents. Mutation is accomplished by reshuffling resource allocation by swapping randomly selected classes at two different time slots, again checking for violation.

Considering random initialization of the MOEA population, many infeasible solutions would be generated and would need repair. Thus, in order to improve computational efficiency for this scheduling problem, the authors suggest a heuristic technique for generating feasible solutions. The approach initially assigns classes to rooms, then assigns rooms to time-slots respecting constraints. Results using a modified version of the NSGA-II reflected better scheduling than the current manual approach.

The other problem address is a land-use management problem where the three objectives are: maximize net economic return from land use, maximize amount of carbon sequestration (global warming), and minimize amount of soil erosion. Regarding land use optimization, the physical and ecological constraints are: (a) assign land use based upon soil permitting (aridity index, topographical soil wetness index etc.), (b) assign land use within permitted range of physical slope, (c) assign land use must be within permitted range of global spatial coherence, (d) total area of specific land use must be within permitted range of total land use allocation.

The MOEA solution to this problem also uses a local search approach on the solution boundary by replacing the land use by one its adjacent units if fitness improves. Instantiating this type of RAP with a real-world Portuguese land management problem provides additional insight to developing such a complex plan. In reality, the assigned land use is permanent agriculture across the entire area, with specific types generally allocated to different regions (patches) based upon their environment.

Again, the two generic problem domains addressed are similar in their models, yet diverse as well due to specific constraints. Also, the discussed MOEA solutions via unique crossover and mutation operators have many similarities. As the authors stated MOEA approaches are able to handle the type of complex RAPs discussed as compared to linear and integer programming techniques.

Other Multi-Objective Assignment Problem Instances

A variety of assignment operators have been briefly discussed. This section lists other assignment problems for completeness that have been solved using MOEAs.

Rachmawati and Srinivasan (2005) proposed a hybrid fuzzy EA for solving a multi-objective resource allocation problem. The specific problem they solved was the student allocation problem.

They found that their algorithm was able to solve the problem with a good success rate.

The constructive genetic algorithm (CGA) mentioned in Section 2.1 was also used to solve a generalized multi-objective assignment problem (GAP) (Lorena, Narciso, & Beasley, 1999), namely, the 0-1 knapsack problem. A set of 24 knapsack problem instantiations of various sizes were used as benchmark problems and the results of the CGA were compared to the best known solution. The results were very close to the best known solutions solved with other evolutionary methods. This is promising considering it is conjectured that the CGA's computational efforts are much smaller than the comparison algorithm.

Palaniappan, Zein-Sabatto, and Sekmen (2001) used an adaptive genetic algorithm for the war resource multi-objective allocation problem. A war simulation program called THUNDER was used to determine the fitness of the generated solutions. The adaptive GA was able to produce solutions that enabled superior performance in all the measured objectives.

MOEA OPERATORS FOR ASSIGNMENT PROBLEMS

MOEA operators play an important role in the evolutionary process. The chromosome representation of the problem must be done in a logical manner and the operators must pair with the representation in order to have efficient execution. For example, if the chromosome is a permutation of individuals, then a two-point crossover may be a problem because it would tend to create invalid results that would have to be repaired. Assignment problems are concerned with putting entities into fixed locations or areas. This can lead to chromosome representations and MOEA operators that are different from some of the more standard operators used on benchmark problems or other optimization problems. This section examines some of the chromosome representations used by application researchers in Section II as well as associated crossover, mutation, and selection operators.

Chromosome Representations

This section examines some of the ways researchers have represented their problem in their chromosome structure. This section is divided into two subsections. The first subsection looks at variable length chromosome representations and the second subsection presents fixed length chromosome representations.

Variable Length Chromosomes

There are a variety of reasons why a researcher may choose to have a variable length chromosome. Often, the problem domain is what dictates the necessity of a variable length chromosome. An example of this is the frequency assignment problem by Weiker et al. (2003). A variable chromosome length is needed since the number of transmitters is not fixed. Each transmitter requires multiple alleles to define its configuration. For every transmitter a value is needed for the following: transmitting power, capacity of the transmitter, position of the transmitter inside the service area, and the set of channels assigned to the transmitter. Figure 3 shows an example of the chromosome.

Not only does the problem domain dictate the necessity of a variable length chromosome, but some algorithm domains also require variable length chromosomes. For example, in the multi-objective quadratic assignment problem research (Kleeman et al., 2004) the algorithm used, the MOMGA-II, a variable length chromosome. The MOMGA-II allows for both under and over specification of the allele values, which means there can be a variable number of alleles for each individual. The algorithm utilizes a template that can fill in any missing values not specified in the chromosome and it has rules that determine which

Figure 3. Example of a chromosome representation for the frequency assignment problem (Weiker, 2003) (©2003, IEEE, Used with Permission)

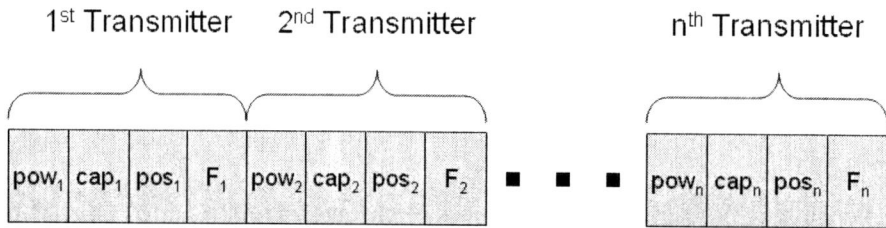

Figure 4. Example of the chromosome representation for the quadratic assignment problem (Kleeman, 2004) (© 2004, IEEE, Used with permission)

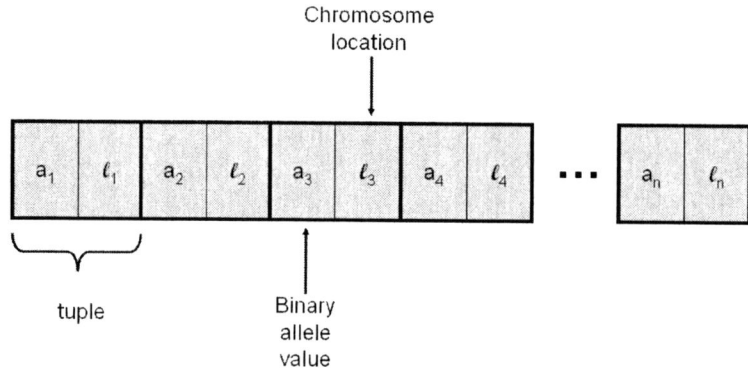

values to use when more than one chromosome location is present. The chromosome consists of two parts—the allele value and the location of the allele in the chromosome. This type of instantiation allows building blocks from anywhere in the chromosome to be matched. The chromosome is encoded in binary, where chromosome location is translated into an integer value and the allele value is rank ordered depending on the integer value of each allele. This type of representation avoided the necessity of having to generate a permutation for the facilities and then to have a repair operator every time a crossover or mutation invalidated the permutation. The disadvantage to this representation is that it increases the search space size because multiple binary values will map to the same solution as opposed to having one unique solution for each binary representation. Figure 4 shows an example of the chromosome, where n varies from one individual to the next.

Fixed Length Chromosomes

Fixed length chromosomes are more common than variable length chromosomes. A fixed length chromosome can be viewed as the default chromosome type, with the variable length chromosome only used as needed. This subsection discusses the fixed length chromosome structures used in the assignment problems discussed in Section II.

In the linear gate assignment problem (Oliveira, Smith, & Holland, 2001), the chromosome is a fixed size and consists of a proportion of random positions receiving a unique gate number for the linear gate assignment problem. The rest of the positions in the chromosome receive the schemata label #. Figure 5 shows an example of the chromosome representation used in the linear gate assignment problem. In this example gate number 8 is in the first position, gate 12 is in the 4th position, and gates 3 and 5 are in the final positions. The other schemata positions can be filled with any of the remaining gate values. The goal of this representation is to attempt to explicitly find good building blocks for the problem. This type of representation is great to determine linkages and epistasis in the chromosome. A disadvantage is determining what values should be used to fill the empty portions of the chromosomes for evaluation purposes.

For the airman assignment problem (Kleeman & Lamont, 2007), the fixed length chromosome represents each airman that requires a job. The jobs are labeled as integers and are used to fill up the chromosome. A repair operator is used to ensure that no duplicate jobs are assigned. This representation is good to use when assigning two disproportionate groups. The chromosome locations should typically represent the smallest group and the largest group should be assigned to the various locations. This allows for smaller chromosome sizes and can lead to increased algorithm efficiency.

Many fixed length chromosomes use binary values for their alleles. The chromosome representation for the causality assignment problem (Wong et al., 2002) consists of each element in the chromosome representing a bond within the bond graph. Every bond has two causal labels (one on each end), which are complimentary. As such, a binary representation for the bonds (0 = flow causality, 1 = effort causality) is sufficient to represent the full causality assignment of the bond graph.

In the fixed channel assignment problem (Jin et al., 2001) binary values are also used. But what is different is that the chromosome is a matrix. The elements of each row (the columns) of the chromosome are the frequencies and the rows are the cells. The values for each element are binary. A one signifies that the frequency is assigned to that particular cell while a zero states otherwise. Figure 6 shows an example of the chromosome used for the fixed channel assignment problem. Note that the columns represent frequencies and the rows represent cells. Using this representation allows the algorithm to compare neighboring cells for the same frequencies and determine if

Figure 5. Example of the chromosome representation of the linear gate assignment problem (Oliveira, 2001)

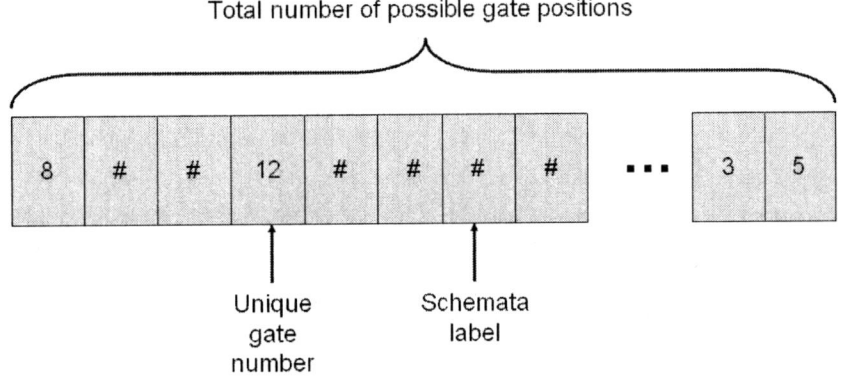

there is a problem in the assignment. This type of representation is good when comparisons are needed to avoid conflicts.

The chromosome in the multilevel generalized assignment problem (Hajri-Gabouj, 2003) is a set of metalevel cells that reflects the number of the different machine types with each cell characterized by a set of identical machines. The cell length is equal to the number of tasks executed on the machines of that cell. While the cell lengths can be variable, the overall chromosome length is fixed. A set of qualified operators is also affected to each cell. Each operator belongs to only one cell, although it can be applied many times in one cell. Specific tasks are associated with each machine in each cell. Note that this encoding allows the finding of an assignment which satisfies constraints. This chromosome representation is problem specific, but it is a good example of how a chromosome can be created to best meet the requirements of a problem.

The target allocation problem by Erdem and Ozdemirel (2003) uses an unconventional representation scheme for the chromosome. For this problem, there are two opposing sides, the blue unit (good) and the red unit (bad). The goal is to allocate resources from various blue units to support battle plans against the red units. As such, blue units can be decomposed into smaller subunits of 2/3, 1/2, or 1/3 of full strength. The chromosome is composed of genes that represent each blue unit. Each gene is a vector, whose size is determined by the first digit of the unit's division code. Each member of a vector is a pair that indicates which red unit the blue unit is assigned to and the allocation fraction allotted to that unit. As such the chromosome can be viewed as either a fixed length (each individual has the same number of genes) or a variable length chromosome (the genes can be various sizes, depending on the random allocation of units). So this chromosome representation does not fit neatly into either category.

The chromosome for the resource allocation problem (Datta et al., 2007) is a three dimensional array where two dimensions represent the physical land area assignment and the third dimension is time (crop years). Figure 7 shows an example of the chromosome representation used for problem. This is another good example of how a chromosome is built to meet the specific problem domain requirements.

Figure 6. Example of the fixed channel assignment problem chromosome representation (Jin, 2001) (© 2001, IEEE, Used with permission)

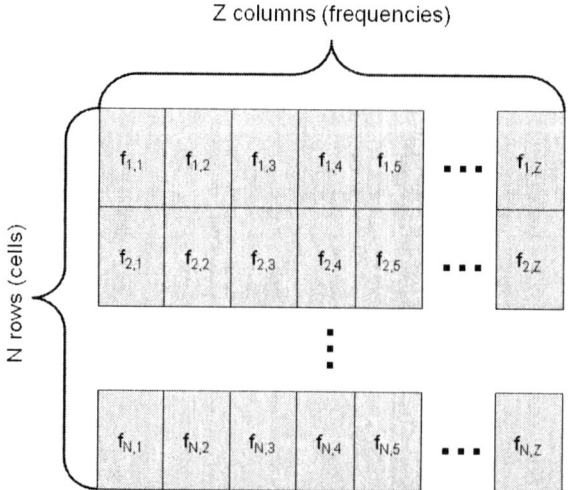

Mutation Operators

Mutation operators are typically used with a small probability in evolutionary algorithms. But these variation operators still play an important role in the outcome of the algorithm. As such, there are several different mutation operators that are used in the Section II applications.

For problems that implement chromosomes with binary representations, quadratic assignment problem (Kleeman, 2004) and causality assignment problem (Wong et al., 2002), a simple bit-flip operator was used. Kleeman et al. (2004) implemented the bit-flip with a low probability using an underlying uniform probability distribution while Wong et al. (2002) based his on a Gaussian probability distribution. The underlying probability distribution used is of course largely problem dependent. This type of mutation operator is one of the easiest to implement and is typically effective in meeting the desired goal of varying the population members. But for some chromosome representations, such as real-valued or permutation representations, this type of mutation method is not practical.

For problems that have chromosome values that are not binary, other mutation methods were employed. One common method was simply randomly selecting an allele or gene to be mutated and then randomly changing that value to another value in the allowed data set. For the target allocation problem (Erdem & Ozdemirel, 2003), a gene is randomly selected using the probability of mutation. The selected gene is replaced by a randomly selected alternative assignment from a generation table that is created upon algorithm initialization. For the airman assignment problem (Kleeman & Lamont, 2007) an allele is randomly selected and the allele value is changed to another job (integer) using a uniform distribution. For the frequency assignment problem by Cotta and Troya (2001), mutation is done via a swap operator. This type of mutation is an extension of the bit-flip mutation, where the chromosome values are not binary, though commonly used by researchers.

For the multilevel generalized assignment problem (Hajri-Gabouj, 2003) the mutation is based on a neighborhood operator and immigration. The neighborhood operator is used to group successive tasks and minimize communication costs. The immigration is used when the neighborhood operator does not produce a new solution. In that instance, a new individual is generated. This immigration procedure has been shown to play an important role in preventing premature convergence. The mutation operation is a four-step process:

- Select a random parent.
- Select a random cell in the parent.
- Starting at the first position in the cell, consider the task and operator for that position. If there are more neighbors in that cell, swap alleles with the next neighbor. Continue through the entire cell.

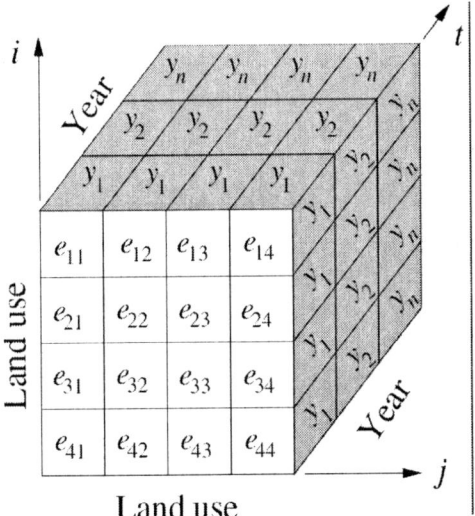

Figure 7. Chromosome representation for the resource allocation problem (Datta, 2007) (© 2007, IEEE, Used with permission)

- If the cell values remain the same after the mutation, then randomly generate an entirely new chromosome.

Some researchers use a mutation operator that was intended to perform more of a local search. For the fixed channel assignment problem (Jin, 2001), the mutation operator is called a local search operator because mutations are done until a user defined "stagnation" limit is reached. The mutation is basically a swap between two randomly chosen positions in the parent. If the swap improves the fitness of the individual, the stagnation limit is set to zero. If the swap does not improve the fitness, the stagnation counter is increased by one. Then, the next swap is implemented. This process continues until a user defined stagnation limit is reached.

Likewise, in the linear gate assignment problem (Oliveira & Lorena, 2001), a local search mutation is used. The local search mutation is always applied to structures no matter how they are created. The algorithm uses a 2-opt neighborhood for the mutation. The algorithm inspects a constant, pre-defined number of neighbors until the best is found. The neighbors are generated by all the two move changes in a constant length part of the structure. The position is chosen at random and from there all possible two move changes in the structure are inspected. Local search mutation methods are effective in discovering better solutions in a localized area of the search space. For some problems, where the search space is fairly smooth, this can be a good method to employ. But for problems that are more deceptive or the search space is more rugged, this type of method may not perform as well as a more globalized version of mutation (such as random mutation).

For the frequency assignment problem by Weicker et al. (2003), multiple mutation operators were used. These operators were grouped into two categories: direct mutations and random mutations. A description of each is:

- **Directed mutations:** These mutation operators include rules of thumb used by experts to get better solutions. These mutations use additional information and their application is limited to situations that satisfy certain preconditions.
- **Random mutations:** Directed mutations cannot guarantee that the entire search space can be reached, as such, random mutations are also used.

Table 1 lists the six directed mutations and five random mutations used by Weiker et al. (2003).

Using multiple mutation operators is a great way to navigate the search space in a variety of ways. A disadvantage would be if one mutation operator works better than the others and it is only used a limited number of times, then the search could be hindered. Using multiple operators is good in unknown problem domains.

The mutation operator for the resource allocation problem (Datta et al., 2007) focuses on random replacement on the array boundary. Another mutation operator finds minimum patchsizes that violate constraints and then steers these infeasible solutions to feasible solutions. Patches are collections of continuous land use. Again, the initial population needs to be feasible. This type of mutation operator is an example of a problem specific operator.

The mutation operators discussed in this chapter range from the more common bit-flip operator to the implementation of eleven mutation operators. Determining which operator to use depends largely on the problem domain, the chromosome representation, the crossover operator, and the selection method chosen. The operators used for a problem need to be matched in such a way that they provide for adequate exploration of the search space while exploiting the good solutions in order to achieve convergence.

Crossover Operators

Crossover operators are typically the primary variation operator used in evolutionary algorithms. There are exceptions (such as the causality assignment problem (Wong et al., 2002) which does not use a crossover operator), but for the most part, this operator is executed with a high probability.

Some researchers use more conventional crossover methods. For the fixed channel assignment problem (Jin, 2001), the crossover method used is essentially a uniform crossover, where two parents are chosen and the child is created from the parents by choosing randomly which values to use from each parent. This method is fairly easy to implement and it limits the disruption of good building blocks that are found at opposite ends of the chromosome.

For the frequency assignment problem by Cotta and Troya (2001) the researchers use classical recombination operators. Specifically, three different recombination operators are employed: cycle crossover (CX) (Goldberg, 1989; Oliver et al., 1987), order crossover (OX) (Davis 1985; Davis 1991; Syswerda 1991), and partially mapped crossover (PMX) (Goldberg & Lingle, 1985). The results of these three operators are compared with each other and all appear to generate similar results. These results are also compared to three heuristic operators and these were found to outperform the heuristic operators as well.

For the airman assignment problem (Kleeman & Lamont, 2007) and the target allocation

Table 1. Mutation operators for the frequency assignment problem (Weiker 2003) (©2003, IEEE, Used with Permission)

Mutation operator	Precondition	Action	Comment
DM1	Transmitters with unused freq. channels exist	Reduce the capacity	Goal is to reduce cost
DM2	Transmitters with maximal capacity that use all freq. channels exist	Put a transmitter with default power and capacity in neighborhood	Goal is to introduce micro-cells in areas with high number of calls
DM3	Transmitters with big overlapping regions exist	Remove such a transmitter	Goal is to reduce interference by reducing overlap
DM4	Transmitters with big overlapping regions exist	Decrease power of the transmitter in a way that all calls remain satisfied	Goal is to reduce cost and interference
DM5	Interference Occurs	Change one of a pair of interfering freq. channels	Goal is to reduce interference
DM6	Transmitters satisfying only a small number of calls exist	Delete the transmitter	Goal is to reduce cost
RM1	N/A	Change position of randomly chosen transmitter	Needed since placement of transmitters are not randomly chosen
RM2	N/A	Introduce new randomly generated individual	Brings fresh genetic material into the optimization
RM3	N/A	Randomly change the power of a random transmitter	Necessary to keep a balance to the directed mutation DM4
RM4	N/A	Randomly change the capacity of a random transmitter	Necessary to keep a balance to the directed mutation DM1
RM5	N/A	Randomly change the frequency channels allocated of a random transmitter	Necessary to keep a balance to the directed mutation DM5

problem (Erdem & Ozdemirel, 2003) a standard two-point crossover method was used. For the latter problem, selection of parents depends upon how many crossover operations are to be applied in each generation. If only one is done, the most fit individual is selected along with another individual from the population. For more than one crossover operation per generation, the first parent of the first crossover operation is always the most fit individual. After that, the rest of the parents are selected via a roulette wheel selection.

Some crossover methods utilize problem domain knowledge. For the frequency assignment problem by Weicker et al. (2003), problem domain knowledge is used in order to increase the probability of combining good characteristics of the parents. The service area is decomposed into two halves by either a horizontal or vertical line. For each half, the fitness of the parents are evaluated and the children inherit the best configuration from each subarea of the parent that was most fit for that subarea. By examining the search space in halves, there can be some undesired effects along the cut line of the service area. To overcome these effects, a margin is drawn on both sides of the cut line and only transmitter configurations outside the margins of each parent are used in the crossover operation. Since this operator is problem dependent, its utility beyond this problem is limited.

The algorithm employed for the multilevel generalized assignment problem [Haj03] also employs a crossover operator utilizing problem domain knowledge. It explores the search space with two crossover operators: the operator/operator and the cell/cell crossover operators. Operator/Operator crossover takes two parents and produces two offspring and allows exchanging at least one task-operator assignment between two parents. A cell/cell crossover operator takes two parents and produces only one offspring. This operator allows transmitting to offspring the task-operator assignments of a selected cell. The mutation is based on a neighborhood operator and immigration.

The resource allocation problem (Datta et al., 2007) also uses a crossover method designed specifically for the problem. The modified crossover operator for this problem requires the decomposition of the chromosome into "blocks" by selecting randomly a pair of rows and columns of land use. Then a "similar" block within the array is chosen at random and it is exchanged with another chromosome (based upon the third dimension - crop years).

Some crossover methods are designed to best fit their algorithm domain. For the linear gate assignment problem (Oliveira & Lorena, 2001), the CGA algorithm is used. This algorithm uses schemata for the population of individuals. To accommodate this representation, the crossover method uses a rule set to determine how the child inherits the parental traits. For this operator, two parents, the base and the guide, are selected from the population. After the two parents are selected, their labels, #, are compared. The new child is generated by the following sequence of operations:

- If a position in both parents contains a # label, then the child receives a # label for that position.
- If only one parent has a # label, then check to see if the gate number of the parent has already been assigned to a position in the child. If it has not been used, then the child receives that gate number. If the gate number has already been used, then the child receives a # label.
- If neither parent has a # label, then first check to see if the base parent's gate number has already been assigned to the child. If it has not, then the child receives base parent's gate number for that position. If that gate number has already been used, then verify if the guide parent's gate number has already been assigned. If it has not then use the guide parent's gate number. If both gate numbers have already been used by the child, then insert a # label into that position.

Another crossover operator designed to better match the algorithm is presented in the quadratic assignment problem (Kleeman et al., 2004). The crossover variation used is called cut-and-splice operator and it was designed to efficiently integrate into the MOMGA-II MOEA. Cut-and-splice is good with variable sized chromosomes because the cut point for each parent can be at a different location. There is a probability associated with both the cut and splice operator. So there is a chance that one parent may be cut but not the other parent and one child may be spliced but not the other. The probabilities of these events occurring are typically low, but they can occur. Figure 8 shows an example of the cut-and-splice operator.

Thus, the range and variety of MOEA mutation operators permit with proper insight to the specific problem's multidimensional fitness landscape, a high performance algorithm design.

In this section, a variety of crossover operators were discussed. Some were more generic crossover methods (two-point crossover, uniform crossover, etc.) that have been applied across many diverse problems. Some crossover methods were designed specifically to meet the needs of the problem being studied. While other methods were designed to best match the algorithm. Deciding which crossover operator to use depends on a variety of factors. Simple problem domains can typically make use of the more common crossover methods. More complex problem domains may require some inventiveness on the researcher in order to design a method that best explores the search space. But the crossover method must be matched effectively with the other operators in order to ensure good convergence and diversity.

Selection Methods

For a stochastic algorithm to be effective, it is crucial to have the right balance of exploration of the search space and exploitation of promising regions in the search space. Therefore, choosing the right selection method is very important in creating effective problem domain / algorithm domain integration. The selection method needs to be selected is such a manner that it is complimentary to the other variation operators. The right balance of exploration and exploitation is largely problem dependent, so there are various

Figure 8. Example of the cut-and-splice operator (Kleeman 2004) (© 2003, IEEE, Used with permission)

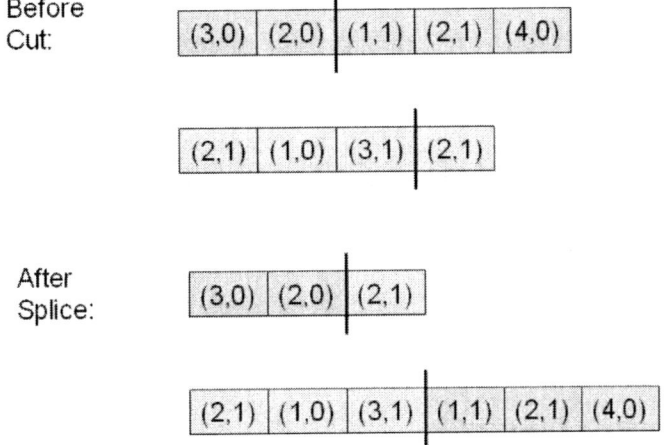

selection methods used for assignment problems discussed in this chapter. Additionally, since these algorithms are multi-objective, the selection mechanism for choosing parents for crossover is often different than the selection mechanism used for determining the next generation of individuals. With that being the case, this section is divided into two subsections and the various selection operators are discussed.

Selection for Recombination

Most of the assignment problems examined in this chapter used traditional selection operators for selecting the parents for crossover. For some, such as the airman assignment problem (Kleeman & Lamont, 2007) and the resource allocation problem (Datta, 2007), they use the selection operator that is embedded in the MOEA (NSGA-II) that they used. In this case, it was tournament selection. Tournament selection was also used for the quadratic assignment problem (Kleeman et al., 2004) and the frequency assignment problem by Weicker et al. (2003). For Weicker, parental selection and replacement are based on a ranking strategy based on dominance. If multiple individuals are dominated by the same number of individuals, preference is given to the ones that dominate the fewest individuals. This favors individuals from less crowded regions.

For the linear gate assignment problem (Oliveira & Lorena, 2001) the selection for crossover is done in the following manner. The population is maintained in an ascending order. So individuals with more genetic information (fewer # labels) are ranked higher than the others. The first parent, or base, is randomly selected out of the first positions of the population. The second parent, called the guide, is randomly selected out of the total population.

For the multilevel generalized assignment problem (Hajri-Gabouj, 2003), parental selection is done in a totally random fashion. For the target allocation problem (Erdem & Ozdemirel, 2003), parental selection uses a combination of elitism and roulette wheel selection. The first parent picked in the first crossover operation for a new generation is always the most fit individual. After that, a roulette wheel selection method is used to find the rest of the parents.

Generational Selection

Generational selection has a slightly different objective than selection for recombination, particularly in multi-objective problems that utilize a Pareto based ranking technique. With selection for recombination, the goal is to combine good building blocks from two or more parents. Probabilistically speaking, an individual with a high fitness value, more than likely poses good building blocks. But there are occasions when individuals with a lower fitness contain good building blocks as well. Therefore, selection operators are geared to favor high fitness solutions, while at the same time, allowing the opportunity for the lower fitness individuals to contribute to the recombination process.

Generational selection is different. First generation multi-objective algorithms performed poorly when standard selection techniques were used. Once elitist selection methods were used, the MOEAs showed significant improvement. Since that time, most MOEAs have employed elitist generational selection techniques, particularly when Pareto based algorithms are used. For example, the airman assignment problem (Kleeman et al., 2007) and the resource allocation problem (Datta et al., 2007) both use the NSGA-II to optimize their problems. The generational selection is done using a Pareto ranking system. Nondominated individuals are set at a rank of zero; individuals dominated by one individual are set at a rank of 1, and so on. The lowest ranking individuals are selected to fill the next generation. If there are too many individuals to fit into the next generation, a crowding operator is used to determine which individuals should be selected based on how dense

Table 2. Summary of assignment problems reviewed in this chapter

Specific Assignment Problem	MOEA Employed	Chromosome Representation	Mutation Operator	Crossover Operator	Selection Method
Linear Gate Assignment Problem	CGA	Schemata	Local search mutation	Rule based	Probabilistic Selection
Multi-objective Quadratic Assignment Problem	MOMGA-II	Binary	Bit flip	Cut-and-splice	Tournament
Airman Assignment Problem	NSGA-II	Integers	Uniform mutation	Two-point	Nondominated Ranking
Causality Assignment Problem	PAES	Binary	Bit flip	None	Nondominated Ranking
Fixed Channel Assignment Problem	Jin GA	Binary Matrix	Local search mutation	Uniform crossover	Probabilistic Selection
Frequency Assignment Problem	stEAPT	Transmitter Parameters	Multiple	Problem Based Elitist Technique	Nondominated Ranking
Frequency Assignment Problem	Cotta GA	Not Given	Swap operator	Multiple	Not Given
Multilevel Generalized Assignment Problem	FGMOA	Meta-level cells	Neighbor swap and immigration	Multiple	Elitist Selection
Resource Allocation Problem	NSGA-II	Two-dimensional matrix	Multiple	"Block" crossover	Nondominated Ranking

of region the individual belongs. An individual in a sparsely populated region would be chosen before an individual in a densely populated region. This allows for more diversity in the solutions.

For the quadratic assignment problem (Kleeman & Lamont, 2004) uses the explicit building block MOEA MOMGA-II, and it probabilistically generates a population of individuals with a specific building block size. There is no selection of individuals between generations since each generation builds individuals based on building block sizes.

For the frequency assignment problem, Weicker et al. (2003) chooses the child only if there is improvement to the overall population. So if a generated child dominates no other individual, and is dominated by at least one individual, it is discarded. If the child does dominate at least one individual, or is not dominated by an individual, the child is kept and the worst individual in the population (based on fitness and rank) is removed. The selection method is based on the cost and interference of the individuals in the population. In order to input new members immediately into the population and for a faster evolution speed, a steady-state selection operator was developed. It works in conjunction with the replacement strategy and its time complexity. The approach is called a steady state evolutionary algorithm with Pareto tournaments (stEAPT).

The multilevel generalized assignment problem (Hajri-Gabouj, 2003) uses a weighted vector algorithm, and not a Pareto based algorithm, and it uses an elitist selection technique. The selection operator simply picks the best solutions to advance to the next generation. Using this type of elitist technique requires care in matching the other operators with this one. This type of technique is more exploitive and as such, the other operators should ensure that enough exploration is being done for the problem.

The causality assignment problem Wong et al. (2002) uses more of a rule-based approach. The next generation is chosen between the parent and the offspring generated by that parent. In each instance the two individuals are compared with each other. If one dominates the other then that individual is kept as a parent. If the child is the one that dominates the parent, then it is also copied into the archive. If the child and parent are both nondominated, then the child is compared to the archive. If the child is dominated by a member of the archive, then it is rejected. If the child dominates some members of the archive, then those individuals are removed from the archive and the child is selected as the parent for the next generation and placed in the archive. If the child is not dominated by any member of the archive and it does not dominate any member either, then it is added to the archive as long as there is still an empty slot.

Table 2 contains a summary of the multi-objective assignment problems discussed in this Chapter. The table lists the specific multi-objective assignment problem, the MOEA used to solve the problem, and the MOEA operators.

SUMMARY

This chapter has touched on the application of MOEAs to various multi-objective assignment problems. The similarities of these types of combinatoric problems allude to the similarity of mathematical fitness models, but with variety in the form of the constraints (Kleeman & Lamont, 2007). Differences, then, are reflected in the search landscapes which are in general very dissimilar over the variety of models. As indicated in this chapter, different MOEA search operators generate quite different results over the specific multi-objective assignment problem landscapes. As discussed, the individual chromosome formulations have a direct impact on the landscape geometry and associated MOEA performance. Selection of MOEA operators and parameters therefore requires one to understand their generic search landscape in order to obtain "good" solutions in an efficient manner. As shown, MOEAs can produce good solutions to a variety of multi-objective assignment problem categories. In the design of experiments for these types of problems, the results of other approaches should also be statistically compared for proper performance evaluation. The chapter's discussion and references present a foundation for the user's application of MOEAs to multi-objective assignment problems.

REFERENCES

Cotta, C. & Troya, J.M. (2001). A comparison of several evolutionary heuristics for the frequency assignment problem. In J. Mira & A. Prieto (Eds), *Connectionist models of neurons, Learning processes, and artificial intelligence. Lecture notes in computer science* (Vol. 2084, pp. 709-716). Berlin, Heidelberg: Springer-Verlag.

Datta, D., Deb, K., & Fonseca, C. M. (2007). Multi-objective evolutionary algorithms for resource allocation problems. In S. Obayashi, K. Deb, C. Poloni, T. Hiroyasu & T. Murata (Eds.), *Evolutionary multi-criterion optimization. In Proceedings of the Fourth International Conference, EMO 2007. Lecture notes in computer science* (Vol. 4403, pp. 401-416). Berlin: Springer.

Day, R. O., Kleeman, M. P., & Lamont, G. B. (2003). Solving the multi-objective quadratic assignment problem using a fast messy genetic algorithm. *Congress on Evolutionary Computation (CEC'2003)* (Vol. 4, pp. 2277–2283). Piscataway, New Jersey: IEEE Service Center.

Deb, K., Agarwal, S., Pratap, A., & Meyarivan, T. (2000). A fast and elitist multi-objective genetic algorithm: NSGA-II. In *Proceedings of Parallel Problem Solving from Nature VI*, (pp. 849-858).

Deb, K., Pratap, A., Agarwal, S., & Meyarivan, T. (2002). A fast and elitist multi-objective genetic algorithm: NSGA–II. *IEEE Transactions on Evolutionary Computation, 6*(2), 182–197.

Davis, L. (1985). Applying adaptive algorithms to epistatic eomains. In *Proceedings of the International Joint Conference on Artificial Intelligence*, (pp 162 – 164). Morgan Kaufmann.

Davis, L. (1991). *Handbook of Genetic Algorithms*.

Erdem, E. & Ozdemirel, N. E. (2003). An evolutionary approach for the target allocation problem. *Journal of the Operational Research Society, 54*(9), 958-969.

Garey, M. R. & Johnson, D. S. (1979). *Computers and intractability: A guide to the theory of NP-completeness*. San Francisco, CA: W. H. Freeman and Co.

Garrett, D., Vannucci, J., Silva, R., Dasgupta, D., & Simien, J. (2005). Genetic algorithms for the sailor assignment problem. In H. G. Beyer & U. M. O'Reilly (Eds.), In *Proceedings of Genetic and Evolutionary Computation (GECCO 2005)*, (pp. 1921-1928). ACM.

Garrett, D., & Dasgupta, D., (2006). Analyzing the Performance of Hybrid Evolutionary Algorithms for the Multi-objective Quadratic Assignment Problem. *IEEE Congress on Evolutionary Computation, (CEC 2006)*, (pp. 1710- 1717). IEEE.

Goldberg, D. E. & Lingle, R. (1985). Alleles, loci, and the traveling salesman problem. In *Proceedings of the First International Conference on Genetic Algorithms and Their Applications*, (pp. 154-159).

Goldberg, D. E. (1989). *Genetic algorithms is search, optimization, and machine learning*. Reading, Massachusetts: Addison-Wesley Publishing.

Hajri-Gabouj, S. (2003). A fuzzy genetic multi-objective optimization algorithm for a multilevel generalized assignment problem. *IEEE Transactions on Systems, Man and Cybernetics, Part C: Applications and Reviews, 33*(2), 214 – 224.

Holder, A. (2005). Navy personnel planning and the optimal partition. *Operations Research, 53*, 77-89).

Jin, M. H., Wu, H. K., Horng, J. T., & Tsai, C. H. (2001). An evolutionary approach to fixed channel assignment problems with limited bandwidth constraint. In *Proceedings of the 2001 IEEE International Conference on Communications, ICC 2001, Vol. 7*, (pp. 2100 – 2104).

Kelemen, A., Kozma, R., & Liang, Y., (2002). Neuro-fuzzy classification for the job assignment problem. *International Joint Conference on Neural Networks IJCNN02, World Congress on Computational Intelligence WCCI2002*, (pp. 630-634). Honolulu, Hawaii: IEEE.

Kleeman, M. P. (2004). *Optimization of heterogeneous UAV communications using the multi-objective quadratic assignment problem*. Unpublished master's thesis, Graduate School of Engineering and Management, Air Force Institute of Technology, Wright-Patterson AFB, Dayton, OH.

Kleeman, M. P., Day, R. O., & Lamont, G. B., (2004). Multi-objective evolutionary search performance with explicit building-block sizes for NPC problems. *Congress on Evolutionary Computation (CEC'2004)* (Vol. 2, pp. 728–735). Piscataway, New Jersey: IEEE Service Center.

Kleeman, M. P. & Lamont, G. B., (2006). The multi-objective constrained assignment problem. In *Proceedings of Genetic and Evolutionary Computation (GECCO 2006)* (Vol. 1, pp. 743-744). ACM.

Kleeman, M. P. & Lamont, G. B. (2007). The multi-objective constrained assignment problem. In *Proceedings of 2007 SPIE Symposium on Defense & Security: Evolutionary and Bio-inspired Computation: Theory and Applications*, Orlando, FL: SPIE.

Knowles, J. D. & Corne, D. W. (1999). The Pareto archived evolution strategy: A new baseline algorithm for Pareto multi-objective optimisation. In *Proceedings of the 1999 Congress on Evolutionary Computation (CEC'99)*, (pp. 98-105).

Knowles, J. D. & Corne, D.W. (2000). Approximating the nondominated front using the Pareto Archived Evolution Strategy. *Evolutionary Computation, 8*(2), 149-172.

Knowles, J. D. & Corne, D. W. (2002). Towards landscape analyses to inform the design of a hybrid local search for the multi-objective quadratic assignment problem. In A. Abraham, J. Ruiz-del-Solar, & M. Koppen (Eds.), *Soft computing systems: Design, management and applications*, (pp. 271—279). Amsterdam: IOS Press.

Knowles, J. D. & Corne, D. W. (2003). Instance generators and test suites for the multi-objective quadratic assignment problem. In *Proceedings of Evolutionary Multi-Criterion Optimization (EMO 2003) Second International Conference*, (pp 295-310). Faro, Portugal.

Lewis, M. W., Lewis, K. R., & White, B. J. (in press). Guided design search in the interval-bounded sailor assignment problem. *Computers and Operations Research*. Elsevier.

Liang, Y., Lin, K. I., & Kelemen, A. (2002). Adaptive generalized estimation equation with bayes classifier for the job assignment problem. In *PAKDD '02: Proceedings of the 6th Pacific-Asia Conference on Advances in Knowledge Discovery and Data Mining*, (pp. 438-449). London, UK: Springer-Verlag.

Lorena, L. A. N., Narciso, M. G., & Beasley, J. E, (1999). *A constructive genetic algorithm for the generalized assignment problem*. Technical report.

Oliveira, A. C. M. & Lorena, L. A. N. (2001). A constructive evolutionary approach to linear gate assignment problems. *ENIA 2001 – Encontro Nacional de Inteligência Artificial*. Fortaleza, Brazil.

Oliver, I. M., Smith, D. J., & Holland, J. R. C. (1987). A study of permutation crossover operators on the traveling salesperson problem. In *Proceedings of the Second International Conference on Genetic Algorithms and their Applications*, (pp. 224 – 230).

Palaniappan, S., Zein-Sabatto, S., & Sekmen, A. (2001). Dynamic multi-objective optimization of war resource allocation using adaptive genetic algorithms. In *Proceedings of the IEEE Southeast Conf.*, (pp. 160-165).

Rachmawati, L. & Srinivasan, D. (2005). A hybrid fuzzy evolutionary algorithm for a multi-objective resource allocation problem. In *Proceedings of the Fifth International Conference on Hybrid Intelligent Systems (HIS'05)*, (pp. 55-60).

Syswerda, G. (1991). Schedule optimization using genetic algorithms. *Handbook of genetic algorithms*.

Weicker, N., Szabo, G., Weicker, K., & Widmayer, P. (2003). Evolutionary multi-objective optimization for base station transmitter placement with frequency assignment. *IEEE Transactions on Evolutionary Computation, 7*(2), 189 – 203.

West, D. B. (2001). *Introduction to graph theory* (2nd ed.). Englewood Cliffs, NJ: Prentice-Hall.

Wong, T., Bigras, P., & Khayati, K. (2002). Causality assignment using multi-objective evolutionary algorithms. In *Proceedings of the 2002 IEEE International Conference on Systems, Man and Cybernetics, vol 4*.

FUTURE RESEARCH DIRECTIONS

The multi-objective assignment problems discussed in this chapter obviously cover a variety of models and applications. Of course, there are many other multi-objective assignment problems that could be discussed in fine detail including variations of the container assignment problem, the traffic assignment problem, the channel assignment problem, the file assignment problem, and the faculty-course-time slot assignment problem with preferences. Each of these as well as variations of those discussed require individual problem domain analysis as to ascertaining the associated unique structure of the fitness search landscape and the appropriateness of the MOEA operators in effectively and efficiently searching this landscape.

Because many of the decision variables in real-world assignment problems are real valued, researchers in addressing such a specific multi-objective assignment problem should consider the variety of real-valued crossover and mutation operators reflected in the literature. Statistical evaluation of these operators and selection operator types on the specific fitness search landscape provides appropriate insight in solving the specific MOP. Parallel and distributed MOEAs via an island model, farming model, or a master/slave could provide a more efficient computational environment.

Extending many of the assignment applications discussed to three or more objectives is reflected of more realistic models (larger dimensions, realistic environmental constraints, visualization techniques). Research should include the integration of the decision maker as to the focus of the search in the many multi-objective space in these cases. This is required in order to reduce the exponential computation in attempting to solve the problem in a local region of the Pareto front.

ADDITIONAL READING

Aleman, R., Hill, R., & Zhang, X. (2006, November). Application of vehicle routing and multiperiod assignment problem to UAV planning. INFORMS International Meeting.

Boyce, D., Lee, D., & Ran, B. (2001). Analytical models of the dynamic traffic assignment problem. *Networks and Spatial Economics, 1*(3).

Capone, A. & Trubian, M. (1999). Channel assignment problem in cellular systems: A new model and a tabu search algorithm. *IEEE Trans. On Vehicular Technology, 48*(4).

Dowdy, L. & Foster, D. (1982). Comparative models of the file assignment problem. *ACM Computing Surveys, 14*(2).

Ismayilova, N., Ozdemir, M. S., & Gasimov, R. N. (2005). A multi-objective faculty-course-time slot assignment problem with preferences. In *Proceedings of 8th International Symposium of the Analytic Hierarchy Process.*

Jesus, J., d Hanafi, S., & Semet, F. (2003). The container assignment problem: Models and solution methods. In *Proceedings of Odysseus.*

Liefooghe, A., Basseur, M., Jourdan, L., & Talbi, E. (2007). Multi-objective combinatorial optimization for stochastic problems: An application to the flow-shop scheduling problem. In *Proceedings of the Fourth International Conference on Evolutionary Multi-Criterion Optimization (EMO).*

Przybyiski, A., Gandibleux, X. & Ehrgott, M. (2005). *The biobjective assignment problem.* LINA, Research Report, no. 05.07.

Xu, J. & Bailey, G. (2001). The airport gate assignment problem: Mathematical model and a tabu search. In *Proceedings of the 34th Hawaii Intl Conf on System Sciences.*

ENDNOTE

*   The views expressed in this chapter are those of the authors and do not reflect the official policy or position of the Department of Defense or the United States Government.

Chapter XIV
Evolutionary Multi-Objective Optimization in Military Applications*

Mark P. Kleeman
Air Force Institute of Technology, USA

Gary B. Lamont
Air Force Institute of Technology, USA

ABSTRACT

Evolutionary methods are used in many fields to solve multi-objective optimization problems. Military problems are no exception. This chapter looks at a variety of military applications that have utilized evolutionary techniques for solving their problem.

INTRODUCTION

Many real world problems in the military are inherently multi-objective problems (MOPs). Quite often, the problem contains competing objectives, where the optimization of one objective degrades the value of another such as mission success vs. resource survival. To solve some of these problems, researchers have applied numerous optimization techniques. The technique applied usually depends on the complexity of the problem. For a simple single objective optimization problem, a deterministic method such as depth-first search, the simplex technique or Tabu search might be the most appropriate method. But for a highly complex, high dimensional NP-complete problem, a stochastic algorithm may be the better choice in finding an acceptable solution in a reasonable amount of time. Multi-objective Evolutionary Algorithms (MOEAs) are a stochastic search method with the ability to find sets of acceptable tradeoff solutions. Also, their performance as addressed in this chapter is less susceptible to the shape of the search landscape and the associated Pareto front (Coello, Van Veldhuizen, & Lamont 2002).

For the modern military there are many complex MOPs that require effective solutions to be provided in an efficient manner. Military MOPs come from a variety of disciplines but usually can be symbolically formulated with objectives and constraints and thus, are reflected in a mathematical or computational model (Coello et al., 2002). In this chapter we consider a variety of explicit military applications including military communication networks (design, routing and layout), resource management (facilities, engine maintenance), mission planning, dynamic simulation and technical resource design optimization (low energy laser, autopilot). Other applications are briefly mentioned. Through these problem domain and MOEA discussions, we wish to motivate the use of MOEA stochastic search techniques to find efficiently "good" solutions to complex multi-objective military problems.

COMMUNICATION NETWORKS

Because of the impact of military communication networks on overall performance, various network problems are addressed. For example, consider a network design problem that attempts to find the best network configuration with respect to total cost and average number of hops. Another presented example develops routing optimization possibilities and layout optimizations of wireless sensor networks. Network sensor layout for wireless sensors and associated management are other important military applications which are discussed.

Network Design

Computer networks are vital for the military in order to relay information quickly. Kleeman (2007a) research the network design problem, which is a critical piece for network centric warfare. The MOP was derived from the single objective problem introduced by Erwin (2006). The problem is a variation of the **multicommodity capacitated network design problem (MCNDP)**. For this problem, a network consists of nodes and arcs. Additionally, each node can have a number of interfaces (interfaces can be different types of connection points in the network—such as satellite, infrared or hardwired connections). Each interface can be connected to every other node (through the same interface type) via an arc, but it does not have to be a fully connected graph. The arcs are unidirectional and each has a fixed capacity. The capacities for each arc can be different. Each node can have a commodity (messages, packets, etc.) that it needs to send to every other node in the network. Each commodity has a bandwidth requirement. This problem is detailed enough that the optimization process can determine where bottlenecks may be in the network and find routes to overcome the bottlenecks. We let u_{if} denote the number of interfaces of type f at node i. The fixed cost of including an arc from node i to node j via interface type f in the network is denoted c_{ijf}. The capacity of each arc is given by cap_{ijf}. In the following arc representation we let the number of interface types be fixed at 2. We use solid and dashed arcs to distinguish between the different interface

Figure 1. Modified Monte Carlo results for the 2nd instance of a 10 node problem (Kleeman, 2007a)

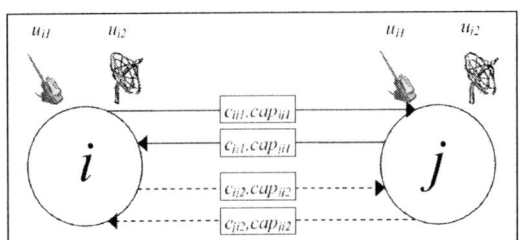

types. We assume if node *i* is connected to node *j* by interface type *f*, then node *j* is connected to node *i* by the same interface type. The fixed cost and capacity associated with each link are not assumed to be equal. These assumptions are made to consider an intentionally broad and general case of this NDP. The variable cost per unit flow for each commodity over each arc is omitted, but not forgotten, from the representation for simplicity. Satellite links and a local wireless network model are reflected in Figure 1. For the generic problem, two objectives are to be optimized: total network cost and average number of hops.

For evaluation, ten different network instances with 10 nodes, 3 interfaces per node, and 90 commodities were randomly generated in order to see how well the MOEA performed (Kleeman, 2007a). The results were compared to a Monte Carlo approach and the previous single objective approach done by Erwin (Erwin, 2006). Erwin aggregated NDP fitness functions into a single objective model and applied a Mixed-Integer Linear Program (MILP) formulation and two heuristic strategies.

The network problem formulation is complex including constraints and thus, can scale to larger realistic networks, but it does have its disadvantages. For example, attempting to generate valid solutions via a standard Monte Carlo approach yielded no valid solutions with 10,000,000 instances. To overcome this obstacle, the Monte Carlo search (and subsequently the MOEA), had to be modified in such a way to meet the constraints and generate feasible or valid solutions. In this case, the node balance constraint was causing the most problems because the probability of meeting the node balance constraint for just one commodity was very slim and to be able to randomly generate a solution where all the commodities met the constraint was astronomical. Once the Monte Carlo and the MOEA were modified to meet the node balance constraint, the algorithms were able to generate valid solutions. The modified Monte Carlo method was used to get an idea of the search landscape and to compare with the MOEA results. Figure 2 shows the results of the modified Monte Carlo method run 50,000 times for the 2nd instance of the 10 node problem. Note that with the new method, approximately 80% of the solutions generated are valid. Of the valid solutions, only 15 are nondominated and make up the Pareto front.

Figure 2. Modified Monte Carlo results for the 2nd instance of a 10 node problem (Kleeman, 2007a)

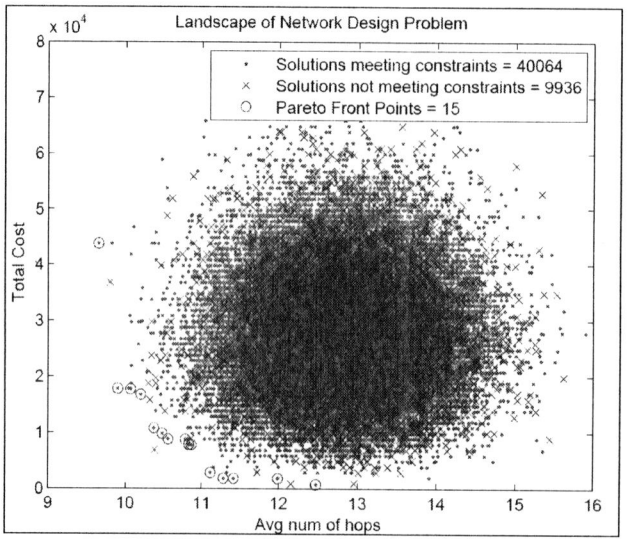

The MOEA chosen to solve this problem was the second generation nondominated sorting algorithm (NSGA-II), developed by Deb, Pratap, Agarwal, and Meyarivan (2002). The NSGA-II is similar to most MOEAs, in that it utilizes recombination, mutation, and tournament selection operators. The niching operator that it uses is a rank based niching which is based on Pareto dominance and a crowding operator. The algorithm gathers results for all population members and then runs through the entire population to find the individuals that are nondominated. These individuals are assigned a rank of 0 and are removed from the search population. Then the algorithm finds the next group of nondominated individuals and gives them a rank of 1 and removes them from the population. The algorithm continues in this fashion until it has sorted all the members based on their Pareto dominance. To determine the next generation, the algorithm pulls individuals with the lowest Pareto ranking into the population. The crowding operator comes into play when the algorithm must pull in a portion of a ranked set of individuals into the population. In this case, the algorithm accepts only the least crowded points in that ranking. A density estimator picks the two nearest points on either side of the point being measured and creates a cuboid. The crowding distance for the point is the average side length of the cuboid. For this problem, a new initialization process and mutation operator had to be implemented in order to ensure the generation of valid solutions. The mutation operator was called propagation mutation. This operator ensured that the node balance constraint would be met for each mutation. For this problem, 200 individuals were created and 250 generations were run. This equated to 50,000 fitness evaluations and allowed for a fair comparison with the modified Monte Carlo approach. No crossover operator was used, but mutation was set at a rate of 10%.

Figure 3 shows how the modified NSGA-II compared with the modified Monte Carlo approach. Note how the initial 200 individuals were dominated by the best Monte Carlo points, but the evolution process was able to find points that dominated every Monte Carlo point.

The modified NSGA-II was run 30 times for each instance and the best total cost results from each run were compared to those generated by

Figure 3. Comparison of the modified NSGA-II with the modified Monte Carlo technique (Kleeman, 2007a)

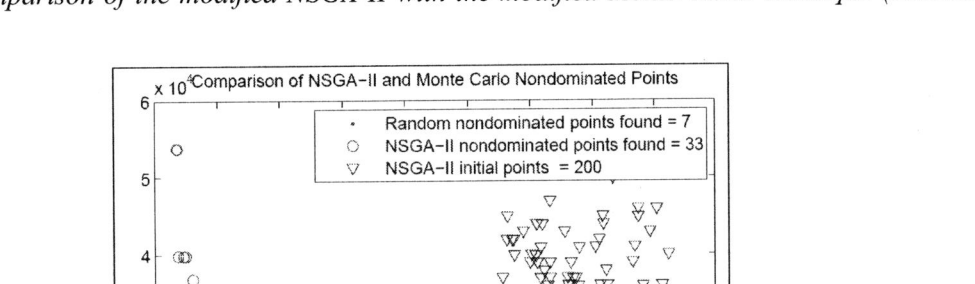

Table 1. Comparison of Modified NSGA-II total cost results with results published by Erwin (Kleeman, 2007a)

Trial	M-NSGA-II (30 runs each trial)			Erwin's [4]
	mean / std dev	best run	worst run	best run
1	**585.19** / 10.63	567.80	620.60	815.9
2	**516.21** / 12.24	493.40	535.00	823.45

Erwin (Erwin, 2006) using the MILP. Table 1 shows how the MOEA approach fared. Note that not only did the MOEA have the best mean for all 10 instances, but even the worst runs of the 30 generated results that were better than Erwin's.

This network research shows that an MOEA can be a viable option to generating realistic network designs. It also shows that an MOEA can play a vital role in the development of network centric systems using only a mutation operator. Continuing efforts should focus on larger networks, use of other MOEA structures, employment of MOEA comparative metrics for performance evaluation, and extended comparison to other fitness aggregated approaches.

Network Routing

Rajagopalan et al. (2005a) have studied mobile agent routing in wireless sensor networks (WSNs). The WSNs are deployed for target detection and are viewed as distributed detection problems. In these problems, the sensors transmit their data to a node called a fusion center. These papers propose a Mobile Agent based Distributed Sensor Network (MADSN) (Qi, Iyengar, & Chakrabarty, 2001), shown in Figure 4, which uses a mobile agent that visits the sensors selectively and fuses the data incrementally. This type of network was chosen because it helps to circumvent the use of battery power and excessive bandwidth for noncritical data.

Multi-Objective Mobile Agent Routing in Wireless Sensor Networks

The research attempts to optimize three objectives: (1) minimization of energy consumption, (2) minimization of path loss, and (3) maximization of the total detected signal energy. Since sensors are battery powered, limiting energy consumption is critical in maintaining the effectiveness of the sensor. In this problem, heterogeneous sensors are used. This allows for sensors to have different capabilities and battery life. For the path loss objective, the wireless communication links must be established between sensors when the mobile

Figure 4. The hierarchical MADSN architecture (Rajagopalan, 2005) (© 2005, IEEE, Used with permission)

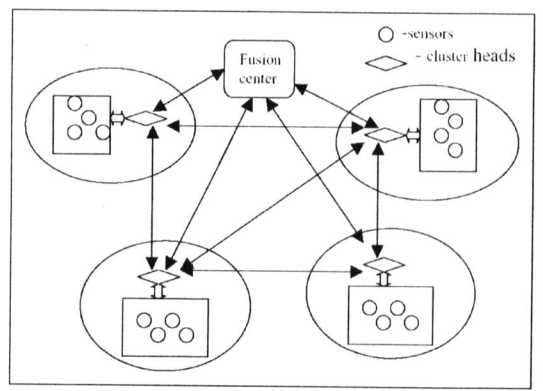

agent moves through the route. Path loss measures the attenuation of the signal on a link. The path loss objective function is an aggregate of all those link losses. Being able to accurately detect targets is another important job of a WSN. Each sensor is capable of detecting a certain amount of energy produced by a target. The mobile agent's goal is to gather the information from each sensor in order to develop accurate target detection and classification. The total detected signal energy objective function is a sum of the energy values from each of the sensors. These energy values are calculated two different ways: randomized median filtering and randomized censored averaging. These two approaches are evaluated in the research as well.

The three objectives are competing objectives. As the number of sensors along the path increases, the detection signal increases, which is good, but the energy consumption and path loss increase as well, which is bad. It is initially not known whether the true Pareto front is convex or not so an MOEA was chosen to solve this MOP since it can efficiently generate trade-off solutions in non-convex regions of the Pareto front. In fact, two MOEAs and a weighted GA were run and their results were compared. The algorithms were: An evolutionary multi-objective crowding algorithm (EMOCA) (Rajagopalan et al., 2004a, Rajagopalan et al., 2004b), the Nondominated Sorting GA-II (NSGA-II) (Deb, Agarwal, Pratap, & Meyarivan, 2000), and the Weighted GA (WGA) (Wu, Rao, Barhen, Iyengar, Vaishnavi, & Qi, 2004). Table 2 shows a comparison of the two MOEAs and the weighted GA. The big difference is in the external archive used by EMOCA and the selection criteria for future generations. The external archive used by EMOCA allows the MOEA to keep more viable solutions. The external archive can grow to accommodate the good solutions whereas the NSGA-II MOEA must keep track of the good solutions with its population members. The selection criterion for the NSGA-II is rank based with a crowding operator. The EMOCA selection process concerns only the parents and the children. If the child dominates the parent, it is selected. If the child is dominated by the selected parent and it has a larger crowding distance than the parent, then the child is added with a probability based on the two crowding distances. If the child does not dominate the parent, than the one with the largest crowding distance is selected. Note that this type of selection criteria rewards diversity more than the NSGA-II rank-based selection.

To compare the results of the two MOEAs, three metrics were used. The set coverage metric (also known as the two-set coverage metric) (Zitzler, 1999) and a domination metric (Rajagopalan et al., 2004a) (which is a slight modification of the two-set coverage metric) were used as convergence metrics. The spacing metric (Schott, 1995) was used as a diversity metric. The EMOCA outperformed the WGA in all test cases using the defined metrics. Figure 5 shows the results between the EMOCA and NSGA-II. Again, for these metrics, the EMOCA appears to outperform the NSGA-II.

Table 2. Comparison of MOEAs and WGA used in (Rajagopalan, 2005) (© 2005, IEEE, Used with permission)

	Mating Selection	Archiving	Generation selection	Crossover operator	Mutation operator
EMOCA	Binary tournament	External archive	Uses policy to reward diversity	Two-point	Swap
NSGA-II	Nondomination ranking	No archiving	Pareto dominance	Two-point	Swap
WGA	Binary tournament	External archive	Elitist steady-state replacement	Two-point	Swap

Figure 6 displays the projection of nondominated points onto two dimensions as generated by the EMOCA and NSGA-II. The left side displays the results of the EMOCA and the right side displays the results of the NSGA-II. Two-point crossover and swap mutation are adequate for generating good results for this type of problem. Note that the EMOCA found many more nondominated points in one trial.

In this research, they also compare randomized median filtering (RMF) and randomized censored averaging (RCA) using the same metrics used to compare the algorithms. Figure 7 shows these results. Based on these results with EMOCA, the RCA method outperforms the RMF method.

This MOEA effort indicates that a multi-objective approach to optimizing agent routing in low power networks provides interesting and acceptable results. New effort should focus on larger networks and incorporating real-world constraints.

Figure 5. EMOCA (E) vs. NSGA-II (N) using set covering (C), domination (Dom), and spacing (S) metrics (Results are over 30 trials) (Rajagopalan, 2005) (© 2005, IEEE, Used with permission)

Problem parameters: (no of targets, clusters, sensors per cluster)	Randomized median filtering					Randomized censored averaging				
	C(N,E)	C(E,N)	Dom(E,N)	S(E)	S(N)	C(N,E)	C(E,N)	Dom(E,N)	S(E)	S(N)
1,5,20	0.005	0.95	0.67	0.002	0.07	0.0047	0.81	0.70	0.005	0.26
2,10,20	0.16	0.84	0.85	0.02	0.09	0.10	0.78	0.73	0.012	0.16
2,10,30	0.11	0.86	0.93	0.006	0.02	0.05	0.76	0.86	0.011	0.14
3,10,40	0.16	0.87	0.75	0.01	0.13	0.18	0.75	0.75	0.008	0.09
3,20,25	0.08	0.83	0.72	0.02	0.38	0.13	0.82	0.77	0.035	0.18
4,30,20	0.11	0.77	0.77	0.06	0.10	0.21	0.86	0.81	0.05	0.13
5,20,35	0.09	0.83	0.84	0.03	0.26	0.19	0.84	0.74	0.03	0.55
5,20,40	0.15	0.86	0.79	0.02	0.27	0.06	0.81	0.79	0.05	0.28
5,30,30	0.28	0.74	0.68	0.05	0.14	0.23	0.82	0.72	0.06	0.25

Figure 6. Projections showing nondominated solutions obtained by EMOCA (left graph) and NSGA-II (right graph) for two dimensions for a 200 node MADSN in one trial (Rajagopalan, 2005) (© 2005, IEEE, Used with permission)

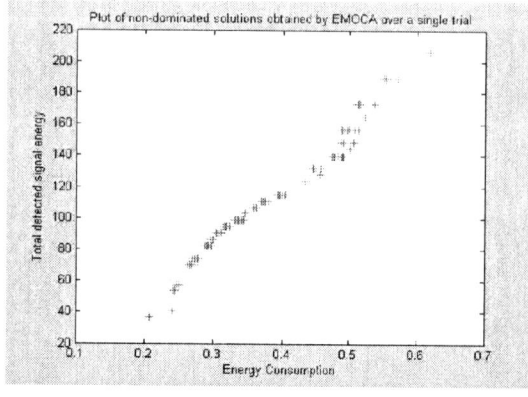
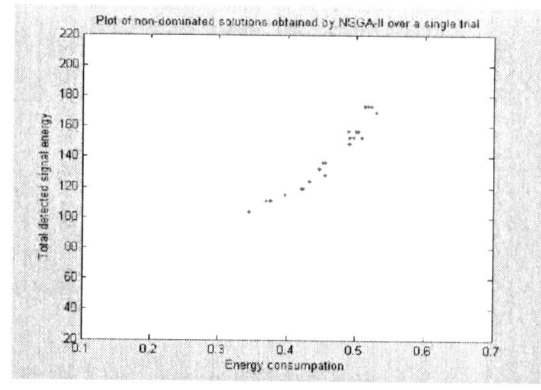

Figure 7. RCA vs. RMF method using set covering (C), domination (Dom), and spacing (S) metrics (Results are over 30 trials) (Rajagopalan, 2005) (© 2005, IEEE, Used with permission)

Problem parameters : (no of targets, clusters and sensors/cluster	C(RMF,RCA)	C(RCA,RMF)	Dom(RCA, RMF)	S(RCA)	S(RMF)
1,5,20	0	0.96	1	0.008	0.023
2,10,20	0.34	0.82	0.66	0.011	0.087
2,10,30	0.17	0.90	0.84	0.005	0.054
3,10,40	0.01	0.80	0.98	0.016	0.097
3,20,25	0.12	0.68	0.68	0.071	0.124
4,30,20	0	0.92	1	0.016	0.942
5,20,35	0.23	0.73	0.58	0.034	0.087
5,20,40	0	0.92	1	0.064	0.091
5,30,30	0.23	0.73	0.58	0.013	0.064

Network Sensor Layout

Wireless sensor networks (WSNs) are important in many fields, particularly in military situations, where an ad hoc communication network is required. But these networks typically have a small geographical footprint. In the military, WSNs may need to be deployed in a large geographical region. For these networks careful sensor deployment (layout optimization and placement) is necessary in order conserve resources so they can be used later in other regions.

Layout Optimization for a Wireless Sensor Network

The WSNs presented by Jourdan and de Weck (2004b) are capable of sensing and communicating. The sensors are assumed identical but can be any type of sensor, such as optical, chemical, or acoustic—depending on the application. Each small sensor is assumed to be able to communicate wirelessly and have a limited communication range. To transmit their information to a home base for analysis, a high energy communication node (HECN) is needed to relay the data to an aircraft or satellite. Figure 8 shows an example of a WSN. The sensors must be positioned strategically in order to ensure all information can be transmitted to the HECN. Since the sensors are likely to be placed behind enemy lines, in a variety of terrains, an airdrop is perceived as the deployment method. An automated planning system for the placement process is presented that uses an idealized domain model based on communication coverage and sensing radius.

In solving this MOP, Jourdan optimizes over two objectives: coverage and lifetime of the network. The coverage is the area of the union of the sensor radii of each connected sensor, divided by the total area of the network. The lifetime is the ratio of time to the first sensor failure divided by the maximum lifetime of a sensor. The two nonlinear objectives are competing: maximizing coverage creates networks that have minimum sensor overlap but maximizing lifetime requires networks where all the sensors are able to communicate with the HECN. An MOEA was used to determine Pareto fronts for the network designs and to demonstrate the relationship the sensor/communication ratio and the final Pareto front layouts. The MOEA uses Pareto dominance (Fonseca & Fleming, 1998) for its fitness measure. The MOEA does implement crossover and muta-

Figure 8. Example of a WSN to monitor a region, with a HECN in the vicinity of the sensors to relay information to a UAV and then to the home base (Jourdan, 2004b) (© 2004, IEEE, Used with permission)

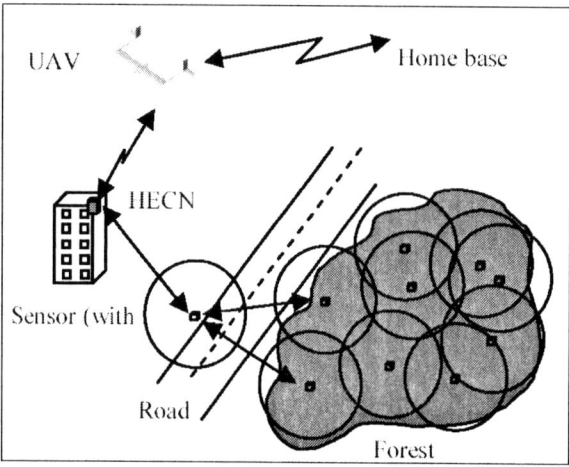

Figure 9. Jourdan's research results for 10 sensors and $R_{Sensor} = R_{COMM} = 2$. Pareto front on the left, the nondominated 5-spoke layout in the center, and the nondominated 3-spoke layout on the right (Jourdan de Weck, 2004b) (© 2004, IEEE, Used with permission)

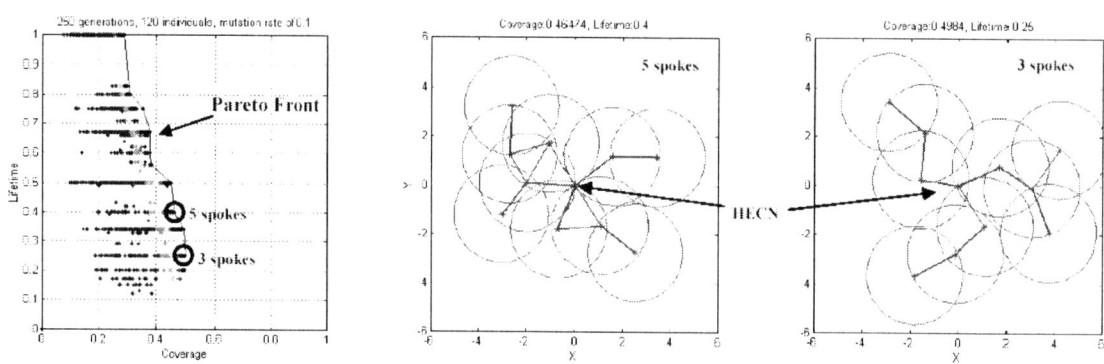

tion, but the authors do not mention the specific type of operators that were used and if elitism or if any niching technique was employed.

The results for a WSN of 10 sensors are shown in Figure 9. Figure 9 shows the Pareto front generated by the MOEA, the known Pareto front (PF_{known}), with respect to the sensor lifetime and network coverage. The center and right figure display the 5-spoke and 3-spoke networks that are circled in the left figure and are on the PF_{known}. These figures are displayed to illustrate the variety of options found along the PF_{known}. Note how the 3-spoke network has better coverage, but the 5-spoke network has a longer lifetime.

The researchers also focused on the sensing and communication radius of each sensor and

Figure 10. Example of a WSN monitoring a facility, using a high energy communication node (HECN) located at the top of a building (Jourdan, 2004a) (©2004, SPIE. Used with permission)

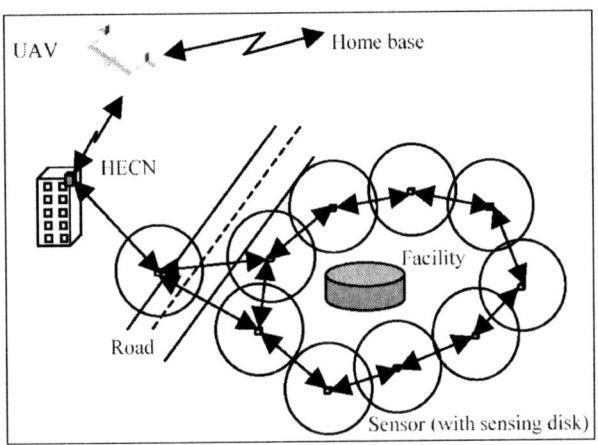

Table 3. Objectives optimized for each case study

Case 1	Case 2	Case 3
Maximize coverage	Maximize coverage	Maximize coverage
Minimize # of sensors	Minimize # of sensors	Minimize # of sensors
Maximize survivability		

their affect on the extremes of the PF_{known}. When comparing the best lifetime results from each PF_{known}, they found that the WSN layouts were identical. The results were more interesting when they compared the best coverage results from the three ratios. The results show that when the communication radius and the sensing radius are identical, the network achieves maximum coverage. This can be expected because when $R_{Sensor} < R_{COMM}$, the sensing area reduced and therefore cannot achieve the same area when the radii are equal. Likewise, when $R_{Sensor} > R_{COMM}$, the sensors must placed closer together in order to communicate with each other. An analysis of these ratios and layouts confirms that the MOEA has also discovered WSN layout patterns associated with the ratio of R_{Sensor}/R_{COMM}.

Possible future efforts include using the number of sensors as a design variable, modeling uncertainty of sensor positions due to airdrop variability, exploring different sensing objectives, and evaluating a heterogeneous set of sensors with various sensing and communication radii and ratios. The costs of the heterogeneous sensors would probably be different, so a third objective, cost, could be added. Finally, performance evaluation using more definitive MOEA metrics would be appropriate.

Automated Placement of Wireless Sensor Network Nodes

Automated planning of a WSN to monitor a critical facility was investigated by Jourdan and de

Weck (Jourdan & de Weck, 2004a) from a multi-objective perspective. Their discussion of layout optimization of WSNs via area coverage and sensor radii is discussed in the previous section. Here, the automated placement of WSN Nodes is highlighted. Their work specifically examines the optimal placement of nodes for a WSN to monitor a critical facility in a hostile region. Figure 10 shows an example of a WSN being used to monitor a facility.

Three case studies are conducted in the research:

1. **Case 1:** Monitor a facility that has two approaching roads. The goal in this case study is to monitor movement, in a hostile region, around a facility of interest and the two approaching roads. In order to ensure sensor survivability, the sensors need to be placed in location where they will not be easily discovered.
2. **Case 2:** Detect movements in and out of a circular area. For this case study, sensor placement is not crucial to their survival. This is similar to the first case study, but in a lower threat environment.
3. **Case 3:** Sensors uniformly cover an entire square area. Again, sensor placement does not affect their survivability. Chemical sensors examining soil in a particular region is an example of where this case could be put into practice.

The objectives of the MOEA depend on the case study. Table 3 shows a list of the case studies and the objectives that the MOEA attempts to optimize. Note that only case study 1 has three objectives while the other two have two objectives.

The design space for Case 1 was found to be non-linear. Further analysis revealed discontinuities in the search space when using five sensors for coverage. The MOEA is the same one used in the previous section. The results from case study 1 are shown in Figure 11. Figure 11(a) shows a plot of all individuals generated by the MOEA with respect to the three objective functions. The nondominated points are circled. Figures 11 (b) – (d) show three different nondominated individuals that were located on the Pareto front (by inspection, one can see that the three points circled in Figure 11(a) are the ones displayed in Figure 11 (b)-(d)). These points attempt to illustrate some of the designs given different trade-offs. The results show that good coverage can be obtained with 5 to 9 sensors but the important trade-off is between limiting the number of sensors and trying to increase the survivability rate. To limit the number of sensors used in the problem, the sensors must be placed closer to the facility. But if the sensors are placed close to the facility, their survivability rate drops. So a decision maker needs to determine the relative importance of these two objectives in order to select the most appropriate solution.

The results for case study 2 are shown in Figure 12. Figure 12(a) shows the Pareto front generated by the MOEA and Figure 12(b) shows an example of one of the results along the Pareto front. These results (as well as the results for case study 3, which are very similar to these) are as expected. In order to get good sensor coverage, enough sensors need to be placed in order to cover the area required. So the Pareto front shows how much coverage is sacrificed as fewer sensors are used.

Each of the case studies was run only once with 300 generations and a population size of 100. One-point crossover and uniform mutation supported the generation of excellent results. The MOEA took between 20-25 minutes to finish the optimization of each one of the case studies. Additional efforts should include evaluation of MOEA metrics, comparisons of results from different MOEA instantiations, and consideration of real-world terrain constraints.

Using a MOEA for placement of wireless network sensors provides considerable insight to solving the associated optimization problem. Further effort should focus on realistic environmental constraints.

Resource Management in Wideband CDMA Systems

According to Chan, Man, Tang, and Kwong (2005), "Resource management is an important issue of the 3G systems to allocate the resources optimally while the quality of service (QoS) requirement of each connecting user can still be satisfied so that the radio spectrum can be efficiently utilized" (Cho, 2005). The QoS was measured using the received bit energy-to-noise density ratio. If a minimum threshold was met for a user for a specified media type, then the QoS requirement was considered to be met. QoS for a user is typically related to three elements: transmission power, transmission rate, and multiple access interference. These three elements are used as the three objective functions of this problem. The goal is to minimize the total transmission power and maximize the total transmission rate of all the users simultaneously while minimizing the total number of violating users.

Chan et al proposed a new MOEA called the Jumping Gene GA (JGGA) in order to solve this multi-objective resource management problem. The algorithm was created to emulate the "jumping gene" phenomenon. The resource management problem is in wideband code division multiple access (CDMA) systems that are used be the military. An innovative MOEA was developed for this problem because it is multifaceted. An MOEA can generate multiple Pareto-optimal solutions

Figure 11. Results for Case 1. Note that the solid circles around the sensors indicate the communication radius and the dashed circles indicate the sensing radius of a sensor (Jourdan, 2004a) (©2004, SPIE. Used with permission)

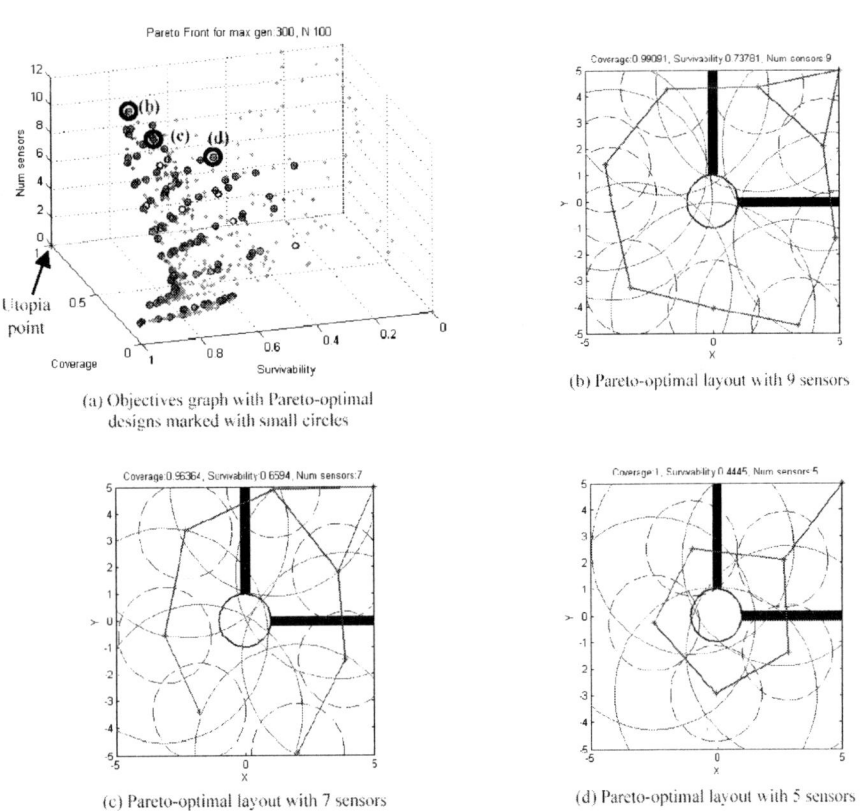

Figure 12. Results for Case 2. Pareto front is shown on the left and a 6 sensor layout from the Pareto front is shown to the right. (Jourdan, 2004a) (©2004, SPIE. Used with permission)

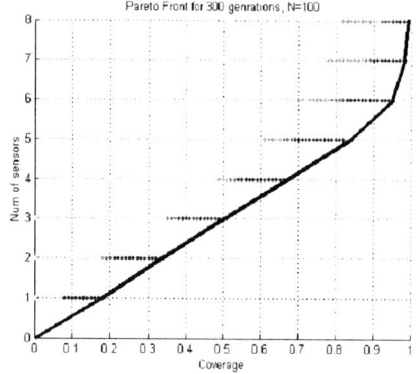
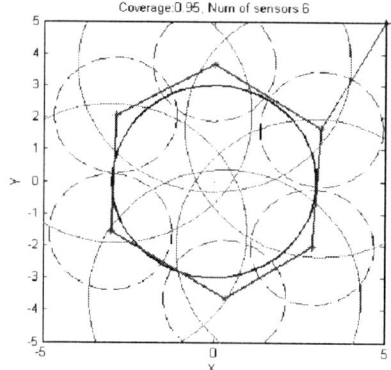

without limiting the search space. Plus, the search space of the problem is large, so a deterministic method would not be appropriate. Because of the unique characteristics of the JGGA, it is presented in further detail.

The JGGA is based on the jumping gene phenomenon. Also known as transposons, they are a sequence in a chromosome that can mover around to different positions within the chromosome. This process is called transposition. There are two types of transposition: the cut-and-paste transposition and the copy-and-paste (or replicate) transposition. Cut-and-paste transposition, shown in Figure 13, can occur two different ways. The first way, Figure 13(a), is to cut a transposon, a set of consecutive genes (one or more) in a chromosome, from the parent and paste it back into the parent in a new, random location. Note that there can be more than one transposon in a chromosome. The second method, Figure 13(b), is to use two parents and cut a transposon from each of the parents and place them into the other parent at a random insertion point.

The copy-and-paste transposition operator can also occur in two different respects. The first method uses one parent. A transposon is copied and is pasted into a different area of the chromosome. The paste location is selected at random and the allele values in those gene positions are replaced with the pasted values. For the second method, two parents are chosen and transposons are copied from each parent. Then, the transposons are pasted into the other parent at a randomly determined location. Since this is a random process, a transposon does not have to be selected every time.

These operators are combined with a crossover (uniform crossover) and a case-based mutation operator. Additionally, the sorting procedure, crowding procedure, and elitism strategy of the NSGA-II algorithm are also used to create the MOEA. The chromosome is composed of real-valued alleles and can be decamped into two segments. The first segment of the chromosome is for the transmission power of each user. The second segment is the transmission rate for each user. Figure 14 displays an example of a chromosome.

The JGGA was compared to a variety of MOEAs (MOGA (Fonseca & Fleming,1998), NPGA2 (Erickson, 2001), NSGA-II (Deb, 2000), and SPEA2 (Zitzler, Laumanns, & Thiele, 2001)). The parameter settings for the MOEAs are shown

Figure 13. Example of the cut-and-paste transposition operator for (a) one parent and (b) two parents (Chan et al., 2005) (©2005, Oxford University Press. Used with permission)

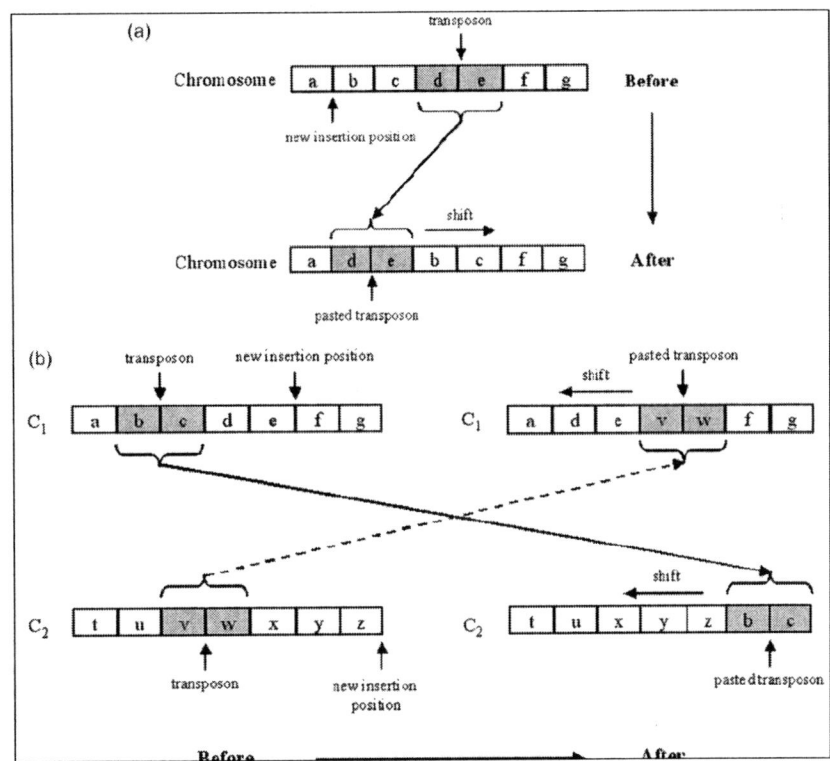

Figure 14. Example of a chromosome encoded for the JGGA (Chan, 2005) (©2005, Oxford University Press. Used with permission)

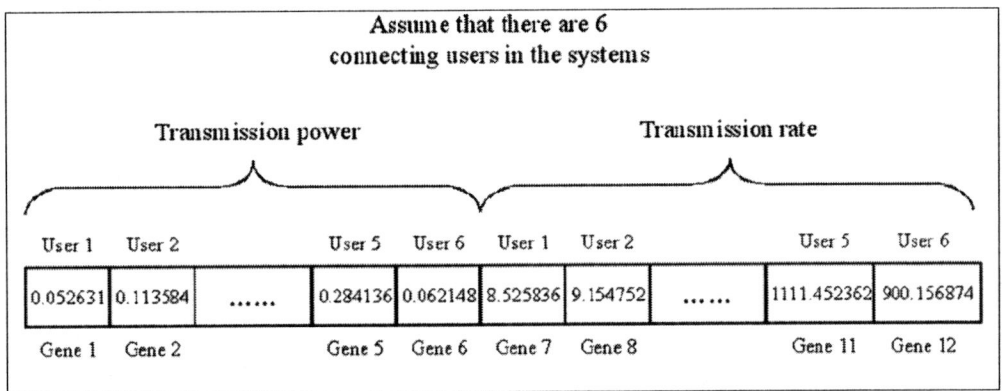

in Table 4. Two metrics were used for comparing the results of the various MOEAs. The first was simply to count the total number of nondominated solutions. Chan calls this the |S| metric (Ishibichi, Yoshida, & Murata, 2003), but it is also known as the overall nondominated vector generation (ONVG) metric (Schott, 1995). While this metric may show that more nondominated points have

Table 4. Parameters of the Compared MOEAs (Cho, 2005) (©2005, Oxford University Press. Used with permission)

Parameter	MOEAs affected	Value / Type
Population Size	All	50
Number of generations	All	100
Crossover type	All	Uniform Crossover
Crossover Probability	All	0.8
Mutation Probability	All	0.02 (25 users) 0.01 (50 users)
Jumping Probability	JGGA	0.02
# of transposons used	JGGA	4
Length of transposon	JGGA	1
Archive size	SPEA2	100

Table 5. Mean and std. dev. for the number of nondominated points found by each MOEA for the 25 user scenario (Chan, 2005) (©2005, Oxford University Press. Used with permission)

Algorithm	MOGA	NPGA2	NSGA2	SPEA2	JGGA
Set 1	8.46 (3.232398)	7.60 (**2.489980**)	8.34 (3.265639)	8.78 (3.074345)	**8.84** (3.780794)
Set 2	7.92 (2.567801)	6.88 (2.895790)	6.40 (**2.505993**)	**8.28** (2.926021)	7.96 (3.117435)
Set 3	7.32 (**2.185772**)	6.70 (2.736786)	7.24 (2.902137)	7.60 (2.814249)	**7.68** (2.679104)
Set 4	9.42 (**3.341197**)	8.24 (3.391519)	9.20 (3.888444)	9.56 (3.661475)	**10.42** (4.190895)
Set 5	7.24 (3.524543)	7.56 (4.123882)	8.02 (4.216586)	8.02 (3.619337)	**8.74** (3.637637)
Set 6	**7.28** (3.340898)	7.04 (3.549422)	6.86 (3.376448)	6.98 (2.817730)	6.26 (**2.762680**)
Set 7	**7.42** (2.341709)	6.68 (2.866636)	6.94 (**2.452835**)	7.12 (2.511095)	7.76 (2.949983)
Set 8	7.00 (2.638181)	6.64 (**2.123770**)	**7.04** (2.449163)	6.58 (2.993927)	7.02 (2.517856)
Set 9	**7.94** (3.437499)	7.34 (2.724775)	6.54 (2.426603)	7.72 (3.137132)	6.98 (**2.353635**)
Set 10	7.20 (**2.244994**)	6.46 (2.316981)	6.68 (2.894408)	8.02 (3.402881)	**8.42** (3.262453)

The value in bracket represents the standard deviation.

been found by one MOEA, it does not measure the quality (convergence) of the points. The second metric, $D1_R$ (Ishibishi et al., 2003), measures the average distance between each solution in a reference set with its nearest solution from the solution set. The reference set is composed of the nondominated solutions derived from all the MOEA runs. The $D1_R$ metric attempts to quantify both the convergence and diversity of the nondominated solutions.

Table 5 lists the results for the MOEAs with to the |S| metric for the 25 user scenario. The JGGA produced the most nondominated points 60% of the time, but the MOGA typically generated the most stable results. The 50 user scenario had similar results. Given the mean and standard deviation, the results in the table appear to be statistically similar.

For the $D1_R$ metric, the JGGA outperformed the other 80 % of the time, with respect to the mean. The NSGA-II and the JGGA both had the best std dev 40% of the time. The 50 user scenario had similar results.

Statistical testing using the binary ε-indicator (Zitzler, Thiele, Laumanns, Fonseca, & Grunert da Fonseca 2003) found the JGGA to score better against the other MOEAs 33 out of 40 (25 users) and 34 out of 40 (50 users) times. There was only one time in each scenario where the JGGA performed worst than another MOEA (both times it was with set 5 and the NPGA2 MOEA). The jumping gene concept provides for effective solutions. Extending this research to use other MOEA operators is suggested.

MANAGEMENT OF MILITARY RESOURCES

Military projects typically have many tradeoff possibilities for development of resources. However, it is usually desirable to find an acceptable approach to ensure the resources last as long as possible. This section presents two efforts that analyze such projects. The first uses an MOEA to increase the lifetime of a military platform as long as possible while keeping the costs down. The second focuses on how to find the best engine maintenance schedule that can get the most engines repaired in the quickest amount of time while ensuring that each engine can stay in service for the longest possible time.

Lifetime Management of Military Platforms

Thie, Chitty, and Reed (2005) compare how well an MOEA and dynamic programming methods resolve obsolete components found throughout a military platform. Obsolete components, such as microelectronics, are often critical components in a military platform. Due to long production cycles for some platforms, some components can even become obsolete before the production process finishes. There are several options that the military has with respect to an obsolete component (such as a last time buy or a redesign of the system containing the obsolete component). There are many factors that the decision maker needs to keep in mind when resolving how to handle an obsolete component. Some factors include acquisition costs, reliability, system availability, and time to implement. These factors need to be analyzed in order to determine the cost-effectiveness of the various options. This leads into the two objectives that are optimized for this problem. The first objective is to maximize the benefits of the chosen option while the second objective is to minimize the costs. Each of these objectives are an aggregation of the multiple costs and benefits associated with the problem. To add to the complexity of this problem, the criteria values are considered uncertain. A Bayesian Belief Network (BBN) is used to model the uncertainty and dependencies associated with the criteria that are used to assess the options for handling obsolete components. In order to fully utilize the information generated by the BBN, measures of effectiveness (MOEs) are used to measure the actual cost compared to the budget, system availability, and implementation time scales. These MOEs operate on the probability density functions generated by the BBN and take into account any dependencies between criteria. MOEs are a measure of how observed values match with the defined user requirements. A user function can vary based on different choices of delta. The slope of the curve determines the rate at which the user's acceptability of the criteria under consideration changes. So a smaller delta equates to a sudden decrease in acceptability whereas a large delta equates to a slower progression from acceptability to rejection.

Initial experiments using an undisclosed EA and dynamic programming are promising. In the initial experiments, information about each component on each circuit board and the number of years they have until becoming obsolete is assumed to be known. Two scenarios were evaluated.

The first scenario is a two-objective problem with each option for resolving an obsolete part having a single cost and benefit. The second scenario has multiple costs and benefits associated with each option. For each of these scenarios, a user function with a medium slope was used. The EA used two populations (one to minimize costs, the other to maximize benefits) with 20 individuals each. The EA was run for 100,000 generations with a random migration of solutions from one population to the other every 10 generations. For the instances run, the dynamic programming method was found to perform slightly better than the EA. But the author states that the problem was relatively simple and larger problems could pose a problem for the dynamic programming method because it is computationally intensive and does not scale well. Future work includes testing the algorithms with real scenarios of large dimension and including constraints.

Military Aircraft Engine Maintenance Scheduling

Many processes in the military can be viewed as a type of scheduling problem. Getting new recruits trained as quickly as possible, setting up effective schedules for aircraft sorties in mission planning, and setting up rendezvous points for multiple military units all require accurate, advanced scheduling. Kleeman et al. (2005; 2006; 2007b) use an MOEA for finding good trade-off options when scheduling aircraft engines for repair. The aircraft engine scheduling problem is an example of a multi-component scheduling problem (Kleeman et al., 2007b). It deals with aircraft engine maintenance at a depot level. The engines are received based on contractual schedules from various organizations. They follow the multi-component scheduling model in that the engines follow a higher level flow-shop through what is called the assembly shops: where the engine is broken down into components for repair and pieced back together and tested. A job-shop model occurs inside the upper-level flow-shop. After the components are broken down, they are repaired in the backshops, where they follow more of a job-shop model, until they are reattached to the engine. For this problem, a list of engines is read in, with each engine listing its arrival time, due time, priority (weight), and mean time before failure (MTBF) for each of its components.

When an engine comes into a logistics workcenter for repair, it is first logged into the system. Aircraft engines are commonly divided into smaller subcomponents which can be worked on individually and then recombined. For this problem, the engine is divided into five logical subcomponents: fan, core, turbine, augmenter, and nozzle. It is assumed that the maintenance shop has one specific work area, or backshop, for each of the components. In reality, an engine component may visit several backshops. For simplicity, it is assumed that they only visit one but varying times for repair are added to take the other backshop visits into account. This is an example of the job-shop problem, but with a twist. After all maintenance is completed on an engine, each engine component's MTBF is compared with other components on the engine. If there is a large disparity among the MTBFs then a component swap may be initiated with another engine in an effort to ensure the MTBFs of the components of a particular engine are similar. This is done so that the engine can have more "time on wing" (TOW) and less time in the shop. Once the swaps are done, the engine is reassembled and tested as a whole to ensure functionality. This represents a flow-shop problem in that each engine has to have maintenance done first, followed by swapping and then testing. So the problem is a representation of the multi-component scheduling problem. Figure 15 shows an example of the flow for two engines. Note how the engines flow from one stage to the next and the subcomponents are repaired in a job-shop paradigm.

This problem has two objectives that need to be optimized. The first objective is to find a schedule that results in repairing the engines in the quickest manner. This is called the makespan. The makespan, which is to be minimized, determines which schedule has a faster process. The second objective is to attempt to keep the MTBF values within a predetermined range for all engines. This may require a number of component swaps from multiple engines. Consequently, these two objectives are conflicting. The first objective attempts to get the engines out as quickly as possible, while the second objective slows down the process by swapping components.

The MOEA used to solve this problem was the General Multi-objective Parallel Evolutionary Algorithm (GENMOP) (Knarr, Goltz, Lamont, & Huang, 2003). GENMOP is an implicit building block MOEA that attempts to find good solutions with a balance of exploration and exploitation. It is a Pareto-based algorithm that utilizes real values for crossover and mutation operators. The MOEA is an extension of the single objective Genetic Algorithm for Numerical Optimization Problems (GENOCOP) (Michaelwicz & Janikow, 1996). Constraint processing is added to enable the software to handle the multi-component scheduling problem. The algorithm was modified to be able to handle permutations, which are common in most scheduling problems. Since chromosomes are generated randomly, a repair mechanism or penalty function must be used in order to elicit a valid permutation. For this implementation, a repair operator was chosen.

The GENMOP algorithm flow is similar to most MOEAs. First, the input is read from a file. Next, the initial population is created and each chromosome is evaluated. The population is then ranked based on the Pareto-ranking of the individuals. Then a mating pool is created and only the most fit individuals are chosen to be in the mating pool. Crossover and mutation are performed on the members of the mating

Figure 15. Example of the maintenance flow for two engines. The first number in each block is the engine number and the second number is the component number (Kleeman, 2007b).

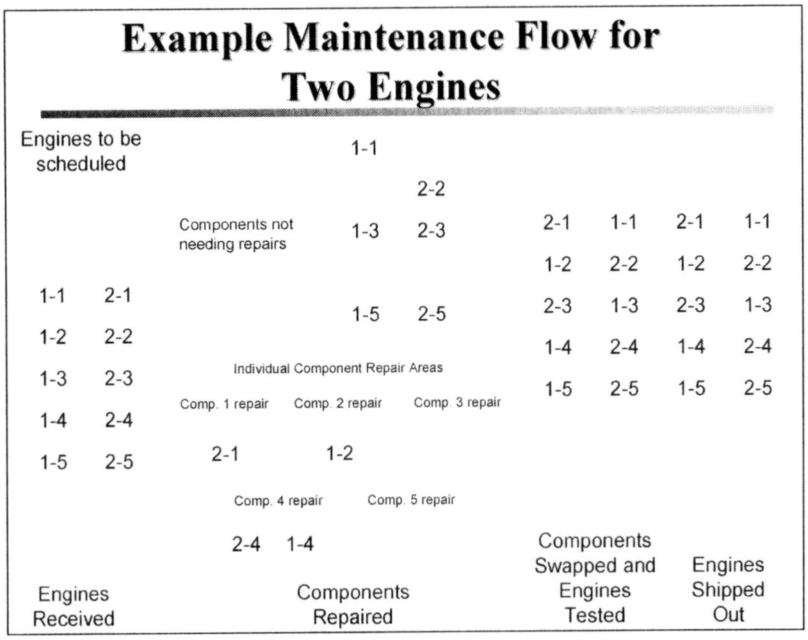

pool. The children created are then evaluated and saved. These children are then combined with the rest of the population. After the children are combined with the parents, the population is then put into Pareto-rank order and the best solutions propagate to the next generation as parents. The program then checks to see if the program has run through its allotted amount of generations. If it has, the program exits. If it has not, the program creates another mating pool and goes through the process again.

The GENMOP MOEA was run using two different approaches. The first approach, or baseline approach, used a fixed chromosome where the permutation of how the engines would be scheduled was at the front of the chromosome and a fixed number of swaps (some of which could be turned off) were listed at the end of the chromosome. The second approach utilized a chromosome with a variable length. If more swaps were needed, the chromosome length was expanded. These two approaches were compared with problem sizes of 5 and 10 engines and with multiple population sizes and numbers of generations. With respect to aggregate swap count and makespan, Table 6 shows the results for 10 engines. Each instance was run 30 times and the mean and standard deviation were compared. This shows that the variable chromosome produces better results for the makespan in every instance and mixed results for the swap count.

This MOEA scheduling effort provides insight to better engine maintenance procedures. The use of a variable length chromosome provided efficiency and utility for this particular problem. A probabilistic combination of GENMOP crossover (Whole arithmetic crossover, simple crossover, heuristic crossover, and pool crossover) and mutation operators (uniform mutation, boundary mutation, and non-uniform mutation) were effective in finding quality solutions. Continuing work should focus on the reality of including "back-room" job-shop (tool and die shop) scheduling of low-level engine elements based in part on probabilities.

Also, the development of a graphical user interface for tool would be of interest.

MISSION PLANNING

Mission planning is another problem that is of high importance to the military. Creating good mission plans are essential in meeting objectives, but also limiting loss of equipment and life (risk). This section lists several efforts where MOEAs have been applied to mission planning.

Planning

Regarding the execution of a given operational military mission, the required process includes mission tasking description, feasibility assessment, target intelligence, mission action plan of execution, scheduled path execution, and other documentation as required or desired. With that said the optimization of military mission action planning and path planning is addressed here using multi-objective evolutionary algorithms (MOEAs). In particular, contemporary aspects of two military missions are presented. A high level course of action (COA) optimization is considered along with path planning development for a terrain following UAV swarm.

Mission planning is a complex and very high dimensional effort; it requires consideration of environmental information, predictions, start and end points, targets and resource constraints. In general, such problems can be modeled as a multi-objective resource-constrained project/task scheduling (RCPS) problem. In general, these types of problems are defined as multi-objective optimization problems (MOPs). As indicated, two detailed MOP models are examples of generic military missions and solved using MOEAs. Table 7 presents an overview of these and some other associated mission tasking discussions. Of course, a variety of other references could be included with focus on MOEAs applied to generic vehicle

Table 6. Testing results for 10 engines (Kleeman et al., 2007b)

Number of engines	Generation size	Population Size	Avg/Std Dev of Component Swaps		Avg/Std Dev of Agg. Swap Count		Avg/Std Dev Makespan	
			Baseline Results	Variable Chromosome	Baseline Results	Variable Chromosome	Baseline Results	Variable Chromosome
10	10	10	3.51 / 2.57	11.6 / 2.01	27.5 / 2.17	28.9 / 2.71	2165.5 / 83.1	2086.4 / 82.8
10	10	100	5.6 / 2.72	9.42 / 4.42	27.0 / 2.40	29.7 / 5.05	2148.1 / 50.2	2023.4 / 136.3
10	10	1000	7.32 / 1.74	12.3 / 1.53	25.6 / 1.29	28.3 / 3.79	2144.9 / 56.4	1979.7 / 85.9
10	25	25	3.55 / 2.00	11.0 / 1.73	26.4 / 1.57	28.8 / 3.42	2142.2 / 43.5	1937.6 / 79.2
10	100	10	3.72 / 1.79	11.4 / 2.19	25.7 / 1.23	24.3 / 2.69	2139.0 / 29.1	1832.4 / 50.5
10	100	100	4.01 / 1.97	13.9 / 0.49	26.5 / 1.63	23.1 / 0.67	2119.1 / 32.7	1893.4 / 0.67
10	100	500	4.03 / 2.30	9.49 / 2.89	25.4 / 1.16	23.8 / 0.87	2128.8 / 36.0	1925.9 / 222.4
10	100	1000	4.45 / 1.98	13.5 / 1.12	24.7 / 0.91	24.8 / 0.43	2133.8 / 53.5	1678.3 / 106.3
10	1000	1000	4.16 / 2.08	13.9 / 0.65	24.8 / 0.64	23.7 / 0.55	2105.5 / 4.53	1638.5 / 54.3

navigation and routing including robots. Future efforts include more real-world constraints, other MOEA structures, and an appropriate spectrum of MOEA metrics, and statistical comparisons.

Courses of Action Planning

During mission planning, the assigned and implied tasks are identified to perform the mission with tasks decomposed into subtasks. Tasks and subtasks can be represented by means of a hierarchical divide and conquer tree structure. Leafs of this hierarchical structure are called elementary tasks. A synchronization analysis requires the identification of temporal and spatial relationships between these elementary tasks. Elementary tasks include starting and ending temporal and spatial activities and task interaction. Available resources and capabilities are assigned to the tasks (a generic assignment problem). Thus, synchronizing a course of action (COA) requires scheduling starting and ending times of all tasks according to resource availability, deployment constraints and task relationships. Any resource or capability has temporal and spatial availability, costing, required preparations, etc. The challenge is to generate complex, spatially and temporally interdependent activities with constrained precedence relationships, subject to resource constraints, and satisfy multiple incommensurable and often conflicting objectives; a NP-complete problem.

A vector of fitness evaluations is proposed to control the proportion of infeasible solutions. Crossover and mutation operators are designed to diversify the search space (exploration) and improve solutions (exploitation) on all objectives from one generation to another. In the generational replacement strategy, a selection procedure, based on the dominance concept and a multi-criteria filtering method, is used. Such a strategy is applied when the population reaches a critical size. Different MOEA schemes are compared and their strengths and weaknesses discussed. The multi-criteria filtering procedure used in the replacement strategy proved very efficient in the diversification of the Pareto front.

The *Multi-objective COA formal model* is explicitly defined by a set of tasks, a set of resources, precedence relationships, resources availability constraints and global performance functions (criteria). Constraints ensure that each task is processed once in its time interval and a precedence condition are fulfilled (feasible tasks) and reflects the availability of resources. Constraints are considered as functions to be optimized as well. Boolean penalty coefficients are used for each resource constraint regarding task execution. The *chromosome structure*, representing a COA network, is represented in the following form: x_i = $[(t_1, R_1, 1), (t_2, R_2, 4)..., (t_n, R_n, 1)]$, for $i=1,...$popsize, where popsize is the population size. t_j is the jth task to be scheduled and R_j, k= $R_k(t_j)$ is one of the sets of resources available to accomplish this task. The objectives considered are quantitative such as cost, reliability, make-span, or qualitative such as the impact of a COA.

The *MOEA operators* consist of crossover and mutation. Selection of two parents for crossover is done using the roulette wheel selection. Two *crossover procedures* are considered, to be used alternatively, in order to explore a greater number of search spaces. The first one is the uniform crossover operator (Syswerda, 1989) which has been shown to be superior to traditional crossover strategies for combinatorial problems. When two chromosomes are selected for crossover, a random mask is generated and their genes are exchanged according to the mask. This mask is simply a binary string with the same length as a COA vector. The parity of each bit determines which genes are exchanged. The second operator is the partial mapped crossover (PMX) proposed by (Goldberg & Lingle, 1985) and is an extension of two-point crossover to permutation representation. A crossover repairing procedure is used, in both operators, to resolve illegitimacy (feasibility) of the offspring if some activities are missing or duplicated by simply transferring these activities from one child to the other one.

The *mutation procedure* is applied randomly on the population and the probability of mutation is inversely proportional to the population size as recommended by De Jong (1975). The two operators used for the mutation consist of: (1) Exchanging, with a probability AND a randomly selected combination of resources between two COA individuals. The offspring, which received the combination with the best criterion, is retained. (2) Switching the quantity of two resources in a combination of resources associated to a randomly selected task.

The *generational replacement strategy* relates to when the population size attains or exceeds a critical value. Individuals are selected, based on their fitness vector, among the parents and the offspring using a replacement procedure. Otherwise, new offspring are generated. Three strategies are tested for the replacement: (1) The

Table 7. MOEA mission planning and routing applications

Specific Application	Problem and Solution Structures
Course of Action (Belfares & Guitouni, 2003)	COA task-scheduling planning MOPS with resource constraints. Their MOEA employs two crossover operators (masked, PMX) and mutation (exchanging resources and tasks) and a repair operator for resulting infeasible individuals. Three selection strategies (a filtering procedure, nondominated sorting, and combined) are compared. Large population sizes and the combined selection approach generated better results for various resource-constrained tasks.
3D UAV Route Planning (Slear, 2006)(Slear, 2006a)(Lamont, Slear, & Melendez, 2007)	Mission path planning design and implementation of a comprehensive system for swarms of autonomous aerial vehicles (UAVs). The objectives are time and fuel consumption and risk. Along with approximated vehicle dynamic constraints, terrain following is required for each mission. Original MOEA mutation and crossover operators are integrated in a parallel computation with excellent results.
COA Planning (Guitouni, Bélanger, & Berger, 2000)	Modeled COA planning as multiple mode resource-constraint project scheduling; COA modeled as a time-space graph (TSG)
Plans of Action (Urli, Lo, & Guitouni, 2003)	Using the TSG model employed a heuristic technique with a CPlex for large dimensional problems.
UAV Path Planning (Don, 2004)	Development of a parallel evolutionary algorithm for unmanned aerial vehicles using multiple objectives (fuel consumption, risk of loss, and reward for success) subject to the UAV physical constraints (speed, acceleration, turn radius), state and end points. A weighted aggregated fitness model is used. Visual and performance metrics indicate acceptable performance

multicriteria filtering procedure (MFP) (Guitouni, 2001) returns (a user defined) nondominated diversified individuals. MFP is based on multi-criteria dynamic conjunctive and disjunctive procedures. The retained solutions are characterized by at least one best-scored objective or by all objectives achieving minimal threshold values, (2) the nondominated sorting approach (NDS) (Srinivas & Deb, 1995), (3) the combined approach: NDS+MFP procedure.

The efficiency of each method is investigated using the example of courses of action with four objectives: the cost and the make-span to be minimized, the resource reliability and the impact on the enemy, to be maximized. The impact is measured on a qualitative scale.

Resource availability and tasks precedence constraints are considered. Three examples are studied to examine the effect of the problem size. The performance indicators of an algorithm are compiled from 5 to 10 runs of each test application. Since the objectives are the cost, the make-span, the reliability, and the impact, the diversity coverage of the approximated Pareto set is defined as COV = (covcost, covreliabilty, covimpact, covmakespan).

Comparison between the three methods is presented in Table 8 using the mean values of the metrics for a six task problem. The replacement strategy (MFP+NDS) clearly outperforms the MFP and the NDS procedures regarding the number of nondominated solutions Ns as well as the extent of coverage COV. The multicriteria-filtering procedure does not generate all nondominated solutions because some of these solutions are eliminated by the conjunctive procedure. More performance metrics need to be evaluated as well as inclusion of additional selection operators.

Mission Planning and Routing

The purpose of this mission path planning research is to design and implement a comprehensive system for swarms of autonomous aerial vehicles (Lamont, 2007). The system consists of a parallel, multi-objective evolutionary algorithm-based path planner and a genetic algorithm-based vehicle router with terrain following. *Path planning* is the process of designing a sequence of states which an object must assume in order to travel from an initial state to a goal state. Path planning optimization is a process that proscribes a particular plan for reaching a goal (end) state from an initial (start) state at a minimal cost. A foundation of this problem description is the vehicle routing problem (VRP), a NP-Complete problem. It is defined as the task of assigning a set of vehicles, each with a limited range and capacity, to a set of locations or targets that must be visited.

A path-planning algorithm is a sequence of steps taken to calculate a path plan given knowledge of the path environment and a set of conditions or constraints. Many successful path-planning algorithms have been developed over the years. These algorithms vary in their effectiveness and efficiency based primarily on the specific formulation of the path planning problem and the number of variables and constraints required to solve the problem.

Representing cost as a fixed objective is adequate for routing problems in which distances between targets are large enough to ignore the added path lengths resulting from having to make series of turns in order to change heading from one location to another. However, when the target layout is such that the distances between the targets are a near as several turn radii of an aircraft apart, then the cost of traveling between any two targets must consider the heading at which the aircraft arrived at the initial location and the heading the aircraft must assume to vector itself towards the next target. Taking this into account, algorithms that solve the VRP would have to calculate the cost of every assignment from scratch in order to accurately represent the cost associated with that assignment. In this research, *a path planning algorithm is developed that calculates the optimal route from a start node to an end node, through a mid point.* This path through a triplet of locations can then be concatenated with other triplets to quickly and accurately calculate the actual cost of a vehicle assignment. This information can be tabularized and fed in as inputs to programs such as the Genetic Vehicle Router where "good" assignments can be made but this time; the costs associated with these assignments are more representative. The goal is not merely to calculate the true cost of a particular assignment made by the router but to influence the router to make better assignments using the more complete cost information.

Terrain Following (TF) is a mode of flight in which an aircraft maintains a fixed altitude above ground level and flies low (on the order of a few hundred feet) through an area of interest. Naturally, this type of flying involves a great deal of climbing and descending, a costly operation.

The first design goal concerns the development of a robust path-planning algorithm for terrain following missions. Since all routes have both *a cost and a risk* associated with them, path planning can naturally be expressed as a multi-objective minimization problem. Most often, decreasing the cost of the path, i.e. the path length and the amount of climbing required to navigate the terrain, results in increasing the risk associated with enemy air defenses. Likewise, a path generated to avoid intersection with all enemy air defense radar systems results in increased path cost.

Because of the common disadvantage of aggregated approaches, a multi-objective objective approach is selected because it provides a choice of routes with cost proportional to their level of risk. Due to the intractability of the path-planning problem, an evolutionary approach is developed to produce low cost routes in a reasonable amount of time. Validation of the path-planning component is accomplished through a set of experiments aimed at testing the planner's ability to produce feasible routes, to avoid terrain and minimize exposure. Analysis of this data accompanies visualizations of solutions to various problem instances.

A *Genetic Vehicle Representation* (GVR) is used for UAV routing. GVR consists of a novel data representation, and original *mutation* and *crossover* operators. The key element of the encoding is that solutions explicitly provide the number of routes and their locations without significant decoding. For *crossover*, two individuals $C1$ and $C2$ are chosen for selection. A sub route r from $C1$ is inserted into a copy of $C2$. The position of the insertion is such that the distance between the insertion location and the first location r is minimized. There are a total of four *mutation* operators used. In the first, *swap mutation*, two locations within a solution are exchanged. The second mutation operator is *inversion*. The third mutation operator is *displacement*. Similar to crossover, a sub route is removed from a solution and moved to a new location. Unlike the crossover operator, however, no effort is made to place the sub route in an insertion point that minimizes distance. The final mutation operator is *insertion*.

Restructuring the path planning problem.

Table 8. mGA performance using the three replacement strategies in the 6t-problem (Belfares, 2003) (© 2003, IEEE, Used with permission)

Method	Ns	Ds	COV
mGA- MFP	3.6	0.33	(18.7; 18.4; 0; 19)
mGA- NDS	4.7	0.70	(20; 10.5; 7; 21.7)
mGA- MFP+NDS	6.8	0.79	(26.3; 30; 25; 39)

Despite the many definitions of the path-planning problem in the literature, nearly all of them structure the problem as the minimization of cost in traveling between a start and goal node. As a result, the output from any good path-planning algorithm can provide the set of link weights for any algorithm that solves the routing problem. however, the locations or targets in a UAV routing problem are confined to a single city; the distances between the targets may be as close as a few aircraft turn radii. In this case, turns which can be made abruptly in a large-scale problem now become factors in the minimization of costs for a tour. A point-to-point link cost is no longer sufficient to represent the true cost of the link. In order to account for the cost associated with turning, the cost of a link must consider the heading of the aircraft when approaching the first node and the destination heading when leaving the target node. By reformulating the path planning problem with the goal of minimizing the cost of traveling from a starting point to a destination point through an intermediate point, a full account of the added distance incurred by making feasible turns can be made. A path planner with this capability would then take as its input three points representing targets, terrain and threat data corresponding to the planning area and return a path containing a complete set of points representing a path that travels through the three points while negotiating threats and minimizing cost.

The general *Multi-objective Problem Formulation* has five objectives which are measures of merit that can be grouped logically into two categories: those that describe the cost of the path in terms of time and fuel consumption, (*path* and *climb*), and those that measure the risk of a given path (*terrain*, *detect*, and *kill*).

When an insertion, deletion or alteration operation is done on the path, the feasibility constraint is often violated. If there is sufficient space between the points of the invalid segment, then a *repair function* adds additional intermediate points to smooth the turns. The repair operator returns a value of *true* if the repair is successful. When *false* is returned, the calling module cancels the operation and returns the path to its previous state. Since the repair function is called only after the location of the point in question is known, no searching is required by this method. The number of operations needed to validate the heading changes between the points is constant.

The intersection between the path and both threat and kill rings are determined exactly the same way as the climbing function. The costs of crossing through a single grid space in either a threat detection or kill zone is a parameter that is passed to the path planner at runtime. A hideability score (risk function) is calculated by summing the number of visible points associated with each grid space the path intersects. The relative weight of hideability versus detection is also parameterized.

The MOEA design includes the design of specific methods and data structures.

The path planner consists of a domain-specific genetic algorithm and a low-overhead parallel architecture that allows for moderate scalability in the size of the routing problem. The specific methods and data structures used in the planner are defined. The data structures of the path planner are contained in a hierarchy. The main program has a population object, which consists of a number of path objects, which consist of a number of point objects. A single terrain object is created in the main program. The terrain object stores the DTED data and threat location and range information. Pointers to the terrain object are passed to population and to the individual routes.

In the path planner, a population consists of an array of 50 path objects. The array data structure facilitates access to individual members of the population. Many of the evolutionary operators used in the algorithm iterate through the population so an array was a logical choice. In addition to the current population, a similar array structure is used to store the Pareto front archive. Once the population is initialized, all nondominated members are copied and stored in the archive. With each evolutionary cycle, the current population is compared to the archive and dominated members are removed from the archive while new nondominated solutions are added. MOEA methods on the population include *Init* (), *Evaluate* (), *Evolve* () *Sort* (), *and Determine Dominance* ().

The path object is the chromosomal unit representing complete, individual solutions to the path planning problem. The path ADT consists of a linked list of point objects representing the flight plan, a set of statistical data including number of points and evaluation function scores, and a set of fixed data which includes the start, middle, and end points and a pointer to the terrain object. Methods of the Path ADT include a constructor, copy constructor, add and delete point operations, point retrieval operators, repair operator, and a set of evaluation functions.

In computational testing, analysis of tradeoffs between cost and risk is required. In this experiment, a real-world route is planned over Nevada in the vicinity of Nellis Air Force Base. The path planner is run first to minimize the cost of the route by minimizing distance and the amount of climbing associated with navigating the route. Then, the route is optimized to reduce risk. Hideability, the degree to which vehicles remain out of site of potential unknown threats is used as the optimization criterion. For completeness, the Pareto front (cost vs. risk) for this problem is shown in Figure 16.

The path planner results were integrated into a parallel swarm simulation with 3D visualization that provide considerable insight into the swarm routing process (Slear, 2006a).

Future improvements to the path planner are needed regarding its ability to explore larger-sized areas for terrain and threat avoidance. Consider more exploratory crossover and mutation operators. Possibly increase the search space through the use of "migrant" population members. Develop a three multi-objective model along with a more realistic vehicle model and timing constraints.

PERSONNEL ASSIGNMENT

In order to function effectively, the military requires considerable personnel. There are many jobs in the military and in order to keep a diverse force, where different individuals can step into another person's job, reassigning people to different jobs is important. But the reassignment process can be quite burdensome. In order to help streamline the process, several researchers have applied evolutionary concepts to the problem. In this section, two assignment efforts are dis-

Figure 16. Pareto front trade-offs for Nellis AFB (Slear, 2006)

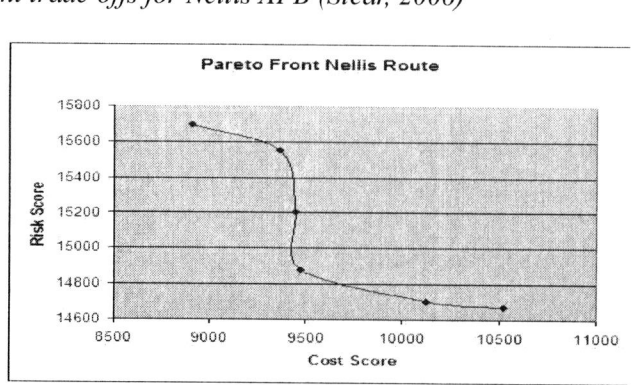

cussed. The first discusses the sailor assignment problem and solves it in a single-objective manner, but points to using an MOEA in the future. The second effort addresses the related airman assignment problem. This problem was designed with multiple objectives in mind. The goal is to find airmen who best fit the job while limiting the costs of sending them to a particular job.

Sailor Assignment Problem

The sailor assignment problem (SAP) deals with the problem that the United States Navy has with assigning new jobs to their sailors. Sailors move around about every two years. As such, it can be time consuming trying to match sailors with jobs that are available. The goal of the problem is to and qualified people for the necessary jobs, while at the same time, trying to keep the sailors happy with their assignment. Several researchers have attacked this problem over the last few years (Garrett, Vannucci, Silva, Dasgupta, & Simien, 2005; Holder, 2005; Kelemen, Kozma, & Liang, 2002; Lewis, Lewis, & White, 2004;Liang, Lin, & Kelemen, 2002; McCauley & Franklin, 2002).

There is also the multi-objective sailor assignment problem (mSAP) which adds another objective into the mix. The first objective is to minimize the discontent that the sailors may have with their respective assignments. The second objective is to minimize the costs associated with moving the sailors to their next job. This problem was mentioned briefly in (Garrett et al., 2005) and more closely matches the real-world problem since it takes costs into account as well. This section focuses on that problem, the next section presents a similar assignment problem that was designed as a MOP and uses an MOEA for solving the problem.

In Garrett's et al. (2005) research, he equally weights the two objectives (fitness and PCS cost) in order to derive a single optimal point. This solution would be only one of the many trade off solutions typically found using an MOEA that employs a Pareto front. And since each objective is equally weighted, the point would be found in the middle of the Pareto front. Four different algorithms are compared: the CHC adaptive search algorithm (Eshelman, 1991), a steady-state GA, a generational GA, and the Gale-Shapley stable marriage algorithm (Gale, 1962). The problem formulation is very similar to the stable marriage formulation, in which the goal is to produce the best cumulative matches among a set of men and women. As such, the Gale-Shapley algorithm is compared with the other algorithms. The problem was set-up in such a way that preprocessing is required. First, every sailor is assigned a set of jobs that he is qualified to fill. A repair operator is also required in order to fix any problems where one job was assigned to multiple sailors. The GAs used in the experiment use stochastic universal sampling for the selection operator and uniform crossover for the recombination operator. Additionally, tournament selection and one and two-point crossover were also tried, but uniform crossover was found to work best in most instances. CHC is another type of GA that attempts to avoid premature convergence by performing cataclysmic mutation when convergence has slowed beyond a specified rate. CHC also employs a crossover operator called HUX, which attempts to ensure that children are not too similar to the parents that produced them. Each of the algorithms were run on nine problem instances—five using real world data and four generated by a random problem generator. The real world data does not include moving costs, only the cumulative fitness of the sailor job matches, whereas the generated data includes those costs.

The results of the real data with only one objective show that the deterministic Gale-Shapley algorithm outperforms the GAs. The results of the algorithms when applied to the randomly generated data, which includes a second objective function, the Gale-Shapely only optimizes on the fitness so it does well with that objective but poorly with minimizing the PCS costs. It would be interesting to see how well the algorithm would have done if it were modified to handle both objectives. The CHC GA is able to find solutions that dominate the other two GAs with respect to both objectives. For future work, the goal is to find a way to maintain multiple different solutions. This can obviously be done with an MOEA that utilizes a Pareto front and ranking in order to find multiple trade-off solutions.

Airman Assignment Problem

Similar to the sailor assignment problem is the Air Force version called the Airman Assignment problem (AAP). The AAP is a multi-objective constrained assignment problem that attempts to match Air Force personnel with open jobs. Unlike the SAP, this problem was initially designed as a MOP. Kleeman et al (2006; 2007c) use an MOEA to solve this problem.

In the Air Force, personnel moves are common; typically an airman is moved every three years. The moves are highly choreographed, where an airman's previous assignments and jobs can play a role in what job is assigned. The goal of the Air Force assignment system is to first meet the needs of the Air Force by filling all the necessary jobs with qualified individuals. The secondary goal is to try to put people into jobs that they want. The problem has two objectives. The first objective is a measurement of how well each assignment meets the needs of the Air Force and at the same time satisfies the desires of the individual. This objective is met through the use of hard constraints and soft constraints. The hard constraints are the ones that must be satisfied for an assignment to be valid. For this problem, an example of a hard constraint is the security clearance that is required for a job. The soft constraints are basically penalty functions. These penalties are applied when an assignment deviates from the ideal candidate or if the person is not given their ideal assignment. These penalties are weighted differently depending on their importance in the eyes of the decision maker. For example, if a person is married to another military member, the air force has a program that attempts to assign both members to the same location. Assigning a husband and wife to two different bases would be extremely detrimental to their morale and could possibly affect their work. As such, if a husband and wife are not assigned together at the same base, this receives a larger penalty than most other penalties. For this problem, there are 3 hard constraints (proper job training, rank, and security clearance) and 11 soft constraints, each with a user defined penalty function. The second objective function is the cost it takes to move each person from one duty location to another. Obviously, the goal is to keep spending down, but as with many multi-objective problems, this objective can run counter to the other objective being optimized.

The goal is to minimize both objectives. For the initial runs of this problem, realistic data was generated that was deemed to best fit the distribution for a typical assignment process in the Air Force. Air force assignments are decomposed into groups and then into subgroups. Typically, the assignment teams have more jobs than individuals. For this problem, problem instances with 20 individuals requiring assignment and 30 jobs available to be filled, and one with 30 individuals and 50 jobs were used. Some of the individuals may not get an assignment, because their constraints prohibit it. In these cases, an assignment is withheld and it would be up to the assignment team to decide the best assignment for that individual. These two instances were chosen because they represent the average problem. Given that the problem is NP-complete, and the landscape is rugged, a MOEA, the NSGA-II, was chosen to solve this problem. The NSGA-II is run with a standard "out of the box" configuration with a crossover probability of 0.9 and a mutation probability of 0.033. A spacing algorithm and the two-set coverage metric were used to determine the algorithm diversity and progression.

The spacing metric was chosen because it was easy to implement and provided a good measurement of the spacing of the points. A value of zero indicates that all members of the known Pareto front are equidistantly spaced. A zero may not be achievable if the vectors in the true Pareto front are not equidistant. The two-set coverage metric compares the nondominated points generated for multiple known Pareto fronts. If one set of solutions dominate the other sets the metric would score a maximum value of one. But if a set of solutions were all dominated, it would get the lowest score of zero. The metric is essentially a ratio of all nondominated points of one algorithm with respect to the other. This metric is used to see how fast the algorithm took to converge toward our final known Pareto front. Experiments were done with population sizes of 200 and 400. Table 9 shows the results of experiments with a population size of 400. Little change occurs after generation 700 because the algorithm has converged. The spacing remained fairly constant for each generation.

The results were also compared graphically. The known Pareto front from generation 100 and generation 1000 were plotted on the same graph and compared with each other. Figure 17 shows the results of the comparison for a population size of 200. The plot shows how the MOEA continued to converge toward the true Pareto front and it also showed how the algorithm first found the points along the interior of the Pareto front and then found the exterior points in the later generations.

As this research indicates, MOEAs can be employed to improve the decision making process for military personnel assignment. Continuing research would emphasize the real-world use of an improved multi-objective assignment system with embedded realistic constraints.

MOEA INTEGRATED MILITARY SIMULATION

Bingül et al. (2000a; 2000b) have done research on integrating an MOEA with a military simulation package called THUNDER. THUNDER is a large campaign simulation model, based on Monte-Carlo simulation. The software was designed in an effort to examine the issues, utility, and effectiveness associated with air and ground forces in a theater-level joint warfare scenario. It judges the outcomes of military actions, incorporates the results, and then uses this infor-

Table 9. Results for population size 400 (Kleeman, 2007c)

Num gens	Avg PF pts	Two Set Coverage		Spacing	
		Mean	Std. Dev.	Mean	Std. Dev.
100	16.900	0.2480	0.1523	4.2628	1.7973
200	19.067	0.3847	0.1729	3.9340	1.8225
300	20.133	0.4955	0.1601	3.6073	1.5946
400	22.167	0.5527	0.1623	3.8493	1.9997
500	23.433	0.6187	0.1703	3.8051	1.8324
600	23.767	0.6622	0.1949	4.1348	2.0679
700	24.200	0.7264	0.1814	4.5595	2.2423
800	23.467	0.8163	0.1597	4.4843	2.6253
900	23.767	0.8932	0.1031	4.5889	2.7065
1000	23.567	1.0000	0.0000	4.5595	2.7029

Figure 17. Comparison of PF known generated with a population size of 200 at 100 and 1000 generations (Kleeman, 2007c)

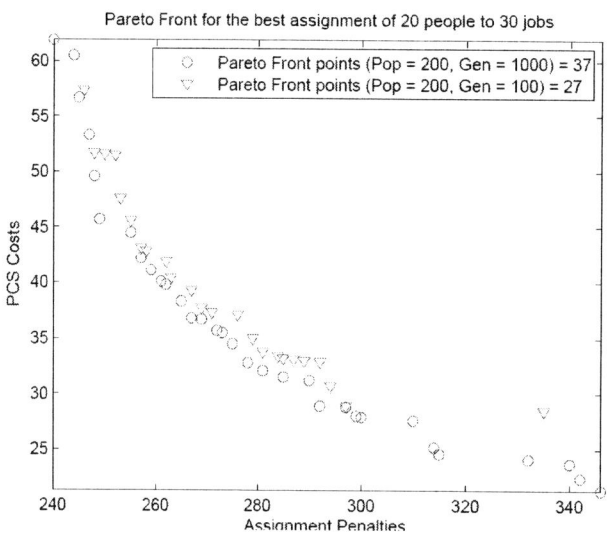

mation to further plan and execute the ongoing operations. It is a two-player simulation with a red team and a blue team. Each team can deploy a variety of air missions to attack various enemy assets or to protect their own assets. After each turn (each turn represents one day) of the mission the software outputs territory lost, aircraft lost, number of strategic targets destroyed, and the number of enemy armor destroyed. From these outputs, the GA was given four objectives: (1) Minimize the amount of territory lost to the enemy, (2) Minimize the number of aircraft lost, (3) Maximize the number of enemy strategic targets destroyed, and (4) Maximize the number of enemy armor destroyed. The objectives are weighted in a variety of manners in order to get a single fitness value.

The GA used in this research uses crossover and mutation, but the specific operator types are never discussed. Some general examples in the papers suggest that 1-point crossover and bit-flip mutation is used, but the paper never explicit states that these are the types of operators he used. The mutation and crossover rates were handled two different ways. In (Bingül, 2000a) the mutation rate was varied between the values of 0.001 and 0.1 while the crossover rate was held steady at 0.7. From these experiments, the researchers determined that for this problem a mutation rate of 0.02 produced the best results. Then, the crossover rate was varied between the values of 0.1 and 0.9 while the mutation rate was held to 0.02. The researchers determined crossover rates of 0.6 and 0.7 seemed to work best for this problem. In (Bingül, 2000b) the authors implemented a fuzzy logic system that adapted the crossover and mutation rates based on the best fitness value and the mean and variance of all the individuals in the population. This adaptive GA was compared to a GA with a fixed mutation rate (while not stated in the paper, the rates are believed to be 0.02 and 0.7 for mutation and crossover, respectively). Figure 18 shows how the rates varied as the GA progressed. The results indicated that after 50 generations (population size not given), the adaptive GA was able to achieve a higher weighted fitness value with a faster rate of convergence.

Since the researchers chose to weight the objectives in order to come to a single solution (instead of using a Pareto-based MOEA), three different weighting methods were developed. The first method, F_1, weights the objectives so that the worst score gets the highest weighting and the best score gets the lowest weighting. The second method, F_2, simply squares each objective value and sums the results. The third method, F_3, uses a squared-error based fitness assignment. Table 10 shows both the best fitness value for each weighting method and the corresponding inputs that the results recommend for the simulation. Note that the abbreviations OCA (offensive counter air), INT (long range air interdiction), DSEAD (lethal direct air defense suppression), and STI (strategic target interdiction) are all percentages on how resources should be applied to each mission type.

The results of each allocation method are shown in Table 11. It shows that while the first method is able to best limit the territory lost, it does the worst in the three other objectives. The last two methods appear to perform in about the same manner, with the second method providing slightly better results in three of the four categories. Note that the last two methods are similar to each other; while the first method is worst than the other two. Crossover and mutation variations are suggested for finding improved results.

DESIGN OF INNOVATIVE EQUIPMENT WITH MOEAS

The military is always involved in the development of innovative weapons and equipment. This section presents two instances where MOEAs are being used to design military equipment. The first effort uses an MOEA to find good designs for a low-power laser using laser physics models. The second uses an MOEA to design an autopilot controller.

Figure 18. Variations of the mutation and crossover rates over 50 generations using the fuzzy logic system (Bingül, 2000b) (© 2000, IEEE, Used with permission)

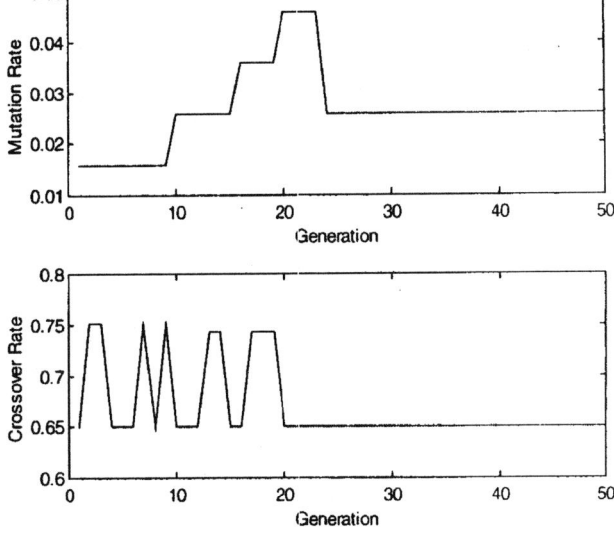

Table 10. Maximum fitness values found using the three weighted fitness functions and their corresponding input allocations for the simulation (Bingül, 2000a) (© 2000, IEEE, Used with permission)

Method	Max fitness	OCA	INT	DSEAD	STI
F_1	14.033	20	27	53	0
F_2	11.893	0	20	40	40
F_3	15.502	14	0	80	6

Table 11. Simulation results based on the best allocation for each weighted fitness function (Bingül, 2000a)

Method	Territory Lost	Enemy Strat Targets Destroyed	Enemy Armor Destroyed	Aircraft Lost
F_1	87.1	482	1796	144
F_2	96.3	500	2061	136
F_3	108.9	491	2060	135

Low-Power Laser Design

The military is involved in many high-tech applications. Advanced laser designs are an example of this type of application. Several people from the Air Force Institute of Technology have been using MOEAs to find designs for a quantum cascade laser (QCL) (Kelemen, 2004; 2007d; Rodriguez, Keller, Lamont, & Nelson, 2005). This section focuses only on the latest work done on this problem.

QCLs are semiconductor lasers that are not based on the heterostructure design, but on quantum mechanics. The QCL does not have the same limitations of the double heterostructure design. As such, QCLs are used in applications where the standard double heterostructure cannot be utilized. Since QCLs operate at room temperature (and in the mid-infrared spectrum) they are ideal candidates to be used as sensors. Many pollutants, explosives, industrial chemicals, and medical substances can only be detected with high accuracy with mid-infrared lasers. Given the wide range of capabilities listed, QCLs can be applied in the environmental, military, security, and medical fields. This research focuses on developing good QCL designs in the terahertz frequency range. As alluded to earlier, a terahertz QCL can have potential applications in spectroscopy, astronomy, medicine, free-space communication, near-space radar, and possibly chemical/biological detection. Of particular interest is its potential use as a sensor for security purposes, particularly in the realm of homeland security.

The QCL problem utilizes two fitness functions that attempt to model two of the most important properties of a QCL. The first fitness function determines how well the energy levels are lining up. The goal is to have good injection of electrons at the top of each quantum well, but at the same time, have good drainage at the bottom of the well. If a laser has good injection, but poor drainage, then the electrons at the top of the well will not be able to jump to the next energy state since it drains slower than the injection process.

The second fitness function determines the overlap ratios. This describes how electrons jump from one state to another. In essence, the fitness function is a measure of how close states are and the ability of the electron to transfer between the two states.

For the QCL problem, the general multi-objective parallel (GENMOP) algorithm was selected. For comparison purposes, the algorithm is extended to include two local search procedures - a simple neighborhood search and a new multitiered neighborhood search.

GENMOP has been applied successfully to a broad range of problems ranging from in-situ bioremediation of contaminated groundwater (Knarr, 2003) to solving the aircraft engine maintenance scheduling problem (Kleeman, 2005; 2007b). The GENMOP MOEA was applied to the QCL problem twice before (Keller & Lamont, 2004; Rodriguez, 2005), but with mixed results. The solutions received in the earlier research obtained good solutions, but they required tedious tweaking in order to find better, more stable solutions. This was due to the algorithm providing a good global search, but inadequate local search. To alleviate this problem, a local search technique was added to the algorithm as indicated.

The multi-tiered local search addition to GENMOP, nicknamed GENMOP-MLTS, focuses the first search on the electrical field. The neighborhood search in this tier uses a neighborhood size that is 4% the size of the actual electrical field search space. This neighborhood size was chosen because it balances efficiency (limit the number of fitness evaluations) with effectiveness. This first tier of local search is run after generations 50 and 100. The local search was chosen to run at these intervals because it provided the algorithm with a good balance of local search and global search. The goal in this first tier of local search is to focus the attention, and fitness evaluations, on the search region that has the most influence on creating good solutions. Through previous experimentation and problem domain knowledge, we determined that the electrical field had the biggest impact on creating good solutions. The second tier of GENMOP-MLTS applies the neighborhood search first to the width of the quantum wells and then to the electrical field. The neighborhood for the wells is 20% of the size of the wells. This neighborhood is larger because the actual search area for the quantum wells is much smaller than the electrical field. The electrical field is then varied with a much smaller neighborhood (1%) than used in the first tier. This second tier is run after generations 150 and 200.

The second tier of neighborhood searches are more for fine-tuning the solutions that are generated in the earlier portion of the algorithm. So the first tier is used for larger adjustments in the solution and the second tier is used to fine-tune the results. This is similar to the principles of simulated annealing, but this approach also directs the search to different regions of the decision space based on what stage the algorithm has reached.

Each implementation of memetic GENMOP is run 100 times in order to be able to effectively compare the results with previous results found. The Pareto front generated by the best results is compared to the other runs. Each implementation is run for 200 generations and starts with 25 individuals. These numbers were chosen in order to better compare the research results with previous results. To compare GENMOP-LS to the multitiered GENMOP-MTLS, each MOEA is run with local search applied every 50 generations (local search applied a total of 4 times during the run). In all instances, the GENMOP-MTLS was able to find high quality solutions (which are designs that can be effectively fabricated into a stable QCL). Figure 19 shows graph comparing GENMOP-LS with GENMOP-MTLS. The values in the graph are overlap ratios and energy level differences. The overlap ratios are unitless while the energy level difference is measured in Angstroms. A zero level is considered the best while one is the worst. The research is interested in finding solutions that are at roughly 0.25 or less. Any values that reach 0.1 are highly desirable. As Figure 19 shows, numerous values from both algorithms are considered acceptable solutions. But it is easy to note that all 11 points generated by GENMOP-MTLS were nondominated while only 1 out of 34 point were nondominated using the baseline GENMOP-LS. This figure empirically confirms that the GENMOP-

MTLS is more effective at finding higher quality solutions. One disadvantage is that fewer points are found along the GENMOP-MTLS Pareto front. This is probably due to the search landscape, where multiple solutions may lead to the same nondominated point. Future efforts should reflect on the inclusion of local search because of the rugged search landscape along with use of modified selection, crossover, and mutation operators.

Autopilot Controller

Blumel, Hughes, and White (2001) use an MOEA to evolve fuzzy logic trajectory controllers in the design of a fuzzy autopilot controller for a missile. A main requirement of designing an autopilot system is to generate a fast response while minimizing the overshoot. This allows the missile to respond quickly to commands and avoid overcorrection. The amount of overshoot that is tolerable depends on the number of g's the missile is pulling. Small amounts of overshoot are typically acceptable for low g's, but any overshoot is usually unacceptable for high g's. The autopilot needs to optimize four objectives in order to gener-

Figure 19. Comparison of GENMOP-LS with local search applied every 50 generations and the improved, multi-tiered, GENMOP-MTLS (Kleeman, 2007d)

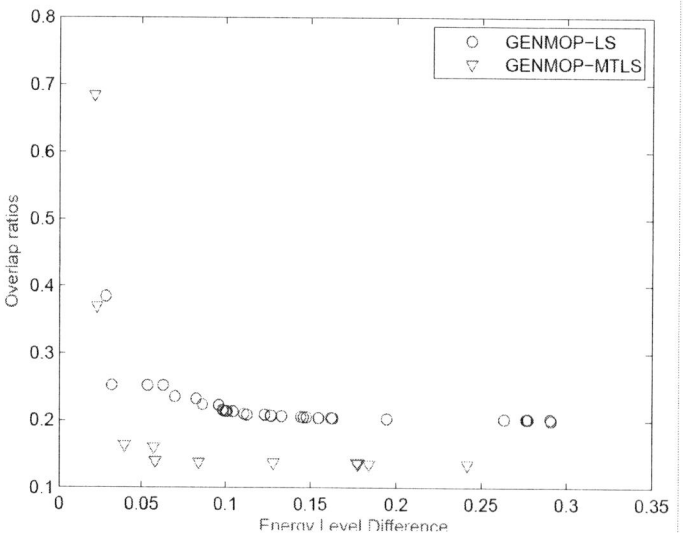

Table 12. The closed loop performance criteria used to find the four objective values (Blumel, 2001) (©2001, Springer-Verlag. Used with permission)

Steady State Error(%)	Settling time(sec)	Rising time(sec)	Overshoot(%)
$Er^* = 0.0$	$Ts^* = 0.15$	$Tr^* = 0.08$	$Os^* = 4.5$
$Er_{max} = 2.0$	$Ts_{max} = 0.25$	$Tr_{max} = 0.14$	$Os_{max} = 25.0$
$Er_{min} = 0.0$	$Ts_{min} = 0.1$	$Tr_{min} = 0.07$	$Os_{min} = 2.0$

ate an accurate and instantaneous response. The four objectives are: side-slip velocity steady state error, overshoot, rise time, and settling time. Table 12 shows the reference points used in calculating the four objectives.

The researchers chose to optimize their fuzzy controller using the original NSGA MOEA (Srinivas & Deb, 1995). Recall that the NSGA is a first generation algorithm that did not incorporate elitism into the algorithm. Since that time improvements have been made and the NSGA-II, as well as other second generation MOEAs that include elitism, have been found to outperform those without elitism. The NSGA selects individuals for the next generation based on a non-dominated ranking process. The algorithm is run with a population size of 100 for 250 generations. Stochastic universal sampling is used to select 20 parents, of which 20 children are created using uniform multipoint crossover and mutation. The 20 children are then combined with the other 100 individuals and the best 100 advance to the next generation.

Since the four objectives are competing, the results can be very diverse. Figure 20 shows a set of lateral acceleration responses derived from different fuzzy controllers that were optimized by the NSGA. Note that some are bad with high overshoot values and some are very slow on rise time and settling time. But others are good, in that they have little steady state error and no overshoot.

Since there are four objectives, plotting a Pareto front for visualization cannot be done. But two objectives can be plotted to show the trade-offs between the various solutions with respect to each objective. Figure 21 show a set of these trade-off plots. The results show that MOEAs can produce a good set of results that allow the system designer to choose between a variety of trade-off solutions. Again, the incorporation of MOEA local search would be useful in fine-tuning the design generating robust control parameter values.

OTHER APPLICATIONS

There are also many other areas where MOEAs were used to solve problems for the military. This section briefly touches upon three diverse areas where MOEAs were used. These papers discuss such things as groundwater remediation, UAV communication optimization and radar waveform optimization.

Groundwater Remediation (Knarr, 2003) (Singh & Minsker, 2004)

Groundwater remediation research has been done by several researchers using MOEAs. This problem is important to the military because they have been attempting to clean-up many of the environmental hazards that were created in the past due to poor disposal methods for unused chemicals. Groundwater cleanup is a big piece of this effort. Knarr (2003) used the GENMOP algorithm to determine design parameter values for horizontal flow treatment wells in order to maximize perchlorate destruction while minimiz-

Figure 20. A set of lateral acceleration responses from different fuzzy controllers found using the MOEA (Blumel, 2001) (©2001, Springer-Verlag. Used with permission)

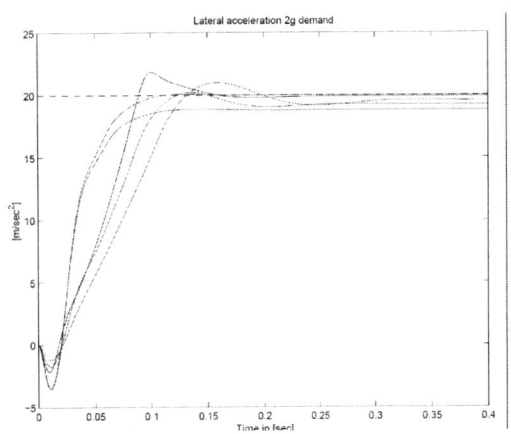

ing cost. Singh (2004) uses a "noisy' NSGA-II MOEA to maximize clean-up while minimizing costs for the clean-up of the Umatilla Chemical Depot. Both papers show that the MOEAs performed well and were able to provide the decision maker with many valid trade-off alternatives the various clean-up projects.

Optimization of UAV Communications (Kleeman, 2004) (Day, 2005)

This problem addresses the future problem of optimizing the communication between multiple, autonomous, heterogeneous UAVs flying in a formation. The goal is to determine the best location in the formation for each type of UAV in order to minimize the total distance that the communication packets have to flow before reaching the desired UAV. It is assumed that there are multiple communication frequencies for each UAV so this makes the problem a multi-objective problem. An explicit building block MOEA (MOMGA-II) was used to optimize this problem. The results show that MOEA is able to find good results, but additional enhancements to the code enabled the algorithm to find even better results (Day, 2005).

Figure 21. Trade-off between the four objectives for the final population (Blumel, 2001) (©2001, Springer-Verlag. Used with permission)

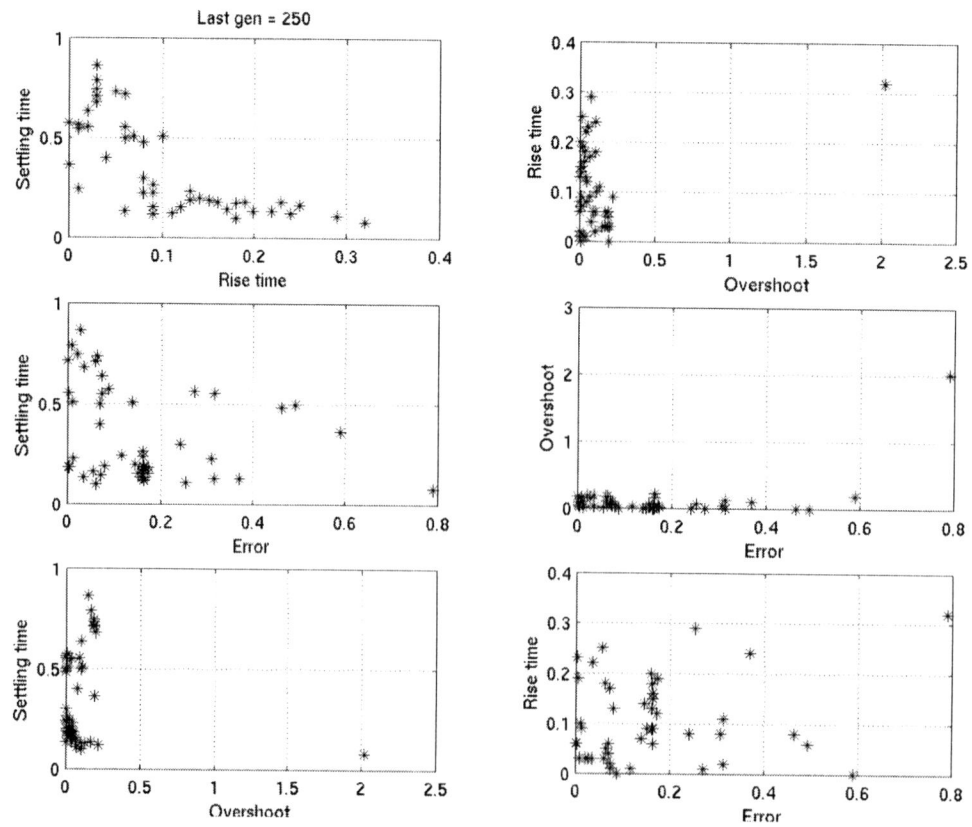

Many-Objective Radar Waveform Optimization (Hughes, 2007)

This problem addresses the waveform design for a pulsed Doppler radar, typical of many airborne fighter radar systems. The intent is to measure both target range and velocity which is impossible for large ranges and high velocities with a single waveform. Multiple waveforms are thus combined in order to resolve target ambiguities. The problem domain includes a generic radar model which has four to twelve integer decision variables with nine objectives. Developing the associated waveform set is accomplished using three multi-objective evolutionary algorithms (NSGA-II, MSOPS, and a prototype MOEA). Initial results indicate that the multi-dimensional search landscapes are very complex and require decision maker focus in order to obtain satisfactory designs. Note that the author provides the underlying software for applying these MOEA techniques to other radar models.

SUMMARY

In this chapter, we have attempted to provide a spectrum of military multi-objective optimization problems whose characteristics imply that an MOEA approach is appropriate. The choice of selected operators indicates that good results can be achieved for these problems. Selection and testing of other operators and associated parameters may generate "better" solutions. It is not intended that these problems represent the totality or even the complete spectrum of all military optimization problems. However, the examples discussed are very complex with high-dimensionality and therefore reflect the many difficulties the military has in achieve their goals. MOEAs with local search are another method of attacking these complex problems that should provide effective and efficient solutions.

REFERENCES

Belfares, L. & Guitouni, A. (2003). Multi-objective genetic algorithms for courses of action planning. In *Proceedings of IEEE Congress on Evolutionary Computation (CEC'2003), Vol 3*, (pp. 1543–1551).

Bingül, Z., Sekmen, A. Ş., Palaniappan, S. & Zein-Sabatto, S. (2000). Genetic algorithms applied to real time multi-objective optimization problems. In *Proceedings of the IEEE Southeastcon*, (pp. 95-103).

Bingül, Z., Sekmen, A. Ş., & Zein-Sabatto, S. (2000). Evolutionary approach to multi-objective problems using adaptive genetic algorithms. In *Proceedings of 2000 IEEE International Conference on Systems, Man, and Cybernetics, vol. 3*, (pp. 1923-1927).

Blumel, A. L., Hughes, E. J., & White, B. A. (2001). Multi-objective evolutionary design of fuzzy autopilot controller. *First International Conference on Evolutionary Multi-Criterion Optimization* (pp. 668-680). *Lecture notes in computer science No. 1993*. Springer-Verlag.

Chan, T. M., Man, K. F., Tang, K. S., & Kwong, S. A. (2005). A jumping gene algorithm for multi-objective resource management in wideband CDMA systems. *The Computer Journal, 48*(6), 749-768.

Coello, C. A. C., Van Veldhuizen, D. A., & Lamont, G. B. (2002). *Evolutionary algorithms for solving multi-objective problems*. Norwell, MA: Kluwer Academic Publishers.

Day, R. O. (2005). *Explicit building block multi-objective evolutionary computation: Methods and applications*. Unpublished doctoral Dissertation, Air Force Institute of Technology, Wright-Patterson AFB, Dayton, OH.

Deb, K., Agarwa,l S., Pratap, A., & Meyarivan, T. (2000). A fast and elitist multi-objective genetic algorithm: NSGA-II. In *Proceedings of the Parallel Problem Solving from Nature VI*, (pp. 849-858).

Deb, K., Pratap, A., Agarwal, S., & Meyarivan, T. (2002). A fast and elitist multi-objective genetic algorithm: NSGA–II. *IEEE Transactions on Evolutionary Computation, 6*(2), 182–197.

Erickson, M., Mayer, A., & Horn, J. (2001). The niched Pareto genetic algorithm 2 applied to the design of groundwater remediation systems. In E. Zitzler, K. Deb, L. Thiele, C. A. Coello Coello, & D. Corne (Eds.), In *Proceedings of the First International Conference Evolutionary Multi-Criterion Optimization*, (pp. 681–695). Springer.

Erwin, M. C. (2006). *Combining quality of service and topology control in directional hybrid wireless networks*. Unpublished master's thesis, Graduate School of Engineering and Management, Air Force Institute of Technology, Wright-Patterson AFB, Dayton, OH.

Eshelman, L. (1991). The CHC adaptive search algorithm. *Foundations of genetic algorithms 1* (pp. 265–283). Morgan Kaufmann.

Fonseca, C. M. & Fleming, P. J. (1998). Multi-objective optimization and multiple constraint handling with evolutionary algorithms—Part I: A unified formulation. *IEEE Transactions on Systems, Man, and Cybernetics A, 28*, 26–37.

Gale, D. & Shapley, L. S. (1962). College admissions and the stability of marriage. *The American Mathematical Monthly, 69*(1), 9–15.

Garrett, D., Vannucci, J., Silva, R., Dasgupta, D., & Simien, J. (2005). Genetic algorithms for the sailor assignment problem. In *Proceedings of the 2005 Genetic and Evolutionary Computation Conference (GECCO)*, (pp 1921-1928).

Goldberg, D. E. & Lingle, R. (1985). Alleles, loci, and the traveling salesman problem. In *Proceedings of the International Conference on Genetic Algorithms and their Applications*, (pp 154-159).

Guitouni, A., Bélanger, M., & Berger, J., (2000). *Report on final lance exercise* (Tech. Rep. DREV-TM-2000-21). Canadian Forces College.

Holder, A. (2005). Navy personnel planning and the optimal partition. *Operations Research, 53* 77-89.

Hughes, E. J. (2007). Radar waveform optimization as a many-objective application benchmark. In *Proceedings of 4th International Conference on Evolutionary Multi-Criterion Optimization (EMO)*, (pp. 700-714).

Ishibuchi, H., Yoshida, T., & Murata, T. (2003). Balance between genetic search and local search in memetic algorithms for multi-objective permutation flowshop scheduling. *IEEE Transactions on Evolutionary Computing, 7*, 204–223.

Jia, D. & Vagners, J. (2004). Parallel evolutionary algorithms for UAV path planning. In *Proceedings of the AIAA 1st Intelligent Systems Technical Conference*.

Jourdan, D. B. & de Weck, O. L. (2004). Multi-objective genetic algorithm for the automated planning of a wireless sensor network to monitor a critical facility. In *Proceedings of the SPIE Defense and Security Symposium, Vol. 5403*, (pp. 565-575).

Jourdan, D. B. & de Weck, O.L. (2004). Layout optimization for a wireless sensor network using a multi-objective genetic algorithm. In Proceedings of the *IEEE Semiannual Vehicular Technology Conference*.

Kelemen, A., Kozma, R., & Liang, Y. (2002). Neuro-fuzzy classification for the job assignment problem. *International Joint Conference on Neural Networks IJCNN02, World Congress on Computational Intelligence WCCI2002*, (pp. 630-634). IEEE.

Keller, T. A. & Lamont, G. B. (2004). Optimization of a quantum cascade laser operating in the terahertz frequency range using a multi-objective evolutionary algorithm. In *Proceedings on 17th International Conference on Multiple Criteria Decision Making (MCDM 2004). Vol 1.*

Kleeman, M. P. (2004). *Optimization of heterogeneous UAV communications using the multi-objective quadratic assignment problem.* Unpublished master's thesis, Graduate School of Engineering and Management, Air Force Institute of Technology, Wright-Patterson AFB, Dayton, OH.

Kleeman, M. P. & Lamont, G. B. (2005). Solving the aircraft engine maintenance scheduling problem using a multi-objective evolutionary algorithm. In *Proceedings of Evolutionary Multi-Criterion Optimization (EMO 2005), LNCS 3410*, (pp. 782-796). Berlin Heidelberg: Springer-Verlag.

Kleeman, M. P. & Lamont, G. B. (2006). The multi-objective constrained assignment problem. In *Proceedings of Genetic and Evolutionary Computation (GECCO 2006)* (Vol. 1, pp. 743-744). ACM.

Kleeman, M. P., Lamont, G. B., Hopkinson, K. M., & Graham, S. R., (2007). Solving multicommodity capacitated network design problems using a multi-objective evolutionary algorithm. In *Proceedings of 2007 IEEE Symposium on Computational Intelligence for Security and Defense Applications (CISDA 2007)*, (pp. 33-41).

Kleeman, M. P. & Lamont, G. B. (2007). Scheduling of a combined flow-shop, job-shop scheduling problem using an MOEA with a variable length chromosome. *Evolutionary scheduling.* Springer Verlag.

Kleeman, M. P. & Lamont, G. B. (2007). The multi-objective constrained assignment problem. In *Proceedings of SPIE Symposium on Defense & Security 2007: Evolutionary and Bio-inspired Computation: Theory and Applications.*

Kleeman, M. P., Lamont, G. B., Cooney, A., & Nelson, T. R. (2007). A multi-tiered memetic multi-objective evolutionary algorithm for the design of quantum cascade lasers. In *Proceedings of Evolutionary Multi-Criterion Optimization (EMO 2007), LNCS 4403*, (pp 186-200). Springer-Verlag.

Knarr, M. R., Goltz, M. N., Lamont, G. B., & Huang, J. (2003). In situ boremediation of perchlorate-contaminated groundwater using a multi-objective parallel evolutionary algorithm. In *Proceedings of IEEE Congress on Evolutionary Computation (CEC'2003)* (Vol. 1, pp. 1604–1611).

Lamont, G. B., Slear, J., & Melendez, K., (2007). UAV swarm mission planning and routing using multi-objective evolutionary algorithms. In *Proceedings of 2007 IEEE Symposium on Intelligent Computation in Multi-Criteria Decision Making.*

Lewis, M. W., Lewis, K. R., & White, B. J. (2004). Guided design search in the interval-bounded sailor assignment problem. *Computers and operations research.* Elsevier.

Liang, Y., Lin, K.-I., & Kelemen, A. (2002). Adaptive generalized estimation equation with bayes classifer for the job assignment problem. In *Proceedings of the 6th Pacific-Asia Conference on Advances in Knowledge Discovery and Data Mining (PAKDD '02)*, (pp. 438-449). Springer-Verlag.

McCauley, L. & Franklin, S. (2002). A large-scale multi-agent system for navy personnel distribution. *Connect. Sci., 14*(4), 371-385.

Michalewicz, Z. & Janikow, C. Z. (1996). Genocop: A genetic algorithm for numerical optimization problems with linear constraints. *Commun. ACM, 39*(12), 223–240.

Qi, H., Iyengar, S. S., & Chakrabarty, K. (2001). Multiresolution data integration using mobile agents in distributed sensor networks. *IEEE Transactions on Systems, Man and Cybernetics Part C: Applications and Rev., 31*(3), 383-391.

Rajagopalan, R. (2004). *Path planning with evolutionary algorithms*. Unpublished master's thesis, Department of Electrical Engineering & Computer Science, Syracuse University.

Rajagopalan, R., Mohan, C. K., Mehrotra, K. G. & Varshney, P. K. (2004). Evolutionary multi-objective crowding algorithm for path computations. In *Proceedings of the Fifth International Conference on Knowledge Based Computer Systems*, (pp. 46-65).

Rajagopalan, R., Mohan, C., Varshney, P., & Mehrotra, K. G. (2005). Multi-objective mobile agent routing in wireless sensor networks. In *Proceedings of 2005 IEEE Congress on Evolutionary Computation (CEC'2005)* (Vol. 2, pp. 1730—1737).

Rajagopalan, R., Varshney, P. K., Mehrotra, K. G., & Mohan, C. K. (2005). Fault tolerant mobile agent routing in sensor networks: A multi-objective optimization approach. In *Proceedings of the 2nd IEEE Upstate NY workshop on Comm. and Networking*.

Rodriguez, A. F., Keller, T. A, Lamont, G. B., & Nelson, T. R. (2005). Using a multi-objective evolutionary algorithm to develop a quantum cascade laser operating in the terahertz frequency range. In *Proceedings of 2005 IEEE Congress on Evolutionary Computation (CEC'2005)* (Vol. 1, pp. 9-16).

Schott, J. R., (1995). *Fault tolerant design using single and multi-criteria genetic algorithm optimization*. Master's Thesis, Department of Aeronautics and Astronautics, Massachusetts Institute of Technology.

Slear, J. N., Melendez, K., & Lamont, G. B. (2006). Parallel UAV swarm simulation with optimal route planning. In *Proceedings of the 2006 Summer Computer Simulation Conference (SCSC'06)*.

Slear, J. N. (2006). *AFIT UAV swarm mission planning and simulation system*. Unpublished master's thesis, Graduate School of Engineering and Mangement, Air Force Institute of Technology, Wright-Patterson AFB, Dayton, OH.

Singh, A. & Minsker, B. S. (2004). Uncertainty based multi-objective optimization of groundwater remediation at the Umatilla Chemical Depot. In *Proceedings of the American Society of Civil Engineers (ASCE) Environmental & Water Resources Institute (EWRI) World Water & Environmental Resources Congress 2004 & Related Symposia*.

Srinivas, N. & Deb, K. (1995). Multi-objective optimization using nondominated sorting in genetic algorithms. *Evolutionary Computation, 2*(3), 221-248.

Thie, C. J., Chitty, D. M., & Reed, C. M. (2005). Using evolutionary algorithms and dynamic programming to solve uncertain multi-criteria optimization problems with application to lifetime management for military platforms. In F. Rothlauf (Ed.), *GECCO workshops* (pp. 181-183). ACM.

Urli, B., Lo, N., & Guitouni, A. (2003). Une approche d'optimisation dans la génération de Plans d'Actions (COA). *31st Annual ASAC Conference*. Halifax, Nova Scotia, Canada.

Wu, Q., Rao, N. S. V., Barhen, J., Iyengar, S. S., Vaishnavi, V. K., Qi, H. & Chakrabarty, K. (2004). On computing mobile agent routes for data fusion in distributed sensor networks. *IEEE Trans. Knowledge and Data Engineering, 16*(6), 740-753.

Zitzler, E. (1999). *Evolutionary algorithms for multi-objective optimization: Methods and applications*. Unpublished doctoral thesis, Swiss Federal Institute of Technology, Zurich, Switzerland (Dissertation ETH No:13398).

Zitzler, E., Laumanns, M. & Thiele, L. (2001). *SPEA2: Improving the strength Pareto evolutionary algorithm* (Tech. Rep. TIK-Report 103). Swiss Federal Institute of Technology, Lausanne, Switzerland.

Zitzler, E., Thiele, L., Laumanns, M., Fonseca, C. M., & Grunert da Fonseca, V. (2003). Performance assessment of multi-objective optimizers: An analysis and review. *IEEE Transactions on Evolutionary Computation, 7*, pp.117–132.

FUTURE RESEARCH DIRECTIONS

Using a MOEA in a military application requires some focus on computational efficiency and ease of use. Also, one can consider the use of non-Pareto approaches in real-world military applications that have a multitude of constraints. What alternative algorithms are available and how do they compare to a MOEA approach statistically? One can examine the integration of a MOEA with other stochastic and deterministic technique in solving military real-world nonlinear constrained problems. What attributes of the MOEA are advantageous as well as supportive of such a multiple search approach?

Continuing research efforts of MOEAs applied to military applications should also employ larger networks, use real-world constraints including environmental, evaluation of other MOEA structures, employment of many and varied MOEA comparative metrics for performance evaluation, and extended comparison to fitness aggregated approaches (single objective models). With regard to the example military problems presented including network optimization, sensor placement, maintenance scheduling, mission planning and routing, and military personnel management, many avenues of research are available via the suggested generic MOEA directions. Consideration of exploratory crossover, mutation and selection operators along with local search techniques is paramount. For example, crossover operators beyond uniform, 1-point and 2-point for evaluation include UNDX, BLX, FR, PNX, and SBX. Modeling uncertainty in the problem domain model, dynamically changing environments, and exploring different objectives are included.

New MOEA military research should include the integration of the decision maker as to the focus of the search in the many multi-objective space. This is required in order to reduce the exponential computation in the global domain by attempting to solve the problem in a local region of the Pareto front.

Again, new and exciting application areas for innovative MOEA military optimization approaches include Microelectrical Mechanical Systems (MEMS) design, knowledge extraction from very large military databases, cryptography and cyber-warfare. Regarding specific military multi-objective problems with MOEA opportunities, the publications and conferences of the Military Application Society as part of the Institute of Operations Research and Management Sciences (INFORMS) are of interest. Of course, the many international evolutionary algorithm journals and conferences should also be perused for possible military relevance.

ADDITIONAL READING (MOEA MILITARY RELEVANCE)

Berro, A. & Duthen, Y. (2001). Search for optimum in dynamic environment: A efficient agent-based method. In *Proceedings of the 2001 Genetic and Evolutionary Computation Conference. Workshop Program* (pp. 51-54).

Bozma, H. I. & Duncan, J. S. (1994). A game—Theoretic approach to integration of modules. *IEEE Transactions on Pattern Analysis and Machine Intelligence, 16*,(11), 1074-1086.

Deb, K. Bhaskara, U. R. N., & Karthik, S. 2007). Dynamic multi-objective optimization and decision-making using modified NSGA-II: A case study on hydro-thermal power scheduling. In *Proceedings of the Fourth International Conference on Evolutionary Multi-Criterion Optimization (EMO).*

Kamalian, R., Takagi, H., & Agogino, A. M. (2004). Optimized design of MEMS by evolutionary multi-objective optimization with interactive evolutionary computation. Genetic and Evolutionary Computation (GECCO 2004), pages 1030--1041.

Kewley, R. H. & Embrechts, M. J. (2002). Computational military tactical planning system. *IEEE Transactions on Systems, Man, and Cybernetics, Part C, 32*(2), 161–171.

Khosla & Nichol (2006). Hybrid evolutionary algorithms for network-centric command and control. SPIE

Kleeman, M. P., Lamont, G. B., Cooney, A., & Nelson, T. R. (2007). A multi-tiered memetic multi-objective evolutionary algorithm for the design of quantum cascade lasers. In Evolutionary Multi-Criterion Optimization (EMO 2007), LNCS 4403, pages 186-200, March 2007. Springer-Verlag.

Kleinmuntz, D. (2007). Risk-based multi-objective resource allocation for infrastructure protection. In *Proceedings of the NFORMS International Meeting.*

Knighton, S., Boyd, J., Cunningham, C., Gray, D., & Parker, J. (2007). Network flow model for optimizing fighter squadron scheduling. In *Proceedings of the INFORMS International Meeting.*

Lawrence, M. (2006). Multi-objective genetic algorithms for materialized view selection in OLAP data warehouses. In *Proceedings of the 2006 Genetic and Evolutionary Computation Conference (GECCO'2006)* (pp. 699-706).

Pankanti, S. & Jain, A. K. (1995). Integrating vision modules: Stereo, shading, grouping, and line labeling. *IEEE Transactions on Pattern Analysis and Machine Intelligence, 17*(8), 831-842.

Parreiras, R. O. & Vasconcelos, J. A. (205). Decision making in multi-objective optimization problems, Real-world multi-objective system engineering. New York: Nova Science Publishers.

Ridder, J. P. & HandUber, J. C. (2005). Mission planning for joint suppression of enemy air defenses using a genetic algorithm. In *Proceedings of Genetic and Evolutionary Computation Conference (GECCO)* (pp. 1929–1936).

Rosenberg, B., Burge, J., & Gonsalves, P. (2005). Applying evolutionary multi-objective optimization to mission planning for time-sensitive targets. In F. Rothlauf (Ed.), In *Proceedings Late breaking paper at Genetic and Evolutionary Computation Conference (GECCO)*

Tirat-Gefen, Y. (2007). Distributed optimization algorithms for multi-target and multi-sensor allocation and scheduling. In *Proceedings of the INFORMS International Meeting.*

Valdes, J. J. & Barton, A. J. (2006). Multi-objective evolutionary optimization for visual data mining with virtual reality spaces. In *Proceedings of the 2006 Genetic and Evolutionary Computation Conference (GECCO'2006)* (pp. 723-730).

Wagner, T., Beume, N., & Naujoks, B. (2007). Pareto-, aggregation-, and indicator-based methods in many-objective optimization. In *Proceedings of the Fourth International Conference on Evolutionary Multi-Criterion Optimization (EMO).*

Yamasaki, K. (2001). Dynamic Pareto optimum GA against changing environments. In *Proceedings of the 2001 Genetic and Evolutionary Computation Conference, Workshop Program* (pp. 47-50).

Yang, A., Abbass, H. A., & Saker. R. (2006). Combat scenario planning: A multi-objective approach. LNCS, Vol. 4247, Springer Verlag, pages 837-844, October, 2006

Zhang, Y., Kamalian, R., Agogino, A. M., & Sequin, C. H. (2006). Design synthesis of microelectromechanical systems using genetic algorithms with component-based genotype representation. *In Proceedings of the 2006 Genetic and Evolutionary Computation Conference (GECCO)* (pp. 731-738).

ENDNOTE

* The views expressed in this chapter are those of the authors and do not reflect the official policy or position of the Department of Defense or the United States Government.

Compilation of References

Abbas, A. K., Lichtman, A. H., & Pober, J. S. (2000). Cellular and molecular immunology (4th ed.). New York: W B Saunders Co.

Abbass, H. A. & Sarker, R. (2002). The Pareto differential evolution algorithm. *International Journal on Artificial Intelligence Tools, 11*(4), 531-552.

Abbass, H. A. (2002). The self-adaptive Pareto differential evolution algorithm. In *Proceedings of the 2002 Congress on Evolutionary Computation (CEC 2002)* (pp. 831-836). Honolulu, HI: IEEE Service Center.

Abbass, H. A. (2003). Speeding up back-propagation using multi-objective evolutionary algorithms. *Neural Computation, 15*(11), 2705–2726.

Abbass, H. A. (2006). An economical cognitive approach for bi-objective optimization using bliss points, visualization, and interaction. *Soft Computing, 10*(8), 687-698.

Abbass, H. A., Sarker, R., & Newton, C. (2001). PDE: A Pareto-frontier differential evolution approach for multi-objective optimization problems. In *Proceedings of the 2001 Congress on Evolutionary Computation (CEC 2001)* (pp. 971-978). Seoul, South Korea: IEEE Service Center.

Abraham, S. G., Rau, B. R., & Schreiber, R. (2000, July). *Fast design space exploration through validity and quality filtering of subsystem designs* (Tech. Rep. No. HPL-2000-98). HP Laboratories Palo Alto.

Akyldiz, I., Su, W., Sankarasubramanian Y., & Cayirci E. (2002). A survey on sensor networks. *IEEE Communications Magazine, 40*(8), 102-14.

Alvarez-Benitez, J. E., Everson, R. M., & Fieldsend, J. E. (2005). A MOPSO algorithm based exclusively on Pareto dominance concepts. *Lecture notes in computer science* (Vol. 3410, pp. 459-473). Springer-Verlag.

Alvarez-Benitez, J. E., Everson, R. M., & Fieldsend, J. E. (2005, March). A MOPSO algorithm based exclusively on Pareto dominance concepts. In C. A. C. Coello, A. H. Aguirre, & E. Zitzler (Eds.), *Evolutionary multi-criterion optimization*. In *Proceedings of the Third International Conference, EMO 2005* (pp. 459–473), Guanajuato, México: Springer.

Alvarez-Benitez, J., Everson, R., & Fieldsend, J. (2005). A MOPSO algorithm based exclusively on Pareto dominance concepts. In C. Coello Coello, A. Aguirre & E. Zitzler (Eds.), *Evolutionary multi-criterion optimisation: Vol. 3410. Lecture notes in computer science* (pp. 459–473). Berlin: Springer-Verlag.

Amos, M., Paun, G., Rozenberg, G., & Salomaa, A. (2002). Topics in the theory of DNA computing. *Theoretical Computer Science, 287*, 3-38.

Angeline, P. J., Saunders, G. M., & Pollack, J. B. (1994). An evolutionary algorithm that constructs recurrent neural networks. *IEEE Transactions on Neural Networks, 5*(1), 54–65.

Angus, D. (2006). Crowding population-based ant colony optimisation for the multi-objective travelling salesman problem. In P. Sloot, G. van Albada, M. Bubak, & A. Referthen (Eds.), *2nd IEEE international e-science and grid computing conference (Workshop on biologically-inspired optimisation methods for parallel and distributed architectures: Algorithms, systems and applications)*. Piscataway: IEEE-Press.

Aquilante, C. L., Langaee T. Y., Anderson P. L., Zineh, I., & Fletcher, C. V. (2006). Multiplex PCR-pyrosequencing assay for genotyping CYP3A5 polymorphisms. *Clinica Chimica Acta, 372*(102), 195-198.

Arita, M., & Kobayashi, S. (2002). DNA sequence design using templates. *New Generation Computing, 20*, 263-277.

Ascia, G., Catania, V., & Palesi, M. (2004, August). A GA based design space exploration framework for parameterized system-on-a-chip platforms. *IEEE Transactions on Evolutionary Computation, 8*(4), 329–346.

Ascia, G., Catania, V., & Palesi, M. (2005, April). A multi-objective genetic approach for system-level exploration in parameterized systems-on-a-chip. *IEEE Transactions on Computer-Aided Design of Integrated Circuits and Systems, 24*(4), 635–645.

Ascia, G., Catania, V., Palesi, M., & Patti, D. (2003, October 3–4). EPIC-Explorer: A parameterized VLIW-based platform framework for design space exploration. In *First workshop on embedded systems for real-time multimedia (ESTIMEDIA)* (pp. 65–72). Newport Beach, California.

Austin, T., Larson, E., & Ernst, D. (2002, February). SimpleScalar: An infrastructure for computer system modeling. *IEEE Computer, 35*(2), 59–67.

Babu, B. V. & Jehan, M. M. L. (2003). Differential evolution for multi-objective optimization. In *Proceedings of the 2003 Congress on Evolutionary Computation (CEC 2003)* (pp. 2696-2703), Canberra, Australia: IEEE Service Center.

Back, T. (1996). *Evolutionary algorithms in theory and practice.* New York: Oxford University Press.

Bak, P. & Sneppen, K. (1993). Punctuated equilibrium and criticality in a simple model of evolution. *Physical Review Letters, 71,* 4083–4086.

Bak, P. (1996). *How nature works.* New York: Springer-Verlag.

Bak, P., Tang, C., & Wiesenfeld, K. (1987). Self-organized criticality: An explanation of 1/f noise. *Physical Review Letters, 59,* 381–384.

Balling, R. (2003). The maximin fitness function; Multi-objective city and regional planning. *Lecture notes in computer science* (Vol. 2632, pp. 1-15). Springer-Verlag.

Barlow, G. J. & Oh, C. K. (2005). Transference of evolved unmanned aerial vehicle controllers to a wheeled mobile robot. In *2005 IEEE International Conference on Robots & Automation (ICRA 2005)* (pp. 2087-2092). Piscataway, NJ: IEEE Press.

Barlow, G. J. & Oh, C. K. (2006). Robustness analysis of genetic programming controllers for unmanned aerial vehicles. In *2006 ACM Genetic & Evolutionary Computation Conference (GECCO 2006)* (pp. 135-142). New York: ACM Press.

Barlow, G. J., Oh, C. K. & Grant, E. (2004). Incremental evolution of autonomous controllers for unmanned aerial vehicles using multi-objective genetic programming. In *2004 IEEE International Conference on Systems, Man & Cybernetics* (pp. 689-694). Piscataway, NJ: IEEE Press.

Bartz-Beielstein, T., Limbourg, P., Mehnen, J., Schmitt, K., Parsopoulos, K. E., & Vrahatis, M. N. (2003). Particle swarm optimizers for Pareto optimization with enhanced archiving techniques. In *Proceedings of the IEEE 2003 Congress on Evolutionary Computation* (pp. 1780-1787). IEEE Press.

Bartz-Beielstein, T., Limbourg, P., Parsopoulos, K. E., Vrahatis, M. N., Mehnen, J., & Schmitt, K. (2003, December). Particle swarm optimizers for Pareto optimization with enhanced archiving techniques. In *Proceedings of the 2003 Congress on Evolutionary Computation (CEC'2003)* (Vol. 3, pp. 1780–1787), Canberra, Australia: IEEE Press.

Baumgartner, U., Magele, C., & Renhart, W. (2004). Pareto optimality and particle swarm optimization. *IEEE Transactions on Magnetics, 40*(2), 1172-1175.

Baumgartner, U., Magele, C., & Renhart, W. (2004, March). Pareto optimality and particle swarm optimization. *IEEE Transactions on Magnetics, 40*(2), 1172–1175.

Beasley, J. (2007). *OR-library.* Retrieved February 10, 2008, from http://people.brunel.ac.uk/ mastjjb/jeb/info.html.

Belew, R. K., McInerney, J. & Schraudolph, N. N. (1992). Evolving networks: Using the genetic algorithm with connectionist learning. In C. G. Langton, C. Taylor, J. D. Farmer, & S. Rasmussen (Eds.), *Artificial Life II: Proceedings of the Second International Workshop on the Synthesis & Simulation of Living Systems* (pp. 511–547). Redwood City, CA: Addison-Wesley.

Belfares, L. & Guitouni, A. (2003). Multi-objective genetic algorithms for courses of action planning. In *Proceedings of IEEE Congress on Evolutionary Computation (CEC'2003), Vol 3,* (pp. 1543–1551).

Benedetti, A., Farina, M., & Gobbi, M. (2006) Evolutionary multi-objective industrial design: The case of a racing car tire-suspension systems. *IEEE Transactions on Evolutionary Computation, 10*(3), 230-244.

Benini, E., & Toffolo A. (2002a). Development of high-performance airfoils for axial flow compressors using evolutionary computation. *Journal of Propulsion and Power, 18*(3), 544-554.

Benini, E., & Toffolo, A. (2002b). Optimal design of horizontal-axis wind turbines using blade-element theory and evolutionary computation. *Journal of Solar Energy Engineering, 124*(4), 357-363.

Bergey, P. K. (1999). An agent enhanced intelligent spreadsheet solver for multi-criteria decision making. In *Proceedings of the Fifth Americas Conference on Information Systems (AMCIS 1999)* (pp. 966-968), Milwaukee, WI.

Berkovits, S., Guttman, J. D., & Swarup, V. (1998) Authentication for mobile agents mobile agents and security. In G. Vigna (ed.), (pp. 114- 136), Springer-Verlag.

Beyer, H. G. & Schwefel, H. P. (2002). Evolution strategies: A comprehensive introduction. *Journal Natural Computing, 1*(1), 3-52.

Bierwirth, C., Mattfeld, D. C., & Kopfer, H. (1996). On permutation representations for scheduling problems. In H. M. Voigt, W. Ebeling, I. Rechenberg, & H.-P. Schwefel (Eds.), *Parallel problem solving from nature -- PPSN IV, Lecture notes in computer science* (pp. 310-318). Berlin, Germany: Springer-Verlag.

Bingül, Z., Sekmen, A. Ş., & Zein-Sabatto, S. (2000). Evolutionary approach to multi-objective problems using adaptive genetic algorithms. In *Proceedings of 2000 IEEE International Conference on Systems, Man, and Cybernetics, vol. 3*, (pp. 1923-1927).

Bingül, Z., Sekmen, A. Ş., Palaniappan, S. & Zein-Sabatto, S. (2000). Genetic algorithms applied to real time multi-objective optimization problems. In *Proceedings of the IEEE Southeastcon*, (pp. 95-103).

Bleuler, S., Laumanns, M., Thiele, L., & Zitzler, E. (2003). Pisa: A platform and programming language independent interface for search algorithms. *Evolutionary multi-criterion optimisation. Lecture notes in computer science*, (Vol. 2632, pp. 494-508). Springer.

Blumel, A. L., Hughes, E. J., & White, B. A. (2001). Multi-objective evolutionary design of fuzzy autopilot controller. *First International Conference on Evolutionary Multi-Criterion Optimization* (pp. 668-680). *Lecture notes in computer science No. 1993*. Springer-Verlag.

Boettcher, S. & Percus, A. (1999). Extremal optimisation: Methods derived from co-evolution. In W. Banzhaf, J. Daida, A. Eiben, M. Garzon, V. Honavar, M. Jakiela, & R. Smith (Eds.), *Genetic and evolutionary computation conference* (pp. 825–832). San Francisco: Morgan Kaufmann.

Boettcher, S. & Percus, A. (2000). Nature's way of optimizing, *Artificial Intelligence, 119*, 275–286.

Boulis, A., Ganeriwal, S., & Srivastava, M. B. (2003). Aggregation in sensor networks: An energy-accuracy tradeoff. *Ad Hoc Networks, 1*, 317-331.

Bourneman, J., Chrobak, M., Vedova, G. D., Figueroa, A., & Jiang, T. (2001). Probe selection algorithms with applications in the analysis of microbial communities. *Bioinformatics, 17*(Supplement 1), 39-48.

Branke, J. & Mostaghim, S. (2006). About selecting the personal best in multi-objective particle swarm optimisation. In T. Runarsson, H. Beyer, E. Burke, J. Merelo Guervos, L. Darrell Whitley, & X. Yao (Eds.), *Parallel problem solving from nature: Vol. 4193. Lecture notes in computer science* (pp. 523–532). Berlin: Springer-Verlag.

Branke, J. (2002). *Evolutionary optimization in dynamic environments*. Massachusetts: Kluwer Academic Publishers.

Branke, J., & Mostaghim, S. (2006, September). About selecting the personal best in multi-objective particle swarm optimization. In T. P. Runarsson, H-G. Beyer, E. Burke, J. J. Merelo-Guervós, L. D. Whitley, & X. Yao (Eds.), *Parallel problem solving from nature—PPSN IX*, In *Proceedings of the 9th International Conference* (pp. 523–532). Reykjavik, Iceland: Springer. *Lecture notes in computer science* (Vol. 4193).

Brennan, L., Gupta, S. M., & Taleb, K. N. (1994). Operations planning issues in an assembly/disassembly environment. *International Journal of Operations and Production management, 14*(9), 57-67.

Brennenman, A. & Condon, A. (2002). Strand design for biomolecular computation. *Theoretical Computer Science, 287*, 39-58.

Bui, L. T. (2007). *The role of communication messages and explicit niching in distributed evolutionary multi-objective optimization*. PhD Thesis, University of New South Wales.

Bui, L. T., Abbass, H. A., & Essam, D. (2005a). Fitness inheritance for noisy evolutionary multi-objective optimization. *Proceedings of the Genetic and Evolutionary Computation Conference (GECCO-2005)* (pp. 779-785). Washington, DC: ACM Press.

Bui, L. T., Abbass, H. A., & Essam, D. (2007). Local models. An approach to distributed multi-objective optimization. *Journal of Computational Optimization and Applications*, In press. DOI: 10.1007/s10589-007-9119-8

Bui, L. T., Branke, J., & Abbass, H. A. (2005b). Multi-objective optimization for dynamic environments. *Proceedings of the Congress on Evolutionary Computation (CEC)* (pp. 2349-2356). Edinburgh, UK: IEEE Press.

Burnet, F. M. (1959). *The clonal selection theory of acquired immunity*. Cambridge University Press.

Buyuksahin, K. M. & Najm, F. N. (2005, July). Early power estimation for VLSI circuits. *IEEE Transactions on Computer-Aided Design, 24*(7), 1076–1088.

Cai, Z., Gong, W., & Huang, Y. (2007). A novel differential evolution algorithm based on ε-domination and orthogonal design method for multi-objective optimization. In *Proceedings of the 4th International Congress on Evolutionary Multi-Criterion Optimization (EMO 2007)* (pp. 286-301). Matsushima, Japan: Springer.

Campelo, F., Guimaraes, F. G., & Igarashi, H (2007). Overview of artificial immune systems for multi-objective optimization. In *Proceedings of the 4th International Conference on Evolutionary Multi-Criterion Optimization, EMO 2007. Lecture notes in computer science* (Vol. 4403, pp. 937–951). Springer

Campelo, F., Guimaraes, F. G., Saldanha, R. R., Igarashi, H., Noguchi, S., Lowther, D. A., & Ramirez, J. A. (2004). A novel multi-objective immune algorithm using nondominated sorting. In *Proceedings of the 11th International IGTE Symposium on Numerical Field Calculation in Electrical Engineering*, Seggauberg, Austria.

Cantuz-Paz, E. (2000). *Efficient and accurate parallel genetic algorithms*. Boston, MA: Kluwer Academic Publishers.

Cardei, M. & Du, D.Z. (2005). Improving wireless sensor network lifetime through power aware organization. *ACM Wireless Networks, 11* (3), 333-40.

Cardei, M. & Wu, J. (2006). Energy efficient coverage problems in wireless ad hoc sensor networks. *Computer Communications, 29*(4), 413-420.

Cardei, M., MacCallum, D., Cheng, X., Min, M., Jia, X., Li, D., & Du, D. Z. (2002). Wireless sensor networks with energy efficient organization. *Journal of Interconnection Networks, 3*(3-4), 213-229.

Carpenter, W. & Barthelemy, J.-F. (1994). *A comparison of polynomial approximation and artificial neural nets as response surface* (Tech. Rep. 92 – 2247). AIAA.

Carter, J. H. (2000). The immune system as a model for pattern recognition and classification. *Journal of the American Medical Informatics Association, 7*(3), 28–41.

Chan, H. & Perrig, A. (2004). ACE: An emergent algorithm for highly uniform cluster formation. In *Proceedings of 2004 European Workshop on Sensor Networks* (pp.154-171).

Chan, T. M., Man, K. F., Tang, K. S., & Kwong, S. A. (2005). A jumping gene algorithm for multi-objective resource management in wideband CDMA systems. *The Computer Journal, 48*(6), 749-768.

Chang, C. S. & Xu, D. Y. (2000). Differential evolution based tuning of fuzzy automatic train operation for mass rapid transit system. *IEE Proceedings on Electric Power Applications, 147*(3), 206-212.

Chang, C. S., Xu, D. Y., & Quek, H. B. (1999). Pareto-optimal set based multi-objective tuning of fuzzy automatic train operation for mass transit system. *IEE Proceedings on Electric Power Applications*, 146(5), 577-583.

Chang, H., Cooke, L., Hunt, M., Martin, G., McNelly, A., & Todd, L. (1999). *Surviving the SOC revolution a guide to platform-based design*. Kluwer Academic Publishers.

Chang, T.-T. & Chang, H.-C. (1998). Application of differential evolution to passive shunt harmonic filter planning. In *8th International Conference on Harmonics and Quality of Power* (pp. 149-153). Athens, Greece.

Charnes, A. & Cooper, W. W. (1961). *Management models and industrial applications of linear programming*. New York: John Wiley and Sons.

Charnes, A., Cooper, W. W., & Ferguson, R. O. (1955). Optimal estimation of executive compensation by linear programming. *Management Science, 1*(2), 138-151.

Chow, C.-K. & Tsui, H.-T. (2004). Autonomous agent response learning by a multi-species particle swarm optimization. In *Proceedings of the 2004 IEEE Con-*

gress on *Evolutionary Computation* (pp. 778-785). IEEE Service Center.

Clerc, M. & Kennedy, J. (2002). The particle swarm-explosion, stability, and convergence in a multidimensional complex space. *IEEE Trans. Evol. Comput., 6*(1), 58-73.

Clouqueur, T., Phipatanasuphorn, V., Ramanathan, P., & Saluja, K.K. (2003). Sensor deployment strategy for detection of targets traversing a region. *Mobile Networks and Applications, 8*(4), 453-61.

CM Labs. (2007). Retrieved February 12, 2008, from http://www.cm-labs.com/software/vortex/

Coello Coello, C. & Lechuga, M. (2002). MOPSO: A proposal for multiple objective particle swarm optimisation. In D. Fogel, M. El-Sharkawi, X. Yao, G. Greenwood, H. Iba, P. Marrow, & M. Shackleton (Eds.), *Congress on evolutionary computation* (pp. 1051–1056). Piscataway: IEEE-Press.

Coello Coello, C. A. & Cortes, N. C. (2005). Solving multi-objective optimization problems using an artificial immune system. *Genetic Programming and Evolvable Machines, 6*, 163-190.

Coello Coello, C. A. & Pulido, G. T. (2001). Multi-objective optimization using a micro-genetic algorithm. In *Proceedings of the Genetic and Evolutionary Computation Conference (GECCO-2001)* (pp. 274-282). San Francisco: Morgan Kaufmann Publishers.

Coello Coello, C. A. (2003). Evolutionary multi-objective optimization: Current and future challenges. *Advances in soft computing-engineering, design and manufacturing* (pp. 243-256). Springer-Verlag.

Coello Coello, C. A., & Cortes, N. C. (2002, September 9-11). An approach to solve multi-objective optimization problems based on an artificial immune system. In *Proceedings of the First International Conference on Artificial Immune Systems, ICARIS2002* (pp. 212-221), University of Kent at Canterbury, UK.

Coello Coello, C. A., & Cruz Cortés, N. (2005, June). Solving multi-objective optimization problems using an artificial immune system. *Genetic Programming and Evolvable machines, 6*(2), 163–190.

Coello Coello, C. A., & Salazar Lechuga, M. (2002, May). MOPSO: A proposal for multiple objective particle swarm optimization. In *Proceedings of the Congress on Evolutionary Computation (CEC'2002)* (Vol. 2, pp. 1051–1056), Piscataway, New Jersey: IEEE Service Center.

Coello Coello, C. A., Christiansen, A. D., & Aguirre, A. H. (1998). Using a new GA-based multi-objective optimization technique for the design of robot arms. *Robotica, 16*, 401–414.

Coello Coello, C. A., Rivera, D. C., & Cortes, N. C. (2003). Use of an artificial immune system for job shop scheduling. In *Proceedings of the Second International Conference on Artificial Immune Systems (ICARIS)*, Napier University, Edinburgh, UK.

Coello Coello, C. A., Toscano Pulido, G., & Salazar Lechuga, M. (2004, June). Handling multiple objectives with particle swarm optimization. *IEEE Transactions on Evolutionary Computation, 8*(3), 256–279.

Coello Coello, C. A., van Veldhuizen, D. A. & Lamont, G. B. (2002). *Evolutionary algorithms for solving multi-objective problems*. New York: Kluwer Academic.

Coello, C. (2006a). *EMOO repository*. Retrieved February 5, 2008 from, http://delta.cs.cinvestav.mx/ccoello/EMOO/

Coello, C. A. & Salazar Lechuga, M. (2002). MOPSO: A proposal for multiple objective particle swarm optimization. In *Proceedings of the 2002 IEEE Congress of Evolutionary Compututation* (pp. 1051-1056). IEEE Service Center.

Coello, C. A. C. (2006b). Evolutionary multi-objective optimization: A historical view of the field. *IEEE Computational Intelligence Magazine, 1*(1), 28-36.

Coello, C. A. C., Pulido, G. T., & Lechuga, M. S. (2004). Handling multiple objectives with particle swarm optimization. *IEEE Transactions one Evolutionary Computation, 8*(3), 256-279.

Coello, C. A., Toscano Pulido, G., & Salazar Lechuga, M. (2004). Handling multiple objectives with particle swarm optimization. *IEEE Trans. Evol. Comput., 8*(3), 256-279.

Cohon, J. L. (1983). *Multi-objective programming and planning*. New York: Academic Press.

Corne, D. W., Jerram, N. R., Knowles, J. D., & Oates, M. J. (2001). PESA-II: Region-based selection in evolutionary multi-objective optimization. In *Proceedings of the Genetic and Evolutionary Computation Conference (GECCO-2001)* (pp. 283-290). San Francisco: Morgan Kaufmann Publishers.

Corne, D. W., Knowles, J. D., & Oates, M. J. (2000). The Pareto-envelope based selection algorithm for multi-objective optimization. Parallel problem solving from nature-PPSN VI, Lecture notes in computer science (pp. 869-878). Springer

Cotta, C. & Troya, J.M. (2001). A comparison of several evolutionary heuristics for the frequency assignment problem. In J. Mira & A. Prieto (Eds), *Connectionist models of neurons, Learning processes, and artificial intelligence. Lecture notes in computer science* (Vol. 2084, pp. 709-716). Berlin, Heidelberg: Springer-Verlag.

Cristescu, R., Beferull-Lozano, B., & Vetterli, M. (2004). On network correlated data gathering. *IEEE INFOCOM, 4*(4), 2571-82.

Cutello, V., Narzisi, G., & Nicosia, G. (2005). A class of Pareto archived evolution strategy algorithms using immune inspired operators for ab-initio protein structure prediction. In *Proceedings of the Third European Workshop on Evolutionary Computation and Bioinformatics, EvoWorkshops 2005-EvoBio 2005*, Lausanne, Switzerland. *Lecture notes in computer science* (Vol. 3449, pp. 54-63).

Cutello, V., Narzisi, G., & Nicosia, G. (2006). A multi-objective evolutionary approach to the protein structure prediction problem. *Journal of the Royal Society Interface, 3*(6), 139-151.

Cutello, V., Narzisi, G., Nicosia, G., & Pavone, M. (2005). Clonal selection algorithms: A comparative case study using effective mutation potentials. In *Proceedings of 4th International Conference on Artificial Immune Systems, ICARIS 2005*, Banff, Canada. *Lecture notes in computer science* (Vol. 3627, pp. 13-28).

Cutello, V., Nicosia, G., & Pavone, M. (2004). Exploring the capability of immune algorithms: A characterization of hypemutation operators. In *Proceedings of Third International Conference on Artificial Immune Systems, ICARIS2004*, Catania, Italy. *Lecture notes in computer science* (Vol. 3239, pp. 263-276).

Cyberbotics. (2007). Retrieved February 12, 2008, from http://www.cyberbotics.com/products/robots/e-puck.html

Das, I. & Dennis, J. E. (1998). Normal-boundary intersection: A new method for generating the Pareto surface in nonlinear multicriteria optimization problems. *SIAM J. Optimization, 8*, 631-657.

Dasgupta, D. (1998). *Artificial immune systems and their applications*. Berlin, Germany: Springer.

Datta, D., Deb, K., & Fonseca, C. M. (2007). Multi-objective evolutionary algorithms for resource allocation problems. In S. Obayashi, K. Deb, C. Poloni, T. Hiroyasu & T. Murata (Eds.), *Evolutionary multi-criterion optimization.* In *Proceedings of the Fourth International Conference, EMO 2007. Lecture notes in computer science* (Vol. 4403, pp. 401-416). Berlin: Springer.

Davis, L. (1985). Applying adaptive algorithms to epistatic eomains. In *Proceedings of the International Joint Conference on Artificial Intelligence*, (pp 162 – 164). Morgan Kaufmann.

Davis, L. (1991). *Handbook of Genetic Algorithms*.

Day, R. O. (2005). *Explicit building block multi-objective evolutionary computation: Methods and applications*. Unpublished doctoral Dissertation, Air Force Institute of Technology, Wright-Patterson AFB, Dayton, OH.

Day, R. O., Kleeman, M. P., & Lamont, G. B. (2003). Solving the multi-objective quadratic assignment problem using a fast messy genetic algorithm. *Congress on Evolutionary Computation (CEC'2003)* (Vol. 4, pp. 2277–2283). Piscataway, New Jersey: IEEE Service Center.

de Castro, L. N. & Timmis, J. (2002b). An artificial immune network for multimodal function optimization. In *Proceedings of the 2002 Congress on Evolutionary Computation, CEC' 02* (Vol. 1, pp. 699-704).

de Castro, L. N. & Von Zuben, F. J. (2002). Learning and optimization using the clonal selection principle. *IEEE Transactions on Evolutionary Computation, 6*(3), 239-251.

de Castro, L. N., & Timmis, J. (2002a). Artificial immune systems: A new computational intelligence approach. Heidelberg, Germany: Springer-Verlag.

Deaton, R., Chen, J., Bi, H., Garzon, M., Rubin, H., & Wood, D. H. (2002). A PCR-based protocol for in vitro selection of non-crosshybridizing oligonucleotides. *Lecture notes in computer science* (Vol. 2568, pp. 196-204).

Deaton, R., Garzon, M., Murphy, R. C., Rose, J. A., Franceschetti, D. R., & Stevens, S. E., Jr. (1998). Reliability and efficiency of a DNA-based computation. *Physical Review Letters, 80*(2), 417-420.

Deb, K. & Agrawal, R. B. (1995). Simulated binary crossover for continuous search space. *Complex Systems, 9*, 115–148.

Deb, K. & Beyer, H. G. (2001). Self-adaptive genetic algorithms with simulated binary crossover. *Evolutionary Computation, 9*(2), 197-221.

Deb, K. & Jain, S. (2002). *Running performance metrics for evolutinary multi-objective optimization* (Tech. Rep. No. 2002004). KanGAL, Indian Institute of Technology, Kanpur 208016, India.

Deb, K. & Reddy, A. R. (2003). Reliable classification of two-class cancer data using evolutionary algorithms. *Biosystems, 72*(1-2), 111-129.

Deb, K. & Saxena, D. K. (2006). Searching for Pareto-optimal solutions through dimensionality reduction for certain large-dimensional multi-objective optimization problems. In *Proceedings of the 2006 Congress on Evolutionary Computation (CEC 2006)* (pp. 3353-3360), Vancouver, BC, Canada: IEEE Service Center.

Deb, K. (1999). Multi-objective genetic algorithms: Problem difficulties and construction of test problems. *Evolutionary Computation, 7*(3), 205-230.

Deb, K. (1999). Multi-objective genetic algorithms: Problem difficulties and construction of test problems. *Evolutionary Computation, 7*(3), 205-230.

Deb, K. (2000). An efficient constraint handling method for genetic algorithms. *Computer Methods in Applied Mechanics and Engineering, 186*(2-3), 311-338.

Deb, K. (2001). *Multi-objective optimisation using evolutionary algorithms*. New York: John Wiley and Sons.

Deb, K., & Goldberg, D. E. (1989). An investigation of niche and species formation in genetic function optimization. In *Proceedings of the 3rd International Conference on Genetic Algorithms* (pp. 42-50). Morgan Kaufmann Publishing.

Deb, K., Agarwa, l S., Pratap, A., & Meyarivan, T. (2000). A fast and elitist multi-objective genetic algorithm: NSGA-II. In *Proceedings of the Parallel Problem Solving from Nature VI*, (pp. 849-858).

Deb, K., Mohan, M., & Mishra, S. (2003). Towards a quick computation of well-spread Pareto-optimal solutions. In G. Goos et al. (Eds.), In *Proceedings of the Second International Conference on Evolutionary Multi-Criterion Optimization* (pp. 222-236). Springer-Verlag.

Deb, K., Mohan, M., & Mishra, S. (2005). Evaluating the epsilon-domination based multi-objective evolutionary algorithm for a quick computation of Pareto-optimal solutions. *Evolutionary Computation, 13*(4), 501-525.

Deb, K., Pratap, A., & Moitra, S. (2000). Mechanical component design for multiple objectives using elitist non-dominated sorting GA. In *Proceedings of the Parallel Problem Solving from Nature VI (PPSN-VI)* (pp. 859-868), Paris, France: Springer.

Deb, K., Pratap, A., Agarval, S., & Meyarivan, T. A. (2002). Fast and elitist multi-objective genetic algorithm: NSGA-II. *IEEE Transactions on Evolutionary Computing, 6*(2), 182–197.

Deb, K., Thiele, L., Laumanns, M., & Zitzler, E. (2001). *Scalable multi-objective optimization test problems* (Tech. Rep. No. 112). Computer Engineering and Networks Laboratory (TIK), Swiss Federal Institute of Technology (ETH), Zurich, Switzerland.

DeJong, K. A. (1975). *An analysis of the behavior of a class of genetic adaptive systems*. Unpublished doctoral thesis, University of Michigan, Ann Arbor.

Ding, M., Cheng, X., & Xue, G. (2003). Aggregation tree construction in sensor networks. *IEEE 58th Vehicular Technology Conference, 4*(4), 2168-2172.

Doerner, K., Gutjahr, W., Hartl, R., & Strauss, C. (2004). Pareto ant colony optimisation: A metaheuristic approach to multi-objective portfolio selection. *Annals of Operations Research, 131*, 79–99.

Dorigo, M. & Di Caro, G. (1999). The ant colony optimisation meta-heuristic. In D. Corne, M. Dorigo, & F. Glover (Eds.), *New ideas in optimisation* (pp. 11–32). London: McGraw-Hill.

Dorigo, M. & Stutzle, T. (2004). *Ant colony optimization*. MIT Press.

Dozier, G., McCullough, S., Homaifar, A., Tunstel, E., & Moore, L. (1998). Multi-objective evolutionary path planning via fuzzy tournament selection. In *Proceedings of the IEEE International Conference on Evolutionary Computation (ICEC'98)* (pp. 684–689). Piscataway, NJ: IEEE Press.

Drmanac, S., Stravropoulos, N. A., Labat, I., Vonau, J., Hauser, B., Soares, M. B., & Drmanac, R. (1996). Gene representing cDNA clusters defined by hybridization of 57,419 clones from infant brain libraries with short oligonucleotide probes. *Genomics, 37*, 29-40.

Du, H. F., Gong, M. G., Jiao, L. C., & Liu, R. C. (2005). A novel artificial immune system algorithm for high-dimensional function numerical optimization. *Progress in Natural Science, 15*(5), 463–471.

Eberhart, R. & Kennedy, J. (1995). A new optimizer using particle swarm theory. *6th international symposium on micro machine and human science* (pp. 39–43). Piscataway: IEEE-Press.

Eberhart, R. C. & Kennedy, J. (1995). A new optimizer using particle swarm theory. In *Proceedings of the Sixth Symposium on Micro Machine and Human Science* (pp. 39-43). Piscataway, NJ: IEEE Service Center.

Eberhart, R. C. & Shi, Y. (1998). Comparison between genetic algorithms and particle swarm optimization. In V. W. Porto et al. (Eds.), *Evolutionary programming: Vol. VII* (pp. 611-616). Springer.

Eeckhout, L., Nussbaum, S., Smith, J. E., & Bosschere, K. D. (2003, September-October). Statistical simulation: Adding efficiency to the computer designer's toolbox. *IEEE Micro, 23*(5), 26–38.

Ehrgott, M. (2005). *Multicriteria optimisation* (2nd ed.). Berlin, Germany: Springer.

Elsaycd, E. A. & Boucher, T. O. (1994). *Analysis and control of production systems*. Upper Saddle River, New Jersey: Prentice Hall.

Engelbrecht, A. (2005). *Fundamentals of computational swarm intelligence*. New York: John Wiley and Sons.

Erdem, E. & Ozdemirel, N. E. (2003). An evolutionary approach for the target allocation problem. *Journal of the Operational Research Society, 54*(9), 958-969.

Erel, E. & Gokcen, H. (1964). Shortest-route formulation of mixed-model assembly line balancing problem. *Management Science, 11*(2), 308-315.

Erickson, M., Mayer, A., & Horn, J. (2001). The niched Pareto genetic algorithm 2 applied to the design of groundwater remediation systems. *Lecture notes in computer science* (Vol. 1993, pp. 681-695). Springer-Verlag.

Erwin, M. C. (2006). *Combining quality of service and topology control in directional hybrid wireless networks*. Unpublished master's thesis, Graduate School of Engineering and Management, Air Force Institute of Technology, Wright-Patterson AFB, Dayton, OH.

Eshelman, L. (1991). The CHC adaptive search algorithm. *Foundations of genetic algorithms 1* (pp. 265–283). Morgan Kaufmann.

Eshelman, L. J. & Schaffer, J. D. (1993). Real-coded genetic algorithms and interval-schemata. In L. D. Whitley, (Ed.), *Foundations of genetic algorithms 2*, (pp. 187–202). California: Morgan Kaufmann Publishers.

Eyerman, S., Eeckhout, L., & Bosschere, K. D. (2006). Efficient design space exploration of high performance embedded out of-order processors. In *Date '06: Proceedings of the conference on design, automation and test in europe* (pp. 351–356).

Feldkamp, U., Saghafi, S., Banzhaf, W., & Rauhe, H. (2001). DNASequenceGenerator – A program for the construction of DNA sequences. *Lecture notes in computer science* (Vol. 2340, pp. 179-188).

Feoktistov, V. & Janaqi, S. (2004). New strategies in differential evolution. In *Proceedings of the 6th International Conference on Adaptive Computing in Design and Manufacture (ACDM 2004)* (pp. 335-346), Bristol, United Kingdom: Springer.

Ferentinos, K. P. & Tsiligiridis, T. A. (2007). Adaptive design optimization of wireless sensor networks using genetic algorithms. *Computer Networks: The International Journal of Computer and Telecommunications Networking, 51*(4), 1031-51.

Fieldsend, J. & Singh, S. (2002). A multi-objective algorithm based upon particle swarm optimisation, An efficient data structure and turbulence. In X. Tao (Ed.), *The U.K. workshop on computational intelligence* (pp. 34–44).

Fieldsend, J. E. & Singh, S. (2002). A multi-objective algorithm based upon particle swarm optimisation, An efficient data structure and turbulence. In *Proceedings of the 2002 UK Workshop on Computational Intelligence* (pp. 34-44). Birmingham, UK.

Fieldsend, J. E. & Singh, S. (2002, September). A multi-objective algorithm based upon particle swarm optimisation, An efficient data structure and turbulence. In *Proceedings of the 2002 U.K. Workshop on Computational Intelligence* (pp. 37-44), Birmingham, UK.

Fieldsend, J. E., Everson, R. M., & Singh, S. (2003). Using unconstrained elite archives for multi-objective optimization. *IEEE Trans. Evol. Comp., 7*(3), 305-323.

Fieldsend, J., Everson, R. M., & Singh, S. (2003). Using unconstrained elite archives for multi-objective optimization. *IEEE Transactions on Evolutionary Computation, 7*(3), 305-323.

Fishburn, P. C. (1974). Lexicographic orders, utilities, and decision rules: A survey. *Management Science, 20*(11), 1442-1471.

Fisher, J. A. (1983, June). Very long instruction word architectures and the ELI512. In *Tenth annual international symposium on computer architecture* (pp. 140–150).

Fisher, J. A., Faraboschi, P., Brown, G., Desoli, G., & Homewood, F. (2000, June). LX: A technology platform for customizable VLIW embedded processing. In *International symposium on computer architecture* (pp. 203–213).

Flikka, K., Yadetie, F., Laegreid, A., & Jonassen, I. (2004). XHM: A system for detection of potential cross hybridization in DNA microarrays. *BMC Bioinformatics, 5*(117).

Fogel, D. B., Fogel, L. J., & Porto, V. W. (1990). Evolving neural networks. *Biological Cybernetics, 63*(6), 487–493.

Fogel, G. B. & Corne, D. W. (2002). *Evolutionary computation in bioinformatics*. Morgan Kaufmann.

Fogel, L. (1962). Autonomous automata. *Industrial Research, 4*, 14–19.

Foli, K., Okabe, T., Olhofer, M., Jin, Y., & Sendhoff, B. (2006). Optimization of micro heat exchanger: CFD, analytical approach and multi-objective evolutionary algorithms. *International Journal of Heat and Mass Transfer, 49*(5-6), 1090-1099.

Fonseca, C. & Fleming, P. (1993). Genetic algorithms for multi-objective optimization: Formulation, discussion and generalization. In *Proceedings of the Fifth International Conference on Genetic Algorithms, San Mateo, California* (pp. 416-423). Morgan Kauffman Publishers.

Fonseca, C. & Fleming, P. (1996). On the performance assessement and comparision of stochastic multi-objective optimizers. In H.-M. Voigt, W. Ebeling, I. Rechenberg, and H.-P. Schwefel (Eds.), *Parallel problem solving from nature - PPSN IV, Lecture Notes in Computer Science* (pp. 584-593). Berlin, Germany: Springer Verlag.

Fonseca, C. M. & Fleming, P. J. (1995). An overview of evolutionary algorithms in multi-objective optimization. *Evolutionary Computation, 3*(1), 1-16.

Fonseca, C. M. & Fleming, P. J. (1998). Multi-objective optimization and multiple constraint handling with evolutionary algorithms-Part I: A unified formulation. *IEEE Transactions on Systems, Man, and Cybernetics-Part A: Systems and Humans, 28*(1), 26-37.

Fonseca, C. M. & Fleming, P. J. (1998). Multi-objective optimization and multiple constraint handling with evolutionary algorithms—Part I: A unified formulation. *IEEE Transactions on Systems, Man, and Cybernetics A, 28*, 26–37.

Fonseca, C. M., & Fleming, P. J. (1993). Genetic algorithms for multi-objective optimization: formulation, discussion and generalization. In S. Forest (Ed.), In *Genetic Algorithms: Proceedings of the Fifth International Conference* (pp. 416–423). San Mateo, CA: Morgan Kaufmann.

Fornaciari, W., Sciuto, D., Silvano, C., & Zaccaria, V. (2002). A sensitivity-based design space exploration methodology for embedded systems. *Design Automation for Embedded Systems, 7*, 7–33.

Forrest, S., Perelson, A. S., Allen, L., & Cherukuri, R. (1994). Self-nonself discrimination in a computer. In *Proceedings of the IEEE Symposium on Research in Security and Privacy* (pp. 202-212). Los Alamitos, CA: IEEE Computer Society Press.

Freschi, F. & Repetto, M. (2005). Multi-objective optimization by a modified artificial immune system algorithm. In *Proceedings of the 4th International Conference on Artificial Immune Systems, ICARIS 2005. Lecture notes in computer science* (Vol. 3627, pp. 248-261). Springer.

Friss, H. T. (1946). A note on a simple transmission formula. In *Proceedings of the Institute of Radio Engineers, Vol. 34* (pp. 254-56).

Fukuda, T., Mori, K., & Tsukiyama, M. (1993). Immune networks using genetic algorithm for adaptive production scheduling. In *Proceedings of the 15th IFAC World Congress* (Vol. 3, pp. 57-60).

Gacogne, L. (1997). Research of Pareto set by genetic algorithm, application to multicriteria optimization of fuzzy controller. In *Proceedings of the 5th European Congress on Intelligent Techniques & Soft Computing (EUFIT'97)* (pp. 837–845), Aachen, Germany.

Gacogne, L. (1999). Multiple objective optimization of fuzzy rules for obstacles avoiding by an evolution algorithm with adaptative operators. In *Proceedings of the Fifth International Mendel Conference on Soft Computing (Mendel'99)* (pp. 236–242), Brno, Czech Republic.

Gale, D. & Shapley, L. S. (1962). College admissions and the stability of marriage. *The American Mathematical Monthly, 69*(1), 9–15.

Galski, R., de Sousa, F., Ramos, F., & Muraoka, I. (2007). Spacecraft thermal design with the generalized extremal optimisation algorithm. *Inverse Problems in Science and Engineering, 15*, 61–75.

Gambardella, L., Taillard, E., & Agazzi, G. (1999). MACS-VRPTW - A multiple ant colony system for vehicle routing problems with time windows. In D. Corne, M. Dorigo, & F. Glover (Eds.), *New ideas in optimisation* (pp. 63–76). London: McGraw-Hill.

Garcia-Martinez, C., Cordón, O., & Herrera, F. (2004). An empirical analysis of multiple objective ant colony optimisation algorithms for the bi-criteria TSP. In M. Dorigo, M. Birattari, C. Blum, L. Gambardella, F. Mondada, & T. Stützle (Eds.), *4th international workshop on ant colony optimisation and swarm intelligence: Vol. 3172. Lecture notes in computer science* (pp. 61–72). Berlin: Springer-Verlag.

Garcia-Martinez, C., Cordón, O., & Herrera, F. (2007). A taxonomy and an empirical analysis of multiple objective ant colony optimisation algorithms for bi-criteria TSP. *European Journal of Operational Research, 180*, 116–148.

Garey, M. & Johnson, D. (1979). *Computers and intractability: A guide to the theory of NP completeness.* San Francisco, CA: W. H. Freeman and Company.

Garey, M. R. & Johnson, D. S. (1979). *Computers and intractability: A guide to the theory of NP-completeness.* San Francisco, CA: W. H. Freeman and Co.

Garrett, D., & Dasgupta, D., (2006). Analyzing the Performance of Hybrid Evolutionary Algorithms for the Multi-objective Quadratic Assignment Problem. *IEEE Congress on Evolutionary Computation, (CEC 2006),* (pp. 1710- 1717). IEEE.

Garrett, D., Vannucci, J., Silva, R., Dasgupta, D., & Simien, J. (2005). Genetic algorithms for the sailor assignment problem. In H. G. Beyer & U. M. O'Reilly (Eds.), In *Proceedings of Genetic and Evolutionary Computation (GECCO 2005),* (pp. 1921-1928). ACM.

Garrett, D., Vannucci, J., Silva, R., Dasgupta, D., & Simien, J. (2005). Genetic algorithms for the sailor assignment problem. In *Proceedings of the 2005 Genetic and Evolutionary Computation Conference (GECCO),* (pp 1921-1928).

Garrett, S. M. (2004). Parameter-free, Adaptive clonal selection. In *Proceedings of IEEE Congress on Evolutionary Computing, CEC 2004* (pp. 1052-1058), Portland, Oregon.

Garrett, S. M. (2005). How do we evaluate artificial immune systems. *Evolutionary Computation, 13*(2), 145-178.

Garzon, M. H. & Deaton, R. J. (1999). Biomolecule computing and programming. *IEEE Transactions on Evolutionary Computation, 3*(3), 236-250.

Garzon, M. H. & Deaton, R. J. (2004). Codeword design and information encoding in DNA ensembles. *Natural Computing, 3*, 253-292.

Gaspar-Cunha, A. & Vieira, A. S. (2004, August). A hybrid multi-objective evolutionary algorithm using an inverse neural network. In *Hybrid metaheuristics, workshop at ECAI 2004.*

Gaweda, A. & Zurada, J. (2001, July 16-19). Equivalence between neural networks and fuzzy systems. In *Proceedings of international joint conference on neural networks* (p. 1334-1339).

Geoffrion, A. M., Dyer, J. S., & Feinberg, A. (1972). An interactive approach for multi-criterion optimization, with an application to the operation of an academic department. *Management Science, 19*(4), 357-368.

Ghosh, A. & Givargis, T. (2004, October). Cache optimization for embedded processor cores: An analytical approach. *ACM Transactions on Design Automation of Electronic Systems, 9*(4), 419–440.

Gibbons, J. D. (1985). *Nonparametric statistical inference* (2nd ed.). M. Dekker.

Gies, D. & Rahmat-Samii, Y. (2004). Vector evaluated particle swarm optimization (VEPSO): Optimization of a radiometer array antenna. In *Proceedings of the AP-S IEEE International Symposium (Digest) of Antennas and Propagation Society, Vol. 3* (pp. 2297-2300).

Givargis, T., Vahid, F., & Henkel, J. (2000). A hybrid approach for core-based system-level power modeling. In *Asia and South Pacific Design Automation Conference.*

Givargis, T., Vahid, F., & Henkel, J. (2002, August). System-level exploration for Pareto-optimal configurations in parameterized System-on-a-Chip. *IEEE Transactions on Very Large Scale Integration Systems, 10*(2), 416–422.

Glover, F. (1977). Heuristic for integer programming using surrogate constraints. *Decision Sciences, 8*, 156–166.

Glover, F. (1994). Tabu search for nonlinear and parametric optimization (with links to genetic algorithms). *Discrete Applied Mathematics, 49*(1-3), 231–255.

Glover, F. (1998). A template for scatter search and path relinking. In *AE '97: Selected papers from the third European conference on artificial evolution*, (pp. 13–54). London, UK: Springer-Verlag.

Goldberg, D. (1989). *Genetic algorithms in search, optimisation and machine learning*. Reading, MA: Addison Wesley.

Goldberg, D. (2002). *The design of innovation: Lessons from and for competent genetic algorithms*. Massachusetts: Kluwer Academic Publishers.

Goldberg, D. E. & Lingle, R. (1985). Alleles, loci, and the traveling salesman problem. In *Proceedings of the First International Conference on Genetic Algorithms and Their Applications*, (pp. 154-159).

Goldberg, D. E. & Lingle, R. (1985). Alleles, loci, and the traveling salesman problem. In *Proceedings of the International Conference on Genetic Algorithms and their Applications*, (pp 154-159).

Goldberg, D. E. (1989). *Genetic algorithms is search, optimization, and machine learning*. Reading, Massachusetts: Addison-Wesley Publishing.

Golinski J. (1970). Optimal synthesis problems solved by means of nonlinear programming and random methods. *Journal of Mechanisms, 5*, 287 – 309.

Gong, M. G., Jiao, L. C., Du, H. F., & Wang, L. (2005). An artificial immune system algorithm for CDMA multiuser detection over multi-path channels. In *Proceedings of the Genetic and Evolutionary Computation Conference (GECCO-2005)* (pp. 2105-2111), Washington, D.C.

Gonzalez, F., Dasgupta, D., & Kozma, R. (2002). Combining negative selection and classification techniques for anomaly detection. In *Proceedings of the Special Sessions on Artificial Immune Systems in Congress on Evolutionary Computation, IEEE World Congress on Computational Intelligence*, Honolulu, Hawaii.

Gordon, P. M. K. & Sensen, C. W. (2004). Osprey: A comprehensive tool employing novel methods for design of oligonucleotides for DNA sequencing and microarrays. *Nucleic Acid Research, 32*(17), 133.

Grierson, D. & Pak, W. (1993). Optimal sizing, geometrical and topological design using genetic algorithms. *Journal of Structured Optimization, 6*, 151–159.

Guan, L. & Kamel, M. (1992). Equal-average hyperplane portioning method for vector quantization of image data. *Pattern Recognition Letters, 13*(10), 693-699.

Guitouni, A., Bélanger, M., & Berger, J., (2000). *Report on final lance exercise* (Tech. Rep. DREV-TM-2000-21). Canadian Forces College.

Güngör, A. & Gupta, S. M. (1999a). A systematic solution approach to the disassembly line balancing problem. In *Proceedings of the 25th International Conference on Computers and Industrial Engineering* (pp. 70-73), New Orleans, Louisiana.

Güngör, A. & Gupta, S. M. (1999b). Disassembly line balancing. In *Proceedings of the 1999 Annual Meeting of the Northeast Decision Sciences Institute* (pp. 193-195), Newport, Rhode Island.

Güngör, A. & Gupta, S. M. (1999c). Issues in environmentally conscious manufacturing and product recovery: A survey. *Computers and Industrial Engineering, 36*(4), 811-853.

Güngör, A. & Gupta, S. M. (2001). A solution approach to the disassembly line problem in the presence of task failures. *International Journal of Production Research, 39*(7), 1427-1467.

Güngör, A. & Gupta, S. M. (2002). Disassembly line in product recovery. *International Journal of Production Research, 40*(11), 2569-2589.

Guntsch, M. & Middendorf, M. (2003). Solving multi-criteria optimisation problems with population-based ACO. In G. Goos, J. Hartmanis, & J. van Leeuwen (Eds.), *Second international conference on evolutionary multi-criterion optimisation: Vol. 2632. Lecture notes in computer science* (pp. 464–478). Berlin: Springer-Verlag.

Gupta, S. & Najm, F. N. (2000a, July). *Analytical models for RTL power estimation of combinational and sequential circuits*.

Gupta, S. & Najm, F. N. (2000b, February). Power modeling for high-level power estimation. *IEEE Transactions on Very Large Scale Integration Systems, 8*(1), 18–29.

Gupta, S. M. & Taleb, K. (1994). Scheduling disassembly. *International Journal of Production Research, 32*(8), 1857-1866.

Gutjahr, A. L. & Nemhauser, G. L. (1964). An algorithm for the line balancing problem. *Management Science, 11*(2), 308-315.

Hackman, S. T., Magazine, M. J., & Wee, T. S. (1989). Fast, effective algorithms for simple assembly line balancing problems. *Operations Research, 37*(6), 916-924.

Haimes, Y. Y., Lasdon, . S., & Wismer, D. A. (1971). On a bicriteriion formulation of the problem of integrated system identification and system optimization. *IEEE Transactions on Systems, Man, and Cybernetics, 1*(3), 296-297.

Hajela, P. & Lin, C.Y. (1992). Genetic search strategies in multicriterion optimal design. *Structural Optimization, 4*, 99–107.

Hajela, P., Yoo, J., & Lee, J. (1997). GA based simulation of immune networks-applications in structural optimization. *Journal of Engineering Optimization*.

Hajri-Gabouj, S. (2003). A fuzzy genetic multi-objective optimization algorithm for a multilevel generalized assignment problem. *IEEE Transactions on Systems, Man and Cybernetics, Part C: Applications and Reviews, 33*(2), 214 – 224.

Handl, J. (2006). *Multi-objective approaches to the data-driven analysis of biological systems*. Unpublished doctoral dissertation, University of Manchester, Manchester, UK.

Hansen, N. & Ostermeier, A. (1996). Adapting arbitrary normal mutation distributions in evolutionary strategies: the covariance matrix adaptation. In *Proceedings of the 1996 IEEE International Conference on Evolutionary Computation (ICEC '96)* (pp. 312-317), Nayoya, Japan: IEEE Service Center.

Hart, E. & Timmis, J. (2005). Application areas of AIS: The past, the present and the future. In *Proceedings of the 4th International Conference on Artificial Immune Systems, ICARIS 2005. Lecture notes in computer science* (Vol. 3627, pp. 483-497). Springer

Hart, E., & Ross, P. (1999). The evolution and analysis of a potential antibody library for use in job-shop scheduling. *New ideas in optimization* (pp. 185–202). McGraw-Hill.

Hartemink, D. K., Gifford, D. K., & Khodor, J. (1999). Automated constraint-based nucleotide sequence selection for DNA computation. *Biosystems, 52*(1-3), 227-235.

Heinzelman, W. R., Chandrakasan, A. P., & Balakrishnan, H. (2002). An application-specific protocol architecture for wireless microsensor networks. *IEEE Trans Wireless Communications, 1*(4), 660-670.

Heinzelman, W., Chandrakasan, A., & Balakrishnan, H. (2000). Energy-efficient communication protocol for wireless micro sensor networks. In *Proceedings of Hawaii Conference on System Sciences*.

Hekstra, G., Hei, D. L., Bingley, P., & Sijstermans, F. (1999, October 10–13). TriMedia CPU64 design space exploration. In *International conference on computer design* (pp. 599–606). Austin Texas.

Hernández-Díaz, A. G., Santana-Quintero, L. V., Coello Coello, C. A., Caballero, R., & Molina, J. (2006). A new proposal for multi-objective optimization using Differential Evolution and rough sets theory. In *Proceedings of the Genetic and Evolutionary Computation Conference (GECCO 2006)* (pp. 675-682). Seattle, WA: ACM Press.

Hernández-Díaz, A. G., Santana-Quintero, L. V., Coello Coello, C., & Molina, J. (2006, March). *Pareto-adaptive ε-dominance* (Tech. Rep. No. EVOCINV-02-2006). México: Evolutionary computation group at CINVESTAV, Sección de Computación, Departamento de Ingeniería Eléctrica, CINVESTAV-IPN.

Hernández-Díaz, A. G., Santana-Quintero, L. V., Coello Coello, C., Caballero, R., & Molina, J. (2006, July). A new proposal for multi-objective optimization using differential evolution and rough sets theory. In M. K. et al., (Eds.), *2006 genetic and evolutionary computation conference (GECCO'2006)*, (Vol. 1, pp. 675–682). Seattle, Washington: ACM Press.

Hilbert, R., Janiga, G., Baron, R., & Thévenin, D. (2006). Multi-objective shape optimization of a heat exchanger using parallel genetic algorithms. *International Journal of Heat and Mass Transfer, 49*(15-16), 2567–2577.

Hillier, F. S. & Lieberman, G. J. (2005). *Introduction to operations research*. New York: McGraw-Hill.

Ho, S. L., Yang, S., Ni, G., Lo, E. W. C., & Wong, H. C. (2005). A particle swarm optimization-based method for multi-objective design optimizations. *IEEE Trans. Magnetics, 41*(5), 1756-1759.

Holder, A. (2005). Navy personnel planning and the optimal partition. *Operations Research, 53* 77-89.

Holland, J. H. (1975). *Adaptation in natural and artificial systems*. Ann Arbor, MI: University of Michigan Press.

Horn, J. & Nafpliotis, N. (1993). *Multi-objective optimization using the niched Pareto genetic algorithm* (Tech. Rep.) IlliGAL Report 93005, Illinois Genetic Algorithms Laboratory, University of Illinois, Urbana, Champaign.

Horn, J. (1997). Multicriteria decision making. In T. Back, D. B. Gogel, & Z. Michalewicz (Eds.), *Handbook of evolutionary computation*. Institute of Physics Publishing.

Horn, J., Nafpliotis, N., & Goldberg, D. (1994). A niched Pareto genetic algorithm for multi-objective optimization. In *Proceedings of the First IEEE Conference on Evolutionary Computation* (Vol. 1, pp. 82-87). IEEE World Congress on Computational Intelligence, Piscataway, New Jersey.

Horn, J., Nafpliotis, N., & Goldberg, D. E. (1994). A niched Pareto genetic algorithm for multi-objective optimization. In *Proceedings of the 1st IEEE Conference on Evolutionary Computation* (pp. 82-87).

Hu, T. C. & Shing, M. T. (2002). *Combinatorial algorithms*. Mineola, NY: Dover Publications.

Hu, X. & Eberhart, R. (2002). Multi-objective optimisation using dynamic neighborhood particle swarm optimisation. In D. Fogel, M. El-Sharkawi, X. Yao, G. Greenwood, H. Iba. P. Marrow, & M. Shackleton (Eds.), *Congress on evolutionary computation* (pp. 1677–1681). Piscataway: IEEE-Press.

Hu, X. & Eberhart, R. (2002). Multi-objective optimization using dynamic neighborhood particle swarm optimization. In *Proceedings of the 2002 IEEE Congress Evolutionary Computututation* (pp. 1677-1681). IEEE Service Center.

Hu, X., Eberhart, R. C., & Shi, Y. (2003). Particle swarm with extended memory for multi-objective optimization. In *Proceedings of the 2003 IEEE Swarm Intelligence Symposium* (pp. 193-197). IEEE Service Center.

Huang, V. L., Qin, A. K., & Suganthan, P. N. (2006). Self-adaptive differential evolution algorithm for constrained real-parameter optimization. In *Proceedings of the 2006 Congress on Evolutionary Computation (CEC 2006)* (pp. 324-331). Vancouver, BC, Canada: IEEE Service Center.

Hughes, E. (2003a, April). Multi-objective binary search optimization. In *Lecture notes on computer science*. In *Proceedings of Second International Conference on Evolutionary Multi-Criterion Optimization* (pp. 102–117).

Hughes, E. (2003b, December). Multiple single objective pareto sampling. In *Proceedings of IEEE Congress on Evolutionary Computation, 2003* (Vol. 4, pp. 2678–2684).

Hughes, E. J. (2007). Radar waveform optimization as a many-objective application benchmark. In *Proceedings of 4th International Conference on Evolutionary Multi-Criterion Optimization (EMO)*, (pp. 700-714).

Huo, X. H., Shen, L. C., Zhu, H. Y. (2006). A smart particle swarm optimization algorithm for multi-objective problems. *Lecture notes in computer science* (Vol. 4115, pp. 72-80). Springer-Verlag.

Igel, C., Hansen, N., & Roth, S. (2007). Covariance matrix adaptation for multi-objective optimization. *Evolutionary Computation, 15*(1), 1-28.

Ignizio, J. P. (1974). Generalized goal programming: An overview. *Computer and Operations Research, 10*(4), 277-289.

Iorio, A. & Li, X. (2004). Solving rotated multi-objective optimization problems using differential evolution. In *Proceedings of the 17th Australian Joint Conference on Artificial Intelligence (AI 2004)* (pp. 861-872). Cairns, Australia.

Iorio, A. & Li, X. (2006). Incorporating directional information within a differential evolution for multi-objective optimization. In *Proceedings of the Genetic and Evolutionary Computing Conference (GECCO 2006)* (pp. 691-697). Seattle, WA: ACM Press.

Iredi, S., Merkle, D., & Middendorf, M. (2001). Bi-criterion optimisation with multi colony ant algorithms. In E. Zitzler, K. Deb, L. Thiele, C. Coello Coello, & D. Corne (Eds.), *First international conference on evolutionary multi-criterion optimisation: Vol. 1993. Lecture notes in computer science* (pp. 359–372). Berlin: Springer-Verlag.

Ireland, D., Lewis, A., Mostaghim, S., & Lu, J. (2006). Hybrid particle guide selection methods in multi-objective particle swarm optimisation. In P. Sloot, G. van Albada, M. Bubak, & A. Referthen (Eds.), *2nd international e-science and grid computing conference (Workshop on biologically-inspired optimisation methods for parallel and distributed architectures: Algorithms, systems and applications)*. Piscataway: IEEE-Press.

Ishibuchi, H., Yoshida, T., & Murata, T. (2003). Balance between genetic search and local search in memetic algorithms for multi-objective permutation flowshop scheduling. *IEEE Transactions on Evolutionary Computing, 7*, 204–223.

Ishida, Y. (1990). Fully distributed diagnosis by PDP learning algorithm: Towards immune network PDP model. In *Proceedings of the International Joint Conference on Neural Networks: 777–782*

Jacob, C., Pilat, M. L., Bentley, P. J., & Timmis, J. (Eds.) (2005). *Artificial immune systems: Proceedings of the fourth international conference on artificial immune systems, ICARIS 2005*. Lecture notes in computer science (Vol. 3627). Banff, Alberta, Canada: Springer-Verlag.

Janson, S. & Middendorf, M. (2004). A hierarchical particle swarm optimizer for dynamic optimization problems. *Lecture notes in computer science* (Vol. 3005, pp. 513-524). Springer-Verlag.

Jensen, M. T. (2003). Reducing the run-time complexity of multi-objective EAs: the NSGA-II and other algorithms. *IEEE Transactions on Evolutionary Computation, 7*(5), 503-515.

Jia, D. & Vagners, J. (2004). Parallel evolutionary algorithms for UAV path planning. In *Proceedings of the AIAA 1st Intelligent Systems Technical Conference*.

Jiang, R., & Sun, C. (1993). Functional equivalence between radial basis function networks and fuzzy inference systems. *IEEE Transactions on Neural Networks, 4*, 156-159.

Jiao, L. C. & Wang, L. (2000). A novel genetic algorithm based on immunity. *IEEE Transactions on Systems, Man and Cybernetics, Part A, 30*(5), 552-561.

Jiao, L. C., Gong, M. G., Shang, R. H., Du, H. F., & Lu, B. (2005). Clonal selection with immune dominance and anergy based multi-objective optimization. In *Proceedings of the Third International Conference on Evolutionary Multi-Criterion Optimization, EMO 2005*. Guanajuato, Mexico: Springer-Verlag, Lecture notes in computer science (Vol. 3410, pp. 474-489).

Jiao, L. C., Liu, J., & Zhong, W. C. (2006). An organizational coevolutionary algorithm for classification. *IEEE Transactions on Evolutionary Computation, 10*(1), 67-80.

Jin, M. H., Wu, H. K., Horng, J. T., & Tsai, C. H. (2001). An evolutionary approach to fixed channel assignment problems with limited bandwidth constraint. In *Proceedings of the 2001 IEEE International Conference on Communications, ICC 2001, Vol. 7*, (pp. 2100–2104).

Jin, R., Chen, W., & Simpsons, T. (2000). *Comparative studies of metamodeling techniques under multiple modeling criteria* (Tech. Rep. No. 2000–4801). AIAA.

Jin, Y. (2005). A comprehensive survey of fitness approximation in evolutionary computation. *Soft Computing, 9*(1), 3-12.

Jin, Y., Olhofer, M., & Sendhoff, B. (2000). On evolutionary optimization with approximate fitness functions. In *Proceedings of genetic and evolutionary computation conference* (pp. 786–793).

Jin, Y., Olhofer, M., & Sendhoff, B. (2001). Evolutionary dynamic weighted aggregation for multi-objective optimization: Why does it work and how? In *Proceedings of the GECCO 2001 Conference* (pp. 1042-1049), San Francisco, CA.

Jin, Y., Olhofer, M., & Sendhoff, B. (2002). A framework for evolutionary optimization with approximate fitness function. *IEEE Transactions on Evolutionary Computation, 6*(5), 481–494.

Johnston, M. D. (2006). Multi-objective scheduling for NASA's future deep space network array. In *Proceedings of the 5th International Workshop on Planning and Scheduling for Space (IWPSS 2006)* (pp. 27-35). Baltimore, MD.

Jourdan, D. B. & de Weck, O. L. (2004). Layout optimization for a wireless sensor network using a multi-objective genetic algorithm. In *Proceedings of the IEEE 59th Vehicular Technology Conference, Vol. 5* (pp. 2466-70).

Jourdan, D. B. & de Weck, O. L. (2004). Multi-objective genetic algorithm for the automated planning of a wireless sensor network to monitor a critical facility. In *Proceedings of the SPIE Defense and Security Symposium, Vol. 5403*, (pp. 565-575).

Jourdan, D. B. & de Weck, O.L. (2004). Layout optimization for a wireless sensor network using a multi-objective genetic algorithm. In Proceedings of the *IEEE Semiannual Vehicular Technology Conference*.

KanGAL. (2003). *NSGA-II source code (real & binary-coded + constraint handling)*. Retrieved February 12, 2008, from http://www.iitk.ac.in/kangal/code/nsga-2code.tar

Kaplinski, L., Andreson, P., Puurand, T., & Remm, M. (2005). MultiPLX: Automatic grouping and evaluation PCR assay design. *Bioinformatics, 21*(8), 1701-1702.

Kar, K. & Banerjee, S. (2003). Node placement for connected coverage in sensor networks. In *Proceedings WiOpt: Modeling and Optimization in Mobile, Ad Hoc and Wireless Networks.*

Kelemen, A., Kozma, R., & Liang, Y. (2002). Neuro-fuzzy classification for the job assignment problem. *International Joint Conference on Neural Networks IJCNN02, World Congress on Computational Intelligence WCCI2002*, (pp. 630-634). IEEE.

Kelemen, A., Kozma, R., & Liang, Y., (2002). Neuro-fuzzy classification for the job assignment problem. *International Joint Conference on Neural Networks IJCNN02, World Congress on Computational Intelligence WCCI2002*, (pp. 630-634). Honolulu, Hawaii: IEEE.

Keller, T. A. & Lamont, G. B. (2004). Optimization of a quantum cascade laser operating in the terahertz frequency range using a multi-objective evolutionary algorithm. In *Proceedings on 17th International Conference on Multiple Criteria Decision Making (MCDM 2004). Vol 1.*

Kennedy, J. & Eberhart, R. (1995). Particle swarm optimisation. *International conference on neural networks* (pp. 1942–1948). Piscataway: IEEE-Press.

Kennedy, J. & Eberhart, R. C. (1995). Particle swarm optimization. In *Proceedings of IEEE International Conference on Neural Networks* (Vol. 4, pp. 1942-1948).

Kennedy, J. & Eberhart, R. C. (1995). Particle swarm optimization. In *Proceedings of the IEEE International Conference Neural Networks, Vol. IV* (pp. 1942-1948). Piscataway, NJ: IEEE Service Center.

Kennedy, J. & Eberhart, R. C. (2001). *Swarm intelligence*. California: Morgan Kaufmann Publishers.

Kennedy, J. (1999). Small worlds and mega-minds: effects of neighborhood topology on particle swarm performance. In *Proceedings of the IEEE Congress Evolutionary Computation* (pp. 1931-1938). IEEE Press.

Kent, W. J. (2002). BLAT – The BLAST-like alignment tool. *Genome Research, 12*, 656-664.

Khare, V., Yao, X., & Deb, K. (2003). Performance scaling of multi-objective evolutionary algorithms. In *Proceedings of the Evolutionary Multi-Objective Optimization Conference, Lecture notes in computer science* (Vol. 2632, pp. 346-390). Springer.

Khare, V., Yao, X., & Deb, K. (2003). Performance scaling of multi-objective evolutionary algorithms. In *Proceedings of the Second International Conference on Evolutionary Multi-Criterion Optimization, EMO 2003. Lecture notes in computer science* (Vol. 2632, pp. 376-390). Springer-Verlag

Kim, D. E. & Hallam, J. (2002). An evolutionary approach to quantify internal states needed for the Woods problem. In B. Hallam, D. Floreano, G. Hayes, J. Hallam, & J.A. Meyer (Eds.), *From Animals to Animats 7: Proceedings of the Seventh International Conference on the Simulation of Adaptive Behavior (SAB2002)* (pp. 312–322). Cambridge, MA: MIT Press.

Kita, H., Yabumoto, Y., Mori, N., & Nishikawa, Y. (1996, September). Multi-objective optimization by means of the thermodynamical genetic algorithm. In H-M. Voigt, W. Ebeling, I. Rechenberg, & H-P. Schwefel, (Eds.), *Parallel problem solving from nature—PPSN IV* (pp. 504–512), Berlin, Germany: Springer-Verlag.

Kitano, H. (1990). Designing neural networks using genetic algorithms with graph generation system. *Complex Systems, 4*(4), 461–476.

Kleeman, M. P. & Lamont, G. B. (2005). Solving the aircraft engine maintenance scheduling problem using a multi-objective evolutionary algorithm. In *Proceedings of Evolutionary Multi-Criterion Optimization (EMO 2005), LNCS 3410*, (pp. 782-796). Berlin Heidelberg: Springer-Verlag.

Kleeman, M. P. & Lamont, G. B. (2006). The multi-objective constrained assignment problem. In *Proceedings of Genetic and Evolutionary Computation (GECCO 2006)* (Vol. 1, pp. 743-744). ACM.

Kleeman, M. P. & Lamont, G. B. (2007). Scheduling of a combined flow-shop, job-shop scheduling problem using an MOEA with a variable length chromosome. *Evolutionary scheduling*. Springer Verlag.

Kleeman, M. P. & Lamont, G. B. (2007). The multi-objective constrained assignment problem. In *Proceedings of 2007 SPIE Symposium on Defense & Security: Evolutionary and Bio-inspired Computation: Theory and Applications*, Orlando, FL: SPIE.

Kleeman, M. P. & Lamont, G. B. (2007). The multi-objective constrained assignment problem. In *Proceedings of SPIE Symposium on Defense & Security 2007:*

Evolutionary and Bio-inspired Computation: Theory and Applications.

Kleeman, M. P. (2004). *Optimization of heterogeneous UAV communications using the multi-objective quadratic assignment problem*. Unpublished master's thesis, Graduate School of Engineering and Management, Air Force Institute of Technology, Wright-Patterson AFB, Dayton, OH.

Kleeman, M. P., Day, R. O., & Lamont, G. B., (2004). Multi-objective evolutionary search performance with explicit building-block sizes for NPC problems. *Congress on Evolutionary Computation (CEC'2004)* (Vol. 2, pp. 728–735). Piscataway, New Jersey: IEEE Service Center.

Kleeman, M. P., Lamont, G. B., Cooney, A., & Nelson, T. R. (2007). A multi-tiered memetic multi-objective evolutionary algorithm for the design of quantum cascade lasers. In *Proceedings of Evolutionary Multi-Criterion Optimization (EMO 2007), LNCS 4403*, (pp 186-200). Springer-Verlag.

Kleeman, M. P., Lamont, G. B., Hopkinson, K. M., & Graham, S. R., (2007). Solving multicommodity capacitated network design problems using a multi-objective evolutionary algorithm. In *Proceedings of 2007 IEEE Symposium on Computational Intelligence for Security and Defense Applications (CISDA 2007)*, (pp. 33-41).

Knarr, M. R., Goltz, M. N., Lamont, G. B., & Huang, J. (2003). In situ boremediation of perchlorate-contaminated groundwater using a multi-objective parallel evolutionary algorithm. In *Proceedings of IEEE Congress on Evolutionary Computation (CEC'2003)* (Vol. 1, pp. 1604–1611).

Knowles, J D. & Corne, D. W. (2000). Approximating the nondominated front using the Pareto archived evolution strategy. *Evolutionary computation, 8*(2), 149-172.

Knowles, J. & Corne, D. (2000a). Approximating the nondominated front using the pareto archibed evoltion strategy. *Evolutionary Computation, 8*(2), 149-172.

Knowles, J. & Hughes, E. J. (2005, March). Multi-objective optimization on a budget of 250 evaluations. *Lecture notes on computer science*. In *Proceedings of Third International Conference on Evolutionary Multi-Criterion Optimization* (Vol. 3410, p. 176-190).

Knowles, J. (2005). A summary-attainment-surface plotting method for visualizing the performance of stochastic multi-objective optimizers. In *Proceedings of the 5th International Conference on Intelligent Systems Design and Applications* (pp. 552–557).

Knowles, J. (2006, February). ParEGO: A hybrid algorithm with on-line landscape approximation for expensive multi-objective optimization problems. *IEEE Transactions on Evolutionary Computation, 10*(1), 50–66.

Knowles, J. D. & Corne, D. W. (1999). The Pareto archived evolution strategy: A new baseline algorithm for multi-objective optimization. *In Proceedings of the 1999 congress on Evolutionary Computation* (pp. 98-105).

Knowles, J. D. & Corne, D. W. (1999). The Pareto archived evolution strategy: A new baseline algorithm for Pareto multi-objective optimisation. In *Proceedings of the 1999 Congress on Evolutionary Computation (CEC'99)*, (pp. 98-105).

Knowles, J. D. & Corne, D. W. (2000). Approximating the nondominated front using the Pareto archived evolution strategy. *Evolutionary Computation, 8*(2), 149–172.

Knowles, J. D. & Corne, D. W. (2002). Towards landscape analyses to inform the design of a hybrid local search for the multi-objective quadratic assignment problem. In A. Abraham, J. Ruiz-del-Solar, & M. Koppen (Eds.), *Soft computing systems: Design, management and applications*, (pp. 271—279). Amsterdam: IOS Press.

Knowles, J. D. & Corne, D. W. (2003). Instance generators and test suites for the multi-objective quadratic assignment problem. In *Proceedings of Evolutionary Multi-Criterion Optimization (EMO 2003) Second International Conference*, (pp 295-310). Faro, Portugal.

Knowles, J. D. & Corne, D.W. (2000). Approximating the nondominated front using the Pareto Archived Evolution Strategy. *Evolutionary Computation, 8*(2), 149-172.

Knowles, J. D., Thiele, L., & Zitzler, E. (2006, February). *A tutorial on the performance assessment of stochastive multi-objective optimizers* (Tech. Rep. No. 214). ETH Zurich, Swiss: Computer Engineering and Networks Laboratory.

Knowles, J., Thiele, L., & Zitzler, E. (2006). *A tutorial on the performance assessment of stochastic multi-objective optimizers* (Rev. ed.) (Tech. Rep. No. 214), Computer Engineering and Networks Laboratory (TIK), Swiss Federal Institute of Technology (ETH), Zurich, Switzerland.

Koski, J. (1985). Defectiveness of weighting method in multicriterion optimisation of structures. *Communications in Applied Numerical Methods, 1*, 333–337.

Koza, J. R. & Rice, J. P. (1991). Genetic generation of both the weights & architecture for a neural network. In *Proceedings of the 1991 International Joint Conference on Neural Networks: Vol. 2* (pp. 397–404). Piscataway, NJ: IEEE Press.

Kukkonen, S. & Deb, K. (2006a). A fast and effective method for pruning of non-dominated solutions in many-objective problems. In *Proceedings of the 9th International Conference on Parallel Problem Solving from Nature (PPSN IX)* (pp. 553-562). Reykjavik, Iceland: Springer.

Kukkonen, S. & Deb, K. (2006b). Improved pruning of non-dominated solutions based on crowding distance for bi-objective optimization problems. In *Proceedings of the 2006 Congress on Evolutionary Computation (CEC 2006)* (pp. 3995-4002). Vancouver, BC, Canada: IEEE Service Center.

Kukkonen, S. & Lampinen, J. (2004a). Comparison of generalized differential evolution algorithm to other multi-objective evolutionary algorithms. In *Proceedings of the 4th European Congress on Computational Methods in Applied Sciences and Engineering (ECCOMAS 2004)*. Jyväskylä, Finland.

Kukkonen, S. & Lampinen, J. (2004b). A differential evolution algorithm for constrained multi-objective optimization: Initial assessment. In *Proceedings of the IASTED International Conference on Artificial Intelligence and Applications (AIA 2004)* (pp. 96-102). Innsbruck, Austria: ACTA Press.

Kukkonen, S. & Lampinen, J. (2004c). An extension of generalized differential evolution for multi-objective optimization with constraints. In *Proceedings of the 8th International Conference on Parallel Problem Solving from Nature (PPSN VIII)* (pp. 752-761). Birmingham, England: Springer.

Kukkonen, S. & Lampinen, J. (2004d). Mechanical component design for multiple objectives using generalized differential evolution. In *Proceedings of the 6th International Conference on Adaptive Computing in Design and Manufacture (ACDM 2004)* (pp. 261-272). Bristol, United Kingdom: Springer.

Kukkonen, S. & Lampinen, J. (2005a). An empirical study of control parameters for generalized differential evolution. In *Proceedings of the Sixth Conference on Evolutionary and Deterministic Methods for Design, Optimization and Control with Applications to Industrial and Societal Problems (EUROGEN 2005)*. Munich, Germany.

Kukkonen, S. & Lampinen, J. (2005b). GDE3: The third evolution step of generalized differential evolution. In *Proceedings of the 2005 Congress on Evolutionary Computation (CEC 2005)* (pp. 443-450). Edinburgh, Scotland: IEEE Service Center.

Kukkonen, S. & Lampinen, J. (2006a). Constrained real-parameter optimization with generalized differential evolution. In *Proceedings of the 2006 Congress on Evolutionary Computation (CEC 2006)* (pp. 911-918). Vancouver, BC, Canada: IEEE Service Center.

Kukkonen, S. & Lampinen, J. (2006b). An empirical study of control parameters for the third version of generalized differential evolution (GDE3). In *Proceedings of the 2006 Congress on Evolutionary Computation (CEC 2006)* (pp. 7355-7362). Vancouver, BC, Canada: IEEE Service Center.

Kukkonen, S., Jangam, S. R., & Chakraborti, N. (2007). Solving the molecular sequence alignment problem with generalized differential evolution 3 (GDE3). In *Proceedings of the 2007 IEEE Symposium on Computational Intelligence in Multi-Criteria Decision-Making (MCDM 2007)* (pp. 302-309). Honolulu, HI: IEEE Service Center.

Kukkonen, S., Sampo, J., & Lampinen, J. (2004). Applying generalized differential evolution for scaling filter design. In *Proceedings of Mendel 2004, 10th International Conference on Soft Computing* (pp. 28-33). Brno, Czech Republic.

Kulik, J., Heinzelman, W. R., & Balakrishnan, H. (2002). Negotiation-based protocols for disseminating information in wireless sensor networks. *Wireless Networks, 8*, 169-185.

Kursawe, F. (1991). A variant of evolution strategies for vector optimization. *Parallel problem solving from nature-PPSN* I. Lecture notes in computer science (Vol. 496, pp. 193-197). Springer-Verlag

Kursawe, F. (1991, October). A variant of evolution strategies for vector optimization. In H. P. Schwefel & R. Männer, (Eds.), *Parallel problem solving from nature.* In *Proceedings of the 1st Workshop, PPSN I*, (Vol. 496, pp. 193–197), Berlin, Germany: Springer-Verlag.

Kyosho. (2007). Retrieved February 12, 2008, from http://www.kyosho.com/jpn/products/robot/index.html

Laguna, M. & Martí, R. (2003). *Scatter search: Methodology and implementations in C.* Kluwer Academic Publishers.

Lahanas, M. (2004). Application of multi-objective evolutionary optimization algorithms in Medicine. In C. A. Coello Coello & G. B. Lamont (Eds.), *Applications of multi-objective evolutionary algorithms* (pp. 365-391). World Scientific.

Lahanas, M., Baltas, D., & Zamboglou, N. (2003). A hybrid evolutionary algorithm for multi-objective anatomy-based dose optimization in high-dose-rate brachytherapy. *Physics in Medicine and Biology, 48*(3), 339-415.

Lambert, A. D. J. (2003). Disassembly sequencing: A survey. *International Journal of Production Research, 41*(16), 3721-3759.

Lambert, A. J. D. & Gupta, S. M. (2005). *Disassembly modeling for assembly, maintenance, reuse, and recycling.* Boca Raton, FL: CRC Press (Taylor & Francis).

Lamont, G. B., Slear, J., & Melendez, K., (2007). UAV swarm mission planning and routing using multi-objective evolutionary algorithms. In *Proceedings of 2007 IEEE Symposium on Intelligent Computation in Multi-Criteria Decision Making.*

Lampinen, J. & Zelinka, I. (1999). Mechanical engineering design optimization by Differential Evolution. *New ideas in optimization* (pp. 128-146). London: McGraw-Hill.

Lampinen, J. (2001). *DE's selection rule for multi-objective optimization* (Tech. Rep.). Lappeenranta University of Technology, Department of Information Technology.

Lampinen, J. (2002). A constraint handling approach for the differential evolution algorithm. In *Proceedings of the 2002 Congress on Evolutionary Computation (CEC 2002)* (pp. 1468-1473). Honolulu, HI: IEEE Service Center.

Landajo, M., Río, M. J., & Pérez, R. (2001, April). A note on smooth approximation capabilities of fuzzy systems. *IEEE Transactions on Fuzzy Systems, 9,* 229–236.

Lange, D. B. & Oshima, M. (1999). Seven good reasons for mobile agents. *Comm. ACM, 42*(3), 88-89.

Lapierre, S. D., Ruiz, A., & Soriano, P. (2006). Balancing assembly lines with tabu search. *European Journal of Operational Research, 168*(3), 826-837.

Larraanaga, P. & Lozano, J. A. (2002). *Estimation of distribution algorithms: A new tool for evolutionary computation.* Norwell, MA: Kluwer Academic Publishers.

Laumanns, M., Thiele, L., Deb, K., & Zitzler, E. (2002). Combining convergence and diversity in evolutionary multi-objective optimization. *Evolutionary Computation, 10*(3), 263-282.

Laumanns, M., Thiele, L., Deb, K., & Zitzler, E. (2002, Fall). Combining convergence and diversity in evolutionary multi-objective optimization. *Evolutionary Computation, 10*(3), 263–282.

Lazzaretto, A., & Toffolo, A. (2004). Energy, economy and environment as objectives in multi-criterion optimization of thermal systems design. *Energy, 29*(8), 1139-1157.

Lazzaretto, A., & Toffolo, A. (2006), On the synthesis of thermal systems: a method to determine optimal heat transfer interactions. In C. A. Frangopoulos, C. D. Rakopoulos, G. Tsatsaronis (Eds.), In *Proceedings of ECOS06: Vol. 1* (pp. 493-501).

Lazzaretto, A., & Toffolo, A. (2007), Energy system diagnosis by a fuzzy expert system with genetically evolved rules. In A. Mirandola, O. Arnas, A. Lazzaretto (Eds.), In *Proceedings of ECOS07: Vol. 1* (pp. 311-318).

Lee, C., Wu, J.-S., Shiue, Y.-L., & Liang, H.-L. (2006). MultiPrimer: Software for multiplex primer design. *Applied Bioinformatics, 5*(2), 99-109.

Lee, I.-H., Kim, S., & Zhang, B.-T. (2004b). Multi-objective evolutionary probe design based on thermodynamic criteria for HPV detection. *Lecture notes in computer science* (Vol. 3157, pp. 742-750).

Lee, I.-H., Shin, S.-Y., & Zhang, B.-T. (2004c). Experimental analysis of ε-multi-objective evolutionary algorithm. In *Proceedings of International Conference on Simulated Evolution and Learning 2004,* SWP-1/127.

Lee, I.-H., Shin, S.-Y., & Zhang, B.-T. (2007). Multiplex PCR assay design by hybrid multi-objective evolutionary algorithm. *Lecture notes in computer science* (Vol. 4403, pp. 376-385).

Lee, J. Y. & Lee, J. J. (2004). Multi-objective walking trajectories generation for a biped robot. In *Proceedings of the IEEE/RSJ International Conference on Intelligent Robots & Systems (IROS 2004)* (pp. 3853-3858), Sendai, Japan.

Lee, J. Y., Shin, S.-Y., Park, T. H., & Zhang, B.-T. (2004a). Solving traveling salesman problems with DNA molecules encoding numerical values. *BioSystems, 78,* 39-47.

Leger, P. C. (1999). *Automated synthesis & optimization of robot configurations: An evolutionary approach.* Unpublished doctoral dissertation, Carnegie Mellon University, Pennsylvania.

LEGO. (2007). Retrieved February 12, 2008, from http://mindstorms.lego.com/

Lewis, A., Abramson, D., & Peachey, T. (2003). An evolutionary programming algorithm for automatic engineering design. In R. Wyrzykowski, J. Dongarra, M. Paprzycki, & J. Wasniewski (Eds.), *5th international conference on parallel processing and applied mathematics: Vol. 3019. Lecture notes in computer science* (pp. 586–594). Berlin: Springer-Verlag.

Lewis, M. W., Lewis, K. R., & White, B. J. (2004). Guided design search in the interval-bounded sailor assignment problem. *Computers and operations research.* Elsevier.

Leyland, G. B. (2002). *Multi-objective optimisation applied to industrial energy problems.* Unpublished doctoral thesis 2572, Swiss Federal Institute of Technology, Lausanne.

Li, F. & Stormo, G. D. (2001). Selection of optimal DNA oligos for gene expression arrays. *Bioinformatics, 17,* 1067-1076.

Li, H. & Zhang, Q. (2006). A multi-objective differential evolution based on decomposition for multi-objective optimization with variable linkages. In *Proceedings of the 9th International Conference on Parallel Problem Solving from Nature (PPSN IX)* (pp. 583-592). Reykjavik, Iceland: Springer.

Li, X. (2003). A non-dominated sorting particle swarm optimizer for multi-objective optimization. *Lecture notes in computer science, Vol. 2723* (pp. 37-48). Springer-Verlag.

Li, X. (2004). Better spread and convergence: Particle swarm multi-objective optimization using the maximin fitness function. *Lecture notes in computer science, Vol. 3102* (pp. 117-128). Springer-Verlag.

Liang, Y., Lin, K. I., & Kelemen, A. (2002). Adaptive generalized estimation equation with bayes classifier for the job assignment problem. In *PAKDD '02: Proceedings of the 6th Pacific-Asia Conference on Advances in Knowledge Discovery and Data Mining,* (pp. 438-449). London, UK: Springer-Verlag.

Liang, Y., Lin, K.-I., & Kelemen, A. (2002). Adaptive generalized estimation equation with bayes classifer for the job assignment problem. In *Proceedings of the 6th Pacific-Asia Conference on Advances in Knowledge Discovery and Data Mining (PAKDD '02),* (pp. 438-449). Springer-Verlag.

Liao, W. & He, L. (2001, September). Power modeling and reduction of VLIW processors. In *International Conference on Parallel Architectures and Compilation Techniques* (pp. 81–88).

Liao, W., Basile, J., & He, L. (2002, November). Leakage power modeling and reduction with data retention. In *IEEE/ACM International Conference on Computer-Aided Design.*

Lin, Y.-C., Hwang, K.-S., & Wang, F.-S. (2002). Hybrid differential evolution with multiplier updating method for nonlinear constrained optimization problems. In *Proceedings of the 2002 Congress on Evolutionary Computation (CEC 2002)* (pp. 872-877). Honolulu, HI: IEEE Service Center.

Lindsey, S., Raghavendra, C., & Sivalingam, K. M. (2002). Data gathering algorithms in sensor networks using energy metrics. *IEEE Transactions on Parallel and Distributed Systems, 13*(9), 924-35.

Lorena, L. A. N., Narciso, M. G., & Beasley, J. E, (1999). *A constructive genetic algorithm for the generalized assignment problem.* Technical report.

Lucas, J. M., Martinez-Barbera, H., & Jimenez, F. (2005). Multi-objective evolutionary fuzzy modeling for the docking maneuver of an automated guided vehicle. In *2005 IEEE International Conference on Systems, Man & Cybernetics* (pp. 2757-2762). Piscataway, NJ: IEEE Press.

Luh, G. C., Chueh, C. H., & Liu, W. W. (2003). MOIA: Multi-objective immune algorithm. *Engineering Optimization, 35*(2), 143-164.

Luh, G. C., Chueh, C. H., & Liu, W. W. (2004). Multi-objective optimal design of truss structure with immune algorithm. *Computers and Structures, 82,* 829–844.

Lund, H. H. & Hallam, J. (1997). Evolving sufficient robot controllers. In *Proceedings of the 4th IEEE International Conference on Evolutionary Computation* (pp. 495–499). Piscataway, NJ: IEEE Press.

Macki, J. & Strauss, A. (1982). *Introduction to optimal control theory.* New York: Springer-Verlag.

Madavan, N. K. (2002). Multi-objective optimization using a Pareto differential evolution approach. In *Proceedings of the 2002 Congress on Evolutionary Computation (CEC 2002)* (pp. 1145-1150). Honolulu, HI: IEEE Service Center.

Mahfouf, M., Chen, M.-Y., & Linkens, D. A. (2004). Adaptive weighted particle swarm optimisation for multi-objective optimal design of alloy steels. *Lecture notes in computer science* (Vol. 3242, pp. 762-771). Springer.

Mahfouf, M., Chen, M-Y., & Linkens, D. A. (2004, September). Adaptive weighted particle swarm optimisation for multi-objective optimal design of alloy steels. *Parallel problem solving from nature - PPSN VIII*, (pp. 762–771). Birmingham, UK: Springer-Verlag.

Maley, C. C. (1998). DNA computation: Theory, practice, and prospects. *Evolutionary Computation, 6*(3), 201-229.

Marathe, A., Condon, A. E., & Corn, R. M. (1999). On combinatorial DNA word design. In E. Winfree & D. K. Gifford (Eds.), In *Proceedings of 5th International Meeting on DNA Based Computers* (pp. 75-89). AMS-DIMACS Series.

Mariano, C. & Morales, E. (1999). *A multiple objective ant-Q algorithm for the design of water distribution irrigation networks* (Tech. Rep. HC-9904), Mexico City: Instituto Mexicano de Tecnologia del Agua.

Mataric, M. & Cliff, D. (1996). Challenges in evolving controllers for physical robots. *Robotics & Autonomous Systems, 19*, 67-83.

Mathieu, O. (2005). *Utilisation d'algorithmes évolutionnaires dans le cadre des problèmes d'empaquetage d'objets*. Unpublished master's thesis, Facultes Universitaires Notre-Dame de la Paix Namur, Brussels.

Mauri, G. & Ferretti, C. (2004). Word design for molecular computing: A survey. *Lecture notes in computer science* (Vol. 2943, pp. 32-36).

McCauley, L. & Franklin, S. (2002). A large-scale multi-agent system for navy personnel distribution. *Connect. Sci., 14*(4), 371-385.

McGeer, T. (1990). Passive dynamic walking. *International Journal of Robotics Research, 9*(2), 62–82.

McGill, R., Tukey, J. W., & Larsen, W. A. (1978). Variations of boxplots. *The American Statistician, 32*, 12-16.

McGovern, S. M. & Gupta, S. M. (2003). Greedy algorithm for disassembly line scheduling. In *Proceedings of the 2003 IEEE International Conference on Systems, Man, and Cybernetics* (pp. 1737-1744), Washington, D.C.

McGovern, S. M. & Gupta, S. M. (2004). Combinatorial optimization methods for disassembly line balancing. In *Proceedings of the 2004 SPIE International Conference on Environmentally Conscious Manufacturing IV* (pp. 53-66), Philadelphia, Pennsylvania.

McGovern, S. M. & Gupta, S. M. (2005). Local search heuristics and greedy algorithm for balancing the disassembly line. *The International Journal of Operations and Quantitative Management, 11*(2), 91-114.

McGovern, S. M. & Gupta, S. M. (2006a). Computational complexity of a reverse manufacturing line. In *Proceedings of the 2006 SPIE International Conference on Environmentally Conscious Manufacturing VI* (CD-ROM), Boston, Massachusetts.

McGovern, S. M. & Gupta, S. M. (2006b). Performance metrics for end-of-life product processing. In *Proceedings of the 17th Annual Production & Operations Management Conference* (CD-ROM) Boston, Massachusetts.

McGovern, S. M., & Gupta, S. M. (2007). A balancing method and genetic algorithm for disassembly line balancing. *European Journal of Operational Research, 179*(3), 692-708.

McGovern, S. M., Gupta, S. M., & Kamarthi, S. V. (2003). Solving disassembly sequence planning problems using combinatorial optimization. In *Proceedings of the 2003 Northeast Decision Sciences Institute Conference* (pp. 178-180), Providence, Rhode Island.

Meyer-Nieberg, S. & Beyer, H. (2007). Self-adaptation in evolutionary algorithms. In F. Lobo, C. Lima, & Z. Michalewicz (Eds.), *Parameter settings in evolutionary algorithms: Vol. 54. Studies in computational intelligence* (pp. 47–76). Berlin: Springer-Verlag.

Mezura-Montes, E., Coello Coello, C. A., & Tun-Morales, E. I. (2004). Simple feasibility rules and differential evolution for constrained optimization. In *Proceedings of the 3rd Mexican International Conference on Artificial Intelligence (MICAI 2004)* (pp. 707-716). Mexico City, Mexico.

Michalewicz, Z. & Janikow, C. Z. (1996). Genocop: A genetic algorithm for numerical optimization problems with linear constraints. *Commun. ACM, 39*(12), 223–240.

Michalewicz, Z. (1996). *Genetic algorithms + data structures = evolution* programs (3rd ed.). London: Springer-Verlag..

Miettinen, K. (1994). *On the methodology of multi-objective optimization with applications.* Unpublished doctoral thesis (Rep. No. 60), University of JyvÄaskylÄa, Department of Mathematics.

Miettinen, K. (1998). *Nonlinear multiobjective optimization.* Boston: Kluwer Academic Publishers.

Mikut, R., Jäkel, J., & Gröll, L. (2005). Interpretability issues in data-based learning of fuzzy systems. *Fuzzy Sets and Systems, 150,* 179–197.

Miller, G. F., Todd, P. M., & Hegde, S. U. (1989). Designing neural networks using genetic algorithms. In J.D. Schaffer (Ed.), In *Proceedings of the Third International Conference on Genetic Algorithms* (pp. 379–384). San Mateo, CA: Morgan Kaufmann.

Moore, J. & Chapman, R. (1999). *Application of particle swarm to multi-objective optimization.* Unpublished manuscript, Department of Computer Science and Software Engineering, Auburn University.

Mostaghim, S. & Halter, W. (2006). Bilevel optimisation of multi-component silicate melts using particle swarm optimisation. In D. Fogel (Ed.), *Congress on evolutionary computation* (pp. 4383–4390). Piscataway: IEEE-Press.

Mostaghim, S. & Teich, J. (2003). Strategies for finding good local guides in multi-objective particle swarm optimisation. *Swarm intelligence symposium* (pp. 26–33). Piscataway: IEEE-Press.

Mostaghim, S. & Teich, J. (2003, April). Strategies for finding good local guides in multi-objective particle swarm optimization (MOPSO). In *2003 IEEE SIS Proceedings*, (pp. 26–33). Indianapolis, IN: IEEE Service Center.

Mostaghim, S. & Teich, J. (2003a). Strategies for finding good local guides in multi-objective particle swarm optimization (MOPSO). In *Proceedings of the 2003 IEEE Swarm Intelligence Symposium* (pp. 26-33). IEEE Service Center.

Mostaghim, S. & Teich, J. (2003b). The role of ε-dominance in multi objective particle swarm optimization methods. In *Proceedings of the IEEE 2003 Congress on Evolutionary Computation* (pp. 1764-1771). IEEE Press.

Mostaghim, S. & Teich, J. (2004). Covering Pareto-optimal fronts by subswarms in multi-objective particle swarm optimization. In *Proceedings of the IEEE 2004 Congress on Evolutionary Computation* (pp. 1404-1411). IEEE Press.

Mostaghim, S. & Teich, J. (2006). About selecting the personal best in multi-objective particle swarm optimization. *Lecture notes in computer science* (Vol. 4193, pp. 523-532). Springer.

Mostaghim, S. (2005). *Multi-objective evolutionary algorithms: Data structures, Convergence and, diversity.* Unpublished doctoral thesis, University of Paderborn, Paderborn.

Mostaghim, S., Branke, J., & Schmeck, H. (2006). *Multi-objective particle swarm optimisation on computer grids* (Tech. Rep. No. 502). Karlsruhe, Germany: University of Karlsruhem, AIFB Institute.

Nain, P. & Deb, K. (2002). *A computationally effective multi-objective search and optimization technique using coarse-to-fine grain modeling* (Tech. Rep. No. Kangal 2002005). Kanpur, India: IITK.

Nair, P. & Keane, A. (1998). Combining approximation concepts with genetic algorithm-based structural optimization procedures. In *Proceeding of 39th AIAA/AASME/ASCE/AHS/ASC Structures, Structural Dynamics and Materials Conference* (p. 1741-1751).

Najm, F. N. & Nemani, M. (1998). Delay estimation VLSI circuits from a high-level view. In *Conference on Design Automation Conference* (pp. 591–594).

Najm, F. N. (1995, January). A survey of power estimation techniques in VLSI circuits. *IEEE Transactions on Very Large Scale Integration Systems, 2*(4), 446–455.

Nassif, N., Kajl, S., & Sabourin, R. (2005). Evolutionary algorithms for multi-objective optimization in HVAC system control strategy. *International Journal of Heating, Ventilating, Air-Conditioning and Refrigerating Research (ASHRAE), 11*(3), 459-486.

Neema, S., Sztipanovits, J., & Karsai, G. (2002, June). *Design-space construction and exploration in platform-based design* (Tech. Rep. No. ISIS-02-301). Institute for Software Integrated Systems Vanderbilt University Nashville Tennessee.

Nelson, A. L. & Grant, E. (2006). Developmental analysis in evolutionary robotics. In *2006 IEEE Mountain Workshop on Adaptive & Learning Systems* (pp. 201-206). Pistacaway, NJ: IEEE Press.

Nicodeme, P. & Steyaert, J.-M. (1997). Selecting optimal oligonucleotide primers for multiplex PCR. In T. Gaasterland et al. (Eds.), In *Proceedings of the 5th International Conference on Intelligent Systems for Molecular Biology* (pp. 210-213). AAAI.

Nicosia, G., Cutello, V., Bentley, P. J., & Timmis, J. (Eds.) (2004). Artificial immune systems. In *Proceedings of The Third International Conference on Artificial Immune Systems, ICARIS 2004,* Catania, Italy. *Lecture notes in computer science* (Vol. 3239). Springer-Verlag

Nissen, V. & Propach, J. (1998). On the robustness of population-based versus point-based optimization in the presence of noise. *IEEE Transactions on Evolutionary Computation, 2*(3), 107-119.

Niu, R., Varshney, P., & Cheng, Q. (2006). Distributed detection in a large wireless sensor network. *International Journal on Information Fusion, 7*(4), 380-394.

Nolfi, S. & Floreano, D. (2000). *Evolutionary robotics: The biology, intelligence & technology of self-organizing machines.* Cambridge, MA: MIT Press/Bradford Books.

Nolfi, S. (2002). Power & limits of reactive agents. *Neurocomputing, 42,* 119–145.

Oduguwa, A., Tiwari, A., Fiorentino, S., & Roy, R. (2006). Multi-objective optimization of the protein-ligand docking problem in drug discovery. In M. Keijzer et al. (Eds.), In *Proceedings of the 8th Annual Conference on Genetic and Evolutionary Computation* (pp. 1793-1800). ACM Press.

Oh, C. K. & Barlow, G. J. (2004). Autonomous controller design for unmanned aerial vehicles using multi-objective genetic programming. In *2004 IEEE Congress on Evolutionary Computaton (CEC 2004)* (pp. 1538-1545). Piscataway, NJ: IEEE Press.

Oliveira, A. C. M. & Lorena, L. A. N. (2001). A constructive evolutionary approach to linear gate assignment problems. *ENIA 2001 – Encontro Nacional de Inteligência Artificial.* Fortaleza, Brazil.

Oliver, I. M., Smith, D. J., & Holland, J. R. C. (1987). A study of permutation crossover operators on the traveling salesperson problem. In *Proceedings of the Second International Conference on Genetic Algorithms and their Applications,* (pp. 224 – 230).

Osman, I. H. & Laporte, G. (1996). Metaheuristics: A bibliography. *Annals of Operations Research, 63,* 513-623.

Osman, I. H. (2004). Metaheuristics: Models, design and analysis. In *Proceedings of the Fifth Asia Pacific Industrial Engineering and Management Systems Conference* (pp. 1.2.1-1.2.16), Gold Coast, Australia.

Osyczka, A. & Kundu, S. (1995). A new method to solve generalized multicriteria optimization problems using the simple genetic algorithm. *Structural Optimization, 10,* 94–99.

Palaniappan, S., Zein-Sabatto, S., & Sekmen, A. (2001). Dynamic multi-objective optimization of war resource allocation using adaptive genetic algorithms. In *Proceedings of the IEEE Southeast Conf.,* (pp. 160-165).

Papadimitriou, C. H. & Steiglitz, K. (1998). *Combinatorial optimization: Algorithms and complexity.* Mineola, NY: Dover Publications.

Papoulis, A. (1984). *Probability, random variables, and stochastic processes.* McGraw-Hill.

Pareto, V. (1896). *Cours d'e_conomie politique professe_ a_l'universite_ de Lausanne* (Vol. 1,2). F. Rouge, Laussanne.

Pareto, V. (1896). *Cours d'economie politique.* Geneve: Libraire Droz.

Parsopoulos, K. & Vrahatis, M. (2002). Particle swarm optimisation method in multi-objective problems. In B. Panda (Ed.), *Symposium on applied computing* (pp. 603–607). New York: ACM Press.

Parsopoulos, K. E. & Vrahatis, M. N. (2002a). Recent approaches to global optimization problems through particle swarm optimization. *Natural Computing, 1*(2-3), 235-306.

Parsopoulos, K. E. & Vrahatis, M. N. (2002b). Particle swarm optimization method in multi-objective problems. In *Proceedings of the ACM 2002 Symposium on Applied Computing* (pp. 603-607). ACM Press.

Parsopoulos, K. E. & Vrahatis, M. N. (2004). On the computation of all global minimizers through particle swarm optimization. *IEEE Transactions on Evolutionary Computation, 8*(3), 211-224.

Parsopoulos, K. E. & Vrahatis, M. N. (2007). Parameter selection and adaptation in unified particle swarm optimization. *Mathematical and Computer Modelling, 46*(1-2), 198-213.

Parsopoulos, K. E., Tasoulis, D. K., & Vrahatis, M. N. (2004). Multi-objective optimization using parallel vector evaluated particle swarm optimization. In *Proceedings of the IASTED 2004 International Conference on Artificial Intelligence and Applications* (pp. 823-828). IASTED/ACTA Press.

Parsopoulos, K. E., Tasoulis, D. K., Pavlidis, N. G., Plagianakos, V. P., & Vrahatis, M. N. (2004). Vector evaluated differential evolution for multi-objective optimization. In *Proceedings of the 2004 Congress on Evolutionary Computation (CEC 2004)* (pp. 204-211). Portland, OR: IEEE Service Center.

Parsopoulos, K. E., Tasoulis, K. E., & Vrahatis, K. E. (2004, February). Multi-objective optimization using parallel vector evaluated particle swarm optimization. In *Proceedings of the IASTED International Conference on Artificial Intelligence and Applications (AIA 2004)*, (Vol. 2, pp. 823–828). Innsbruck, Austria: ACTA Press.

Pasemann, F., Steinmetz, U., Hulse, M., & Lara, B. (2001). Evolving brain structure for robot control. In J. Mira & A. Prieto (Eds.), In *Proceedings of the International Work-Conference on Artificial & Natural Neural Networks (IWANN'2001): Vol. 2* (pp. 410–417). Berlin: Springer-Verlag.

Pattem, S., Poduri, S., & Krishnamachari, B. (2003). Energy-quality tradeoffs for target tracking in wireless sensor networks. In *Proceedings Information Processing in Sensor Networks* (pp. 32-46).

Patti, D. & Palesi, M. (2003, July). *EPIC-Explorer*. Retrieved February 11, 2008, http://epic-explorer.sourceforge.net/

Penchovsky, R. & Ackermann, J. (2003). DNA library design for molecular computation. *Journal of Computational Biology, 10*(2), 215-229.

Pirjanian, P. (1998). Multiple objective action selection in behavior-based control. In *Proceedings of the 6th Symposium for Intelligent Robotic Systems* (pp. 83–92), Edinburgh, UK.

Pirjanian, P. (2000). Multiple objective behavior-based control. *Robotics & Autonomous Systems, 31*(1-2), 53–60.

Ponnambalam, S. G., Aravindan, P., & Naidu, G. M. (1999). A comparative evaluation of assembly line balancing heuristics. *The International Journal of Advanced Manufacturing Technology, 15*, 577-586.

Price, K. & Storn, R. (1996). Minimizing the real functions of the ICEC'96 contest by differential evolution. In *Proceedings of the 1996 IEEE International Conference on Evolutionary Computation (ICEC '96)* (pp. 842-844). Nagoya, Japan: IEEE Service Center.

Price, K. V. (1999). An introduction to differential evolution. *New ideas in optimization* (pp. 79-108). London: McGraw-Hill.

Price, K. V., Storn, R. M., & Lampinen, J. A. (2005). *Differential evolution: A practical approach to global optimization*. Berlin: Springer-Verlag.

Price, K., Storn, R., & Lampinen, J. (2005). *Differential evolution - A practical approach to global optimization*. Berlin, Germany: Springer.

Purshouse, R. & Fleming, P. (2003). Evolutionary multi-objective optimisation: An exploratory analysis. In R. Sarker, R. Reynolds, H. Abbass, K. Tan, B. McKay, D. Essam, & T, Gedeon (Eds.), *Congress on evolutionary computation* (pp. 2066–2073). Piscataway: IEEE-Press.

Qi, H., Iyengar, S. S., & Chakrabarty, K. (2001). Multi-resolution data integration using mobile agents in distributed sensor networks. *IEEE Transactions on Systems, Man and Cybernetics Part C: Applications and Rev., 31*(3), 383-391.

Qi, H., Iyengar, S. S., & Chakrabarty, K. (2001). Multiresolution data integration using mobile agents in distributed sensor networks. *IEEE Transactions on Systems, Man and Cybernetics Part C: Applications and Rev., 31*(3), 383-391.

Ra, S.-W. & Kim, J.-K. (1993). A fast mean-distance-ordered partial codebook search algorithm for image vector quantization. *IEEE Transactions on Circuits and Systems-II, 40*(9), 576-579.

Rachlin, J., Ding, C., Cantor, C., & Kasif, S. (2005a). MuPlex: Multi-objective multiplex PCR assay design. *Nucleic Acids Research, 33*(web server issue), w544-w547.

Rachlin, J., Ding, C., Cantor, C., & Kasif, S. (2005b). Computational tradeoffs in multiplex PCR assay design for SNP genotyping. *BMC Genomics, 6*(102).

Rachmawati, L. & Srinivasan, D. (2005). A hybrid fuzzy evolutionary algorithm for a multi-objective resource allocation problem. In *Proceedings of the Fifth International Conference on Hybrid Intelligent Systems (HIS'05)*, (pp. 55-60).

Ragsdell, K. E. & Phillips, D. T. (1975). Optimal design of a class of welded structures using geometric programming. *Journal of Engineering for Industry Series B, B*(98), 1021–1025.

Raich, A. M. & Liszkai, T. R. (2003). Multi-objective genetic algorithms for sensor layout optimization in structural damage detection. In *Proceedings of the Artificial Neural Networks in Engineering Conference* (pp. 889-894).

Rajagopalan, R. & Varshney, P. K. (2006). Data aggregation techniques in sensor networks: A survey. *IEEE Communications Surveys and Tutorials, 8*(4), 48-63.

Rajagopalan, R. (2004). *Path planning with evolutionary algorithms*. Unpublished master's thesis, Department of Electrical Engineering & Computer Science, Syracuse University.

Rajagopalan, R., Mohan, C. K., Mehrotra, K. G. & Varshney, P. K. (2004). Evolutionary multi-objective crowding algorithm for path computations. In *Proceedings of the Fifth International Conference on Knowledge Based Computer Systems*, (pp. 46-65).

Rajagopalan, R., Mohan, C. K., Mehrotra, K. G., & Varshney, P. K. (2005a). An evolutionary multi-objective crowding algorithm: Benchmark test function results. In *Proceedings 2nd Indian International Conference on Artificial Intelligence* (pp.1488-1506), Pune, India.

Rajagopalan, R., Mohan, C. K., Mehrotra, K. G., & Varshney, P. K. (2006). EMOCA: An evolutionary multi-objective crowding algorithm. *Journal of Intelligent Systems*.

Rajagopalan, R., Mohan, C. K., Varshney, P. K., & Mehrotra, K. G. (2005b). Multi-objective mobile agent routing in wireless sensor networks. In *Proceedings IEEE Congress on Evolutionary Computation* (Vol. 2, pp.1730-1737).

Rajagopalan, R., Mohan, C. K., Varshney, P. K., & Mehrotra, K. G. (2005c). Sensor placement for energy efficient target detection in wireless sensor networks: A multi-objective optimization approach. In *Proceedings of the 39th Annual Conference on Information Sciences and Systems*, Baltimore, Maryland.

Rajagopalan, R., Mohan, C., Varshney, P., & Mehrotra, K. G. (2005). Multi-objective mobile agent routing in wireless sensor networks. In *Proceedings of 2005 IEEE Congress on Evolutionary Computation (CEC'2005)* (Vol. 2, pp. 1730—1737).

Rajagopalan, R., Varshney, P. K., Mehrotra, K. G., & Mohan, C. K. (2005). Fault tolerant mobile agent routing in sensor networks: A multi-objective optimization approach. In *Proceedings of the 2nd IEEE Upstate NY workshop on Comm. and Networking*.

Rajapakse, M., Schmidt, B., & Brusic, V. (2006). Multi-objective evolutionary algorithm for discovering peptide binding motifs. *Lecture notes in computer science* (Vol. 3907, pp. 149-158).

Rakowska, J., Haftka, R. T., & Watson, L. T. (1991). Tracing the efficient curve for multi-objective control-structure optimization. *Computing Systems in Engineering, 2*(6), 461-471.

Randall, M. & Lewis, A. (2006). An extended extremal optimisation model for parallel architectures. In P. Sloot, G. van Albada, M. Bubak, & A. Referthen (Eds.), *2nd international e-science and grid computing conference (Workshop on biologically-inspired optimisation methods for parallel and distributed architectures: Algorithms, systems and applications)*. Piscataway: IEEE-Press.

Randall, M. (2005). A dynamic optimisation approach for ant colony optimisation using the multidimensional knapsack problem. In H. Abbass, T. Bossamaier, & J. Wiles (Eds.), *Recent advances in artificial life* (pp. 215–226). Singapore: World Scientific.

Raquel, C. R. & Naval, P. C., Jr. (2005). An effecive use of crowding distance in multi-objective particle swarm optimization. In *Proceedings of the GECCO 2005* (pp. 257-264). ACM Press.

Ratle, A. (1999). Optimal sampling stategies for learning a fitness model. In *Proceedings of 1999 congress on evolutionary computation* (Vol. 3, p. 2078-2085). Washington, DC.

Ray, R. O., Zydallis, J. B., & Lamont, G. B. (2002). Solving the protein structure prediction problem through a multi-objective genetic algorithm. In *Proceedings of IEEE/DARPA International Conference on Computational Nanoscience* (pp. 32-35).

Ray, T. & Liew, K. M. (2002). A swarm metaphor for multi-objective design optimization. *Engineering Optimization, 34*(2), 141-153.

Redmond, J. & Parker, G. (1996, August). Actuator placement based on reachable set optimization for expected disturbance. *Journal of Optimization Theory and Applications, 90*(2), 279–300.

Reif, J. H. (2002). The emergence of the discipline of biomolecular computation in the US. *New Generation Computing, 20*(3), 217-236.

Reyes Sierra, M. & Coello Coello, C. A. (2005, June). Fitness inheritance in multi-objective particle swarm optimization. In *2005 IEEE Swarm Intelligence Symposium (SIS'05)* (pp. 116–123). Pasadena, California: IEEE Press.

Reyes-Sierra, M. & Coello Coello, C. (2006). Multi-objective particle swarm optimizers: A survey of the state-of-the-art. *International Journal of Computational Intelligence Research, 2*, 287–308.

Reyes-Sierra, M. & Coello, C. A. (2005). Improving PSO-based multi-objective optimisation using crowding, mutation and ε-dominance. *Lecture notes in computer science* (Vol. 3410, pp. 505-519). Springer-Verlag.

Reyes-Sierra, M. & Coello, C. A. (2006a). Multi-objective particle swarm optimizers: A survey of the state-of-the-art. *International Journal of Computational Intelligence Research, 2*(3), 287-308.

Reyes-Sierra, M. & Coello, C. A. (2006b). On-line adaptation in multi-objective particle swarm optimization. In *Proceedings of the 2006 IEEE Swarm Intelligence Symposium* (pp. 61-68). IEEE Press.

Robič, T. & Filipič, B. (2005). DEMO: Differential evolution for multi-objective optimization. In *Proceedings of the 3rd International Conference on Evolutionary Multi-Criterion Optimization (EMO 2005)* (pp. 520-533). Guanajuato, Mexico: Springer.

Rodriguez, A. F., Keller, T. A, Lamont, G. B., & Nelson, T. R. (2005). Using a multi-objective evolutionary algorithm to develop a quantum cascade laser operating in the terahertz frequency range. In *Proceedings of 2005 IEEE Congress on Evolutionary Computation (CEC'2005)* (Vol. 1, pp. 9-16).

Ronald, E. M. A. & Sipper, M. (2001). Surprise versus unsurprise: Implications of emergence in robotics. *Robotics & Autonomous Systems, 37*, 19–24.

Rönkkönen, J., Kukkonen, S., & Lampinen, J. (2005a). A comparison of differential evolution and generalized generation gap model. *Journal of Advanced Computational Intelligence and Intelligent Informatics, 9*(5), 549-555.

Rönkkönen, J., Kukkonen, S., & Price, K. V. (2005b). Real-parameter optimization with differential evolution. In *Proceedings of the 2005 Congress on Evolutionary Computation (CEC 2005)* (pp. 506-513). Edinburgh, Scotland: IEEE Service Center.

Rosen, K. H. (1999). *Discrete mathematics and its applications*. Boston, MA: McGraw-Hill.

Rouchka, E. C., Khalyfa, A., & Cooper, N. G. F. (2005). MPrime: Efficient large scale multiple primer and oligonucleotide design for customized gene microarrays. *BMC Bioinformatics, 6*(175).

Rouillard, J.-M., Zuker, M., & Gulari, E. (2003). OligoArray 2.0: Design of oligonucleotide probes for DNA micorarrays using a thermodynamic approach. *Nucleic Acids Research, 31*(12), 3057-3062.

Rozen, S. & Skaletsky, H. J. (2000). Primer3 on the www for general users and for biologist programmers. In S. Krawetz & S. Misenser (Eds.), *Bioinformatics and methods and protocols: Methods in molecular biology* (pp. 365-386). Humana Press.

Rudolph, G. & Agapie, A. (2000). Convergence properties of some multi-objective evolutionary algorithms. In *Proceedings of the Congress on Evolutionary Computation* (pp. 1010-1016). IEEE Press.

Rudolph, G. (1998). On a multi-objective evolutionary algorithm and its convergence to the Pareto set. In *Proceedings of the 5th IEEE Congress on Evolutionary Computation, CEC 1998* (pp. 511-516). Piscataway, New Jersey: IEEE Service Center.

Rumelhart, D. E., Hinton, G. E., & Williams, R. J. (1986). Learning internal representations by error propagation. In D.E. Rumelhart & J.L McClelland (Eds.), *Parallel Distributed Processing: Vol. 1* (pp. 381–362). Cambridge, MA: MIT Press.

Runyon, R. P., Coleman, K. A., & Pittenger, D. (1996). *Fundamentals of behavioral statistics*. Boston: McGraw-Hill.

Sahni, S. & Xu, X. (2005). Algorithms for wireless sensor networks. *International Journal on Distributed Sensor Networks, 1*, 35-56.

Salazar Lechuga, M. & Rowe, J. E. (2005). Particle swarm optimization and fitness sharing to solve multi-objective optimization problems. In *Proceedings of the 2005 IEEE Congress on Evolutionary Computation* (pp. 1204-1211). IEEE Service Center.

Sami, M., Sciuto, D., Silvano, C., & Zaccaria, V. (2000). Power exploration for embedded VLIW architectures.

In *IEEE/ACM International Conference on Computer Aided Design* (pp. 498–503). San Jose, California: IEEE Press.

Sander, T. & Tschudin, C. (1998) Protecting mobile agents against malicious hosts mobile agent and security. In G. Vigna (Ed.), (pp. 44-60), Springer-Verlag.

SantaLucia, J., Jr. & Hicks, D. (2004). The thermodynamics of DNA structural motifs. *Annual Review of Biophysics and Biomolecular Structure, 33*, 415-440.

Schaffer, J. (1985). Multiple objective optimization with vector evaluated genetic algorithms. *Genetic algorithms and their applications: Proceedings of the first international conference on genetic algorithms* (pp. 93-100). Hillsdale, New Jersey.

Schaffer, J. D. (1984). *Multiple objective optimization with vector evaluated genetic algorithms*. Unpublished doctoral thesis, Vanderbilt University, Nashville, TN.

Schoske, R., Vallone, P. M., Ruiberg, C. M., & Butler, J. M. (2003). Multiplex PCR design strategy used for the simultaneous amplification of 10 Y chromosome short tandem repeat (STR) loci. *Analytical and Bioanalytical Chemistry, 375*, 333-343.

Schott, J. (1995). Fault tolerant design using single and multicriteria genetic algorithm optimization. Unpublished master's thesis, Department of Aeronaustics and Astronautics, Massachusets Institute of Technology.

Schott, J. R. (1995). *Fault tolerant design using single and multictiteria gentetic algorithm optimization*. Unpublished master's thesis, Massachusetts Institute of Technology, Cambridge.

Schott, J. R. (1995). *Fault tolerant design using single and multi-criteria genetic algorithm optimization*. Unpublished master's thesis, Department of Aeronaustics and Astronautics, Massachusetts Institute of Technology.

Schott, J. R., (1995). *Fault tolerant design using single and multi-criteria genetic algorithm optimization*. Master's Thesis, Department of Aeronautics and Astronautics, Massachusetts Institute of Technology.

Scott, M. & Antonsson, E. (2005). Compensation and weights for trade-offs in engineering design: Beyond the weighted sum. *Journal of Mechanical Design, 127*, 1045–1055.

Shen C., Srisathapornphat C., & Jaikaeo C., (2001). Sensor information networking architecture and applications. *IEEE Personal Communications*, 52–59.

Shin, S.-Y. (2005). *Multi-objective evolutionary optimization of DNA sequences for molecular computing*. Unpublished doctoral dissertation, Seoul National University, Seoul, Korea.

Shin, S.-Y., Lee, I.-H., & Zhang, B.-T. (2006). Microarray probe design using ε-multi-objective evolutionary algorithms with thermodynamic criteria. *Lecture notes in computer science* (Vol. 3907, pp. 184-195).

Shin, S.-Y., Lee, I.-H., & Zhang, B.-T. (submitted). EvoOligo: Oligonucleotide probe design with multi-objective evolutionary algorithms.

Shin, S.-Y., Lee, I.-H., Kim, D., & Zhang, B.-T. (2005a). Multi-objective evolutionary optimization of DNA sequences for reliable DNA computing. *IEEE Transactions on Evolutionary Computation, 9*(2), 143-159.

Shin, S.-Y., Lee, I-H., & Zhang, B.-T. (2005b). DNA sequence design using ε-multi-objective evolutionary algorithms. *Journal of Korea Information Science Society: Software and Application, 32*(12), 1218-1228.

Simpsons, T., Mauery, T., Korte, J., & Mistree, F. (1998). *Comparison of response surface and kringing models for multidisciplinary design optimization* (Tech. Rep. No. 98 – 4755). AIAA.

Singh, A. & Minsker, B. S. (2004). Uncertainty based multi-objective optimization of groundwater remediation at the Umatilla Chemical Depot. In *Proceedings of the American Society of Civil Engineers (ASCE) Environmental & Water Resources Institute (EWRI) World Water & Environmental Resources Congress 2004 & Related Symposia*.

Slear, J. N. (2006). *AFIT UAV swarm mission planning and simulation system*. Unpublished master's thesis, Graduate School of Engineering and Mangement, Air Force Institute of Technology, Wright-Patterson AFB, Dayton, OH.

Slear, J. N., Melendez, K., & Lamont, G. B. (2006). Parallel UAV swarm simulation with optimal route planning. In *Proceedings of the 2006 Summer Computer Simulation Conference (SCSC '06)*.

Slijepcevic, S. & Potkonjak, M. (2001). Power efficient organization of wireless sensor networks. In *Proceedings of the IEEE International Conference on Communications* (pp. 472-476).

Smith, R. E., Dike, B. A., & Stegmann, S. A. (1995). Fitness inheritance in genetic algorithms. *SAC '95: Proceedings of the 1995 ACM symposium on applied computing (pp. 345–350). Nashville, Tennessee: ACM Press.

Spieth, C., Streichert, F., Speer, N., & Zell, A. (2005). Multi-objective model optimization for inferring gene regulatory networks. *Lecture notes in computer science* (Vol. 3410, pp. 607-620).

Srinivas, N. & Deb, K. (1994). Multi-objective optimization using nondominated sorting in genetic algorithms. *Evolutionary Computation, 2*(3), 221-248.

Srinivasan, D. & Seow, T. H. (2003). Particle swarm inspired evolutionary algorithm (PS-EA) for multi-objective optimization problem. In *Proceedings of the IEEE 2003 Congress on Evolutionary Computation* (pp. 2292-2297). IEEE Press.

Steuer, R. E. (1986). *Multiple criteria optimization: Theory, computation, and applications.* John Wiley & Sons, Inc.

Storn, R. & Price, K. V. (1995). *Differential evolution: A simple & efficient adaptive scheme for global optimization over continuous spaces* (Tech. Rep. No. TR-95-012). Berkeley: International Computer Science Institute.

Storn, R. & Price, K. V. (1995). *Differential evolution—A simple and efficient adaptive scheme for global optimization over continuous spaces* (Tech. Rep.). ICSI, University of California, Berkeley.

Storn, R. (1999). System design by constraint adaptation and Differential Evolution. *IEEE Transactions on Evolutionary Computation, 3*(1), 22-34.

Storn, R. and Price, K. (1995). *Differential evolution—A simple and efficient adaptive scheme for global optimization over continuous spaces* (Tech. Rep. No. tr-95-012). ICSI.

Suresh, G., Vinod, V. V., & Sahu, S. (1996). A genetic algorithm for assembly line balancing. *Production Planning and Control, 7*(1), 38-46.

Syswerda, G. (1991). Schedule optimization using genetic algorithms. *Handbook of genetic algorithms.*

Szymanek, R., Catthoor, F., & Kuchcinski, K. (2004). Time-energy design space exploration for multi-layer memory architectures. In *Design, Automation and Test in Europe* (pp. 181–190).

Takagi, T. & Sugeno, M. (1985). Fuzzy identification of systems and its application to modeling and control. *IEEE Transaction on System, Man and Cybernetics, 15*, 116-132.

Tanaka, F., Nakatsugawa, M., Yamamoto, M., Shiba, T., & Ohuchi, A. (2002). Towards a general-purpose sequence design system in DNA computing. In X. Yao (Ed.) In *Proceedings of 2002 Congress on Evolutionary Computation* (pp. 73-84). IEEE Press.

Taniguchi, T., Tanaka, K., Ohtake, H., & Wang, H. O. (2001). Model construction, rule reduction, and robust compensation for generalized form of Takagi-Sugeno fuzzy systems. *IEEE Transactions on Fuzzy Systems, 9*(4), 525–538.

Tarakanov, A. & Dasgupta, D. (2000). A formal model of an artificial immune system. *BioSystems, 55*(1/3), 151-158.

Taylor, T. & Massey, C. (2001). Recent developments in the evolution of morphologies & controllers for physically simulated creatures. *Artificial Life, 7*(1), 77–87.

Teo, J. & Abbass, H. A. (2004). Automatic generation of controllers for embodied legged organisms: A Pareto evolutionary multi-objective approach. *Evolutionary Computation, 12*(3), 355–394.

Thie, C. J., Chitty, D. M., & Reed, C. M. (2005). Using evolutionary algorithms and dynamic programming to solve uncertain multi-criteria optimization problems with application to lifetime management for military platforms. In F. Rothlauf (Ed.), *GECCO workshops* (pp. 181-183). ACM.

Tilak, S., Abu-Ghazaleh, N., & Heinzelman, W. (2002). Infrastructure tradeoffs for sensor networks. In *Proceedings ACM 1st International Workshop on Sensor Networks and Applications* (pp. 49-58).

Timmis, J., Neal, M., & Hunt, J. (2000). An artificial immune system for data analysis. *Biosystems, 55*(1/3), 143–150.

Tobler, J. B., Molla, M. N., Nuwaysir, E. F., Green, R. D., & Shavlik, J. W. (2002). Evaluating machine learning approaches for aiding probe selection for gene-expression arrays. *Bioinformatics, 18*, 164-171.

Toffolo, A., & Benini, E. (2003). Genetic diversity as an objective in multi-objective evolutionary algorithms. *Evolutionary Computation, 11*(2), 151-167.

Toffolo, A., & Lazzaretto, A. (2002). Evolutionary algorithms for multi-objective energetic and economic optimization in thermal system design. *Energy, 27*(6), 549-567.

Torn, A. & Zilinskas, A. (1989). *Global optimization*. Springer-Verlag.

Torres, F., Gil, P., Puente, S. T., Pomares, J., & Aracil, R. (2004). Automatic PC disassembly for component recovery. *International Journal of Advanced Manufacturing Technology, 23*(1-2), 39-46.

Toscano Pulido, G. (2005). *On the use of self-adaptation and elitism for multi-objective particle swarm optimization*. Unpublished doctoral dissertation, Computer Science Section, Department of Electrical Engineering, CINVESTAV-IPN, Mexico.

Toscano Pulido, G., & Coello, C. A. (2004). Using clustering techniques to improve the performance of a particle swarm optimizer. *Lecture notes in computer science* (Vol. 3102, pp. 225-237). Springer.

Tovey, C. A. (2002). Tutorial on computational complexity. *Interfaces, 32*(3), 30-61.

Tubaishat, M. & Madria, S. (2003). Sensor networks: An overview. *IEEE Potentials, 22*(2), 20- 23.

Tušar, T. & Filipič, B. (2007). Differential evolution versus genetic algorithms in multi-objective optimization. In *Proceedings of the 4th International Conference on Evolutionary Multi-Criterion Optimization (EMO 2007)* (pp. 257-271). Matsushima, Japan: Springer.

Urli, B., Lo, N., & Guitouni, A. (2003). Une approche d'optimisation dans la génération de Plans d'Actions (COA). *31st Annual ASAC Conference*. Halifax, Nova Scotia, Canada.

Vahid, F. & Givargis, T. (2001, March). Platform tuning for embedded systems design. *IEEE Computer, 34*(3), 112–114.

Valero, A., Lozano, M. A., Serra, L., Tsatsaronis, G., Pisa, J., Frangopoulos, C. A., & von Spakovsky, M. R. (1994). CGAM problem: Definition and conventional solution. *Energy, 19*(3), 279-286.

Van Veldhuizen, D. A. & Lamont, G. B. (2000a). Multi-objective optimization with messy genetic algorithms. In *Proceedings of the 2000 ACM Symposium on Applied Computing* (pp. 470-476), Villa Olmo, Como, Italy.

Van Veldhuizen, D. A. & Lamont, G. B. (2000b). On measuring multi-objective evolutionary algorithm performance. In *Proceedings of the 2000 IEEE Congress on Evolutionary Computation, CEC 2000* (Vol. 1, pp. 204-211). Piscataway, New Jersey: IEEE Service Center.

Van Veldhuizen, D. A. (1999). *Multi-objective evolutionary algorithms: Classification, analyses, and new innovations*. Unpublished doctoral thesis. Presented to the Faculty of the Graduate School of Engineering of he Air Force Institute of Technology. Air University.

Veldhuizen, D. (1999). *Multi-objective evolutionary algorithms: Classifications, analyses, and new innovation*. Unpublished doctoral thesis, Department of Electrical Engineering and Computer Engineering, Air-force Institute of Technology, Ohio.

Veldhuizen, D. A. V. & Lamont, G. B. (1998). *Multi-objective evolutionary algorithm research: A history and analysis* (Tech. Rep. No. TR-98-03), Wright-Patterson AFB, Ohio: Department of Electrical and Computer Engineering, Graduate School of Engineering, Air Force Institute of Technology.

Veldhuizen, D. A. V. & Lamont, G. B. (2000, July). On measuring multi-objective evolutionary algorithm performance. *2000 congress on evolutionary computation* (Vol. 1, pp. 204–211). Piscataway, New Jersey: IEEE Service Center.

Veldhuizen, D. A. V., Zydallis, J. B., & Lamont, G. B. (2003). Considerations in engineering parallel multi-objective evolutionary algorithms. *IEEE Transactions on Evolutionary Computation, 7*(2), 144-173.

Veldhuizen, D. V. (1999). *Multi-objective evolutionary algorithms: Classification, analyses, and new innovations*. Unpublished doctoral dissertation, Air Force Institute of Technology, Dayton.

Vijaykrishnan, N., Kandemir, M., Irwin, M. J., Kim, H. S., Ye, W., (2003, January). Evaluating integrated hardwaresoftware optimizations using a unified energy estimation framework. *IEEE Transactions on Computers, 52*(1), 59–73.

Villalobos-Aria, M. A., Toscano Pulido, G., & Coello, C. A. (2005). A proposal to use stripes to maintain diversity in a multi-objective particle swarm optimizer. In *Proceedings of the 2005 IEEE Swarm Intelligence Symposium* (pp. 22-29). IEEE Service Center.

Vlachogiannis, J. G. & Lee, K. Y. (2005). Determining generator contributions to transmission system using parallel vector evaluated particle swarm optimization. *IEEE Transactions on Power Systems, 20*(4), 1765-1774.

Walker, J., Garrett, S., & Wilson, M. (2003). Evolving controllers for real robots: A survey of the literature. *Adaptive Behavior, 11*(3), 179–203.

Wang, F.-S. & Chiou, J.-P. (1997). Differential evolution for dynamic optimization of differential-algebraic systems. In *Proceedings of the 1997 IEEE International Conference on Evolutionary Computation (ICEC 1997)* (pp. 531-536). Indianapolis, IN: IEEE Service Center.

Wang, F.-S. & Sheu, J.-W. (2000). Multi-objective parameter estimation problems of fermentation processes using a high ethanol tolerance yeast. *Chemical Engineering Science, 55*(18), 3685-3695.

Wang, L.F., Tan, K. C., & Chew, C. M. (2006). *Evolutionary robotics: From algorithms to implementations*. Singapore: World Scientific Publishing.

Wang, L.-X. & Mendel, J. M. (1992). Generating fuzzy rules by learning from examples. *IEEE Transactions on System, Man and Cybernetics, 22*, 1414–1427.

Wang, X. & Seed, B. (2003). Selection of oligonucleotide probes for protein coding sequences. *Bioinformatics, 19*(7), 796-802.

Wang, X., Xing, G., Zhang, Y., Lu, C., Pless, R., & Gill, C. D. (2003). Integrated coverage and connectivity configuration in wireless sensor networks. In *Proceedings of the First ACM Conference on Embedded Networked Sensor Systems* (pp. 28-39).

Weber, C., Maréchal, F., & Favrat, D. (2006, August). *Network synthesis for district heating with multiple heat plants*. Paper presented at PRES06, Prague, Czech Republic.

Weicker, N., Szabo, G., Weicker, K., & Widmayer, P. (2003). Evolutionary multi-objective optimization for base station transmitter placement with frequency assignment. *IEEE Transactions on Evolutionary Computation, 7*(2), 189–203.

Wernersson, R. & Nielsen, H. B. (2005). OligoWiz 2.0 – Integrating sequence feature annotation into the design of microarray probes. *Nucleic Acids Research, 33*(web server issue), W611-W615.

West, D. B. (2001). *Introduction to graph theory* (2nd ed.). Englewood Cliffs, NJ: Prentice-Hall.

While, L., Bradstreet, L., Barone, L., & Hingston, P. (2005). Heuristics for optimising the calculation of hypervolume for multi-objective optimization problems. *IEEE congress on evolutionary computation* (Vol. 3, pp. 2225-2232). IEEE Press.

While, R. L., Hingston, P., Barone, L., & Huband, S. (2006). A faster algorithm for calculating hypervolume. *IEEE Transactions on Evolutionary Computation, 10*(1), 29-38.

White, J. A. & Garrett, S. M. (2003). Improved pattern recognition with artificial clonal selection. In *Proceedings of the Second International Conference on Artificial Immune Systems (ICARIS)*, Napier University, Edinburgh, UK.

Wierzbiki, A. P. (1980). Optimization techniques, Part 1. *Metholodlogical guide to multi-objective optimisation, Lecture notes in control and information sciences 22*. (pp. 99-123), Berlin, Germany: Springer-Verlag.

Wolpert, D. H. & Macready, W. G. (1997). No free lunch theorems for optimization. *IEEE Transactions on Evolutionary Computation, 1*(1), 67-82.

Wong, T., Bigras, P., & Khayati, K. (2002). Causality assignment using multi-objective evolutionary algorithms. In *Proceedings of the 2002 IEEE International Conference on Systems, Man and Cybernetics, vol 4*.

Wu, Q., Rao, N. S. V., Barhen, J., Iyengar, S. S., Vaishnavi, V. K., Qi, H., & Chakrabarty, K. (2004). On computing mobile agent routes for data fusion in distributed sensor networks. *IEEE Transactions on Knowledge and Data Engineering, 16*(6), 740-753.

Wu, Q., Rao, N. S. V., Barhen, J., Iyengar, S. S., Vaishnavi, V. K., Qi, H. & Chakrabarty, K. (2004). On computing mobile agent routes for data fusion in distributed sensor networks. *IEEE Trans. Knowledge and Data Engineering, 16*(6), 740-753.

Xue, F., Sanderson, A. C., & Graves, R. J. (2003). Pareto-based multi-objective differential evolution. In *Proceedings of the 2003 Congress on Evolutionary Computation (CEC 2003)* (pp. 862-869). Canberra, Australia: IEEE Service Center.

Yamada, T., Soma, H., & Morishita, S. (2006). PrimerStation: A highly specific multiplex genomic PCR primer design server for the human genome. *Nucleic Acid Research, 34*(web server issue), W665-W669.

Yan, L., Srikanthan, T., & Gang, N. (2006). Area and delay estimation for FPGA implementation of coarse-grained reconfigurable architectures. In *ACM SIGPLAN/SIGBED Conference on Language, Compilers and Tool Support for Embedded Systems* (pp. 182–188).

Yao, X. (1999). Evolving artificial neural networks. In *Proceedings of the IEEE, 87*(9), 1426–1447.

Yu, Y., Krishnamachari, B., & Prasanna, V.K. (2004). Energy-latency tradeoffs for data gathering in wireless sensor networks. In *Proceedings IEEE INFOCOM* (pp. 244-55).

Zaharie, D. (2002). Critical values for the control parameters of differential evolution algorithms. In *Proceedings of Mendel 2002, 8th International Conference on Soft Computing* (pp. 62-67). Brno, Czech Republic.

Zaharie, D. (2003a). Control of population diversity and adaptation in differential evolution algorithms. In *Proceedings of Mendel 2003, 9th International Conference on Soft Computing* (pp. 41-46). Brno, Czech Republic.

Zaharie, D. (2003b). Multi-objective optimization with adaptive Pareto differential evolution. In *Proceedings of Symposium on Intelligent Systems and Applications (SIA 2003)*. Iasi, Romania.

Zeleny, M. (1973). Multiple criteria decision making. *Compromise programming* (pp. 262-301). University of South Carolina Press.

Zeng, K., Zhang, N.-Y., & Xu, W.-L. (2000, December). A comparative study on sufficient conditions for takagi-sugeno fuzzy systems as universal approximators. *IEEE Transactions on Fuzzy Systems, 8*(6), 773–778.

Zeng, X.-J. & Keane, J. A. (2005, October). Approximation capabilities of hierarchical fuzzy systems. *IEEE Transactions on Fuzzy Systems, 13*(5), 659–672.

Zeng, X.-J. & Singh, M. G. (1996, February). Approximation accuracy analisys of fuzzy systems as function approximators. *IEEE Transactions on Fuzzy Systems, 4*, 44–63.

Zhang, B.-T. & Shin, S.-Y. (1998). Molecular algorithms for efficient and reliable DNA computing. In J. R. Koza et al. (Eds.), In *Proceedings of the Third Annual Conference on Genetic Programming* (pp. 735-742). Morgan Kaufmann.

Zhang, H. & Hou, J. C. (2003). Maintaining sensing coverage and connectivity in large sensor networks (Tech. Rep. UIUC, UIUCDCS-R- 2003-2351).

Zielinski, K. & Laur, R. (2007). Variants of differential evolution for multi-objective optimization. In *Proceedings of the 2007 Symposium on Computational Intelligence in Multi-Criteria Decision-Making (MCDM 2007)* (pp. 91-98). Honolulu, HI: IEEE Service Center.

Zitzler, E. & Thiele, L. (1998). Multi-objective optimization using evolutionary algorithms—A comparative case study. *Parallel problem solving from nature, Lecture notes in computer science* (Vol. 1498, pp. 292-304). Springer.

Zitzler, E. & Thiele, L. (1999). Multi-objective evolutionary algorithms: A comparative case study and the strength Pareto approach. *IEEE Transactions on Evolutionary Computation, 3*(4), 257–271.

Zitzler, E. & Thiele, L. (1999). Multi-objective evolutionary algorithms: A comparative case study and the strength Pareto approach. *IEEE Transactions on Evolutionary Computation, 3*(4), 257–271.

Zitzler, E. & Thiele, L. (1999, November). Multi-objective evolutionary algorithms: A comparative case study and the strength Pareto approach. *IEEE Transactions on Evolutionary Computation, 3*(4), 257–271.

Zitzler, E. (1998). *Evolutionary algorithms for multi-objective optimization: Methods and applications.* Unpublished doctoral dissertation, Swiss Federal Institute of Technology (ETH), Zuerich, Switzerland.

Zitzler, E. (1999). *Evolutionary algorithms for multi-objective optimization: Methods and applications*, Swiss Federal Institute of Technology Zurich. Submitted for publication.

Zitzler, E. (1999). *Evolutionary algorithms for multi-objective optimisation: Methods and applications.* Unpublished doctoral thesis, Swiss Federal Institute of Technology (ETH).

Zitzler, E. (1999). *Evolutionary algorithms for multi-objective optimization: Methods and applications.* Unpublished doctoral thesis, Swiss Federal Institute of Technology, Zurich, Switzerland (Dissertation ETH No:13398).

Zitzler, E., (1999). *Evolutionary algorithms for multi-objective optimization: Methods and applications.* Unpublished doctoral dissertation, Zurich, Switzerland: Swiss Federal Institute of Technology.

Zitzler, E., Deb, K., & Thiele, L. (1999). Comparison of multi-objective evolutionary algorithms on test functions of different difficulty. In A. Wu (Ed.), *Genetic and evolutionary computation conference (Workshop Program)* (pp. 121–122).

Zitzler, E., Deb, K., & Thiele, L. (2000). Comparison of multi-objective evolutionary algorithms: empirical results. *Evolutionary Computation, 8*(2), 173-195.

Zitzler, E., Deb, K., & Thiele, L. (2000). Comparison of multi-objective evolutionary algorithms: Empirical results. *Evolutionary Computation, 8*(2), 173-195.

Zitzler, E., Deb, K., & Thiele, L. (2000, Summer). Comparison of multi-objective evolutionary algorithms: Empirical results. *Evolutionary Computation, 8*(2), 173–195.

Zitzler, E., Laumanns, M. & Thiele, L. (2001). *SPEA2: Improving the strength Pareto evolutionary algorithm* (Tech. Rep. TIK-Report 103). Swiss Federal Institute of Technology, Lausanne, Switzerland.

Zitzler, E., Laumanns, M., & Thiele, L. (2001). SPEA2: Improving the strength Pareto evolutionary algorithm for multi-objective optimization. In K. C. Giannakoglou, D. T. Tsahalis, J. Periaux, K. D. Papailiou, & T. Fogarty (Eds.), *Evolutionary methods for design optimization and control with applications to industrial problems* (pp. 95-100). International Center for Numerical Methods in Engineering (Cmine).

Zitzler, E., Laumanns, M., & Thiele, L. (2001). *SPEA2: Improving the strength Pareto evolutionary algorithm* (Tech. Rep. No. 103) Swiss Federal Institute of Technology.

Zitzler, E., Laumanns, M., & Thiele, L. (2001, September). SPEA2: Improving the performance of the strength pareto evolutionary algorithm. In *EUROGEN 2001 Evolutionary Methods for Design, Optimization and Control with Applications to Industrial Problems* (pp. 95–100). Athens, Greece.

Zitzler, E., Thiele, L., & Deb, K. (2000). Comparison of multi-objective evolutionary algorithms: Empirical results. *Evolutionary Computation, 8*(1), 173-195.

Zitzler, E., Thiele, L., Laumanns, M., Fonseca, C. M., & da Fonseca, V. G. (2003). Performance assessment of multi-objective optimizersan analysis and review. *IEEE Transactions on Evolutionary Computation, 7*(2), 117-132.

About the Contributors

Lam Thu Bui is a Research Fellow at the School of ITEE, University of New South Wales at Australian Defence Force Academy. He is currently doing research in the field of evolutionary computation, specialized with Evolutionary Multi-Objective Optimization. He holds a Bachelor of Informatics, a Masters Degree in Information Technology, and a PhD in Computer Science. He has been involved with academic area including teaching and researching for over seven years and about 20 refereed journal and conference papers and book chapters related to multi-objective optimization. He has been a member of the program committees of several conferences and workshops in the field of evolutionary computing, such as the IEEE Congress on Evolutionary Computation (CEC) and The Genetic and Evolutionary Computation Conference (GECCO).

Sameer Alam is a Research Fellow at the Defence and Security Applications Research Centre, University of New South Wales at the Australian Defence Force Academy, Canberra, Australia. He holds B.S. in Maths, M.A. in Economics and M.Tech. in Comp. Sc. He recently submitted his Ph.D. to the University of New South Wales. He has published over 9 refereed journal and conference papers mainly in the area of air traffic management. His research interest includes multi-objective optimization, heuristic search and swarm intelligence. He is invited reviewer for a number of journal and conferences including IEEE Transactions on Intelligent Transportation Systems, Journal of Transportation Science-C, Elsevier Science, 2nd International Conference on Bio-Inspired Computing in China, 2007, 6th International Conference on Simulated Evolution and Learning in China, 2006 and 2nd IFIP Conference on Biologically Inspired Collaborative Computing in Italy, 2008. He was also the program committee member for the first IEEE Symposium on Artificial Life 2007 in Honolulu, Hawaii, USA.

* * * * *

Hussein Abbass is the director of the Defence and Security Applications Research Centre (DSARC) at the University of New South Wales at the Australian Defence Force Academy (UNSW@ADFA) in Canberra, Australia. He has a BA, BSc, PG-Dip, and master's degree all from Cairo University Egypt, an MS from Edinburgh University Scotland, and a PhD from QUT Australia. He is an advisory professor at Vietnam National University, Ho-Chi Minh City, a senior member of the IEEE, a senior member of the Australian Computer Society (ACS), the chair of ACS National Committee on Complex Systems, the chair of the IEEE Task Force on Complex Adaptive Systems and Artificial Life, and a member of a number of national and international committees including the IEEE Technical Committee on Data

Mining and the IEEE working group on soft computing in the SMC society. He has 170+ refereed papers and is particularly interested in modelling and simulation of complex systems with a focus on the defence and security domain. On a fundamental level, he works on artificial neural networks, ensemble learning, evolutionary computation, multiagent systems, and multiobjective optimisation. He has been a technical co-chair and a member of the technical committee for many conferences including a PC co-chair for CEC'07, SEAL 06, and IEEE-Alife'07.

Giuseppe Ascia received the Laurea degree in electronic engineering and a PhD in computer science from the Universita` di Catania, Italy (1994 and 1998, respectively). In 1994, he joined the Institute of Computer Science and Telecommunications at the Universita` di Catania. Currently, he is an associate professor at the Universita` di Catania. His research interests are soft computing, VLSI design, hardware architectures, and low-power design.

Vincenzo Catania received the Laurea degree in electrical engineering from the Universita` di Catania, Italy, in 1982. Until 1984, he was responsible for testing microprocessor system at STMicroelectronics, catania, Italy. Since 1985 he has cooperated in research on computer network with the Istituto di Informatica e Telecomunicazioni at the Universita` di Catania, where he is a Full Professor of computer science. His research interests include performance and reliability assessment in parallel and distributed system, VLSI design, low-power design, and fuzzy logic.

Carlos A. Coello Coello received a PhD in computer science from Tulane University (in the USA), in 1996. He has published over 180 papers in international peer-reviewed journals and conferences. He has also co-authored the book *Evolutionary Algorithms for Solving Multi-Objective Problems* (Kluwer Academic Publishers, 2002) and has co-edited the book *Applications of Multi-Objective Evolutionary Algorithms* (World Scientific, 2004). He actually serves as associate editor of the journals *IEEE Transactions on Evolutionary Computation*, *Evolutionary Computation* and *Computational Optimization and Applications* and *the Journal of Heuristics*. His current research interests are: evolutionary multiobjective optimization and constraint-handling techniques for evolutionary algorithms.

Alessandro Di Nuovo received a PhD in computer engineering from the University of Catania, Italy, in 2005. Since 2004 he has cooperated in research with the Department of Computer and Telecommunications at the University of Catania, where he is currently a PhD student. His main activities regard computational intelligence and its applications in computer, medical and social sciences, parallel and distributed systems, hardware/software co-design.

Maoguo Gong received a BS in electronic engineering from Xidan University, Xian, China, in 2003 with the highest honor. He was a master's student in the Institute of Intelligent Information Processing (IIIP), Xidian University, from August 2003 to August 2004 and a research student in the Complex Systems Summer School 2006 of the Santa Fe Institute (SFI). He earned the "Fund of Excellent Doctor" and doctor's degree in April 2007. Now, he is a lecturer of IIIP and a member of IEEE. His research interests are broadly in the area of computational intelligence and hybrid intelligent systems. The areas of special interests include artificial immune systems, evolutionary computation, data mining, optimization and some other related areas. He has published round about 30 papers in journals and conferences.

About the Contributors

Surendra M. Gupta is a professor of mechanical and industrial engineering and director of the Laboratory for Responsible Manufacturing at Northeastern University in Boston. He received his BE in electronics engineering from Birla Institute of Technology and Science, MBA from Bryant University, and MSIE and PhD in industrial engineering from Purdue University. He has authored and co-authored about 350 technical papers published in prestigious journals, books and conference proceedings. He has traveled to all seven continents and presented his work at international conferences there (except Antarctica). His recent activities can be viewed at http://www1.coe.neu.edu/~smgupta/.

Licheng Jiao received the BS from Shanghai Jiao Tong University, Shanghai, China, in 1982, an MS and a PhD from Xi'an Jiao Tong University, Xi'an, China (1984 and 1990, respectively). Now, he is the dean of School of Electronic Engineering (SEE) and the director of Institute of Intelligent Information Processing (IIIP), Xidian University. His current research interests include signal and image processing, natural computation and intelligent information processing. He is an IEEE senior member, member of IEEE Xi'an Section Executive Committee, and the chairman of Awards and Recognition Committee, executive committee member of Chinese Association of Artificial Intelligence, councilor of Chinese Institute of Electronics, committee member of Chinese Committee of Neural Networks, and expert of Academic Degrees Committee of the State Council. He has charged of and completed about 40 important scientific research projects which win many science and technology awards, published more than 10 monographs and a hundred papers in international journals and conferences.

Mark P. Kleeman is a PhD candidate in computer engineering, at the Air Force Institute of Technology, WPAFB, Dayton, OH. He graduated summa cum laude from North Carolina State University (1999) with BS degrees in computer engineering, electrical engineering, and computer science; and was a distinguished graduate from the Air Force Institute of Technology (2004) with an MS in computer engineering. His research interests include: evolutionary computation, parallel and distributed computation, and combinatorial optimization problems (single objective and multi-objective). He has authored over twenty refereed papers, including several book chapters, and has been a conference keynote speaker.

Saku Kukkonen received an MS in computer and information science from the University of Delaware in 2000 and an MS(Eng.) in IT from the Lappeenranta University of Technology in 2002. He is currently a full time PhD student with the Lappeenranta University of Technology and his areas of interest include mainly global optimization, evolutionary computing, differential evolution, constraint handling, and multiobjective optimization.

Gary B. Lamont is a professor in the Department of Electrical and Computer Engineering, Graduate School of Engineering and Management, Air Force Institute of Technology, WPAFB, Dayton, OH; B. of Physics, 1961; MSEE, 1967, PhD, 1970; University of Minnesota. He teaches courses in computer science and computer engineering. His research interests include: evolutionary computation, artificial immune systems, information security, parallel and distributed computation, combinatorial optimization problems (single objective and multi-objective), software engineering, digital signal processing, and intelligent and distributed control. Dr. Lamont has authored several textbooks (Multi-Objective EAs, Computer Control), various book chapters as well as numerous papers.

Jouni Lampinen received MS and DS degrees from University of Vaasa (1998 and 2000, respectively). He is currently a professor of information processing with the Lappeenranta University of Technology. His areas of interest include evolutionary computing, global optimization, constraint handling approaches, and multiobjective optimization, and their applications. In particular he has been involved with the development of the differential evolution algorithm.

In-Hee Lee received a BS in computer engineering from Seoul National University (SNU), Seoul, Korea, in 2001. She is currently working towards a PhD at the School of Computer Science and Engineering, SNU. Her research interests include multiobjective evolutionary computation, DNA computing, bioinformatics.

Andrew Lewis is a senior research specialist with Research Computing Services at Griffith University, also holds an adjunct position as a senior lecturer in the School of Information and Communication Technology, and is a member of Griffith's Institute for Integrated and Intelligent Systems. He has spent over 20 years in computational research and high performance computing, including a decade in industrial applied research. His research interests include parallel optimization algorithms for large numerical simulations, including gradient descent, direct search methods, evolutionary programming and biologically-inspired methods, multiobjective optimization techniques for engineering design, and parallel, distributed and grid computing technologies.

Wenping Ma received a BS in computer science and technology from Xidian University, Xi'an, China, in 2003. From September 2003 to August 2004, she was an MS student, Since September 2004, she has been a PhD student in pattern recognition and intelligent systems, Institute of Intelligent Information Processing, Xidian University. Currently, she is a teacher at Xidian University. Her research interests including artificial immune systems, evolutionary computation, and image processing.

Seamus M. McGovern is a senior-level electronics engineer and Volpe fellow at the U.S. DOT National Transportation Systems Center. He holds a faculty appointment at Northeastern University and is a reserve aerospace engineering duty officer and pilot assigned to the Office of Naval Research. He has co-authored more than two-dozen technical papers and chapters and is the recipient of four fellowships, eleven merit-based scholarships, a national best dissertation prize, and election to three scholastic honor societies. He is a member of the Decision Sciences Institute and the Institute of Industrial Engineers.

Kishan G. Mehrotra received a PhD (statistics) from the University of Wisconsin at Madison, in 1971. He is currently a professor and the Computer and Information Science program director in the Department of Electrical Engineering and Computer Science at Syracuse University, where he has been teaching since 1970. His research interests include pattern recognition, evolutionary algorithms, computer performance evaluation, information theory, and nonparametric statistics. He has co-authored *Elements of Artificial Neural Networks* (MIT Press, 1997), several book chapters, and over 125 journal and conference papers. He has held several offices in the American Statistical Association, and serves on the editorial board of the journal *Applied Intelligence*.

About the Contributors

Zbigniew Michalewicz is an internationally renowned new technologies expert. Michalewicz has published over 200 articles and 15 books on the subjects of business intelligence, predictive data mining, and optimisation. These include *Adaptive Business Intelligence* (www.AdaptiveBusinessIntelligence.com.au) and *Winning Credibility: A Guide for Building a Business from Rags to Riches* (www.Credibility.com.au). Zbigniew is a professor in AI at the University of Adelaide, and serves as chairman of the board for SolveIT Software Pty Ltd (www.SolveITSoftware.com), a company specialising in planning & scheduling optimisation and predictive modelling. Michalewicz has over 25 years of academic and industry experience, and possesses expert knowledge of many Artificial Intelligence methods and modern heuristics. He has led numerous data mining and optimisation projects for major corporations such as General Motors, Pernod Ricard Pacific, Ford Motor Company, Bank of America, ABP, McGuigan Simeon Wines, and Dentsu, and for several government agencies in the United States of America, Australia, and Poland. Michalewicz has also served as the chairman of the Technical Committee on Evolutionary Computation, and later as executive vice president of IEEE Neural Network Council. His scientific and business achievements have been recognised by countless media outlets, including *CNN, TIME Magazine, Newsweek, NBC, New York Times, Forbes,* and *the Associated Press* among others. Zbigniew completed his master's degree at Technical University of Warsaw in 1974 and he received a PhD from the Institute of Computer Science, Polish Academy of Sciences, in 1981. He also holds a Doctor of Science in computer science from the Polish Academy of Science, and in 2002 he received the title of "professor" from the President of Poland, Mr. Alexander Kwasniewski. Michalewicz also holds professor positions at the Institute of Computer Science, Polish Academy of Sciences, the Polish-Japanese Institute of Information Technology, and the State Key Laboratory of Software Engineering of Wuhan University, China. He is also associated with the Structural Complexity Laboratory at Seoul National University, South Korea.

Chilukuri K. Mohan received a PhD (computer science) from the State University of New York at Stony Brook, in 1988, and a BTech (computer science) from the Indian Institute of Technology at Kanpur, in 1983. He is currently a professor in the Department of Electrical Engineering and Computer Science at Syracuse University, where he has been teaching since 1988. He has co-authored *Elements of Artificial Neural Networks* (MIT Press, 1997), and authored *Frontiers of Expert Systems: Reasoning with Limited Knowledge* (Kluwer, 2000). He has also authored/co-authored over 100 research papers in various areas of artificial intelligence. He is a member of an IEEE Task Force on Swarm Intelligence, and serves on several international conference committees.

Sanaz Mostaghim received a PhD in electrical engineering from the University of Paderborn, Germany in 2004. After her PhD, she worked as a post doc at the Swiss Federal Institute of Technology (ETH) in Zürich. During her PhD and post doc, she worked on multiobjective optimization algorithms using evolutionary algorithms and particle swarm optimization, and successfully applied them to several different applications from geology and computational chemistry. She is currently working as an assistant professor at the University of Karlsruhe, Germany. Her research interests are multi-objective optimization, particle swarm optimization, grid computing and visualization of optimal solutions.

Lynnie Dewi Neri received a BS (Hon.) in IT from Universiti Utara Malaysia (UUM) in 2002. Currently, she is a master's student in the IT program, School of Engineering and Information Technology, Universiti Malaysia Sabah (UMS) and as a contract lecturer in Universiti Teknologi Mara (UiTM), teaching subjects information technology and mathematics. Her research interests are in the fields of evolutionary algorithms, evolutionary robotics and neural networks.

Minh Ha Nguyen graduated (with first class honors) from the University of Canberra, Australia in 1999 and was awarded a PhD from the University of New South Wales in 2006. Her work is focusing on evolutionary computation, neural networks and data mining.

Maurizio Palesi received the Laurea degree and the PhD in computer engineering from Universita' di Catania, Italy, in 1999 and 2003, respectively. Since December 2003, he has held a research contract as Assistant Professor at the Dipartimento di Ingegneria Informatica e delle Telecomunicazioni, Facolta' di Ingegneria, Universita' di Catania. His research focuses on Platform based system design, design space exploration, low-power techniques for embedded systems, and Network-on-Chip architectures.

Konstantinos E. Parsopoulos is with the Department of Mathematics, University of Patras, Greece, where he received the Diploma (1998), MSc (2001) and PhD (2005) degrees. He was a visiting research fellow at the Collaborative Research Center "Computational Intelligence" (SFB 531), Department of Computer Science, University of Dortmund, Germany (2001), and at INRIA (Institut National de Recherche en Informatique et en Automatique), France (2003 and 2006). He is co-author of more than 50 publications in refereed international journals and conferences and his work has received more than 700 citations. His research interests include stochastic optimization algorithms and computational intelligence.

Davide Patti received the Laurea degree and the PhD degree in computer engineering at University of Catania, in 2003 and 2007, respectively. His research focuses on Platform based system design, design space exploration, low-power techniques for embedded systems, and Network-on-Chip architectures.

Ramesh Rajagopalan received an MS (Honors) degree in physics and a BE (Honors) degree in electrical and electronics from the Birla Institute of Technology and Science, Pilani, India in 2002. He received an MS in electrical engineering from Syracuse University, Syracuse, NY in 2004. He is currently a PhD candidate in the Electrical Engineering and Computer Science Department at Syracuse University. He was awarded the Graduate School Masters Prize at Syracuse University in recognition of his research and scholarship. He received the best poster award for his work on path planning algorithms at Nunan Research Day, Syracuse University. His research interests include evolutionary computation, wireless communications, distributed sensor networks, and multi-objective optimization.

Noel Antonio Ramírez-Santiago received a BS in computer systems engineering from the Escuela Superior de Cómputo of the Instituto Politécnico Nacional, and an MS in computer science from CINVESTAV-IPN (both located in México City), in 2003 and 2007, respectively. His current research interests include: scatter search, particle swarm optimization and evolutionary multiobjective optimization.

Marcus Randall is an associate professor in the School of Information Technology, Bond University, Australia. He has written approximately 50 journal articles, conference papers and book chapters in the area of metaheuristic search algorithms. Additionally, he is the author of the book *Algorithms:*

About the Contributors

Machines of the Mind. His research interests include evolutionary computing, parallel programming methods, ant colony and extremal optimisation algorithms.

Luis Vicente Santana-Quintero received a BS in computer systems engineering from the Escuela Superior de Cómputo of the Instituto Politécnico Nacional, and an MS in computer science from CINVESTAV-IPN (both located in Mexico City), in 2002 and 2004, respectively. He is currently working towards a PhD in the Department of Computer Science at the Centro de Investigación y de Estudios Avanzados del Instituto Politécnico Nacional (CINVESTAV-IPN), in Mexico City. His current research interests include: evolutionary multiobjective optimization, particle swarm optimization, differential evolution and evolutionary algorithms in general.

Ronghua Shang received a BS from the School of Science, Xidian University, Xi'an, China, in 2003 and is currently pursuing a PhD in pattern recognition and intelligent information system from the Institute of Intelligent Information Processing, Xidian University. Her research interests include evolutionary computation, artificial immune system, multiobjective optimization, image and video processing, and data mining.

Soo-Yong Shin received BS, MS, and PhD degrees in computer engineering from Seoul National University (SNU), Seoul, Korea, in 1998, 2000, and 2005, respectively. He is guest research at National Institute of Standards and Technology (NIST), Maryland from April 2006. He has been a visiting student at Computer Science and Artificial Intelligence Laboratory (CSAIL), Massachusetts Institute of Technology (MIT) from March 2004 and August 2004. His research interests include evolutionary computation, probabilistic graphical models, DNA computing, bioinformatics, and medical informatics.

Jason Teo is a senior lecturer in computer science at the School of Engineering and Information Technology and the deputy director of the Centre for Artificial Intelligence, Universiti Malaysia Sabah. He received his doctorate in information technology from the University of New South Wales, Australia, researching Pareto artificial evolution of virtual legged organisms. He has over 60 publications in the areas of artificial life, evolutionary robotics, evolutionary computing and swarm intelligence. His current research interests focus on the theory and applications of evolutionary multiobjective optimization algorithms in co-evolution, robotics and metaheuristics.

Andrea Toffolo was born in 1972. Toffolo earned an MS in mechanical engineering 1996. Toffolo is a consultant in system engineering 1997–2000, eanred a PhD in energy engineering 2002, and post-doctoral studies in industrial engineering, 2003–2005. Toffolo is a lecturer in internal combustion engines, energy systems, and turbomachinery design at the Department of Mechanical Engineering, University of Padova. Toffolo is the winner of the ASME Obert Award 2007. Toffolo's main research interests are in turbomachinery design and operation (fans, wind turbines, centrifugal and axial compressors, microturbines), modeling and optimization of energy conversion systems (fuel cells, combined cycle power plants), thermoeconomic diagnostics. He is author or co-author of more than 40 papers published in international journals and conference proceedings.

Pramod K. Varshney received the BS degree in electrical engineering and computer science and the MS and PhD degrees in electrical engineering from the University of Illinois at Urbana-Champaign in 1972, 1974, and 1976 respectively. Since 1976 he has been with Syracuse University, Syracuse, NY where he is currently a professor of electrical engineering and computer science. He serves as a distinguished lecturer for the Aerospace and Electronic Systems (AES) society of the IEEE. He is on the editorial board of *Information Fusion*. He was the president of International Society of Information Fusion during 2001. His current research interests are in distributed sensor networks, communications, signal and image processing and remote sensing.

Michael N. Vrahatis is a professor at the Department of Mathematics, University of Patras, Greece, since 2000, where currently he serves as director of the Division of Computational Mathematics and Informatics. He received the Diploma and PhD degrees in mathematics from the University of Patras, in 1978 and 1982, respectively. He is the author (or co-author) of more than 300 publications (more than 120 of which are published in international refereed journals) in his research areas, including computational mathematics, optimization, computational intelligence, data mining and cryptography. His research publications have received more than 1800 citations.

Byoung-Tak Zhang received a BS and MS in computer science and engineering from Seoul National University (SNU), Seoul, Korea, in 1986 and 1988, respectively, and a PhD in computer science from University of Bonn, Bonn, Germany, in 1992. He is a professor at the School of Computer Science and Engineering at SNU and directs the Biointelligence Laboratory and the Center for Bioinformation Technology (CBIT). He has been a visiting scientist at the Computer Science and Artificial Intelligence Laboratory (CSAIL), Massachusetts Institute of Technology (MIT), Cambridge, from August 2003 to August 2004. His research interests include probabilistic models of learning and evolution, biomolecular/DNA computing, and molecular learning/evolving machines.

Index

Symbols

ε-Dominance 86
ε-Multi-objective Evolutionary Algorithm 246
ε-multi-objective evolutionary algorithm (ε-MOEA) 246, 248

A

Ab-Ab Affinity 110
Ab-Ag Affinity 110
Action Planning 407
Adaptive Pareto DE (APDE) 49
Aerofoil Shape for Axial Compressor Blades 334
airman assignment problem 368
Airman Assignment problem (AAP) 414
AMOPSO 33
ant colony optimisation (ACO) 186
Ant Colony Optimization (ACO) 2
Ant colony optimization (ACO) 187
antibodies 110
Antibody 110
Antibody Population 110
Antigen 110
antigen 110
Arabidopsis Calmodulin (AC) 253
Area Coverage 215
Artificial Immune Systems (AIS) 2, 106
assembly line 149
Assignment Problems 364
Assignment Problems, MOEA operators 373
Atificial Evolution 302
Autopilot Controller 420
Axial Compressor Blades 334

B

B-cell receptors (BCRs) 108
back-propagation (BP) 305
bang-bang weighted aggregation (BWA) 27
Blind search 161

C

C-MOPSOSS 83
Causality Assignment Problem 368
Chromosome Representations 373
CI-based MO 1
CLONALG 108
cloning 119
code division multiple access (CDMA) 399
Combinatorial Production Problem 148
Combinatorial Production Problem, assessment tools 148
Communication Networks 389
Complex Energy Systems 352
Component Details, design of 334
Computational Intelligence 265
Constrained causality 369
Constrained Multi-objective Optimization using Particle Swarm Optimization with Scatter Search (C-MOPSOSS) 83
constructive genetic algorithm (CGA) 366
Control System 355
conventional weighted aggregation (CWA) 27
cost-performance problem 2
Courses of Action Planning 407
crossover 47
Crossover operators 379
crossover procedures 408

D

data accuracy 213
Data aggregation 213
Data transmission 210
Decision Fusion Model 228
decision space 3
decision variable space 3
DE for Multi-objective Optimization (DEMO) 49
Deployment Cost 211
Design space exploration (DSE) 268
Design Space Exploration Approaches 269
Design Space Exploration DSE) 266
Design Space Exploration of Embedded Systems 265
Detection Accuracy 212, 222
Detection Probability 211
Differential Evolution (DE) 2
differential evolution (DE) 43
differential evolution (DE) algorithm 46
Differential Evolution for Multi-objective Optimization with Random Sets (DEMORS) 49
Directed mutations 378
DNA computing 240
DNA Computing Sequence Design 244
DNA Computing Sequence Optimization Results 249
DNA microarrays 245
DNA Sequence Design 239
DNA sequence design, evolutionary multi-objective optimization 239
DNA Sequence Design for DNA Computing 247
DNA sequences 239
Dominance Clonal Selection Operation (DCSO) 111
dominance relation 3
Dominant Antibody 110
dominated tree 30
DSEAD (lethal direct air defense suppression) 417
dynamic channel assignment (DCA) problem 369
dynamic inheritance probability adjuster (DIPA) 31

E

EDA (Electronic Design Automation) 266
EFX (emitter-frequency crossover) 370
elite particle 31
elitism approach 9
Embedded Systems 265
EMO-Based Generation 307
EMO algorithm 300
EMO Algorithms, comparison 322
EMOCA 208, 218
Energy Consumption 211, 212, 221
Energy Conversion Systems 333
energy conversion systems 333
Energy Cost Analysis 229
Energy Systems, design of 344
Energy Systems, operation of 355
EPSOC 189
EPSOC algorithm 190
Estimation of Distribution Algorithms (EDA) 2
evolutionary algorithms (EAs) 2, 43
Evolutionary methods 388
Evolutionary Multi-Objective Optimization 239, 333, 364, 388
evolutionary multi-objective optimization (EMO) techniques 300
Evolutionary Multi-Objective Optimization for Assignment Problems 364
Evolutionary Multi-Objective Optimization in Military Applications 388
Evolutionary Neural Network Algorithm and Controller 304
Evolutionary Objectives 304
Evolutionary Population Dynamics 185
evolutionary population dynamics (EPD) 186
evolutionary programming dynamics (EPD) 185
Evolutionary Robotics 301
Evolved Pareto Controllers for Four-Legged Locomotion 309
Evolved Pareto Controllers for Six-Legged Locomotion 312
Evolved Pareto Controllers for Two-Legged Locomotion 309
EX (emitter crossover) 370
Extremal Optimization 188
Extremal Optimization (EO) 186

Index

F

feasible search region 3
feasible solutions 3
First-Available-Emitter (FAE) local search heuristic 370
First-Available-Frequency (FAF) FAE local search heuristic 370
fixed channel assignment (FCA) problem 369
Fixed Length Chromosomes 374
Four-Legged Locomotion 309
Frequency Assignment Problem (FAP) 370
fusion center 209
Fuzzy Expert Systems 356
Fuzzy Function Approximation 276
fuzzy genetic multi-objective optimization algorithm (FGMOA) 371
FX (frequency crossover) 370

G

GDE1 53
GDE2 53
GDE3 54
Generalized Differential Evolution (GDE) 50
generalized differential evolution (GDE) 43
generalized multi-objective assignment problem (GAP) 373
general multi-objective parallel (GENMOP) algorithm 419
general purpose registers (GPR) 280
generational replacement strategy 408
Generational Selection 382
genetic algorithm (GA) 149, 370
genetic algorithms (GA) 46
Genetic Operators 223, 229
genetic programming (GP) system 302
Genetic Vehicle Representation (GVR) 410
genotype 3
Genotype Representation 305
global Pareto optimal set 4
global variant of PSO 25
Good DNA Sequence 240
Groundwater Remediation 421

H

Heat Exchanger Networks 349
heat exchanger networks (HENs) 349
Heat Exchangers, optimal design 339
Hierarchical Fuzzy Model 280
Hierarchical Fuzzy System (HFS) 276
high energy communication node (HECN) 395
High Level Machine Description Facility (HM-DES) machine specification 280
human immune system (HIS) 106
Human Papillomavirus (HPV) 253
hunter-killer (H-K) general-purpose heuristic 149
Hybrid Multi-objective Evolutionary Design for Multiplex PCR Assay 256

I

Immune Dominance Clonal Multi-Objective Algorithm 111
Immune Dominance Clonal Multi-objective Algorithm (IDCMA) 106, 111, 112
Immune Dominance Clone Operation (IDCO) 111
Immune Dominance Recognizing Operation 111
Immune Dominance Recognizing Operation (IDRO), 111
immune system 110
immunology 110
Indifferent causality 369
Innovative Equipment with MOEAs 417
Instruction Level Parallelism (ILP) 278
INT (long range air interdiction) 417
interactive methods 7

J

Jumping Gene GA (JGGA) 399

L

Latency 213
LEACH protocol 214
Lexicographic Goal Programming 148
Limb Dynamics 317
linear gate assignment problem (LGAP) 365
Line balancing 149
local Pareto optimal set 4
local variants 25

Locomotion 300
Low-Power Laser Design 418

M

magnetic anomaly detector (MAD) hunting circle 162
Mandatory causality 369
many-objective 44
Microarray Probe Design 245
Military Aircraft Engine Maintenance Scheduling 404
Military Applications 388
Military Platforms, lifetime management of 403
Military Resources 403
Military Resources, management of 403
Mission planning 406
Mission Planning and Routing 409
Mobile Agent based Distributed Sensor Networks (MADSNs) 212
Mobile Agent Distributed Sensor Network (MADSN) Architecture 220
Mobile Agent Routing 212
Mobile Agent Routing in Sensor Networks 220
mobile multimedia application domain 266
MOEA Integrated Military Simulation 415
MOEA operators 408
MOEAs 2, 208
MOGA+Fuzzy Approach 272
MOO algorithms 217
MOO problems 209
MOPSO 11
MO techniques 1
multi-objective 44
multi-objective algorithms, traditional 4
multi-objective ant colony optimization (MOACO) 187
Multi-Objective Assignment Problem Instances 372
Multi-objective Assignment Problems 365
Multi-Objective Clonal Selection Algorithm (MOCSA) 109
Multi-objective COA formal model 407
Multi-objective DE (MODE) 49
Multi-Objective Design Space Exploration 265
Multi-objective Differential Evolution based Decomposition (MODE/D) 49
multi-objective EAs (MOEAs) 43
Multi-objective Evolutionary Algorithm 275
multi-objective evolutionary algorithm (MOEA) 77
Multi-Objective Evolutionary Algorithms 208
Multi-objective evolutionary algorithms 209
Multi-Objective Evolutionary Algorithms (MOEAs) 218, 265, 266
Multi-objective Evolutionary Algorithms (MOEAs) 388
multi-objective evolutionary algorithms (MOEAs) 208, 364
Multi-Objective Evolutionary Probe Optimization 253
Multi-Objective Evolutionary Sequence Optimization 248
Multi-Objective Evolution of Robotic Controllers 307
Multi-objective Formulation of DNA Computing Sequence Design 247
Multi-Objective Formulation of Multiplex PCR Assay 255
Multi-Objective Formulation of Oligonucleotide Microarray Probe Design 252
multi-objective Immune Algorithm (MOIA) 109
Multi-Objective Mobile Agent Routing 392
Multi-Objective Mobile Agent Routing in Wireless Sensor Networks 392
Multi-Objective Optimisation Problems 185
Multi-Objective Optimization 77, 106
Multi-objective Optimization 301
multi-objective optimization 1, 20, 43
multi-objective optimization (MOO) techniques 209
Multi-objective Optimization Algorithms 217
multi-objective optimization concepts 21
Multi-objective optimization problem 78
multi-objective optimization problems (MOPs) 44, 406
Multi-objective Optimization Problems in Sensor Networks 210
multi-objective optimization with constraints 44
Multi-objective Oriented Metaheuristics 186

multi-objective particles swarm optimization approaches 20
multi-objective particle swarm optimization (MOPSO) 186
Multi-Objective Particle Swarm Optimizer 76
multi-objective pptimisation using evolutionary algorithms (MOEAs) 185
multi-objective problems (MOPs) 388
multi-objective PSO (MOPSO) 30
multi-objective PSO algorithms, concepts 25
multi-objective PSO approaches 26
multi-objective quadratic assignment problem category (mQAP) 367
Multi-Objective Robotics 300
multicommodity capacitated network design problem (MCNDP) 389
Multicriteria selection procedure 150
Multilevel Generalized Assignment Problem 371
multiobjective evolutionary algorithms (MOEAs) 8
multiobjective optimization (MO) 1
multiobjective optimization problems (MOPs) 1
Multiplex PCR Assay Selection Results 257
Multiplex PCR Primer Design 245
Multiplex Polymerase Chain Reaction 255
mutation 47
Mutation Operators 377
mutation procedure 408

N

naïve search 161
neighborhood topologies 24
Network Design 389
Network lifetime 213
Network Routing 392
Network Sensor Layout 395
no-preference methods 4
non-elitism approach 8
Nondominated Neighbor Immune Algorithm (NNIA) 106, 118
NP-complete combinatorial problems 148
NSGA-II 9, 77, 208

O

objective space 3
OCA (offensive counter air) 417
Oligonucleotide Microarray 252
Oligonucleotide Microarray Probe Design 252
OMOPSO 33
Operational dynamics 314
Operational Dynamics Beyond the Evolutionary Window 315
Operational Dynamics under Noisy Conditions 314
opt-aiNet 109
Optimal Rotors for Horizontal-Axis Wind Turbines 341
Optimal Synthesis of Heat Exchanger Networks 349
Optimization of System Design Parameters 345
Optimized District Heating Networks, design of 353

P

PAES 11
Parameterized System Architecture 278
Pareto(-frontier) Differential Evolution (PDE) algorithm 49
Pareto-based PSO approaches 30
Pareto-optimal 45
Pareto Archived Evolution Strategy (PAES) 369
Pareto controllers 300
Pareto DE Approach (PDEA) 49
Pareto dominance 22, 78
Pareto Evolution of Locomotion Controllers 322
Pareto Front 78
Pareto front 76
Pareto optimal front (POF) 2
Pareto optimality 20, 78
Pareto optimal set 1, 22
Pareto optimal solution 1
Pareto Set Approximations 281
Pareto solutions 300
particles 22

particle swarm inspired evolutionary algorithm (PS-EA) 31
Particle Swarm Optimization 84
particle swarm optimization 20
Particle Swarm Optimization (PSO) 2, 79, 186
particle swarm optimization (PSO) 21, 77
particle swarm optimization (PSO) approach 76
Path Loss 212, 222
path planning problem 410
PDE 10
Personnel Assignment 412
phenotype 3
Planning 406
polymerase chain reaction (PCR) 245
posteriori methods 5
Predicate registers (PR) 280
Preferred causality 369
preliminary pareto decision 28
priori methods 6
probability inheritance tree 31
Probe Design for Oligonucleotide Microarray 252
Probe Selection Results 253
Problem Formulation 221
PSO, Multi-Objective Algorithms 79
PSO-based multi-objective approaches 21
PSO algorithm 21

Q

quantum cascade laser (QCL) 418

R

Radar Waveform Optimization 423
randomized censored averaging (RCA) 394
randomized median filtering (RMF) 394
Random mutations 378
resource-constrained project/task scheduling (RCPS) 406
resource allocation or assignment problems (RAPs) 371
Resource Allocation Problem 371
ring topology 24
Robotics 300

S

sailor assignment problem (SAP) 413
Scatter Search 85
Scatter search (SS) 82
scatter search (SS) 77
search space 3
selection 48
Selection Methods 381
Self-adaptive PDE (SPDE) 49
Sensor Network Design 208
Sensor Network Design, multiple objectives 215
sensor network design problems 208
Sensor networks 210
Sensor nodes 210
Sensor Placement for Energy Efficient Target Detection 227
Sensor Placement Problem 210
Simulated Robot Morphologies 303
Simulation Flow 279
Six-Legged Locomotion 312
SPANN-R Algorithm 307
SPEA2 10
Speed-up Design Space Exploration 272
star topology 25
steady state evolutionary algorithm with Pareto tournaments (stEAPT) 383
STI (strategic target interdiction) 417
strict dominance 3
swarm 22
swarm explosion 23
System-on-a-Chip (SoC) platforms 268
System Design Parameters 345

T

T-cell receptors (TCRs) 108
Target Detection, probability 228
Terrain Following (TF) 410
Two-Legged Locomotion 309

U

UAV Communications 422
uninformed search 161
unmanned aerial vehicles (UAVs) 302

Index

V

Variable Length Chromosomes 373
vector Artificial Immune System (VAIS) 109
Vector Evaluated DE (VEDE) 49
vector evaluated genetic algorithm (VEGA) 29, 187
vector evaluated PSO (VEPSO) 29
vehicle routing problem (VRP) 409
very large scale integration (VLSI) design 366
Very Long Instruction Word (VLIW) microprocessor 266
Very Long Instruction Word (VLIW) processors 278
Virtual Simulation 302
Vortex physics engine 303

W

weak dominance 3
weak search 161
weight based genetic algorithm 218
Wideband CDMA Systems 399
Wideband CDMA Systems, resource management 399
Wireless Sensor Network 395
Wireless Sensor Network, layout optimization 395
Wireless Sensor Network Nodes 397
Wireless Sensor Network Nodes, automated placement 397
Wireless Sensor Networks 392
Wireless sensor networks (WSNs) 209, 395